Fundamentals and Clinics of Deep Brain Stimulation
An Interdisciplinary Approach

脑深部电刺激基础与临床 跨学科技术

原著 [荷] Yasin Temel
[荷] Albert F. G. Leentjens
[荷] Rob M. A. de Bie
[法] Stephan Chabardes
[加] Alfonso Fasano
主译 张建国

中国科学技术出版社
·北京·

图书在版编目（CIP）数据

脑深部电刺激基础与临床：跨学科技术 /（荷）亚辛·泰梅尔 (Yasin Temel) 等原著；张建国主译 . —北京：中国科学技术出版社, 2021.10

ISBN 978-7-5046-9090-6

Ⅰ. ①脑… Ⅱ. ①亚… ②张… Ⅲ. ①神经系统疾病—电疗法 Ⅳ. ① R741.05

中国版本图书馆 CIP 数据核字 (2021) 第 122185 号

著作权合同登记号：01-2021-3606

First published in English under the title
Fundamentals and Clinics of Deep Brain Stimulation: An Interdisciplinary Approach
edited by Yasin Temel, Albert F. G. Leentjens, Rob M. A. de Bie, Stephan Chabardes, Alfonso Fasano
Copyright © Springer Nature Switzerland AG 2020
This edition has been translated and published under licence from Springer Nature Switzerland AG.
All rights reserved.

策划编辑	宗俊琳　焦健姿
责任编辑	孙　超
装帧设计	佳木水轩
责任印制	李晓霖

出　版	中国科学技术出版社
发　行	中国科学技术出版社有限公司发行部
地　址	北京市海淀区中关村南大街 16 号
邮　编	100081
发行电话	010-62173865
传　真	010-62179148
网　址	http://www.cspbooks.com.cn

开　本	889mm×1194mm　1/16
字　数	391 千字
印　张	15
版　次	2021 年 10 月第 1 版
印　次	2021 年 10 月第 1 次印刷
印　刷	天津翔远印刷有限公司
书　号	ISBN 978-7-5046-9090-6 / R·2723
定　价	158.00 元

（凡购买本社图书，如有缺页、倒页、脱页者，本社发行部负责调换）

译校者名单

主　　译　张建国

译 校 者（以姓氏笔画为序）

王　乔　　王　秀　　王　垚　　王慧敏　　尹子霄
石　林　　朱冠宇　　刘钰晔　　刘焕光　　刘德峰
杨岸超　　张　华　　张　凯　　张　弨　　张建国
陈颖川　　孟凡刚　　赵宝田　　胡文瀚　　袁天硕
韩春雷　　解自行

内容提要

本书引进自世界知名的 Springer 出版社，是一部介绍脑深部电刺激（DBS）相关理论和实践的专业参考书。书中所述融合了不同国家不同学科的专家意见，提供了适合 DBS 治疗的神经及精神性疾病的发病机制、脑解剖与功能、症状学方面的最新见解，涵盖了刺激方案的基本概念和最新概念，以及必要的硬件和软件知识等内容，还对特定患者的管理技巧和 DBS 治疗策略进行了总结。本书内容系统全面，深入浅出，图表明晰，非常适合 DBS 领域各层次的神经外科医师参考阅读，亦可作为多学科团队中该领域学者的案头参考书。

译者前言

Benabid 教授及其同事首次将脑深部电刺激（deep brain stimulation，DBS）技术用于治疗震颤并推广开来，DBS 在过去的 30 多年中已成为广泛用于治疗多种疾病的外科方法。近年来，随着神经调控技术基础研究的不断深入，以及对帕金森病、肌张力障碍疾病、癫痫、精神疾病及 PVS 等患者的进一步认识，DBS 已成为治疗运动障碍疾病的一线治疗手段，并在精神外科、疼痛、促醒、阿尔茨海默病、癫痫等领域表现出良好的治疗效果。

本书由多位来自欧美各国的神经内外科及精神科医师共同编写，是一部实用性、可读性很强的跨学科案头参考书，重点介绍了 DBS 基础理论与临床实践方面的内容，并根据已发表的指南提供临床建议。书中论述深入浅出，于"无声处见惊雷"，既是对 DBS 发展至今的很好总结，又是对未来开展 DBS 工作的良好借鉴与指引，旨在为参与 DBS 患者治疗的医生及其他相关专业人士，如心理学家、护士、物理治疗师及神经科学家等提供参考。

随着医学技术及医工、科技的快速发展，DBS 的理念、技术也在迅速发展进步。相信不论是刚刚接触 DBS 领域的青年医师，还是一直在此领域历练多年的功能神经外科专家，都会从书中获益良多。

很荣幸能够翻译此书，并希望借此书与国内同道共勉。

首都医科大学附属北京天坛医院

原书前言

人们对采用脑深部电刺激术（DBS）治疗神经和精神系统疾病的兴趣与日俱增。现代 DBS 应用最早始于 20 世纪 80 年代后期，将其用于治疗以震颤为主的帕金森病患者，但在实验环境下使用电流抑制疾病症状的历史已远远早于这一时期。DBS 已成为治疗多种神经及精神系统疾病的公认治疗方法，因为其他保守药物治疗及心理治疗对这些疾病无效。这些疾病包括特发性震颤、肌张力障碍、癫痫和强迫症等。本书将讨论这些疾病及其他新的正处于评估阶段的 DBS 适应证。

多方面的发展推动了 DBS 的普及。人们对疾病症状的发生机制已有了进一步的了解。我们已经确认神经或精神系统疾病会导致特定脑区或特定神经通路的活动中断，进而引起特定的症状。一个很好的例子就是丘脑底核兴奋性的改变与帕金森病的核心症状有关，DBS 刺激丘脑底核能够抑制该病理性兴奋并改善这些运动症状。另一个例子就是震颤，它与丘脑运动区的震颤细胞有关，而 DBS 刺激该区域可中止震颤。在强迫症的治疗中也利用了同样的机制，DBS 刺激基底核边缘部分可改善严重的强迫症状。令人们对 DBS 兴趣大增的另一个原因是神经和精神性疾病的新药研发不尽人意，主要困难在于血脑屏障的存在，以及大多数药物的非选择性导致药物无法作用于脑内。

来自不同国家不同学科的著者为本书的编写贡献了自己的专业知识和个人经验。书中所述提供了适合 DBS 治疗的神经及精神性疾病的发病机制、脑解剖与功能、症状学方面的最新见解。此外，还对特定患者的管理技巧和 DBS 治疗策略进行了概述。书中还囊括了刺激方案的基本概念和最新概念，以及必要的硬件和软件知识。本书的编写由神经内科、神经外科、精神科医师共同完成，真实反映了该领域的跨学科性质。

我们认为，拥有全面了解 DBS 治疗可能性最新知识的多学科团队，是成功治疗的基本要求。

Yasin Temel
Maastricht, The Netherlands

Albert F. G. Leentjens
Maastricht, The Netherlands

Rob M. A. de Bie
Amsterdam, The Netherlands

Stephan Chabardes
Grenoble, France

Alfonso Fasano
Toronto, ON, Canada

目 录

第一篇 总论

第 1 章 脑深部电刺激的历史 …………………………………………………………… 002
第 2 章 脑深部电刺激的靶点解剖 ……………………………………………………… 011
第 3 章 脑深部电刺激的机制 …………………………………………………………… 023
第 4 章 脑深部电刺激手术和技术 ……………………………………………………… 030
第 5 章 未来展望：自适应脑深部电刺激 ……………………………………………… 039
第 6 章 基底节的神经生理学与脑深部电刺激 ………………………………………… 053
第 7 章 脑深部电刺激手术麻醉 ………………………………………………………… 060
第 8 章 程控：通用特性 ………………………………………………………………… 072
第 9 章 神经心理学评估 ………………………………………………………………… 098
第 10 章 伦理问题 ………………………………………………………………………… 112
第 11 章 脑深部电刺激患者围术期管理 ………………………………………………… 123

第二篇 神经病学

第 12 章 脑深部电刺激治疗帕金森病 …………………………………………………… 130
第 13 章 震颤 ……………………………………………………………………………… 146
第 14 章 肌张力障碍 ……………………………………………………………………… 166
第 15 章 癫痫 ……………………………………………………………………………… 180
第 16 章 抽动秽语综合征 ………………………………………………………………… 191

第三篇 精神病学

第 17 章 强迫症的脑深部电刺激治疗 …………………………………………………… 202
第 18 章 脑深部电刺激治疗抑郁症 ……………………………………………………… 216
第 19 章 脑深部电刺激的其他适应证 …………………………………………………… 226

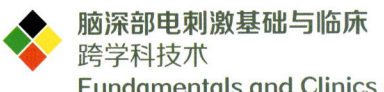

脑深部电刺激基础与临床
跨学科技术
Fundamentals and Clinics of Deep Brain Stimulation
An Interdisciplinary Approach

第一篇

总 论
General Section

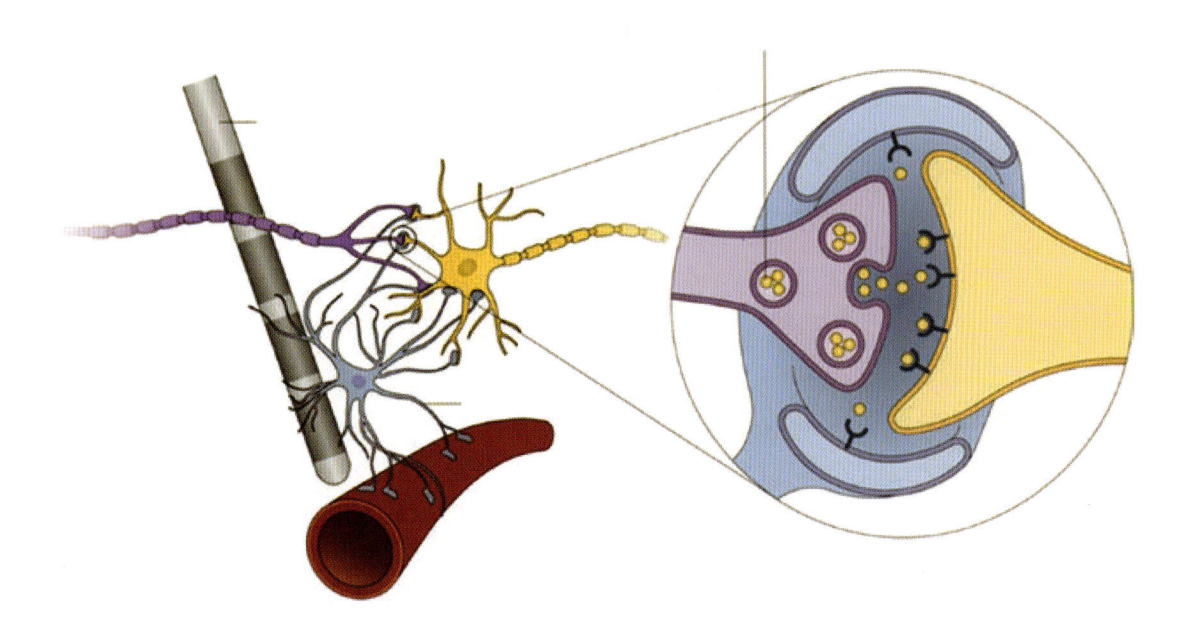

第1章 脑深部电刺激的历史
The History of Deep Brain Stimulation

J. D. Hans Speelman　Rick Schuurman　**著**
解自行　孟凡刚　**译**　刘德峰　杨岸超　张建国　**校**

> **摘要**：脑深部电刺激（deep brain stimulation，DBS）是通过在脑的特定结构进行慢性电脉冲刺激从而达到治疗效果的医疗方式。随着应用于人脑的立体定向装置的发展和可信的立体定向图谱发表，于1947年这种方式开始应用。这两项进步使得通过颅骨钻孔进行脑深部结构的精准毁损得以实现。随后，毁损手术被慢性高频电刺激所取代。20世纪50年代，DBS开始用来治疗精神病患者，但是由于伦理的反对和抗精神病药物的投入使用被废止了。在20世纪60年代，这项技术被用来治疗运动障碍类疾病。1993年，DBS治疗震颤得到认可，其后被许可用于治疗帕金森病、肌张力障碍、强迫症和癫痫。

一、概述

脑深部电刺激（DBS）旨在通过对特定的皮质下结构或传导束进行高频电脉冲刺激，获得某些的神经或精神疾病的症状改善。电刺激的实现是先通过颅骨钻孔植入电极到颅内靶点结构，而后电极通过皮下连接到一个脉冲发生器。通过这项技术，不但可以影响病理生理状态下神经活性，如对运动障碍类疾病的治疗，也可以影响正常生理状态下的神经活性，如对慢性疼痛的治疗。

用来植入脑深部电极的特殊装置，被称为立体定向框架，其误差范围为0.5～1mm，并且已经得到了及时的发展和完善（Guiot等，1962）。此外，手术的关键是颅内结构细节的可视化，以确定相对于立体定向框架的脑内结构的位置，以及对电极尖端位置进行神经生理调控的可能性。这些领域的进展对于DBS治疗神经和精神疾病的发展是十分重要的。

二、第一个发展阶段

英国神经外科医师Victor Horsley最早于1905年使用Clarke-Horsley立体定向框架（以两个创造者名字命名）研究动物脑深部结构的功能。这个装置的出现使得能够对动物脑深部解剖结构进行毁损（图1-1）（Horsley和Clarke，1908）。Clarke医师不仅是生理学先驱，也是"立体定向装置"的设计者，他在1920年以前就建议应用立体定向框架进行人脑肿瘤的手术，采用电解毁损或植入镭元素，以及治疗慢性疼痛（Schur和Merrington，1978）。加拿大神经病学家和神经生理学家Aubrey Mussen对Clarke-Horsley立体定向框架进行了改进，从而可用于人脑深部肿瘤的手术。但是，那时没有外科医师愿意用这个设备（Olivier等，1983）。主要问题是脑内深部结构与外部颅骨特征存在较大的差异，并且缺少一个可靠的立体定向神经解剖图

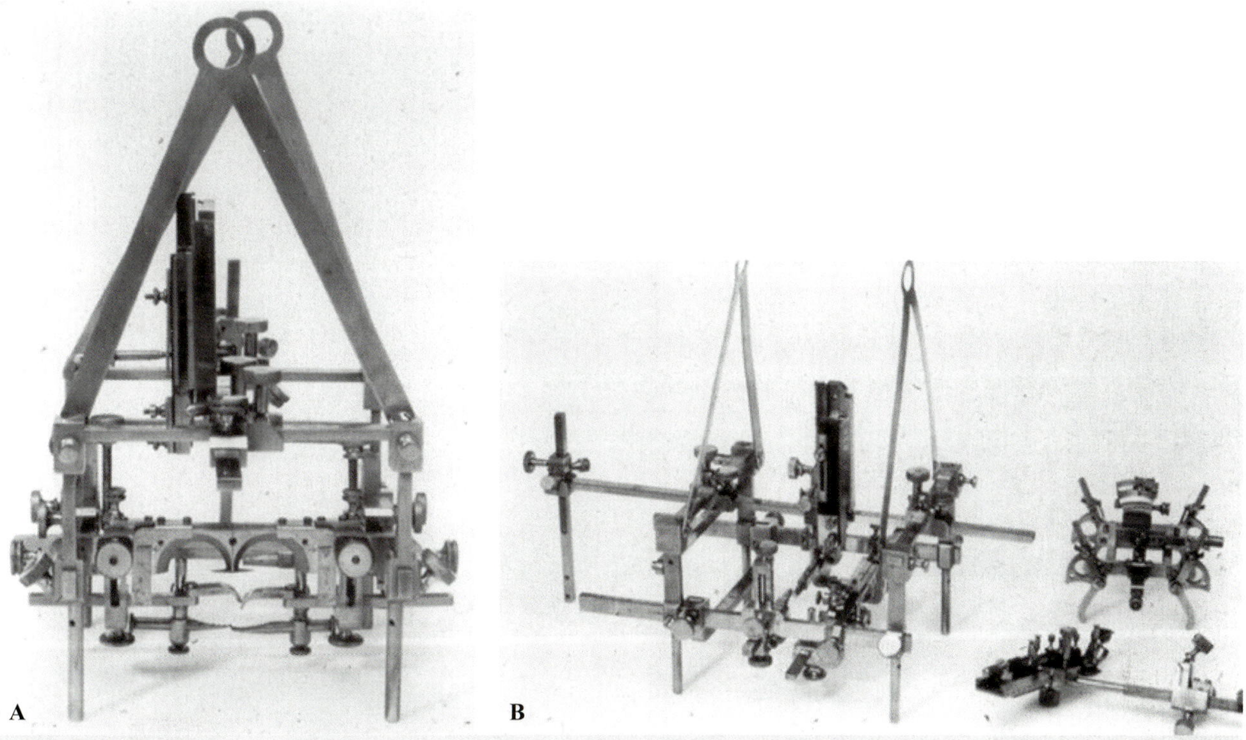

▲ 图 1-1　Clarke 和 Horsley 设计的立体定向框架
前面观（A）和侧面观（B），右侧是脊髓的立体定向穿刺装置

谱。直到 1947 年这项技术才通过改进的立体定向装置用于人类患者（Spiegel 等，1947）。

三、1947 年以前的神经外科手术

（一）精神疾病的外科治疗

瑞典精神病学家 Gottlieb Burckhardt 于 1888 年最早对 6 名具有精神症状和行为障碍的精神病患者进行神经外科手术。在那时针对精神病患者的手术是有很大争议的。在 1935 年于伦敦召开的第二届世界神经病学大会上，对精神疾病的神经外科手术（也被称为精神外科）才被接受为一种医学治疗方法（Heller 等，2006）。同年，葡萄牙神经病学家 Egas Moniz 和神经外科医师 Almeida Lima 首次对一个精神病患者进行了双侧额叶离断手术。Moniz 因此与 Rudolf Walter Hess 共同获得了 1949 年的诺贝尔生理学或医学奖，以表彰其发现额叶离断对某些精神疾病的治疗价值。1936 年，乔治 – 华盛顿大学的神经病学家 Walter Freeman 与神经外科医师 James Watts 一起启动了"前额叶离断项目"（Heller 等，2006；Mashour 等，2005）。他采用了经眶的额叶离断，也被称为"碎冰锥脑叶离断"，这使得神经外科医师的参与变得多余了。这个手术在美国被用于超过 40 000 名具有精神症状和（或）行为障碍的人（Shorter，1997）。1948 年在葡萄牙里斯本召开的国际精神外科大会上报告了 5000 例脑叶离断的结果。由于这个手术被认为是一个试验性的手术，因此这个手术受到了严重的质疑批评（Freed 等，1949）。此外，适应证尚未明确描述，缺乏适当的术前筛查，也没有统一的手术技术。

（二）神经外科治疗运动障碍

1890 年，Horsley 为一名单侧手足徐动症患者首次实施了切除部分运动皮质治疗运动障碍的

神经外科手术，并取得了良好的效果。不幸的是，这一结果被遗忘了（图 1-2）(Horley，1890，1909；Kandel 和 Schavinsky，1972)。1912 年首次报道了对帕金森病患者通过切断颈部传入神经使得僵直得到了改善（Leriche，1921）。在这之后，报道了在脊髓不同的节段通过进行椎体外系传导束的切断，用来治疗手足徐动症和肌张力障碍，而不是帕金森病，并且都取得了一些改善，但是大部分都是短暂的改善（Speelman 和 Bosch，1998）。

从 1937 年开始，对皮质脊髓束的毁损手术被接受，其包括运动皮质（运动前区皮质）、内囊、脑干（中脑大脑脚切断术）和脊髓（Seeplman 和 Bosch，1998）。所有这些中，只有大脑脚切断术持续到 20 世纪 50 年代初。最终这一手术方式也被放弃了，因为手术缓解椎体外系的运动障碍是归结于人为导致的瘫痪，而没有改善帕金森的僵直和运动迟缓（图 1-3 和图 1-4）(Speelman 和 Bosch，1998；Redfern，1989)。1939 年美国爱荷华州大学的神经外科医师 Russell Meyers 开始通过基底神经节手术治疗运动障碍的神经外科手术试验。首位患者是一名女性，患有脑炎后单侧静止性震颤 7 年。她在接受对侧运动前区皮质切断术后没有改善。但是她在接受额外的尾状核前部切除术后，震颤永久地消失了，并且没有不良反应（Meyers，1940）。在 1951 年 Meyers 发表了 58 例震颤麻痹患者的外科手术疗效（表 1-1）。他的结论是通过离断苍白球的传出纤维和（或）切除尾状核的前部并且同时离断内囊前肢，震颤和僵直可以得到明显改善。但是，一半的患者出现了 3 个月至 1 年的短暂性记忆障碍，并且该手术的死亡率高达 15.7%（Meyers，1951a,b）。

四、1947 年开启立体定向神经外科的临床实践

1947 年，天普大学医学中心（宾夕法尼亚州，费城）的神经病学家 Ernest A. Spiegel（图 1-5）和神经外科学家 H. T. Wycis，以及他们的

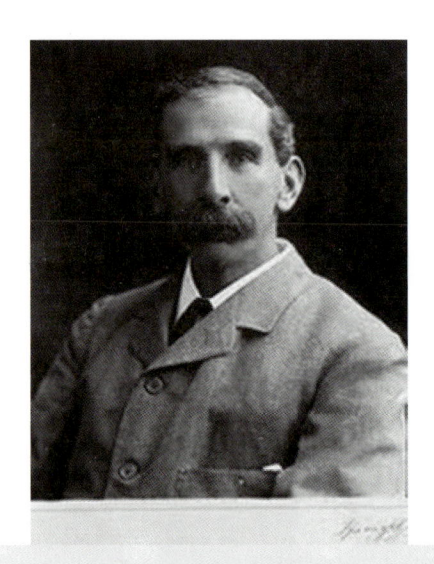

▲ 图 1-2 英国神经外科医师 Victor Alexander Haden Horsley 先生（1867—1916）

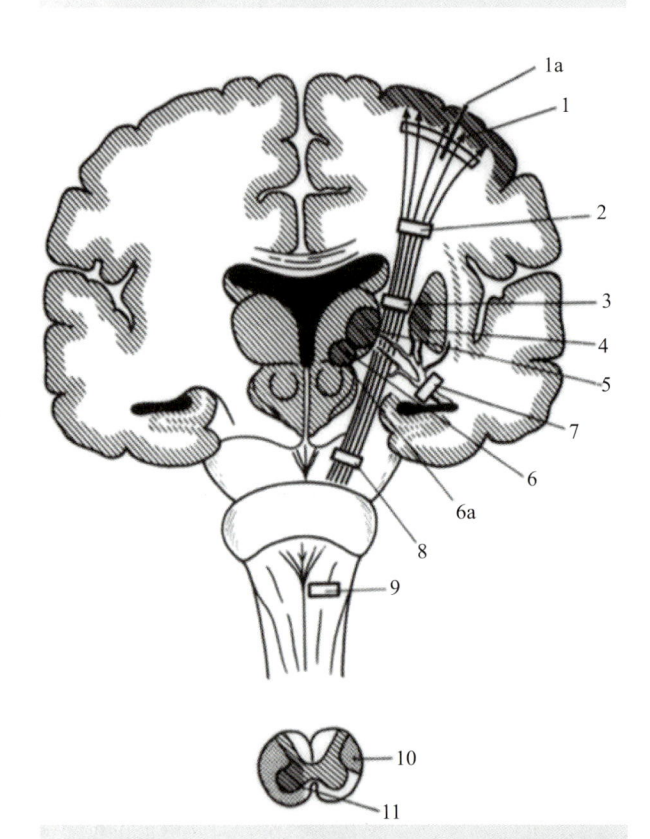

▲ 图 1-3 帕金森病外科手术方式的模式图（Speelman 和 Bosch，1998）

1. 运动前区和运动区皮质切除；2. 在半卵圆中心切断皮质脊髓束；3. 在内囊水平切断皮质脊髓束；4. 苍白球切开术，GPi-DBS 5. 丘脑切开术；6. "雷富尔区切开术"（Cooper 和 Bravo，1958）；7 脉络膜前动脉结扎术（Cooper，1953）；8. 大脑脚切断术；9. 在延髓水平切断红核脊髓束和顶盖脊髓束；10. 在脊髓切断皮质脊髓束；11. 半侧颈髓切断术（Leriche，1912）

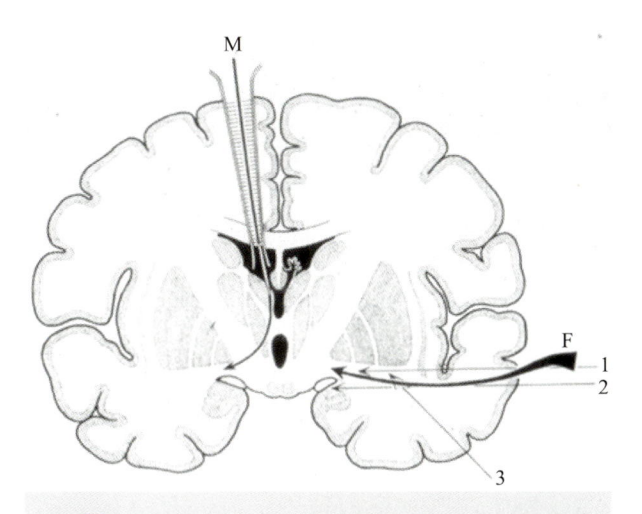

▲ 图 1-4　切断苍白球的传导束，Russell Meyers 方式（M）
法国神经外科医师 Fenelon 介绍一种"盲"切手术方法（F）（Fénelon，1950）

合作者记录："暴露皮质下脑结构需要相当大的手术范围。因为改进的立体定向技术用于人脑手术看起来是可取的""这个装置正被用于精神外科"。他们继续写道："进一步的应用正在被研究，例如，立体定向切断脊髓丘脑束治疗特定的疼痛类型如幻肢痛，进行立体定向苍白球毁损用于治疗不自主运动，以及用于抽吸肿瘤的囊性液体"（Spiegel 等，1947）。2 年后，作者们发表了立体定向丘脑背内侧核团毁损的治疗结果，共有 38 个病例，由于患有精神分裂症、抑郁或严重的强迫症，大部分都在精神病院治疗。他们报告通过丘脑毁损可以获得症状改善，但是没有额叶离断带来的人格改变或癫痫的风险（Freed 等，1949；Spiegel 等，1949）。

两个方面的进展对立体定向手术（Spiegel 等称为脑切开术）的临床实践十分重要：①通过 X 线可以显示颅内的脑结构；②脑立体定向图谱的发展。Spiegel 和 Wycis 通过松果体钙化、缰核连合、空气脑室造影确定后连合，进而确定丘脑和苍白球（GPi）的位置（Schurr 和 Merrington 1978）。巴黎的精神病学家和神经外科学家 Jean Tailarach 同样使用脑室造影，通过前连合或室间孔与后连合的连线作为参考，进而确定颅内的结构（Talairach 等，1949）。在 1952 年 Spiegel 和 Wycis 出版了第一本人脑的立体定向图谱（Spiegel 等，1949；Spiegel 和 Wycis，1952）。在那之后，立体定向神经外科开始在其他各个中心出现，并得到进一步的发展（Talairach 等，1949；Leksell，1949；Riechert 和 Wolff，1951；Hayne 和 Meyers，1950；Narabayashi 等，1956）。虽然立体定向神经外科仍然被认为是一个实验性的操作，但是也给予了研究活体人脑生理和疾病的机会。

在 Russell Meyers 前期试验手术基础上（见

表 1-1　总结 Rusell Meters 治疗震颤麻痹的外科手术试验（1951a）

手术方式	患者数量
尾状核头部切除术	1
切除尾状核，并曲线切断内囊前肢	11
切除尾状核，并曲线切断内囊前肢及壳核前 1/3	6
切除尾状核，并曲线切断内囊前肢及壳核前 1/3，以及苍白球前极	4
豆状襻切断术（切断苍白球纤维）	22
豆状襻切断，以及切除尾状核，切断内囊前肢	10
豆状襻切断，以及切除尾状核，切断内囊前肢，切除壳核前 1/3	3
切除尾状核，以及线性分开"运动"和"运动前区"皮质，并从下部切断运动前区皮质	1
总患者数	58

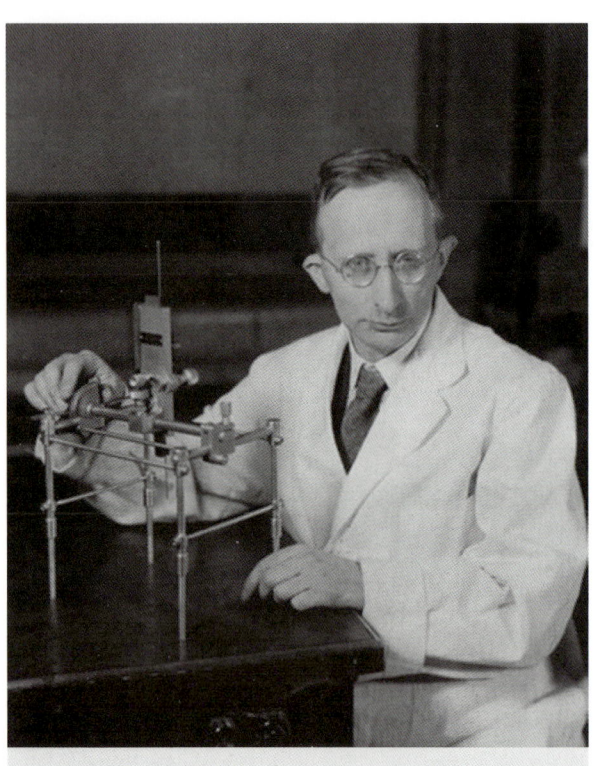

▲ 图1-5　Ernest A. Spiegel（1895—1985）

前面），苍白球和它的传导束、豆状核的柄和传导束被认为是立体定向外科治疗运动障碍疾病的靶点，如帕金森病、舞蹈病、手足徐动症和肌张力障碍（Leksell，1949；Narabayashi 等，1956；Fenelon，1950；Spiegel 和 Wycis，1950；Guiot 和 Brion，1953）。在 1953 年，纽约 St Barnabas 医院的神经外科医师 Irving Cooper，报告了 2 例帕金森病患者在结扎脉络膜前动脉后运动症状得到了改善。他认为这是由于结扎脉络膜前动脉导致了苍白球的坏死的结果（Cooper，1953）。这些结果都支持将苍白球和（或）豆状核柄作为运动障碍病的外科手术靶点。Spiegel 提到在 1948—1961 年，全世界 80 个中心进行了大约 6000 例手术用来治疗锥体外系疾病，其中 90% 进行立体定向苍白球切开术；而在 1948 年以前只有 302 例手术（Spiegel 和 Wycis，1962）。

弗莱堡（德国）的神经解剖学家 Rolf Hassler 和 Irving Cooper 使用丘脑替代苍白球为震颤和帕金森病的首选靶点（Hassler 和 Riechert 1954；Cooper 和 Bravo，1958）。其他脑结构，如丘脑下结构（不定带和 Forel 区域）及底丘脑核，也被尝试用作这些疾病的治疗靶点（Heller 等，2006；Bertrand，1958；Spiegel 等，1963；Andy 等，1963；Spiegel，1969）。

在 1968 年，进行了超过 37 000 例立体定向手术，大部分是用来治疗帕金森病。有人认为，只有 12%～15% 的帕金森患者适合做立体定向手术。因此形成了更严格的手术患者筛查和手术技术规范，并且这时立体定向脑图谱已发布。

（一）左旋多巴的初次使用

1969 年左旋多巴开始用于帕金森病的治疗引起世界性的轰动，进行立体定向手术的患者数量，以及世界各地的该领域的医学中心数量出现急剧减少（Refern，1989）。然而，在 1970 年成立了以促进立体定向外科技术的发展为目标的"欧洲立体定向和功能神经外科学会"。由于放射诊断（特别是 CT 扫描）和计算机技术领域的进展，增大了诊断和治疗颅内深部肿瘤的可能性。由于颅内微电极记录和宏观刺激的进展，增加了对于疼痛、痉挛和癫痫的治疗机会。

（二）立体定向手术的复兴

20 世纪 80 年代初，由于左旋多巴治疗的缺点和不良反应，人们对帕金森病的立体定向神经外科重新产生了兴趣。最初，丘脑切开术和左旋多巴联合用于治疗帕金森病的震颤和僵直（Siegfried，1980；Gildenberg，1984）。芬兰裔瑞典人 Lauri Laitinen 是于默奥和斯德哥尔摩的神经外科医生，他和同事们继续根据瑞典神经外科医生 Leksell 的坐标进行苍白球切开术，并在 1992 年发表了治疗帕金森病运动症状和左旋多巴诱发异动症的苍白球切开术的良好结果（图 1-6）（Laitinen 等，1992a，b）。随后，苍白球内侧部（GPi）变成了帕金森病、舞蹈症和肌张力障碍治疗的一个首选靶点。丘脑仍然是治疗药物难治性震颤患者的靶点。

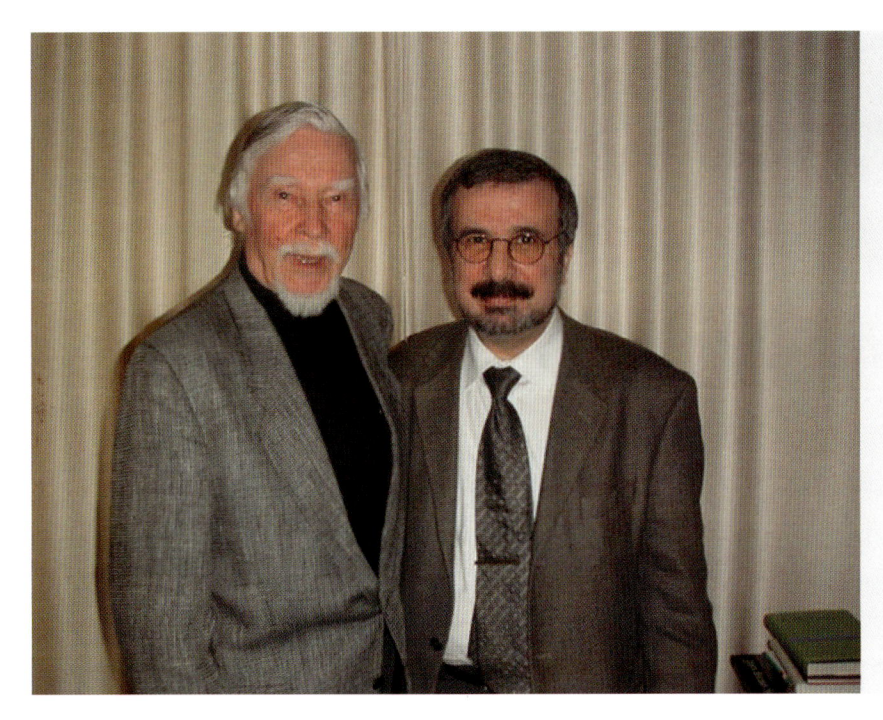

◀ 图 1-6 左侧为神经外科医师 Lauri Laitinen（1928—2005），右侧是他的学生，伦敦和瑞典神经外科医师 Marwan Hariz（1953）

五、脑深部电刺激

自从立体定向用于临床实践之后，在 1947 年就通过植入电极给予电刺激来验证靶点的位置。当观察到症状改善而没有明显的不良反应时，就通过加热、冷冻、化学、电解或机械的方法进行毁损（或切开）（Schurr 和 Merrington，1978；Albe-Fessard 等，1953）。除此之外，还进行体内脑神经生理学研究（Gildenberg，2005）。最初的 DBS 的慢性治疗是通过连接外部导线来实现的。外部电刺激时患者也是可移动的，外部电刺激可使用数月，最长达到 1 年半。因为没有合适的脉冲发生器可以应用，在外部电刺激之后，最终还是要做毁损治疗（Blomstedt 和 Hariz，2010；Hariz 等，2010）。

（一）精神病适应证

20 世纪 50 年代，DBS 已经被用来研究行为障碍和精神病的发病机制和治疗效果（Delgado 等，1952；Sem-Jacobsen，1959）。在那时，新奥尔良市杜兰特大学的精神病学家 Robert C. Heath 开始研究慢性脑深部电刺激治疗精神病、疼痛和癫痫发作的患者（Heath，1963）。他发表的《使用脑起搏器调解情绪：治疗难治性精神性疾病》在 1977 年引起了对精神外科伦理问题的广泛讨论（Baumeister，2000）。这些讨论和抗精神病药物的应用，使得精神病的神经外科治疗适应证被认为是过时的，这种情况一直持续到 20 世纪 90 年代后期（Hariz 等，2010；Baumeister 2000；Krack 等，2010）。

（二）疼痛

自从应用立体定向以后，慢性药物难治性疼痛就成了神经生理学、立体定向神经外科，以及后来的 DBS 的研究目标（Schurr 和 Merrington，1978；Iskander 和 Nashold，1995）。最初，疼痛的治疗聚焦在影响疼痛进程的情绪通路，即进行内侧丘脑的毁损和慢性刺激。但是，20 世纪 60 年代将治疗的靶点改为丘脑躯体感觉区（Tasker，1982；Hosobuchi 等，1973）、导水管周围和脑室旁灰质。

（三）运动障碍

慢性脑深部电刺激作为运动障碍病的一种治疗方法是从 20 世纪 60 年代后期开始的，最早的科学家是列宁格勒（现在称为圣彼得堡）的神经生理学家和神经病学家 Natalia Petrovna Bechtereva（Blomstedt 和 Hariz，2010）。Bechtereva 通过外部刺激器，使用多个电极对基底神经节和运动丘脑进行慢性高频电刺激，持续时间可达 1.5 年。她经常观察到在无刺激间歇期间症状的持续长时间的改善。因为这时还没有可植入的脉冲发生器，所以她认为这是植入电极导致的"微毁损"效应（Bechtereva 等，1975）。

20 世纪 70 年代的早期，通过植入可接收外部信号的皮下脉冲发生器来激活颅内电极，从而使脑深部结构慢性电刺激变成了可能（Blomstedt 和 Hariz 2010；Heath 1963；Iskander 和 Nashold，1995；Gildenberg，2006；Sarem-Aslani 和 Mullett，2011）。1980 年 Irving Cooper 发表了通过慢性电刺激丘脑和苍白球治疗各种运动障碍病的结果（Cooper 等，1980）。同年，南安普敦（英国）的神经外科医师 Brice 和他的合作者发表了对 2 例患有多发性硬化和严重意向性震颤的患者进行丘脑慢性电刺激可以抑制其震颤的报道（Brice 和 McLellan，1980）。密西西比大学（美国）医学院的神经外科医师 Orlando J. Andy，报道了丘脑深部电刺激在 9 例运动障碍病患者中取得了令人满意的结果，其中 5 例表现为帕金森病的静止性震颤（Andy，1983）。Jean Siegfried（瑞士，苏黎世）报道了对 5 例"丘脑综合征"患者，进行丘脑感觉神经核团慢性刺激可减轻疼痛和抑制运动障碍的症状（Siegfried，1986）。法国神经外科医师 G. Mazars（巴黎）和同事之前也报道过类似结果（Tasker，1982）。

六、1980 年至今

DBS 高频刺激对于一些特定的神经病学和精神病学症状是有效的。虽然其疗效和毁损类似，但是 DBS 的优点是在停止刺激后阳性和阴性反应都是可逆的，另外目前高频刺激（>100Hz）的植入性脉冲发生器是可用的，当时主要适应证是慢性疼痛。

1987 年，格勒诺布尔（法国）的 Alim Benabid（图 1-7）和同事发表了他们通过连续丘脑刺激治疗帕金森病震颤的结果，从此开启了 DBS 历史上的一个新时代。他们报道了 4 名患者，其中 1 例因对侧做过丘脑切开术接受单侧丘脑连续刺激，另外 3 例接受单侧慢性丘脑刺激。4 例患者所有的电极都植入在丘脑腹侧中间核（Vim）（Benabid 等，1987）。由于苍白球腹后外侧切开术治疗帕金森病具有较好的效果，这仍然是大多数临床医师的外科治疗选择（Laitinen 等，1992b；Svennilson 等，1960）。"格勒诺布尔团队"在 1991 年发表了他们丘脑 Vim DBS 治疗 26 例帕金森病和 6 例特发性震颤患者的长期疗效（Benabid 等，1991）。1992 年，在这些有效结果的基础上，共有 14 个中心参加了"欧洲多中心丘脑 DBS 研究"（Limousin 等，1999）。在那时，Jean Siegfried 等报道了 GPi DBS 的效果和苍白球切开类似，但是即使在同一手术过程中也可以安全地进行双侧电极植入（Siegfried 和 Lippitz，1994）。

DBS 在帕金森病治疗中的真正突破是 1995 年发表的以底丘脑核（subthalamic nucleus，STN）为靶点的慢性 DBS 取得的良好疗效（Limousin 等，1995）。选择 STN 作为外科靶点是以脑网络的生理学知识为基础的，该知识是通过

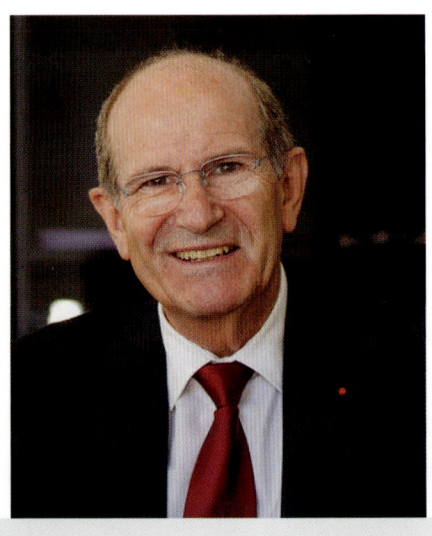

▲ 图 1-7 Alim-Louis Benabid 教授（1972），一位法国格勒诺布尔的神经外科和神经生物学家

DBS手术过程和动物实验中的神经生理结构获得的（Bergman等，1990；Aziz等，1991；Kringelbach等，2007；Benazzouz等，1993）。

再之后的重要进展是刺激装置的改善和ICT领域的知识扩展。磁共振（MRI）扫描和融合术前MRI和CT的技术使得计算靶点结构的坐标变得更可靠。此外，还可以在手术后看到刺激电极的位置与预期靶点结构的关系。微电极记录（MER）技术的引入是神经生理学技术在确定脑内结构位置（特别是STN）方面的一种改进。目前，全世界范围有超过170 000名患者接受了双侧或单侧的DBS电极植入。其中80%的患者是运动障碍病患者，其中主要是帕金森病，其次是震颤和肌张力障碍。对于这些适应证，基于以下临床随机试验（表1-2），DBS作为常规治疗已经获得了美国食品药品管理局（FDA）和欧盟委员会（CE）批准。另外，DBS治疗强迫症和癫痫也是被正式认可的。

目前的研究进展包括进行立体定向放射手术（伽马刀）"毁损"，经颅高聚焦超声治疗，DBS电极和设备的进一步技术改进（见第5章），手术过程中微电极记录（MER）的必要性（见第6章），以及全麻下完成整个手术步骤的可能性（见第7章）（Hariz，2017；Elaime等，2010；Wang等，2015）。

表1-2 在欧洲和美国注册的DBS治疗各种适应证的研究

适应证	CE注册	FDA注册
震颤	1993	1997
帕金森病		
• Vim	1997	1999
• STN/GPi	1998	2002
肌张力障碍	2003	2003（HDE）
强迫症	2009	2008（HDE）
癫痫	2010	—

CE. 欧盟委员会；FDA. 美国食品药品管理局；Vim. 丘脑腹中间核；STN. 底丘脑核；GPi. 苍白球内侧部；HDE. 人道主义器材豁免

参考文献

[1] Akil H, Richardson DE, Hughes J, et al. Enkephalin-like material elevated in ventricular cerebrospinal fluid of pain patients after analgetic focal stimulation. Science. 1978;201:463–5.

[2] Albe-Fessard D, Arfel G, Guiot G. Activités électriques caractéristiques de quelques structures cérébrales chez l'homme. Ann Chir. 1953;17:1185–214.

[3] Andy OJ. Thalamic stimulation for control of movement disorders. Appl Neurophysiol. 1983;46:107–11.

[4] Andy OJ, Jarko MF, Sias FR. Subthalamotomy in treatment of parkinsonian tremor. J Neurosurg. 1963;20:860–70.

[5] Aziz TZ, Peggs D, Sambrook MA, Crossman AR. Lesion of the subthalamic nucleus for the alleviation of 1-methyl-4-phenyl-1,2,3,6-tetrahydropyridine (MPTP)-induced parkinsonism in the primate. Mov Disord. 1991;6:288–92.

[6] Baumeister AA. The Tulane electrical brain stimulation program. A historical case study in medical ethics. J Hist Neurosci. 2000;9:262–78.

[7] Bechtereva NP, Bondarchuk AN, Smirnov VM, Meliutcheva LA, Shandurina AN. Method of electrostimulation of the deep brain structures in the treatment of some chronic diseases. Confin Neurol. 1975;37:136–40.

[8] Benabid AL, Pollak P, Louveau A, Henry S, de Rougement J. Combined (thalamotomy and stimulation) stereotactic surgery of the VIM thalamic nucleus for bilateral Parkinson's disease. Appl Neurophysiol. 1987;50:344–6.

[9] Benabid AL, Pollak P, Gervason C, et al. Long-term suppression of tremor by chronic stimulation of the ventral intermediate thalamic nucleus. Lancet. 1991;337:403–6.

[10] Benazzouz A, Gross C, Feger J, Boraud T, Bioulac B. Reversal of rigidity and improvement in motor performance by subthalamic high-frequency stimulation in MPTP-treated monkeys. Eur J Neurosci. 1993;5:382–9.

[11] Bergman H, Wichmann T, DeLong MR. Reversal of experimental parkinsonism by lesions of the subthalamic nucleus. Science. 1990;249:1436–8.

[12] Bertrand CM. A pneumotaxic technique for producing localized cerebral lesions and its use in the treatment of Parkinson's disease. J Neurosurg. 1958;15:251–64.

[13] Blomstedt P, Hariz MI. Deep brain stimulation for movement disorders before DBS for movement disorders. Parkinsonism Relat Disord. 2010;16:429–33.

[14] Brice J, McLellan LD. Suppression of intention tremor by contingent deep brain stimulation. Lancet. 1980;1:1221–2.

[15] Burckhardt G. Ueber Rindexcisionen, als Beitrag zur operative Therapie der Psychosen. Allg Z Psychiatr Psych Med. 1891;47:463–548.

[16] Cooper IS. Ligation of the anterior choroidal artery for unvoluntary movements; parkinsonism. Psychiatr Q. 1953;27:317–9.

[17] Cooper IS, Bravo GJ. Anterior chorioidal artery occlusion, chemopallidectomy and chemothalamectomy: a consecutive series of 700 patients. In: Fields WS, editor. Pathogenesis and treatment of parkinsonism. Springfield: Thomas; 1958. p. 325–63.

[18] Cooper IS, Upton ARM, Amin I. Reversibility of chronic neurologic deficits. Some effects of electrical stimulation of the thalamus and internal capsule in man. Appl Neurophysiol. 1980;43:244–58.

[19] Delgado JM, Hamlin H, Chapman WP. Technique of intracranial electrode implacement for recording and stimulation and its possible therapeutic value in psychotic patients. Confin Neurol. 1952;12:315–9.

[20] Elaime AL, Arthurs BJ, Lamoreaux WT, et al. Gamma knife radiosurgery form movement disorders: a concise review of the literature. World J Surg Oncol. 2010;8:61.

[21] Fénelon MF. Essais de traitement neurochirurgical du syndrome parkinsonien par intervention directe sur les voies extrapyramidales immédiament sous-striopallidales (anse lenticulaire). Rev Neurol. 1950;83:437–9.

[22] Freed H, Spiegel E, Wycis HT. Somatic procedures for the relief of anxiety. Psychiatr Q. 1949;23:227–35.

[23] Gildenberg PL. The present role of stereotactic surgery in the management of Parkinson's disease. In: Hassler RG, Christ JF, editors. Parkinson-specific motor and mental disorders, vol. 40. New York: Raven; 1984. p. 447–52.

[24] Gildenberg PL. Evolution of neuromodulation. Stereotact Funct Neurosurg. 2005;83:71–9.

[25] Gildenberg PL. Evolution of basal ganglia surgery for movement disorders. Stereotact Funct Neurosurg. 2006;84:131–5.

[26] Guiot G, Brion S. Traitement des mouvements anormaux par la coagulation pallidale. Rev Neurol (Paris). 1953;89:578–80.

[27] Guiot G, Hardy J, Albe-Fessard D. Délimitation precise des structures sous-corticales et identification de noyaux thalamiques chez l'homme par l'éctrophysiologie stéréotaxique. Neurochirurgia (Stuttgart). 1962;5:1–18.

[28] Hariz MI. My 25 stimulating years with DBS in Parkinson's disease. J Parkinsons Dis. 2017;7(Suppl 1):S35–41.

[29] Hariz MI, Blomstedt P, Zrinzo L. Deep brain stimulation between 1947 and 1987: the untold story. Neurosurg Focus. 2010;29:E1.

[30] Hassler R, Riechert T. Indikationen und Lokalisationsmethode der gezielten Hirnoperationen. Nervenarzt. 1954;25:441–7.

[31] Jasper HH, Hunter J (1949) cited in:Hayne R, Meyers R. An improved model of a stereotaxic instrument. J Neurosurg. 1950;7:463–6.

[32] Heath RG. Electrical self-stimulation of the brain in man. Am J Psychiatr. 1963;120:571–7.

[33] Heller AC, Amar AP, Liu CY, Apuzzo ML. Surgery of the mind and mood: a mosaic of issues in time and evolution. Neurosurgery. 2006;59:720–39.

[34] Horsley V. Remarks on the surgery of the central nervous system. Br Med J. 1890;2:1286–92.

[35] Horsley V. The Linacre lecture on the so-called motor area of the brain. Br Med J. 1909;2(2533):121–32.

[36] Horsley V, Clarke RH. The structure and functions of the cerebellum examined by a new method. Brain. 1908;31:45–124.

[37] Hosobuchi Y, Adams JE, Rutkin B. Chronic thalamic stimulation for the control of facial anaesthesia dolorosa. Arch Neurol. 1973;29:158–61.

[38] Iskander BJ, Nashold BS Jr. History of functional neurosurgery. Neurosurg Clin N Am. 1995;6:1–25.

[39] Kandel EI, Schavinsky YV. Stereotaxic apparatus and operations in Russia in the 19th century. J Neurosurg. 1972;37:407–11.

[40] Krack P, Hariz MI, Baunez C, Guridi J, Obeso JA. Deep brain stimulation: from neurology to psychiatry? TINS. 2010;33:474–84.

[41] Kringelbach ML, Jenkinson N, Owen S, Aziz TZ. Translational principles of deep brain stimulation. Nat Rev Neurosci. 2007;8:623–35.

[42] Laitinen LV, Bergenheim AT, Hariz MI. Leksell's posteroventral pallidotomy in the treatment of Parkinson's disease. J Neurosurg. 1992a;76:53–61.

[43] Laitinen LV, Bergenheim AT, Haris MI. Ventroposterolateral pallidotomy can abolish all parkinsonian symptoms. Stereotact Funct Neurosurg. 1992b;58:14–21.

[44] Leksell L. A stereotaxic apparatus for intracerebral surgery. Acta Chirurg Scand. 1949;99:229–33.

[45] Leriche R. Ueber chirurgische Eingriffe bei parkinsonischer Krankheit. Neurol Zbl. 1912;13:1093–6.

[46] Limousin P, Pollak P, Benazzous A, et al. Effects of parkinsonian signs and symptoms of bilateral subthalamic stimulation. Lancet. 1995;345:91–5.

[47] Limousin P, Speelman JD, Gielen F, Janssens M. Multicentre European study of the thalamic stimulation in parkinsonian and essential tremor. J Neurol Neurosurg Psychiatry. 1999;66:289–96.

[48] Mashour GA, Walker EE, Martuza RL. Psychosurgery: past, present, and future. Brain Res Rev. 2005;48:409–19.

[49] Meyers R. Surgical procedure for postencephalitic tremor, with notes on the physiology of premotor fibers. Arch Neurol Psychiatr. 1940;44:455–9.

[50] Meyers R. Surgical experiments in the therapy of certain 'extrapyramidal' diseases: a current evaluation. Acta Psychiatr Neurol Suppl. 1951a;67:7–40.

[51] Meyers R. Dandy's striatal theory of "the center of consciousness". AMA Arch Neurol Psychiatry. 1951b;65:659–72.

[52] Narabayashi H, Okuma T, Shikiba S. Procaine oil blocking of the globus pallidus. AMA Arch Neurol Psychiatry. 1956;75:36–48.

[53] Olivier A, Bertrand G, Picard C. Discovery of the first human stereotactic instrument. Appl Neurophysiol. 1983;46:84–91.

[54] Redfern RM. History of stereotactic surgery for Parkinson's disease. Br J Neurosurg. 1989;3:271–304.

[55] Riechert T, Wolff M. Ueber ein neues Zielgerät zur intrakraniellen elektrischen Ableitung und Ausschaltung. Arch Psychiatr Nervenkr Z Gesamte Neurol Psychiatr. 1951;186:225–30.

[56] Sarem-Aslani A, Mullett K. Industrial perspective on deep brain stimulation: history, current state, and developments. Front Integr Neurosci. 2011;5:46.

[57] Schurr PH, Merrington WR. The Horsley-Clarke stereotaxic apparatus. Br J Surg. 1978;65:33–6.

[58] Sem-Jacobsen CW. Depth-electrographic observations in psychotic patients. Acta Psychiatr Scand Suppl. 1959;34:412–6.

[59] Shorter E. A history of psychiatry: from the era of the asylum to the age of Prozac. Hoboken: Wiley; 1997.

[60] Siegfried J. Is the neurosurgical treatment of Parkinson's disease still indicated? J Neural Transm Suppl. 1980;(16):195–8.

[61] Siegfried J. Effects de la stimulation du noyau sensitive du thalamus sur les dyskinesies et la spasticity. Rev Neurol (Paris). 1986;142:380–3.

[62] Siegfried J, Lippitz B. Bilateral chronic stimulation of ventroposterolateral pallidum: a new therapeutic approach for alleviating all parkinsonian symptoms. Neurosurgery. 1994;35:1126–9.

[63] Speelman JD, Bosch DA. Resurgence of functional neurosurgery for Parkinson's disease: a historical perspective. Mov Disord. 1998;13:582–8.

[64] Spiegel EA. Indications for stereoencephalotomies. A critical assessment. Confin Neurol. 1969;31:5–10.

[65] Spiegel EA, Wycis HT. Thalamotomy and pallidotomy for treatment of choreic movements. Acta Neurochirurgica. 1950;2(3–4):417–22.

[66] Spiegel EA, Wycis HT. Stereoencephalotomy (thalamotomy and related procedures) part 1: methods and stereotaxic atlas of the human brain. New York: Grüne and Stratton; 1952.

[67] Spiegel EA, Wycis HT. Stereoencephalotomy part II: clinical and physiological applications. New York: Grune & Stratton; 1962.

[68] Spiegel EA, Wycis HT, Marks M, Lee J. Stereotaxic apparatus for operations on the human brain. Science. 1947;106:349–50.

[69] Spiegel EA, Wycis HT, Freed H. Thalamotomy: neuropsychiatric aspects. N Y State J Med. 1949;49(19):2273.

[70] Spiegel EA, Wycis HT, Szekely EG, Adams DJ, Flanagan M, Baird HW. Campotomy in various extrapyramidal disorders. J Neurosurg. 1963;20:871–81.

[71] Svennilson E, Torvik A, Lowe R, Leksell L. Treatment of parkinsonism by stereotactic thermolesions in the pallidal region: a clinical evaluation of 81 cases. Acta Psychiatr Scand. 1960;35:358–77.

[72] Talairach J, Hecaen H, David M, Monnier M, de Ajuriaguerra J. Recherches sur la coagulation therapeutique des structure sous-corticales chez l'homme. Rev Neurol. 1949;81:4–24.

[73] Talairach J, Paillas JE, David M. Dyskinésie de type hémiballique traitée par cortectomie frontale limitée, puis par coagulation de l'anse lenticulaire et de la portion interne du globus pallidus. Amélioration importante depuis un an. Rev. Rev Neurol (Paris).1950;83:440–51.

[74] Tasker RR. Thalamic stereotaxic procedures. In: Schaltenbrand G, Walker AE, editors. Stereotaxy of the human brain. New York: Georg Thieme Verlag; 1982.

[75] Wang TR, Dallapiazza R, Elias WJ. Neurological applications of transcranial high intensity focused ultrasound. Int J Hyperthermia. 2015;31:285–91.

第2章 脑深部电刺激的靶点解剖
Anatomy of Targets for Deep Brain Stimulation

Ali Jahanshahi　Juergen K. Mai　Yasin Temel　著
韩春雷　孟凡刚　译　刘德峰　杨岸超　张建国　校

摘要：脑深部电刺激（DBS）通过调节脑内特定解剖结构的兴奋性来改善神经和（或）精神性疾病的临床症状。因此，获悉这些靶区的解剖特点及生理学功能对于开展DBS手术至关重要。基底核和丘脑是DBS的主要靶区。这些结构通过相互独立或联系的投射纤维与高级（皮质）和低级（脑干）脑区相联系。这些投射纤维不仅主要负责运动控制，而且还负责其他功能，如运动学习、联合功能及情感。经典的基底核环路模型认为，信息流经基底核传递至皮质通过两条通路，而新的模型表明，尚有其他的平行环路加强了基底核的经典功能，这些通路涉及大脑的联合及边缘区域。目前，DBS治疗运动障碍性疾病采用的靶点包括底丘脑核的背外侧部、苍白球内侧部的腹后外侧及丘脑的腹外侧核。对于精神性疾病，主要采用腹侧纹状体区域的核团，包括伏隔核、内囊腹侧部、底丘脑核的腹内侧部、苍白球内侧部的前部及丘脑内侧核。Papez环路中的丘脑前核则是DBS治疗难治性癫痫所采用的靶点。本章将讨论这些靶点的解剖细节。

一、概述

DBS旨在通过调节局部解剖结构的兴奋性，进而改善特定神经性和（或）精神性疾病的症状。DBS已经发展成为一些特定疾病的重要治疗手段，包括帕金森病（PD）（Deuschl等，2006）、特发性震颤（Benabid等，1993；Hubble等，1996）、肌张力障碍（Krauss等，1999）、癫痫（Fisher等，2010）及强迫症（OCD）（Nuttin等，1999；Denys等，2010）。此外，研究者对DBS治疗重度抑郁、抽动秽语综合征（GTS）和多种其他精神性疾病的临床疗效也进行了探索（Bewernick等，2010；Lozano等，2012；Ackermans等，2011）。尽管问世已30年，但DBS治疗作用的神经生理学机制仍不明确（Gradinaru等，2009）。了解DBS治疗神经或精神性疾病的作用机制，不仅对于理解DBS是怎样工作的，而且对于如何使DBS变得更有效，以及怎样将其有效地推广至其他神经系统疾病的治疗中是至关重要的。任何机制研究的本质，甚至是那些内在地试图揭示治疗作用或病理生理学背后机制的研究，都是一种解剖学。DBS需要刺激那些与疾病症状相关的解剖网络具有有效投射的区域。尽管与核心精神病理学相关的解剖模型在不断发展，但可以想象，熟悉基底核、丘脑及其他皮质，以及皮质下结构的解剖学关系对于深入了解DBS在神经和精神性疾病中的应用仍是至关重要的。DBS术中精准的植入电极后才能获得理想的疗效。实际上，对解剖学有了清晰的认识后，可以解释DBS的大部分疗效和不良反应。本章旨在阐明那些被认为发挥 DBS 治疗效果的最常用靶点的解剖结构。主要聚焦用于神经及精神性疾病治疗的基底核和丘脑的解剖。接下来开始对皮质 – 基底核 – 丘脑皮质环路及其中的单个的区域进行讨论。

二、皮质 – 基底核 – 丘脑皮质环路

基底核由苍白球复合体、纹状体、黑质和底丘脑核（STN）构成（Alexander 和 Crutcher，1990）。运动环路中，"直接""间接"及"超直接"通路调节皮质至基底核的神经活动，并最终决定了丘脑的整体兴奋性。皮质的投射纤维通过两个输入结构投射至基底核。第一个是纹状体，包括壳核、背侧纹状体的尾状核，以及腹侧纹状体的伏隔核。第二个输入结构是 STN。

将纹状体作为一个输入结构已有一些时间（Albin 等，1989），但提出将 STN 作为一个输入核团的时间还为时尚短（Nambu 等，2002）。皮质 – 底丘脑核投射即超直接通路是谷氨酸能的兴奋性通路（图 2–1）。皮质 – 纹状体传出纤维投射至尾状核、壳核及伏隔核，并进一步在基底核环路中进行处理加工。这些传出纤维来自整个的同侧及对侧的皮质，本质上是兴奋性的，与纹状体神经元树突棘形成的神经末梢以谷氨酸作为神经递质，而且这些投射具有一定的局部定位关系（Gerfen，1984；Donoghue 和 Herkenham，1986）。皮质投射至纹状体的纤维分为两类，一是锥体束神经元（pyramidal tact neurons），它发出皮质 – 锥体束投射并支配同侧纹状体神经元，构成间接通路；二是端脑内神经元（intra-telencephalic neurons），它投射至双侧的纹状体神经元，构成直接通路（Lei 等，2004）。

丘脑 – 纹状体投射纤维构成了支配纹状体的第二大传入纤维，这在过去的几年内被严重地忽视。这些投射纤维主要来自丘脑的中线核和板内核（Berendse 和 Groenewegen，1990），以及丘脑腹侧运动核（McFarland 和 Haber，2001）。丘脑 – 纹状体投射路径与皮质纹状体投射类似。

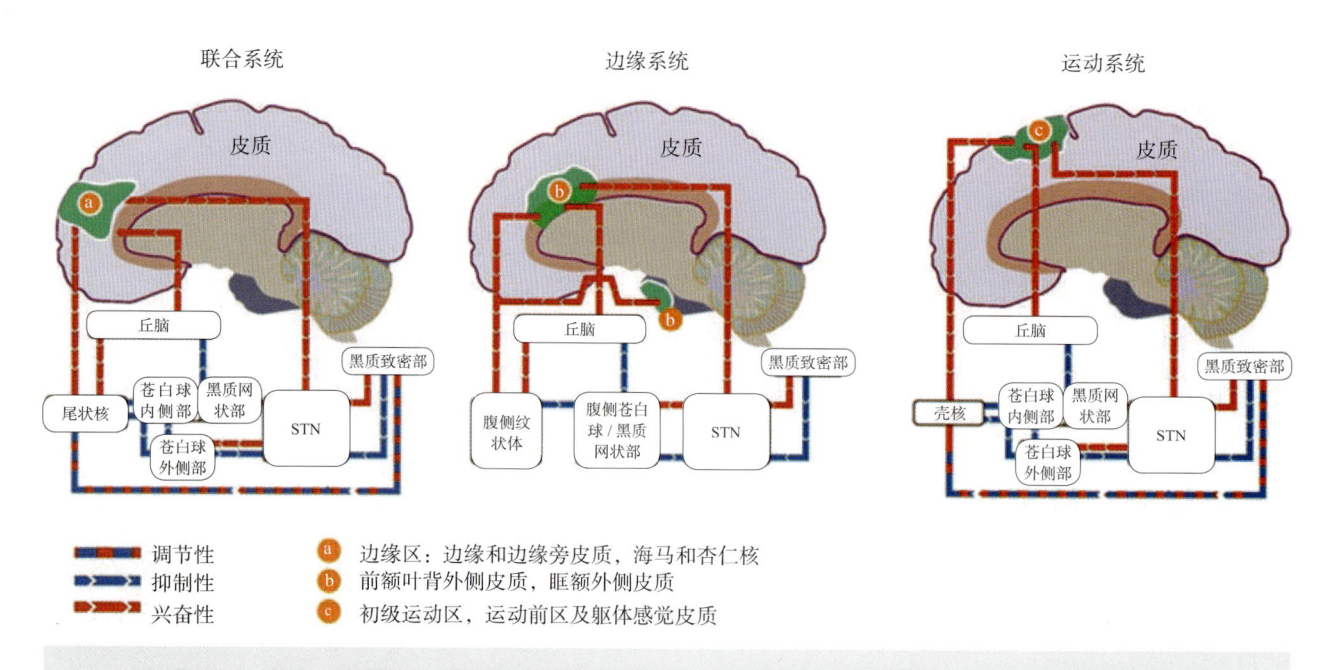

▲ 图 2–1 皮质 – 基底核 – 丘脑皮质投射主要包括 3 个功能通路，即运动通路、联合通路及边缘通路
运动通路的连接如上所述。联合通路中的皮质 – 纹状体投射主要支配尾状核，而其余投射则与运动通路类似。边缘脑区的传出纤维通过 STN 和腹侧纹状体球进入基底核。这些传出纤维通过腹侧苍白球到达丘脑内侧部（Alexander 等，1990），进而返回至相关皮质区域（经许可转载，引自 Temel 等，2005）
STN. 底丘脑核

皮质纹状体投射纤维投射至背侧纹状体并到达苍白球复合体，形成两个主要的纹状体通路。通过直接通路，这些投射纤维到达基底核的输出核团，包括苍白球内侧部（GPi）和黑质网状部（SNr）。直接通路由通过突触投射至 GPi 和 SNr 的中型多棘神经元（MSN）构成，MSN 主要表达 D_1 型多巴胺能受体。而间接通路由表达 D_2 型多巴胺能受体的 MSN 的传出纤维构成。通过间接通路，纹状体首先投射至苍白球外侧部（GPe），然后到达 STN，最后通过 STN 到达基底核的输出核团（GPi 和 SNr）。间接通路还参与了 GPe 到 GPi 间的直接投射。除皮质 - 纹状体和丘脑 - 纹状体投射外，杏仁核复合体也发出谷氨酸能投射纤维至纹状体（Ragsdale 和 Graybiel，1988）。GPi 和 SNr 主要投射至丘脑的腹外侧部，丘脑腹外侧部则反过来投射回大脑皮质（只要是额叶）。丘脑至皮质的投射纤维同样是兴奋性的。GPi 和 SNr 的传出纤维通过轴突侧支与不同的靶区相联系（Parent 和 Hazrati，1995；Parent 等，2000）。基底核中只有 STN 是以谷氨酸作为神经递质的兴奋性核团，除此之外，所有的投射都是抑制性的，以 GABA 作为神经递质。基底核输出核团的投射纤维到达丘脑腹外侧核，并通过丘脑到达皮质；详见综述（Lanciego 等，2012）。

单胺能神经递质系统在调控基底核的功能中发挥着重要的作用。正常的基底核系统功能高度依赖于完整的多巴胺递质释放到输入核团。黑质投射至纹状体的多巴胺能传出纤维主要源自黑质致密部（SNc）中的 A9 类多巴胺能神经元。此外，少部分由位于后红核的 A8 类神经元构成（Dahlstrom 和 Fuxe，1964）。黑质致密部除投射至纹状体的运动及联合区外，还投射至 STN。中脑纹状体和中脑边缘区多巴胺能神经投射纤维来自腹侧被盖区（VTA）的 A10 多巴胺能神经元，支配腹侧纹状体（如伏隔核）和 STN 的腹内侧。多巴胺释放障碍与多种基底核疾病有关，如帕金森综合征（Parkinsonism）、肌张力障碍、舞蹈症及抽动症。除多巴胺能投射外，脑干中缝核的血清素型细胞也发出纤维投射至纹状体背侧和腹侧（Anden 等，1966）。然而，因实验结果存在争议，这些投射纤维的功能尚不明确。

三、解剖结构

（一）纹状体

纹状体是一个具有复杂神经元表型及递质系统的异质性结构。一些组织化学及免疫组织化学染色表明，纹状体主要包含纹状小体（striosomes）和基质（matrix）。纹状小体和基质具有明显的分界，根据两者表达的神经化学标记物很容易将其区分。例如，乙酰胆碱免疫组织化学染色（Graybiel 和 Ragsdale，1978）表明，在强阳性 AChE 染色的背景（基质）中，存在一些零散的淡染区域（纹状小体）。其他标记物的免疫细胞化学染色，如 P 物质、γ- 氨基丁酸（GABA）、神经降压素，同样显示出了这些标记物在纹状体的这两个分区中具有选择性表达的特点（Pert 等，1976；Graybiel 等，1981；Gerfen，1984；Desban 等，1995）。MSN 神经元的轴突侧支和树突分支被局限在纹状体中某一类结构中，要么位于纹状小体，要么位于基质内。例如，纹状小体中 MSN 神经元的树突并不进入邻近基质区，反之亦然。鉴于在传入和传出纤维连接中存在差异，纹状小体和基质在一系列神经系统疾病中的作用也明显不同。位于基质中的 MSN 神经元投射至 GPe、GPi 和 SNr，而纹状小体中的 MSN 神经元则主要支配 SNc。然而，纹状小体和基质中的 MSN 神经元却都发出轴突侧支支配 Gpe、GPi 和 SNr（Gerfen，1984；Bolam 等，1988；Kawaguchi 等，1989；Gimenez-Amaya 和 Graybiel，1990；Fujiyama 等，2011）。就传入纤维而言，源自大脑皮质和丘脑的谷氨酸能神经元，以及源自 SNc 的多巴胺能神经元主要支配基质部分，而来自边缘皮质区域和杏仁核的神经元则选择性投射至纹状小体（Graybiel，1984；Donoghue 和 Herkenham，1986；Ragsdale

和 Graybiel，1988；Gerfen，1992；Sadikot 等，1992a，b；Kincaid 和 Wilson，1996）。纹状小体-基质这种组织方式所产生的确切功能仍待进一步研究（Lanciego 等，2012）。

（二）纹状体神经元

纹状体含有两种不同的神经元，包括投射神经元（90%）和中间神经元（10%）。由于投射神经元具有小到中等的神经元胞体（直径 20μm），因此也被称为中型多棘神经元（MSN）。这些神经元是多极神经元，而且树突上有树突棘。所有的 MSN 神经元都是以 GABA 作为神经递质的抑制性神经元。MSN 神经元可根据其投射模式进一步分为支配 GPe 的神经元和支配 GPi 与 SNr 的神经元。纹状体中投射至 GPe 的 MSN 神经元形成抑制性的间接通路（纹状体-GPe-STN-GPi/SNr），从而抑制靶区的神经元，这些神经元表达多巴胺 D_2 受体（D_2R）。相反，直接投射至 GPi 和 SNr 的 MSN 神经元形成兴奋性直接通路（纹状体-苍白球），这些神经元表达多巴胺 D_1 受体（D_1R）。直接与间接通路的另外一个关键的不同点是直接通路的源头神经元表达神经肽 P 物质，而间接通路的源头神经元表达神经肽、脑啡肽和强啡肽。此外，纹状体还含有几种不同种类的中间神经元，不同于 MSN 神经元，这些中间神经元具有光滑的树突。根据神经化学表型及形态学特点可将这些中间神经元分为以下 4 类（Kawaguchi 等，1995）：①胆碱能神经元，以乙酰胆碱作为神经递质，体形最大，数量最多，具有紧张性放电（tonic firing）模式的电生理特性；②表达小清蛋白（parvalbumin）的 GABA 能神经元，同时具有快速放电（fast-spiking）的电生理放电特点；③表达钙调蛋白的 GABA 能神经元；④另外一种以一氧化氮作为神经递质的 GABA 能神经元，也被称为氮能神经元。这些中间神经元与 MSN 神经元一起构成了复杂的纹状体内环路。例如，紧张性放电和快速放电样 GABA 能中间神经元都会受到多巴胺能神经元的控制，两者也可反过来调节 MSN 神经元的兴奋

性。同时，钙调蛋白和氮能中间神经元也可支配紧张性放电和快速放电样 GABA 能中间神经元（详细参见综述，Lanciego 等，2012）。

（三）腹侧纹状体

腹侧纹状体包括伏隔核、尾状核腹内侧部，以及嗅结节的棘细胞部（spined cell part）（Nauta，1979；Parent 和 Hazrati，1995；Nakano，2000）。其中，伏隔核（NAC）是腹侧纹状体最重要的部分。NAC 位于前连合（AC）后缘的前方，平行于中线，位于尾状核的腹侧和内侧并向背外侧延伸至壳核（图 2-2）。观察 NAC 的结构，矢状位要优于水平位，而冠状位又优于矢状位。在 MRI T_2 像上，NAC 信号要高于尾状核和壳核，使其与两者的边界更容易分别。不同于纹状体，NAC 分为核心区（core）和外周区（shell），其中每区只具有单一的特性。外周区从内侧、腹侧及外侧包绕核心区。众所周知，根据神经化学标记物及电生理特性，很容易将核心区与外周区进行区分。此外，核心区与外周区在传入及传出纤维连接上也有所不同，提示两者在神经系统疾病中也具有不同的功能。95% 以上 NAC 细胞是 GABA 能 MSN 投射神经元。

NAC 也被称为腹侧纹状体，这一概念由 Heimer 和 Wilson（1975）提出，用于区分背侧纹状体。它的特点是接受大量来自边缘区的投射纤维，如杏仁核、海马及前额叶。鉴于此，NAC 已被作为 DBS 治疗精神性疾病的靶点。NAC 直接接受来自下托（海马结构最下方的结构，位于内嗅皮质与海马 CA_1 区之间）、海马、杏仁核、丘脑，以及前额叶前缘皮质的谷氨酸能传出纤维，除此之外，还通过中脑边缘区的多巴胺能神经投射接受来自腹侧被盖区（VTA）、黑质的间接传入纤维。NAC 的主要传出纤维发自其中的 MSN 神经元，并投射至中脑和基底核的多个区域，如苍白球复合体、终纹、视前区、带旁核（nucleus parataenialis）、丘脑背内侧核、外侧缰核、黑质腹侧盖区（substantia nigra-ventral tegmental area）、下丘脑外侧、扣带回、丘脑、

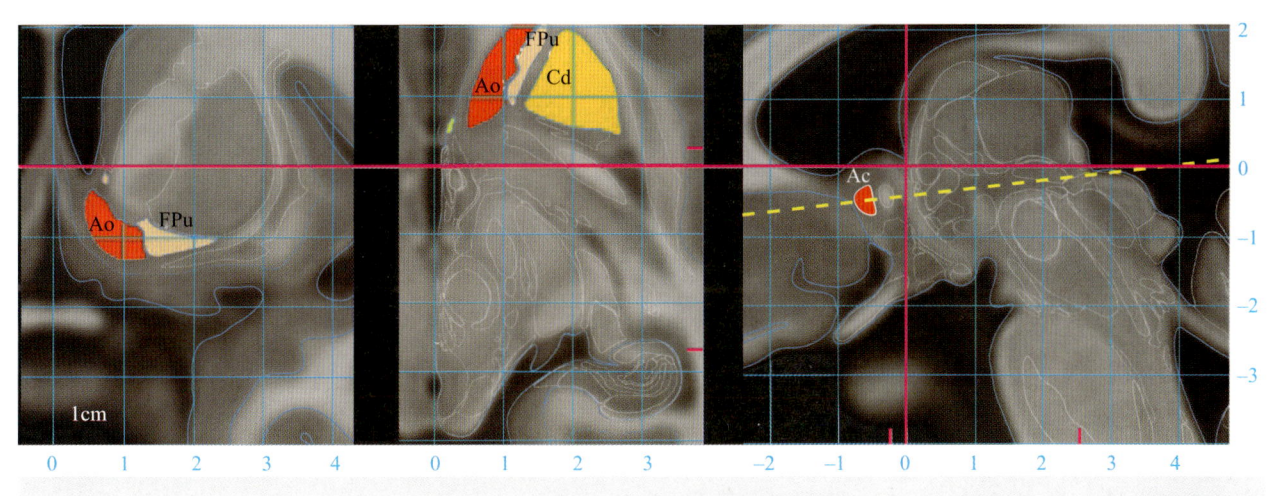

▲ 图 2-2 MNI 空间显示伏隔核的位置
Ac. 伏隔核；FPu. 壳核索；Cd. 尾状核

苍白球及苍白球下区、杏仁核和隔核（详见综述，Salgado 和 Kaplitt，2015）

除 NAC 外，腹侧纹状体还包括嗅觉系统的纹状体成分、尾状核和壳核的腹侧、内侧及尾侧部（Heimer 和 Wilson，1975；Fudge 和 Haber，2002）。NAC 的尾侧是终纹红核（BNST），两者间的解剖界限往往不是很明确。研究表明 BNST 在 OCD 的病理生理中发挥重要的作用，而且刺激该区域可以改善 OCD 患者的临床症状（Luyten 等，2016）。BNST 与 NAC 外周区联系密切。NAC 核心区与外周区的纤维联系不同。在 DBS 中，怎样对待这两分区尚不十分明确。图 2-2 展示了 NAC 在 MNI 空间中的定位。

（四）底丘脑核

底丘脑核（STN），又称 Luysi 体（Corpus Luysi），是一个神经元密集的小核团，它位于间脑与中脑的交界处，恰好位于未定带的腹侧和黑质的背侧（Hameleers 等，2006）。在过去的几年里，STN 是 DBS 治疗 PD 的主要靶点，而且因研究表明它也是一个治疗 OCD 的潜在靶点而引起了更多的关注。

关于 STN 传入和传出纤维的经典模型认为，STN 仅含有源自 GPe（间接通路的第二个中继站）的 GABA 能传入纤维，以及支配基底核输出核团的传出纤维。这个经典模型已受到挑战，研究表明 STN 还接受来自大脑皮质的谷氨酸能纤维投射，即超直接通路，该通路为大脑运动相关皮质提供了一个绕过基底核输入核团，直接到达输出核团的通路。这些投射纤维来着初级运动皮质、辅助运动区、运动前区皮质、额眼区及辅助眼区，而且这些传入纤维在 STN 水平的组织分布具有躯体定位关系（Nambu 等，1996，2002）。超直接通路的特点是其传递速度要快于通过基底核传递的直接和间接通路，因此可以有力地兴奋基底核输出核团。此外，STN 还接受来自丘脑的投射纤维，这些纤维的组织分布具有局部定位关系（Sadikot 等，1992a）。这些丘脑 -STN 投射纤维是双侧性的，但以单侧为主（Castle 等，2005）。STN 投射至基底核的传出纤维表现为具有大量的神经元突起分支，并发出轴突支配 GPi、GPe 和 SNr（Van Der Kooy 和 Hattori，1980）。

尽管 DBS 刺激 STN 可有效缓解严重的运动症状，但也可带来神经精神性不良反应，如情感淡漠、强迫行为、性欲亢进、抑郁症及自杀意念（Temel 等，2005），这些不良反应是由于意外刺激到 STN 的非运动区所致。根据与其联络的不同的神经环路，可以将 STN 分为背外侧运动区、中间联合区及位于腹内侧的边缘区（Lambert

等，2012）（图 2-3）。尽管已有所报道，但是对于这些亚功能分区的功能的了解还不深入，以至于不能针对不同的患者进行分区的个体化治疗。但是，在临床工作中，常常将 DBS 电极置于 STN 的背外侧部，从而仅调控 PD 患者的运动环路（图 2-4）（Kocabicak 和 Temel，2013）。刺激腹内侧部可作用于边缘环路，这已用于 OCD 患者的治疗（Mallet 等，2008）。STN 被重要的结构和投射纤维包绕。上纵束或内侧前脑束位于 STN 的背内侧，它是一个负责情感的重要的单胺能神经投射纤维，刺激该区域可影响情感相关的指标（Schlaepfer 等，2013）。刺激 STN 尾侧的 SNr 也可影响情感反应（Bejjani 等，1999）。另一方面，SNr 又被用来治疗 PD 步态障碍（Weiss 等，2013）。STN 的前内侧面对下丘脑核团，刺激这些区域可引起自主神经性不良反应。其中，刺激 STN 外侧的大脑脚可引起最严重的不良反应。如果电流波及该部位的锥体束，患者可能出现震颤、抽搐和构音障碍（图 2-5）。

最近 MRI 技术方面的进步，如 7T 成像，极大提高了我们对人 STN 的 3 分区的可视化能力。可以想象，这项技术可能会应用到临床工作中用于指导 PD 和 OCD 患者的立体定向电极植入，使 STN 亚分区定位更加可靠。这些技术的进步迫切需要我们对 STN 亚分区要有更加清晰的解剖认识，从而用于确定手术靶点，这样才能促进临床工作的进步。

四、苍白球

（一）苍白球外侧部

GPe 与 GPi、腹侧苍白球一起构成苍白球复合体（图 2-6）。GPe 侧方由壳核包绕。GPe 和 GPi 在细胞及化学构筑方面具有许多相似之处，两核团内都稀疏分布着大胞体的 GABA 能神经元。GPe 和 GPi 的另外一个特点是两核团的神经元都表达丰富的钙离子结合蛋白，即小白蛋白。GPe 接受两个主要的传入系统，一是来自纹状体 D_2 受体型 MSN 神经元的投射纤维，这个抑制性传入纤维构成间接通路的第一个突触中继站。二是来自纹状体的表达 2A 型腺苷受体的投射纤维（Rosin 等，1998）。通过 GPe 与 STN 间的交互联系使得 GPe 接受丰富的谷氨酸能兴奋性投射。GPe 与 STN 间的互相投射提示 GPe 不仅仅是一个简单的纹状体与 STN 间的中继站，它可能在基底核中发挥着重要的作用（Shink 等，1996）。此外，长期以来，我们已经获知 GPe 与 GPi 间也存在交互连接。GPe 还接受另外一个微弱的来自板内核尾侧的谷氨酸能投射纤维（Kawaguchi 等，1990）。

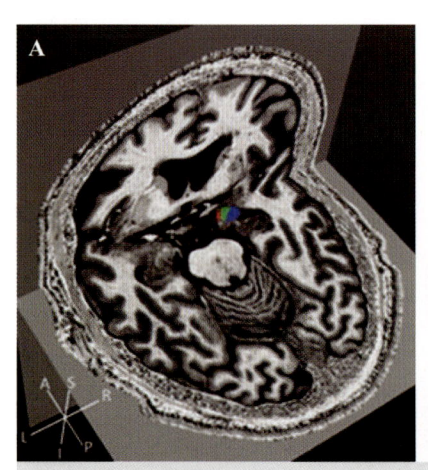

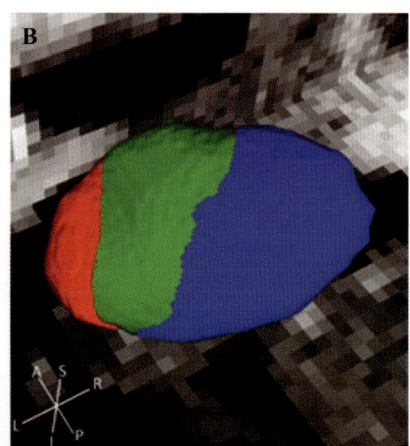

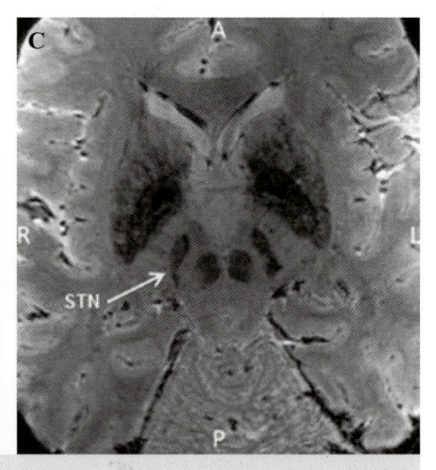

▲ 图 2-3　A. 底丘脑核（STN）的解剖方位；B. 基于不同的神经环路联系可以将 STN 分为 3 个亚功能分区，包括背外侧运动区（蓝色）、中间联合区（绿色）和腹内侧边缘区（红色）；C. 7T 磁共振 T_2 像上显示 STN
（经许可转载，引自 Temel 等，2016）

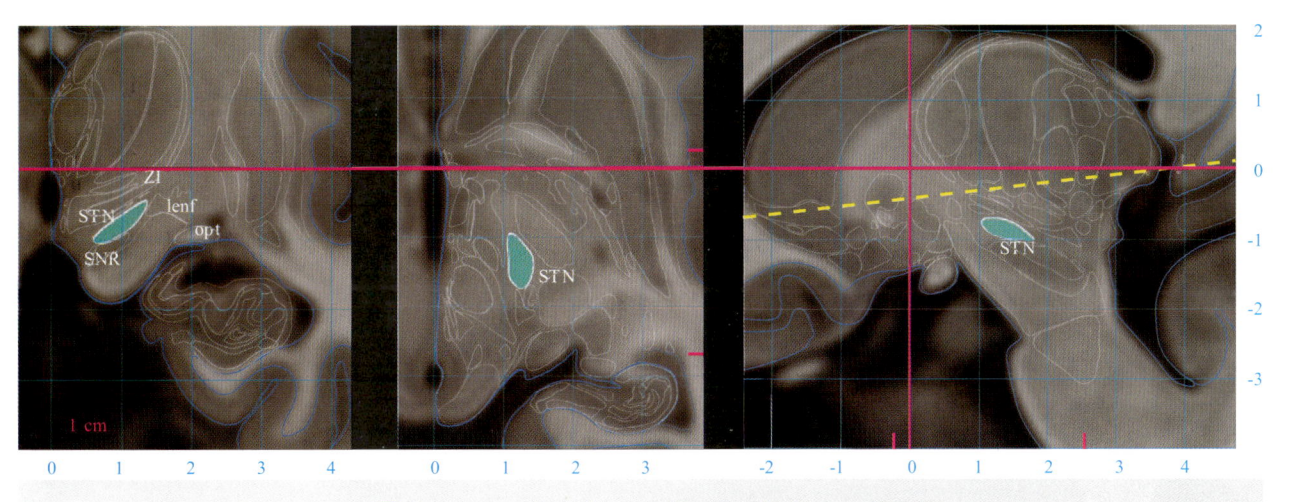

▲ 图 2-4 MNI 空间结合人脑解剖图谱显示 STN 的位置

临床工作中，刺激电极常置于 STN 的背外侧。从左至右，依次为 STN 冠状位、轴位及矢状位图像。红线表示 MNI 空间中的 0 点。MNI 空间与前后连合（黄色虚线）平面相倾斜

STN. 底丘脑核；SNR. 黑质网状部；ZI. 未定带；lenf. 豆状核；opt. 视束

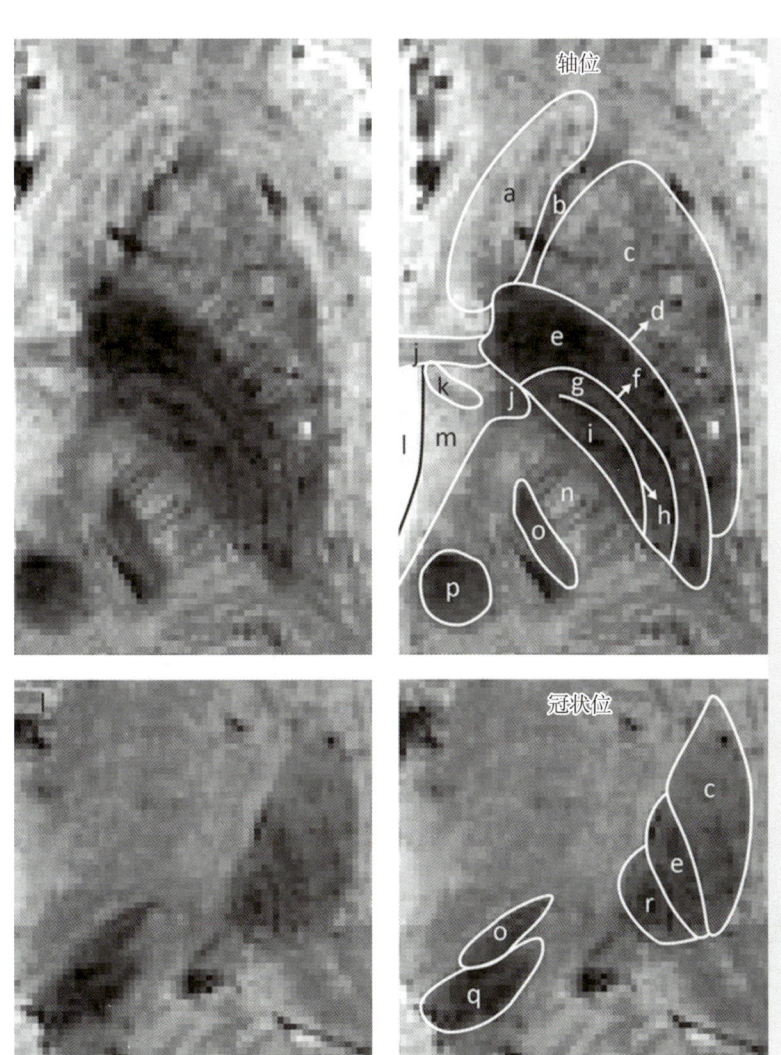

◀ 图 2-5 底丘脑核附近的解剖结构

a. 尾状核；b. 内囊前肢；c. 壳核；d. 外髓板；e. 苍白球外侧部；f. 内髓板；g. 苍白球内侧部外侧带；h. 不全髓板；i. 苍白球内侧部内侧带；j. 前连合；k. 穹窿；l. 第三脑室；m. 下丘脑；n. 内囊后肢；o. 底丘脑核；p. 红核；q. 黑质；r. 苍白球内侧部

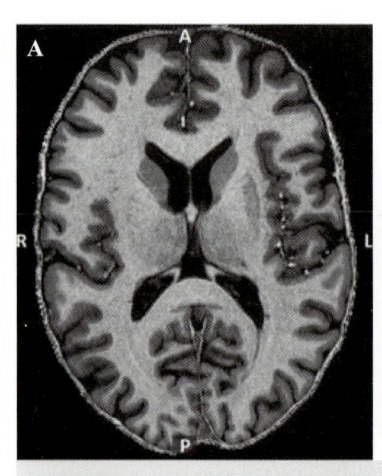

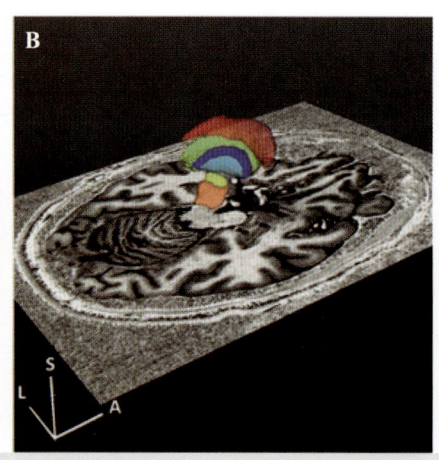

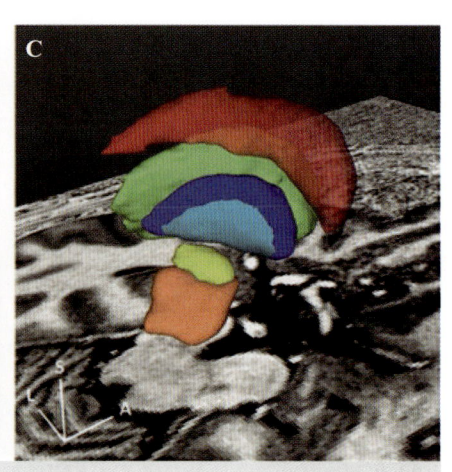

▲ 图2-6　A. 基底核水平面观；B. 去掉周围结构的基底核结构图；C. 放大后的 B 图，基底核的三维方位图，尾状核（红色），壳核（绿色），苍白球外侧部（深蓝），苍白球内侧部（浅蓝），底丘脑核（黄色）及黑质（粉红）（经许可转载，引自 Temel 等，2016）

（二）苍白球内侧部

GPi 是苍白球的内侧部分，位于 GPe 的内侧及内囊后支的外侧（图 2-7）。GPi 与 GPe 以内髓板为界。GPe 与壳核以外髓板为界。有时在 GPi 内也可看到一层薄板，即不全髓板（lamina pallidali incompleta）。在 DBS 手术的微电极电生理记录中，这个板状结构可体现在电信号的静息区上。GPi-DBS 的不良反应多与 GPi 内侧的内囊有关，包括麻木感和构音障碍。很显然，视束经过 GPi 的尾侧，意外刺激到视束会引起视觉不良反应。

人们常将 GPi 和 SNr 看作一组核团，不仅因为两者在功能上都是基底核的输出核团，而且它们在细胞及化学构筑上也存在许多共性，而且两者的传入及传出纤维类型上的差异也很小。苍白球由抑制性的 GABA 能投射神经元组成，这些神经元具有长轴突，且存在高频率放电，通过共振性放电抑制靶核团。GPi 的细胞密度要低于纹状体。此外，GPi 内含有大量交叉的有髓鞘的纹状体传出纤维，使其在 T_2 像上比纹状体更容易识别。GPi 接受来自纹状体背侧的直接通路及来自 STN 的间接通路的投射纤维。直接通路是 GPi 抑制性传入纤维中的主要成分，含有表达 D_1R 的纹状体 MSN 神经元。作为间接通路的一部分，STN

发出兴奋性谷氨酸能投射纤维至 GPi。此外，同侧的底丘脑核-苍白球和底丘脑核-黑质投射发出谷氨酸能的兴奋性传入纤维至 GPi。兴奋性与抑制性的投射纤维汇合于 GPi（和 SNr）的神经元，这些神经元转而支配丘脑及脑干区域。

GPi 主要发出 3 条投射纤维：①豆核襻（ansa lentiformis in older texts），由外侧的 GPi 神经元发出，并沿着内囊的腹内侧及头侧进入红核前区（field H of Forel）。②豆核束（lenticular fasciculus 或 Forel's field H_2），位于 STN 与未定带之间，由内侧的 GPi 神经元的轴突组成，穿经内囊。豆核襻与豆核束在红核前区水平融合在一起，汇入丘脑束（thalamic fasciculus 或 H_1 of Forel），止于腹侧丘脑核及丘脑板内核，形成苍白球丘脑投射。③苍白球中脑被盖投射，支配脑干区域，如上丘和脚桥核（PPN）（Haber 等，2011）。苍白球-丘脑投射纤维支配腹前运动丘脑的致密细胞区和小细胞区（分别称为 VAdc 和 VApc）。作为基底核的 2 个输出核团之一，GPi 已被用作功能神经外科的治疗靶点。Lars Leksell 最早开展 GPi 毁损术用于治疗 PD，Laitinen 进一步发展了该手术（Laitinen 等，1992）。毁损的部位是 GPi 背外侧的感觉运动区。1994 年，GPi-DBS 用于治疗 PD（Siegfried 和 Lippitz，1994）。如今，GPi 的感觉运动区已成为治疗原

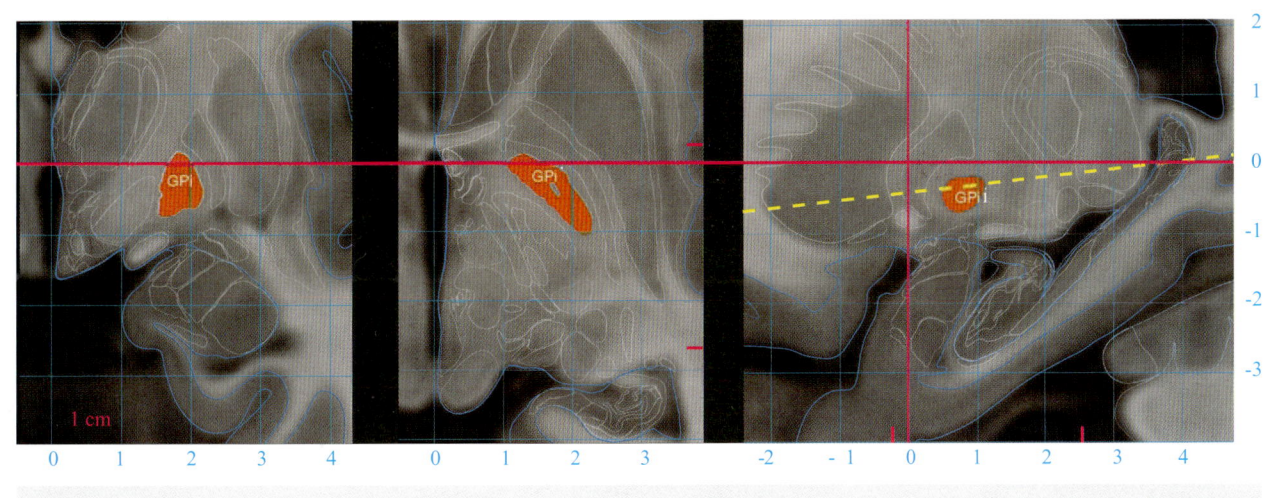

▲ 图 2-7 苍白球在 MNI 空间的定位
GPi. 苍白球内侧部

发性及继发性肌张力障碍的主要靶点。在一些情况下，PD 患者也可以用这种方式进行治疗。近年来，GPi 前部也作为 DBS 刺激靶点用于治疗抽动秽语综合征（Smeets 等，2016）。

五、丘脑

丘脑几乎位于大脑的中央，侧脑室的下方（Ohye，1990）。左右两侧丘脑通过丘脑间黏合相联系。丘脑可接收来自皮质的运动、感觉、边缘环路及联合环路的信息，也可将信息传入至上述部位（Kandel，2000）。丘脑接收并处理感觉和运动性传入信息并与皮质进行交互联系。它将感觉信息传递至皮质并参与了运动、觉醒及情感功能。经典的丘脑分区基于细胞构筑、髓板构筑（myleo-architecture）和解剖位置，主要分为前部、内侧、中线、板内、外侧、后部、背侧和腹侧部核群（Ohye，1990）。丘脑尽管是个异质性的核团，这些核团却能很好地组织在一起。丘脑神经元主要以谷氨酸作为神经递质。

就 DBS 而言，丘脑的 2 个核心核群尤为重要。第一个核群是腹外侧核，其中的腹中间内侧核（Vim 核）最为重要（图 2-8）。Vim 在功能神经外科中用做治疗震颤。另一个重要核团是丘

脑前核（AN），它在立体定向手术中用于治疗难治性癫痫（图 2-9）。Vim 接受来自基底核输出核团的纤维并发出纤维投射至皮质的运动区。此外，它还接受来自小脑的重要传入纤维（Moers-Hornikx 等，2009）。AN 是 Papez 环路中的一个核团，而 Papez 环路是边缘系统中的重要环路，参与情感及记忆控制（Hescham 等，2013）。AN 主要投射至颞叶边缘结构和扣带回。连接乳头体与丘脑前核的乳头体丘脑束是设计电极植入路径的重要参考结构。

六、结论

了解基底节区疾病的解剖学和生理学是现代医学发展的一个新兴领域。这些疾病的神经外科治疗其实就是基于解剖的操作方法。目前 DBS 治疗神经和精神性适应证的主要靶点都位于基底核和丘脑。这些核团均在皮质 - 基底核 - 丘脑皮质的运动、联合及边缘环路中扮演着重要角色。丘脑前核稍有特殊，不在该系统内，用于 DBS 治疗癫痫。深入了解电流刺激下局部及远端部位神经环路改变的本质和程度，将有助于明确是哪些结构起到治疗作用，并有助于了解不同患者间会出现相反效果的机制。

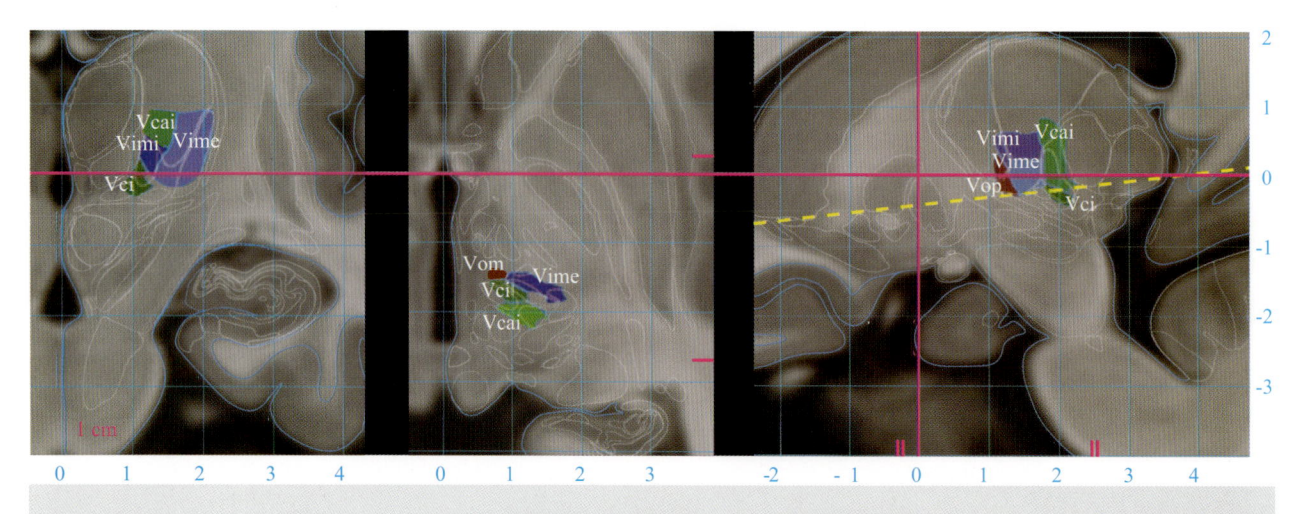

▲ 图 2-8 丘脑腹中间内侧核在 MNI 空间中的定位

Vimi. 丘脑腹中间内侧核内侧部；Vime. 丘脑腹中间内侧核外侧部；Vci. 丘脑腹后内侧核；Vcai. 丘脑腹后前内侧核；Vom. 丘脑腹侧核中部；Vop. 丘脑腹侧核后部

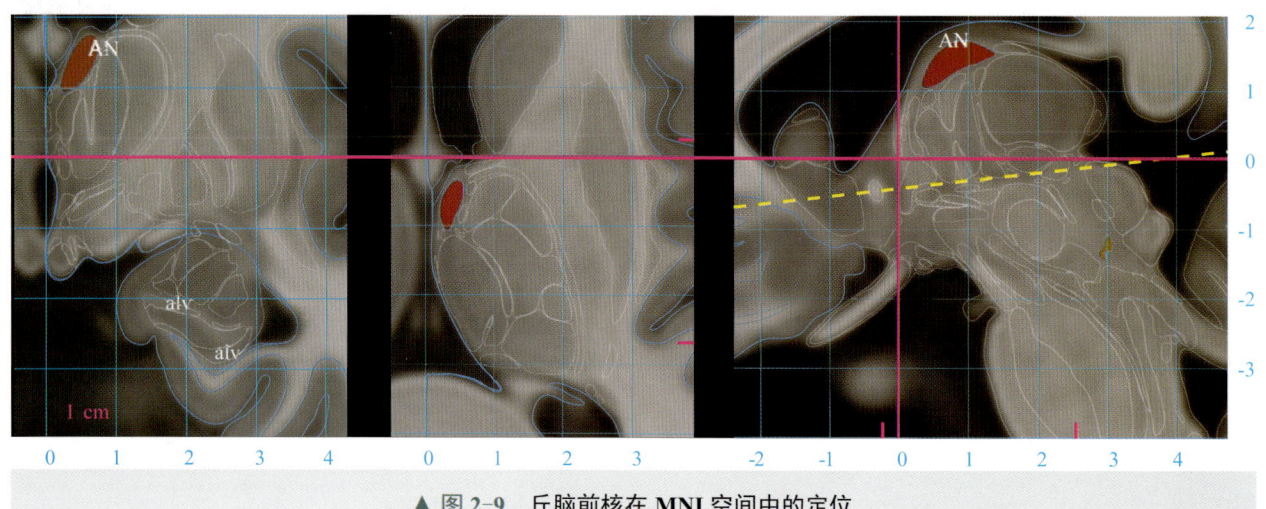

▲ 图 2-9 丘脑前核在 MNI 空间中的定位

AN. 丘脑前核

参考文献

[1] Ackermans L, Duits A, van der Linden C, et al. Double-blind clinical trial of thalamic stimulation in patients with Tourette syndrome. Brain. 2011;134:32–844.

[2] Albin RL, Young AB, Penney JB. The functional anatomy of basal ganglia disorders. Trends Neurosci. 1989;12:366–75.

[3] Alexander GE, Crutcher MD. Functional architecture of basal ganglia circuits: neural substrates of parallel processing. Trends Neurosci. 1990;13:266–71.

[4] Alexander GE, Grutcher MD, DeLong MR. Basal ganglia-thalamocortical circuits: parallel substrates for motor, oculomotor, "prefrontal" and "limbic" functions. Prog Brain Res. 1990;85:119–46.

[5] Anden NE, Dahlstrom A, Fuxe K, et al. Ascending noradrenaline neurons from the pons and the medulla oblongata. Experientia. 1966;22:44–5.

[6] Basar K, Sesia T, Groenewegen H, et al. Nucleus accumbens and impulsivity. Prog Neurobiol. 2010;92:533–57.

[7] Bejjani BP, Damier P, Arnulf I, et al. Transient acute depression induced by high-frequency deep-brain stimulation. N Engl J Med. 1999;340:1476–80.

[8] Benabid AL, Pollak P, Seigneuret E, et al. Chronic VIM thalamic stimulation in Parkinson's disease, essential tremor and extra-pyramidal dyskinesias. Acta Neurochir Suppl. 1993;58:39–44.

[9] Berendse HW, Groenewegen HJ. Organization of the thalamostriatal projections in the rat, with special emphasis on the ventral striatum. J Comp Neurol. 1990;299:187–228.

[10] Bewernick BH, Hurlemann R, Matusch A, et al. Nucleus accumbens deep brain stimulation decreases ratings of depression and anxiety in treatment-resistant depression. Biol Psychiatry. 2010;67:110–6.

[11] Bolam JP, Izzo PN, Graybiel AM. Cellular substrate of the histochemically defined striosome/matrix system of the caudate nucleus: a combined Golgi and immunocytochemical study in cat and ferret. Neuroscience. 1988;24:853–75.

[12] Castle M, Aymerich MS, Sanchez-Escobar C, et al. Thalamic innervation of the direct and indirect basal ganglia pathways

in the rat: ipsi- and contralateral projections. J Comp Neurol. 2005;483:143–53.
[13] Dahlstrom A, Fuxe K. Localization of monoamines in the lower brain stem. Experientia. 1964;20:398–9.
[14] Denys D, Mantione M, Figee M, et al. Deep brain stimulation of the nucleus accumbens for treatment-refractory obsessive-compulsive disorder. Arch Gen Psychiatry. 2010;6:1061–8.
[15] Desban M, Gauchy C, Glowinsk J, Kemel ML. Heterogeneous topographical distribution of the striatonigral and striatopallidal neurons in the matrix compartment of the cat caudate nucleus. J Comp Neurol. 1995;352:117–33.
[16] Deuschl G, Schade-Brittinger C, Krack P, et al. A randomized trial of deep-brain stimulation for Parkinson's disease. N Engl J Med. 2006;355:896–908.
[17] Donoghue JP, Herkenham M. Neostriatal projections from individual cortical fields conform to histochemically distinct striatal compartments in the rat. Brain Res. 1986;365:397–403.
[18] Fisher R, Salanova V, Witt T, et al. Electrical stimulation of the anterior nucleus of thalamus for treatment of refractory epilepsy. Epilepsia. 2010;51:899–908.
[19] Fudge JL, Haber SN. Defining the caudal ventral striatum in primates: cellular and histochemical features. J Neurosci. 2002;22:10078–82.
[20] Fujiyama F, Sohn J, Nakano T, et al. Exclusive and common targets of neostriatofugal projections of rat striosome neurons: a single neuron-tracing study using a viral vector. Eur J Neurosci. 2011;33:668–77.
[21] Gerfen CR. The neostriatal mosaic: compartmentalization of corticostriatal input and striatonigral output systems. Nature. 1984;311:461–4.
[22] Gerfen CR. The neostriatal mosaic: multiple levels of compartmental organization. Trends Neurosci. 1992;15:133–9.
[23] Gimenez-Amaya JM, Graybiel AM. Compartmental origins of the striatopallidal projection in the primate. Neuroscience. 1990;34:111–26.
[24] Gradinaru V, Mogri M, Thompson KR, et al. Optical deconstruction of parkinsonian neural circuitry. Science. 2009;324:354–9.
[25] Graybiel AM. Correspondence between the dopamine islands and striosomes of the mammalian striatum. Neuroscience. 1984;13:1157–87.
[26] Graybiel AM, Ragsdale CW Jr. Histochemically distinct compartments in the striatum of human, monkeys, and cat demonstrated by acetylthiocholinesterase staining. Proc Natl Acad Sci U S A. 1978;75:5723–6.
[27] Graybiel AM, Ragsdale CWJ, Yoneoka ES, Elde RP. An immunohistochemical study of enkephalins and other neuropeptides in the striatum of the cat with evidence that the opiate peptides are arranged to form mosaic patterns in register with the striosomal compartments visible by acetylcholinesterase staining. Neuroscience. 1981;6:377–97.
[28] Haber SN, Adler A, Bergman H. Basal ganglia. Cambridge: Academic Press; 2011.
[29] Hameleers R, Temel Y, Visser-Vandewalle V. History of the corpus Luysii: 1865-1995. Arch Neurol. 2006;63:1340–2.
[30] Heimer L, Wilson R. The subcortical projections of the allocortex: similarities in the neural associations of the hippocampus, the piriform cortex, and the neocortex. In: Santini M, editor. Persepectives in neurobiology, Golgi centennial symposium. New York: Raven Press; 1975. p. 177–93.
[31] Hescham S, Lim LW, Jahanshahi A, et al. Deep brain stimulation in dementia-related disorders. Neurosci Biobehav Rev. 2013;37:2666–75.
[32] Hubble JP, Busenbark KL, Wilkinson S, et al. Deep brain stimulation for essential tremor. Neurology. 1996;46:1150–3.
[33] Kandel ER. The neurobiology of behavior. In: Kandel ER, Schwartz JH, Jessel TM, editors. Principles of neural science. New York: McGraw-Hill; 2000. p. 1–36.
[34] Kawaguchi Y, Wilson CJ, Emson PC. Intracellular recording of identified neostriatal patch and matrix spiny cells in a slice preparation preserving cortical inputs. J Neurophysiol. 1989;62:1052–68.
[35] Kawaguchi Y, Wilson CJ, Emson PC. Projection subtypes of rat neostriatal matrix cells revealed by intracellular injection of biocytin. J Neurosci. 1990;10:3421–38.
[36] Kawaguchi Y, Wilson CJ, Augood SJ, Emson PC. Striatal interneurones: chemical, physiological and morphological characterization. Trends Neurosci. 1995;18:527–35.
[37] Kincaid AE, Wilson CJ. Corticostriatal innervation of the patch and matrix in the rat neostriatum. J Comp Neurol. 1996;374:578–92.
[38] Kocabicak E, Temel Y. Deep brain stimulation of the subthalamic nucleus in Parkinson's disease: surgical technique, tips, tricks and complications. Clin Neurol Neurosurg. 2013;115:2318–23.
[39] Krauss JK, Pohle T, Weber S, et al. Bilateral stimulation of globus pallidus internus for treatment of cervical dystonia. Lancet. 1999;354:837–8.
[40] Laitinen LV, Bergenheim AT, Hariz MI. Leksell's posteroventral pallidotomy in the treatment of Parkinson's disease. J Neurosurg. 1992;76:53–61.
[41] Lambert C, Zrinzo L, Nagy Z, et al. Confirmation of functional zones within the human subthalamic nucleus: patterns of connectivity and sub-parcellation using diffusion weighted imaging. Neuroimage. 2012;60:83–94.
[42] Lanciego JL, Luquin N, Obeso JA. Functional neuroanatomy of the basal ganglia. Cold Spring Harb Perspect Med. 2012;2:a009621.
[43] Lei W, Jiao Y, Del Mar N, Reiner A. Evidence for differential cortical input to direct pathway versus indirect pathway striatal projection neurons in rats. J Neurosci. 2004;24:8289–99.
[44] Lozano AM, Giacobbe P, Hamani C, et al. A multicenter pilot study of subcallosal cingulate area deep brain stimulation for treatment-resistant depression. J Neurosurg. 2012;116:315–22.
[45] Luyten L, Hendrickx S, Raymaekers S, et al. Electrical stimulation in the bed nucleus of the stria terminalis alleviates severe obsessive-compulsive disorder. Mol Psychiatry. 2016;21:1272–80.
[46] Mallet L, Polosan M, Jaafari N, et al. Subthalamic nucleus stimulation in severe obsessive-compulsive disorder. N Engl J Med. 2008;359:2121–34.
[47] McFarland NR, Haber SN. Organization of thalamostriatal terminals from the ventral motor nuclei in the macaque. J Comp Neurol. 2001;429:321–36.
[48] Moers-Hornikx VM, Sesia T, Basar K, et al. Cerebellar nuclei are involved in impulsive behaviour. Behav Brain Res. 2009;203:256–63.
[49] Nakano K. Neural circuits and topographic organization of the basal ganglia and related regions. Brain Dev. 2000;22(Suppl 1):S5–16.
[50] Nambu A, Takada M, Inase M, Tokuno H. Dual somatotopical representations in the primate subthalamic nucleus: evidence for ordered but reversed body-map transformations from the primary motor cortex and the supplementary motor area. J Neurosci. 1996;16:2671–83.
[51] Nambu A, Tokuno H, Takada M. Functional significance of the cortico-subthalamo-pallidal 'hyperdirect' pathway. Neurosci Res. 2002;43:111–7.
[52] Nauta HJ. A proposed conceptual reorganization of the basal ganglia and telencephalon. Neuroscience. 1979;4:1875–81.
[53] Nuttin B, Cosyns P, Demeulemeester H, et al. Electrical stimulation in anterior limbs of internal capsules in patients with obsessive-compulsive disorder. Lancet. 1999;354:1526.
[54] Ohye C. Thalamus. In: Paxinos G, editor. The human nervous system. San Diego: Academic Press; 1990. p. 439–82.
[55] Parent A, Hazrati LN. Functional anatomy of the basal ganglia. I. The cortico-basal ganglia-thalamo-cortical loop. Brain Res Brain Res Rev. 1995;20:91–127.
[56] Parent A, Sato F, Wu Y, et al. Organization of the basal ganglia: the importance of axonal collateralization. Trends Neurosci. 2000;23:S20–7.
[57] Penny GR, Wilson CJ, Kitai ST. Relationship of the axonal and dendritic geometry of spiny projection neurons to the compartmental organization of the neostriatum. J Comp Neurol. 1988;269:275–89.
[58] Pert CB, Kuhar MJ, Snyder SH. Opiate receptor: autoradiographic localization in rat brain. Proc Natl Acad Sci U S A. 1976;73:3729–33.
[59] Plantinga BR, Temel Y, Roebroeck A, et al. Ultra-high field

magnetic resonance imaging of the basal ganglia and related structures. Front Hum Neurosci. 2014;8:876.

[60] Ragsdale CW Jr, Graybiel AM. Fibers from the basolateral nucleus of the amygdala selectively innervate striosomes in the caudate nucleus of the cat. J Comp Neurol. 1988;269:506–22.

[61] Rosin DL, Robeva A, Woodard RL, et al. Immunohistochemical localization of adenosine A2A receptors in the rat central nervous system. J Comp Neurol. 1998;401:163–86.

[62] Sadikot AF, Parent A, Francois C. Efferent connections of the centromedian and parafascicular thalamic nuclei in the squirrel monkey: a PHA-L study of subcortical projections. J Comp Neurol. 1992a;315:137–59.

[63] Sadikot AF, Parent A, Smith Y, Bolam JP. Efferent connections of the centromedian and parafascicular thalamic nuclei in the squirrel monkey: a light and electron microscopic study of the thalamostriatal projection in relation to striatal heterogeneity. J Comp Neurol. 1992b;320:228–42.

[64] Salgado S, Kaplitt MG. The nucleus accumbens: a comprehensive review. Stereotact Funct Neurosurg. 2015;93:75–93.

[65] Schlaepfer TE, Bewernick BH, Kayser S, et al. Rapid effects of deep brain stimulation for treatment-resistant major depression. Biol Psychiatry. 2013;73:1204–12.

[66] Shink E, Bevan MD, Bolam JP, Smith Y. The subthalamic nucleus and the external pallidum: two tightly interconnected structures that control the output of the basal ganglia in the monkey. Neuroscience. 1996;73:335–57.

[67] Siegfried J, Lippitz B. Bilateral chronic electrostimulation of ventroposterolateral pallidum: a new therapeutic approach for alleviating all parkinsonian symptoms. Neurosurgery. 1994;35:1126–9.

[68] Smeets AJM, Duits AA, Plantinga BR, et al. Deep brain stimulation of the internal globus pallidus in refractory Tourette syndrome. Clin Neurol Neurosurg. 2016;142:54–9.

[69] Temel Y, Blokland A, Steinbusch HW, Visser-Vandewalle V. The functional role of the subthalamic nucleus in cognitive and limbic circuits. Prog Neurobiol. 2005;76:393–413.

[70] Temel Y, PLantinga B, Kuijf ML. Anatomie van de gebruikte targets bij diepe hersenstimulatie. In: Temel Y, Leentjens AFG, de Bie RMA, editors. Handboek diepe hersenstimulatie bij neurologische en psyciatrische aandoeningen. Houten: Bohn Stafleu van Loghum; 2016. p. 11–7.

[71] Van Der Kooy D, Hattori T. Single subthalamic nucleus neurons project to both the globus pallidus and substantia nigra in rat. J Comp Neurol. 1980;192:751–68.

[72] Vidailhet M, Jutras MF, Grabli D, Roze E. Deep brain stimulation for dystonia. J Neurol Neurosurg Psychiatry. 2013;84:1029–42.

[73] Weiss D, Walach M, Meisner C, et al. Nigral stimulation for resistant axial motor impairment in Parkinson's disease? A randomized controlled trial. Brain. 2013;136:2098–108.

[74] Wichmann T, Kliem MA, Soares J. Slow oscillatory discharge in the primate basal ganglia. J Neurophysiol. 2002;87:1145–8.

第3章 脑深部电刺激的机制
Mechanisms of Deep Brain Stimulation

Abdelhamid Benazzouz　Clement Hamani　**著**
尹子霄　杨岸超　**译**　王　乔　张建国　**校**

> **摘要**：底丘脑核（subthalamic nucleus，STN）脑深部电刺激（deep brain stimulation，DBS）是目前治疗某些神经及精神障碍性疾病的一种手术疗法，适应证包括帕金森病、震颤、肌张力障碍及强迫症等。然而，其作用机制仍存在争议。在本章中，我们对基于动物模型的实验数据和患者的临床数据描述并探讨 DBS 作用的机制。
>
> 临床常用的刺激频率为 130～185Hz，其包含了一系列非常复杂的神经元抑制和兴奋的交互作用，且不仅在靶点局部起作用，在靶点的远隔位置也有作用。大量研究显示这些刺激频率会通过去极化阻滞机制和（或）刺激神经元（例如，GABA-介导的传入神经元）诱导靶结构的功能性失活。刺激的其他结果还包括神经胶质活动、突触传递的改变，以及通过增加神经发生、增加营养因子水平、改变受体表达和改变大脑结构体积来提高神经可塑性。
>
> 因此，DBS 是通过多种复杂的机制来实现治疗作用的。更好的理解其作用机制有助于改进其应用，提高疗效。

一、概述

脑深部电刺激（DBS）通过植入的电极将电流释放到脑实质中。对伴有运动波动和显著多巴胺能药物不良反应的帕金森病（Parkinson disease，PD）患者而言，底丘脑核（STN）高频刺激（high-frequency stimulation，HFS）是目前非常有效的治疗选择。该神经外科疗法的提出主要是基于对基底节环路生理学及病理生理学机制的更深入的理解，其有助于构建包括不同皮质区、基底节和丘脑在内的运动环路的解剖和功能组织模型（Albin 等，1989；Alexander 和 Crutcher，1990）。在该模型中，通过纹状体和 STN 皮质信号传递到基底节的输出核团，即苍白球内侧部（internal part of globus pallidus，GPi）和黑质网状部（pars reticulata of the substantia nigra，SNr）的两个主要结构。纹状体和 STN 接受来自皮质的直接兴奋性谷氨酸能投射，并对 GPi 和 SNr 产生抑制性与兴奋性相反的作用。因为它们从纹状体接收抑制性 GABA 投射，从 STN 接收兴奋性谷氨酸能投射。STN 常被视为一个中继核团，除了通过直接皮质-STN 通路外，皮质还通过纹状体、苍白球外侧部（external part of globus pallidus，GPe）参与的间接通路调控 STN。除上述的间接（纹状体-GPe-STN-GPi/SNr）通路和超直接（皮质-STN）通路外，还存在直接通路，即纹状体发出的 GABA-介导的抑制信号作用于 GPi/SNr 的输出结构。

该皮质基底节 - 丘脑皮质环路对于理解 STN 在 PD 病理生理学的作用是必不可少的。既往研究主要从两方面探究 STN 在 PD 中的作用，一方面为 STN 的异常电活动（Albin 等，1989；Alexander 和 Crutcher，1990；DeLong，1990；Alexander 等，1990）；另一方面为 STN 的损毁，其可以导致帕金森猴运动症状的缓解及异动症的出现（Bergman 等，1990）。STN HFS 的疗效最初是在偏侧帕金森病非人灵长类动物模型［通过注射 1- 甲基 -4- 苯基 -1,2,3,6- 四氢吡啶（MPTP）构建］中被证实的（Benazzouz 等，1993，1996）。该结果使得 STN HFS 迅速被运用到晚期 PD 患者上（Limousin 等，1995，1998；Krack 等，2003）。

尽管 DBS 作为一种外科疗法能够有效治疗 PD 和其他一些神经精神障碍性疾病，但其疗效的机制仍然还存在争议。我们将在本章中基于动物模型的实验数据和患者的临床数据进行描述并探讨 DBS 作用的复杂机制。

二、DBS 的工作原理

一般来说，单脉冲阴极刺激使包括细胞体、轴突和树突在内的神经结构去极化。一旦动作电位被激活，神经元则倾向于复极化，正常的离子/神经递质基线平衡被重建。这与 HFS 导致的情况相反，因为临床上 DBS 最常使用的频率为 130～185Hz。很重要的一点是神经附属物（而非神经元胞体）才能顺应这种高频率。此外，持续的 HFS 将使得原本用于清除胞外特定离子和递质的机制过载（Hamani 和 Temel，2012）。总体而言，接受长期 HFS 的神经组织可能会建立新的动态平衡（Florence 等，2016）。这就包括非常复杂的神经元抑制和兴奋交互变化，且该作用不仅在刺激靶点局部，在靶点的远隔位置也发挥作用。

（一）DBS 对刺激靶点的作用

最初对于 DBS 机制的假设试图在丘脑、底丘脑核或苍白球损毁术和 HFS 治疗震颤、帕金森病和肌张力障碍的临床前、临床结果中找寻线索（Bergman 等，1990；Benazzouz 等，1993；Benabid 等，1998；Eltahawy 等，2004；Tasker，1998）。其结果表明 HFS 可能通过靶结构的功能失活来发挥作用（Beurrier 等，2001；Magarinos-Ascone 等，2002；Kiss 等，2002；Kringelbach 等，2007；Lozano 等，2002；Vitek，2002）。

支持该理论的电生理研究表明，在正常和 6-OHDA 损伤的大鼠（Benazzouz 等，2000a；Tai 等，2003）、PD 患者（Filali 等，2004；Welter 等，2004），以及 MPTP 处理的非人灵长动物中（Meissner 等，2005）观察到 STN DBS 时神经活动的抑制。与这些电生理研究一致，在实验性帕金森模型中，研究人员通过细胞色素氧化酶（一种神经活动标记物）原位杂交法也同样观察到 STN HFS 能诱导底丘脑核代谢活动正常化。相似的结论也在 GPi DBS 治疗帕金森猴模型和 PD 患者中被观察到。大鼠的大脑中也能观察到 DBS 时静默的 STN 神经元（Anderson 等，2006；Beurrier 等，2001；Filali 等，2004；Kiss 等，2002；Magarinos-Ascone 等，2002；Meissner 等，2005）。

胞外电极的 HFS 可能对局部的细胞群产生直接作用。从神经元的角度而言，触点周围神经元的抑制常常可以用"去极化阻滞"来解释（Beurrier 等，2001；Kringelbach 等，2007；Magarinos-Ascone 等，2002）。它包括刺激引起的电压门控电流激活的改变，阻止了刺激电极附近的神经输出（Beurrier 等，2001）（图 3-1）。这种直接作用是由于电场作用于神经元的膜结构，导致每个神经结构的去极化和超极化。该现象已经在体外 STN 脑切片中被证实，HFS 的静默效应不是由于局部网络的激活也不是通过刺激 STN 的传入纤维实现的（Beurrier 等，2001）。支持这一论断的是，即使在谷氨酸能和 GABA- 介导的离子性突触传递阻滞药物环境中，以及在足以阻断 STN 突触传递的高浓度钴的情况

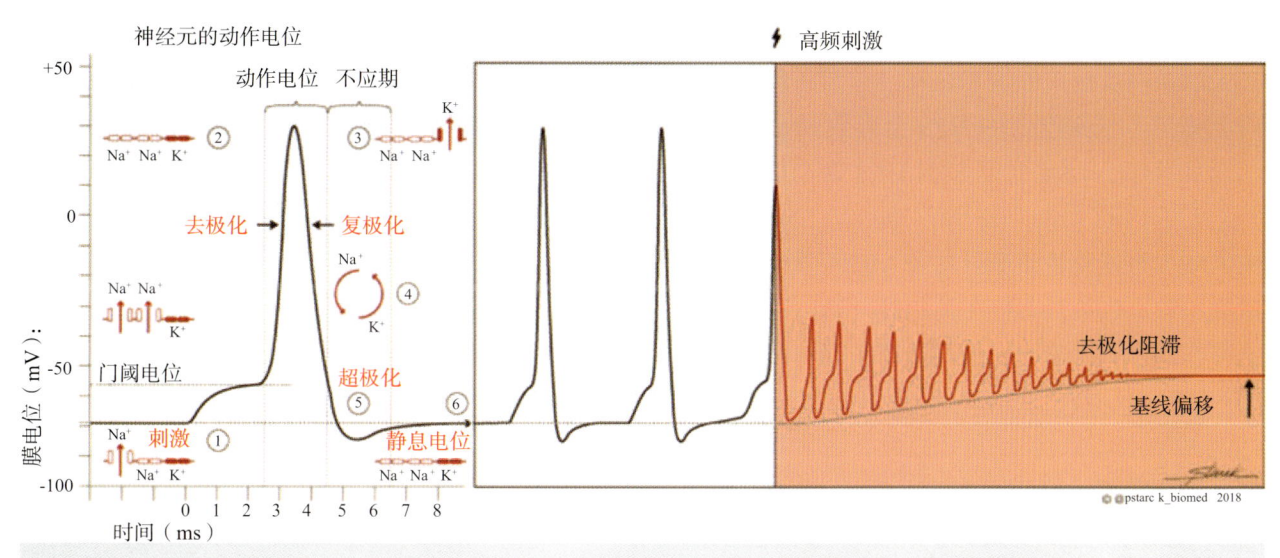

▲ 图 3-1　高频刺激（HFS）通过去极化阻滞导致丘脑底神经元放电的抑制

下，这种静默效应仍然能被观察到（Beurrier 等，2001）。去极化阻滞在抗精神病药物治疗的多巴胺神经元中广泛存在（Grace 和 Bunney，1986；Esposito 和 Bunney，1989；Valenti 等，2011）。在急性激活下，动作电位振幅衰减、放电尖峰变宽，导致动作电位产生失败，最终形成去极化阻滞（Richards 等，1997；Blythe 等，2009）。一项计算模型研究提出，去极化阻滞可能是由于电压门控 Na^+ 通道的累积失活，其导致动作电位阈值的持续增加并最终达到去极化使得动作电位完全无法产生（Kuznetsova 等，2010）。然而值得一提的是，在 STN 中去极化阻滞并非是持续性的，随着时间的推移胞体最终会恢复其复极化机制。此外，即使当膜正向电位增加及动作电位振幅降低时，神经递质仍然能以较小的非量子释放的形式被少量释放（Ammari 等，2011）。在靶点区域内，GABA 介导的中间神经元轴突受到刺激可能导致神经递质释放，进一步抑制主细胞（Filali 等，2004）。同样，丘脑神经元主要接受兴奋性传入，其可以通过刺激来激活（Dostrovsky 和 Lozano，2002）。

但是必须注意的是，去极化阻滞并非是 DBS 的唯一主要机制，已经有在体试验提出被抑制的 STN 神经元仅占全部神经元的一小部分。不过在大部分情况下，STN DBS 会导致啮齿动物（Tai 等，2003）、非人灵长类动物（Meissner 等，2005）和人（Filali 等，2004；Welter 等，2004）的 STN 神经元的部分抑制，表现为放电频率的降低。

对于强迫行为，啮齿动物 STN 或脚内核刺激的作用与局部注射 GABA 激动药的作用类似（Klavir 等，2009；Winter 等，2008），提示电刺激对靶点结构的功能影响主要表现为抑制。这与伏隔核刺激相反，伏隔核刺激能抑制毁损后观察到的强迫行为增加（van Kuyck 等，2003；Winter 等，2008）。

（二）DBS 对下游核团的作用

除直接作用以外，HFS 还能通过激活靶区的传入、传出，以及经过的投射纤维来影响神经元的活动（Kringelbach 等，2007）。通过这种作用，动作电位可以顺行或逆行传播，调节距靶区一定距离的神经结构的活动（Kringelbach 等，2007；Hashimoto 等，2003；Temel 等，2007；Windels 等，2000）。一些电生理研究表明 STN HFS 能引起大鼠 SNr 神经元活动的抑制（Benazzouz 等，2000a；Tai 等，2003）。同样，STN HFS 能够逆转多巴胺去神经化诱导的 SNr 中细胞色素氧化酶 mRNA 表达的变化（Benazzouz 等，2004；Salin 等，2002）。其他研究表明，STN HFS 可能通过激活兴奋性和抑制性突触传入通路，以及投射神经元的逆向激活来影响SNr神经元的活性。已有研究报道，低强度STN HFS会导致SNr神经元活动的降低，而高强度STN HFS则会提高SNr神经元的活动（Maurice等，2003）。SNr细胞放电的减少可能是由于SNr中GABA-介导的递质激活所致，因为局部应用荷包牡丹碱可能会阻止这种作用。该结果与先前的研究结果一致，提示STN-HFS后GP神经元活性增加（Benazzouz等，1995）。6-OHDA损伤大鼠的神经化学微透析研究已经证实了γ-氨基丁酸（gamma-aminobutyric acid，GABA）在SNr的内释放来源于苍白球（Windels等，2005）。结果表明，STN HFS对偏侧帕金森大鼠SNr的细胞外谷氨酸水平无影响，但能显著升高GABA水平。此外，这种GABA水平的增加能被鹅膏蕈氨酸损伤GP所消除，这表明STN HFS的治疗作用可能部分来自于对苍白球黑质纤维的刺激。这种活性的增加可能是由于激活了谷氨酸能的底丘脑黑质投射通路，因为诱发兴奋的潜伏期与底丘脑黑质神经元的传导时间一致（Maurice等，2003）。另一项在MPTP帕金森病猴模型中进行的研究观察到GPi和GPe活性的增加，而两者都接受来自STN的兴奋性谷氨酸能传入纤维（Hashimoto等，2003）。在抑制性传出纤维方面也有类似的发现，GPi刺激能抑制正常猴（Anderson等，2003）和肌张力障碍患者（Montgomery，2006）的丘脑神经元活动，而GPe刺激抑制了STN神经元活动（Vitek，2002）。

至于其他靶点，除局部效应外，伏隔核刺激也被证明可以调节远隔靶点区域的神经元活动（McCracken and Grace，2007）。这其中包括眶额皮质，其代谢活性在强迫症患者中增高，而在腹侧内囊/腹侧纹状体DBS治疗后降低（Abelson等，2005；Nuttin等，2003）。

此外，人体正电子发射断层扫描研究显示，STN DBS会导致GPi血流量的增加（Hershey等，2003），而丘脑DBS可导致皮质血流量增加，两者血流量的增加都与刺激靶点的输出激活一致（Perlmutter等，2002）。同样，功能磁共振研究中也发现，接受STN DBS的患者会出现GPi血氧水平依赖性信号的升高（Jech等，2001）。

然而术中进行的PD患者微透析研究并没有得到STN-HFS时GPi神经元活性增加的结果。他们发现STN-HFS使运动丘脑腹前核的GABA水平降低了30%，运动丘脑腹前核是一个向皮质传递运动信息的关键结构（Stefani等，2011）。且GABA水平的降低与运动症状的改善显著相关，这与基底节输出结构神经元活性的降低一致（Benazzouz等，2000a；Maurice等，2003；Tai等，2003）。

HFS对靶区和远隔结构的其他影响还包括神经胶质活动、突触传递和神经可塑性的改变（Cooperrider等，2014；Hamani等，2012）。神经可塑性的变化具体表现为神经发生增加、营养因子水平增加、受体表达及大脑结构体积等的变化（Chakravarty等，2016；Hamani and Temel，2012；Hamani等，2012；Toda等，2008）。可塑性的变化同样在精神性疾病的临床前模型中被大量报道（Hamani and Temel，2012）。目前还尚不清楚是否是这些变化导致了DBS对患者行为的影响。

（三）DBS对皮质神经元活动的影响

除了对基底节核团的影响外，STN-HFS还可以通过投射到脑干和脊髓的STN正下方的肾上腺轴突，以及投射到STN的"超直接"通路纤维，直接对大脑皮质产生逆向影响。在一项PD患者的研究中，STN-HFS时可观察到极短潜伏期后皮质的激活（Ashby等，2001）。类似的结果同样在麻醉大鼠（Li等，2007）及未麻醉但使用急性多巴胺能阻滞药的大鼠（Dejean等，2009）中被观察到，表现为皮质慢波振荡的减少。另一项研究证实STN-HFS对初级运动皮质（M_1）的V层皮质纤维投射神经元起到了逆向激活作用，其能导致6-OHDA损伤大鼠M_1区异常神经活动的中止并改善运动障碍（Li等，2012）。近期的研究表明，黑质致密部（substantia nigra compacta，SNC）多巴胺能神经元的损伤会导致运动皮质记录到的锥体神经元平均放电率和爆发放电模式的显著增加。此外还能观察到细胞膜放电特性的改变，包括去极化的静息膜电位和输入电阻的增加。应用特定的参数以缓解PD症状时，STN-HFS可使锥体细胞的放电模式规则化，并恢复其膜电特性（Degos等，2013）。总而言之，诸多证据表明，运动皮质的逆向激活是STN-HFS通过减少PD振荡和症状来调节疗效的潜在机制之一。Oswal等（2016）通过使用脑磁图同时记录STN和皮质，提出有治疗效果的STN-HFS不仅能局部抑制STN内的低β振荡，且该抑制程度与运动症状的改善相关，还能选择性地抑制STN与包括辅助运动区在内的运动前区之间的振荡活动耦合。

（四）STN-HFS在调节多巴胺神经递质中的作用

STN-DBS对内源性DA及其代谢物浓度的影响多年来一直争论不休。由于STN-HFS仅对左旋多巴敏感的运动症状有效，且长期STN-HFS治疗下PD患者的多巴胺能药物剂量可降低50%，有学者认为纹状体多巴胺能活动的变化是STN-HFS发挥临床疗效的机制之一（Benabid等，1998；Moro等，1999）。几项实验性研究表明，STN-DBS激活了正常大鼠纹状体的DA神经元（Benazzouz等，2000b），这种激活可导致6-OHDA大鼠PD模型纹状体中DA的释放和多巴胺能代谢活动显著增加（Bruet等，2001；Meissner等，2001，2002，2003；He等，2014）。此外，纹状体胞外的3,4-二羟基苯乙酸（3,4-dihydroxyphenylacetic acid，DOPAC）和高香草酸（homovanillic acid，HVA）含量在STN-DBS治疗中显著增加。这些作用可能是投射到SNC DA神经元上的STN谷氨酸能神经元的直接激活所致（Lee等，2006）。但也有人认为STN-DBS抑制了GABA SNr神经元的活性，减轻了GABA介导的对SNC神经元的抑制作用，从而导致它们的放电频率增加，纹状体DA释放增多。除了多巴胺和代谢物含量的变化外，最近的一项研究（Carcenac等，2015）还评估了麻醉后4h单侧STN-HFS大鼠和去多巴胺能神经大鼠多巴胺能受体表达的变化。他们用 [^{3}H]SCH 23390、[^{125}I] 碘仿和 [^{125}I]OHPIPAT 分别评估 D_1、D_2 和 D_3 受体的密度，结果显示STN-HFS无论是在正常的还是6-OHDA损伤的大鼠中，均增加了纹状体中 D_1 受体的水平。但 D_2 和 D_3 受体水平在STN-HFS下大幅降低，该现象仅限于伏隔核且与动物的多巴胺能状态无关。作者认为STN-HFS对纹状体 D_1 受体表达的影响可能是其改善运动症状的机制，而其对伏隔核 D_2/D_3 受体水平的影响可能是PD患者STN-DBS术后出现神经精神不良反应（如术后淡漠）的原因。然而与上述动物模型研究不同的是，使用 [^{11}C]raclopride结合的PD患者PET研究表明，STN-DBS没有显著改变纹状体尾状核和壳核中DA浓度或DA神经递质水平（Abosch等，2003；Hilker等，2003）。综上所述，STN-HFS对运动症状的疗效不太可能是由于纹状体多巴胺能神经递质增加所致。

三、结论

DBS通过多种复杂的机制发挥治疗作用，这些机制不仅表现为对靶区和下游结构的抑制或兴奋，还表现为改变放电模式和包括神经胶质活动、突触传递、神经可塑性的改变，以及神经发生的增加、营养因子水平增加、受体表达改变和脑结构体积改变等其他现象。更好的理解DBS的作用机制将有助于改进该疗法的应用并提高疗效。

参考文献

[1] Abelson JL, Curtis GC, Sagher O, et al. Deep brain stimulation for refractory obsessive-compulsive disorder. Biol Psychiatry. 2005;57:510–6.
[2] Abosch A, Kapur S, Lang AE, et al. Stimulation of the subthalamic nucleus in Parkinson's disease does not produce striatal dopamine release. Neurosurgery. 2003;53:1095–102.
[3] Albin RL, Young AB, Penney JB. The functional anatomy of basal

ganglia disorders. Trends Neurosci. 1989;12:366–75.
[4] Alexander GE, Crutcher MD. Functional architecture of basal ganglia circuits: neural substrates of parallel processing. Trends Neurosci. 1990;13:266–71.
[5] Alexander GE, Crutcher MD, DeLong MR. Basal ganglia-thalamocortical circuits: parallel substrates for motor, oculomotor, "prefrontal" and "limbic" functions. Prog Brain Res. 1990;85:119–46.
[6] Ammari R, Bioulac B, Garcia L, Hammond C. The subthalamic nucleus becomes a generator of bursts in the dopamine-depleted state. Its high frequency stimulation dramatically weakens transmission to the globus pallidus. Front Syst Neurosci. 2011;5:43.
[7] Anderson ME, Postupna N, Ruffo M. Effects of high-frequency stimulation in the internal globus pallidus on the activity of thalamic neurons in the awake monkey. J Neurophysiol. 2003;89:1150–60.
[8] Anderson TR, Hu B, Iremonger K, Kiss ZH. Selective attenuation of afferent synaptic transmission as a mechanism of thalamic deep brain stimulation-induced tremor arrest. J Neurosci. 2006;26:841–50.
[9] Ashby P, Paradiso G, Saint-Cyr JA, Chen R, Lang AE, Lozano AM. Potentials recorded at the scalp by stimulation near the human subthalamic nucleus. Clin Neurophysiol. 2001;112:431–7.
[10] Benabid AL, Benazzouz A, Hoffmann D, et al. Long-term electrical inhibition of deep brain targets in movement disorders. Mov Disord. 1998;13(Suppl 3):119–25.
[11] Benazzouz A, Gross C, Feger J, Boraud T, Bioulac B. Reversal of rigidity and improvement in motor performance by subthalamic high-frequency stimulation in MPTP-treated monkeys. Eur J Neurosci. 1993;5:382–9.
[12] Benazzouz A, Piallat B, Pollak P, Benabid AL. Responses of substantia nigra pars reticulata and globus pallidus complex to high frequency stimulation of the subthalamic nucleus in rats: electrophysiological data. Neurosci Lett. 1995;189:77–80.
[13] Benazzouz A, Boraud T, Feger J, Burbaud P, Bioulac B, Gross C. Alleviation of experimental hemiparkinsonism by high-frequency stimulation of the subthalamic nucleus in primates: a comparison with L-Dopa treatment. Mov Disord. 1996;11:627–32.
[14] Benazzouz A, Gao DM, Ni ZG, Piallat B, Bouali-Benazzouz R, Benabid AL. Effect of high-frequency stimulation of the subthalamic nucleus on the neuronal activities of the substantia nigra pars reticulata and ventrolateral nucleus of the thalamus in the rat. Neuroscience. 2000a;99:289–95.
[15] Benazzouz A, Gao D, Ni Z, Benabid AL. High frequency stimulation of the STN influences the activity of dopamine neurons in the rat. Neuroreport. 2000b;11:1593–6.
[16] Benazzouz A, Tai CH, Meissner W, Bioulac B, Bezard E, Gross C. High-frequency stimulation of both zona incerta and subthalamic nucleus induces a similar normalization of basal ganglia metabolic activity in experimental parkinsonism. FASEB J. 2004;18:528–30.
[17] Bergman H, Wichmann T, DeLong MR. Reversal of experimental parkinsonism by lesions of the subthalamic nucleus. Science. 1990;249:1436–8.
[18] Beurrier C, Bioulac B, Audin J, Hammond C. High-frequency stimulation produces a transient blockade of voltage-gated currents in subthalamic neurons. J Neurophysiol. 2001;85:1351–6.
[19] Blythe SN, Wokosin D, Atherton JF, Bevan MD. Cellular mechanisms underlying burst firing in substantia nigra dopamine neurons. J Neurosci. 2009;29: 15531–41.
[20] Boraud T, Bezard E, Bioulac B, Gross C. High frequency stimulation of the internal globus pallidus (GPi) simultaneously improves parkinsonian symptoms and reduces the firing frequency of GPi neurons in the MPTP-treated monkey. Neurosci Lett. 1996;215:17–20.
[21] Bruet N, Windels F, Bertrand A, Feuerstein C, Poupard A, Savasta M. High frequency stimulation of the subthalamic nucleus increases the extracellular contents of striatal dopamine in normal and partially dopaminergic denervated rats. J Neuropathol Exp Neurol. 2001;60:15–24.
[22] Carcenac C, Favier M, Vachez Y, et al. Subthalamic deep brain stimulation differently alters striatal dopaminergic receptor levels in rats. Mov Disord. 2015;30:1739–49.
[23] Chakravarty MM, Hamani C, Martinez-Canabal A, et al. Deep brain stimulation of the ventromedial prefrontal cortex causes reorganization of neuronal processes and vasculature. Neuroimage. 2016;125:422–7.
[24] Cooperrider J, Furmaga H, Plow E, et al. Chronic deep cerebellar stimulation promotes long-term potentiation, microstructural plasticity, and reorganization of perilesional cortical representation in a rodent model. J Neurosci. 2014;34:9040–50.
[25] Degos B, Deniau JM, Chavez M, Maurice N. Subthalamic nucleus high-frequency stimulation restores altered electrophysiological properties of cortical neurons in parkinsonian rat. PLoS One. 2013;8(12):e83608.
[26] Dejean C, Hyland B, Arbuthnott G. Cortical effects of subthalamic stimulation correlate with behavioral recovery from dopamine antagonist induced akinesia. Cereb Cortex. 2009;19:1055–63.
[27] DeLong MR. Primate models of movement disorders of basal ganglia origin. Trends Neurosci. 1990;13:281–5.
[28] Dostrovsky JO, Lozano AM. Mechanisms of deep brain stimulation. Mov Disord. 2002;17(Suppl 3):S63–8.
[29] Dostrovsky JO, Levy R, Wu JP, Hutchison WD, Tasker RR, Lozano AM. Microstimulation-induced inhibition of neuronal firing in human globus pallidus. J Neurophysiol. 2000;84:570–4.
[30] Eltahawy HA, Saint-Cyr J, Giladi N, Lang AE, Lozano AM. Primary dystonia is more responsive than secondary dystonia to pallidal interventions: outcome after pallidotomy or pallidal deep brain stimulation. Neurosurgery. 2004;54:613–9.
[31] Esposito E, Bunney BS. The effect of acute and chronic treatment with SCH 23390 on the spontaneous activity of midbrain dopamine neurons. Eur J Pharmacol. 1989;162:109–13.
[32] Filali M, Hutchison WD, Palter VN, Lozano AM, Dostrovsky JO. Stimulation-induced inhibition of neuronal firing in human subthalamic nucleus. Exp Brain Res. 2004;156:274–81.
[33] Florence G, Sameshima K, Fonoff ET, Hamani C. Deep brain stimulation: more complex than the inhibition of cells and excitation of fibers. Neuroscientist. 2016;22:332–45.
[34] Grace AA, Bunney BS. Induction of depolarization block in midbrain dopamine neurons by repeated administration of haloperidol: analysis using in vivo intracellular recording. J Pharmacol Exp Ther. 1986;238:1092–100.
[35] Hamani C, Temel Y. Deep brain stimulation for psychiatric disease: contributions and validity of animal models. Sci Transl Med. 2012;4:142–8.
[36] Hamani C, Machado DC, Hipolide DC, et al. Deep brain stimulation reverses anhedonic-like behavior in a chronic model of depression: role of serotonin and brain derived neurotrophic factor. Biol Psychiatry. 2012;71:30–5.
[37] Hashimoto T, Elder CM, Okun MS, Patrick SK, Vitek JL. Stimulation of the subthalamic nucleus changes the firing pattern of pallidal neurons. J Neurosci. 2003;23:1916–23.
[38] He Z, Jiang Y, Xu H, et al. High frequency stimulation of subthalamic nucleus results in behavioral recovery by increasing striatal dopamine release in 6-hydroxydopamine lesioned rat. Behav Brain Res. 2014;263:108–14.
[39] Hershey T, Revilla FJ, Wernle AR, et al. Cortical and subcortical blood flow effects of subthalamic nucleus stimulation in PD. Neurology. 2003;61:816–21.
[40] Hilker R, Voges J, Ghaemi M, et al. Deep brain stimulation of the subthalamic nucleus does not increase the striatal dopamine concentration in parkinsonian humans. Mov Disord. 2003;18:41–8.
[41] Jech R, Urgosik D, Tintera J, et al. Functional magnetic resonance imaging during deep brain stimulation: a pilot study in four patients with Parkinson's disease. Mov Disord. 2001;16:1126–32.
[42] Kiss ZH, Mooney DM, Renaud L, Hu B. Neuronal response to local electrical stimulation in rat thalamus: physiological implications for mechanisms of deep brain stimulation. Neuroscience. 2002;113: 137–43.
[43] Klavir O, Flash S, Winter C, Joel D. High frequency stimulation and pharmacological inactivation of the subthalamic nucleus reduces 'compulsive' lever-pressing in rats. Exp Neurol. 2009;215:101–9.
[44] Krack P, Batir A, Van Blercom N, et al. Five-year follow-up of bilateral stimulation of the subthalamic nucleus in advanced Parkinson's disease. N Engl J Med. 2003;349:1925–34.

[45] Kringelbach ML, Jenkinson N, Owen SL, Aziz TZ. Translational principles of deep brain stimulation. Nat Rev Neurosci. 2007;8:623–35.

[46] Kuznetsova AY, Huertas MA, Kuznetsov AS, Paladini CA, Canavier CC. Regulation of firing frequency in a computational model of a midbrain dopaminergic neuron. J Comput Neurosci. 2010;28:389–403.

[47] Lee KH, Blaha CD, Harris BT, et al. Dopamine efflux in the rat striatum evoked by electrical stimulation of the subthalamic nucleus: potential mechanism of action in Parkinson's disease. Eur J Neurosci. 2006;23:1005–14.

[48] Li S, Arbuthnott GW, Jutras MJ, Goldberg JA, Jaeger D. Resonant antidromic cortical circuit activation as a consequence of high-frequency subthalamic deep-brain stimulation. J Neurophysiol. 2007;98:3525–37.

[49] Li Q, Ke Y, Chan DC, et al. Therapeutic deep brain stimulation in parkinsonian rats directly influences motor cortex. Neuron. 2012;76:1030–41.

[50] Limousin P, Pollak P, Benazzouz A, et al. Effect of parkinsonian signs and symptoms of bilateral subthalamic nucleus stimulation. Lancet. 1995;345:91–5.

[51] Limousin P, Krack P, Pollak P, et al. Electrical stimulation of the subthalamic nucleus in advanced Parkinson's disease. N Engl J Med. 1998;339:1105–11.

[52] Lozano AM, Dostrovsky J, Chen R, Ashby P. Deep brain stimulation for Parkinson's disease: disrupting the disruption. Lancet Neurol. 2002;1:225–31.

[53] Magarinos-Ascone C, Pazo JH, Macadar O, Buno W. High-frequency stimulation of the subthalamic nucleus silences subthalamic neurons: a possible cellular mechanism in Parkinson's disease. Neuroscience. 2002;115:1109–17.

[54] Maurice N, Thierry AM, Glowinski J, Deniau JM. Spontaneous and evoked activity of substantia nigra pars reticulata neurons during high-frequency stimulation of the subthalamic nucleus. J Neurosci. 2003;23(30):9929–36.

[55] McCracken CB, Grace AA. High-frequency deep brain stimulation of the nucleus accumbens region suppresses neuronal activity and selectively modulates afferent drive in rat orbitofrontal cortex in vivo. J Neurosci. 2007;27:12601–10.

[56] Meissner W, Reum T, Paul G, et al. Striatal dopaminergic metabolism is increased by deep brain stimulation of the subthalamic nucleus in 6-hydroxydopamine lesioned rats. Neurosci Lett. 2001;303:165–8.

[57] Meissner W, Harnack D, Paul G, et al. Deep brain stimulation of subthalamic neurons increases striatal dopamine metabolism and induces contralateral circling in freely moving 6-hydroxydopamine-lesioned rats. Neurosci Lett. 2002;328:105–8.

[58] Meissner W, Harnack D, Reese R, et al. High-frequency stimulation of the subthalamic nucleus enhances striatal dopamine release and metabolism in rats. J Neurochem. 2003;85:601–9.

[59] Meissner W, Leblois A, Hansel D, et al. Subthalamic high frequency stimulation resets subthalamic firing and reduces abnormal oscillations. Brain. 2005;128:2372–82.

[60] Montgomery EB. Effects of GPi stimulation on human thalamic neuronal activity. Clin Neurophysiol. 2006;117:2691–702.

[61] Moro E, Scerrati M, Romito LM, Roselli R, Tonali P, Albanese A. Chronic subthalamic nucleus stimulation reduces medication requirements in Parkinson's disease. Neurology. 1999;53:85–90.

[62] Nuttin B, Gybels J, Cosyns P, Gabriels L, Meyerson B, Andreewitch S, Rasmussen SA, Greenberg B, Friehs G, Rezai AR, Montgomery E, Malone D, Fins JJ. Deep brain stimulation for psychiatric disorders. Neurosurg Clin N Am. 2003;14(2):xv–xvi.

[63] Oswal A, Beudel M, Zrinzo L, et al. Deep brain stimulation modulates synchrony within spatially and spectrally distinct resting state networks in Parkinson's disease. Brain. 2016;139:1482–96.

[64] Perlmutter JS, Mink JW, Bastian AJ, et al. Blood flow responses to deep brain stimulation of thalamus. Neurology. 2002;58(9):1388–94.

[65] Richards CD, Shiroyama T, Kitai ST. Electrophysiological and immunocytochemical characterization of GABA and dopamine neurons in the substantia nigra of the rat. Neuroscience. 1997;80:545–57.

[66] Salin P, Manrique C, Forni C, Kerkerian-Le Goff L. High-frequency stimulation of the subthalamic nucleus selectively reverses dopamine denervation-induced cellular defects in the output structures of the basal ganglia in the rat. J Neurosci. 2002;22:5137–48.

[67] Stefani A, Fedele E, Pierantozzi M, et al. Reduced GABA content in the motor thalamus during effective deep brain stimulation of the subthalamic nucleus. Front Syst Neurosci. 2011;5:17.

[68] Tai CH, Boraud T, Bezard E, Bioulac B, Gross C, Benazzouz A. Electrophysiological and metabolic evidence that high-frequency stimulation of the subthalamic nucleus bridles neuronal activity in the subthalamic nucleus and the substantia nigra reticulata. FASEB J. 2003;17:1820–30.

[69] Tasker RR. Deep brain stimulation is preferable to thalamotomy for tremor suppression. Surg Neurol. 1998;49:145–53.

[70] Temel Y, Boothman LJ, Blokland A, et al. Inhibition of 5-HT neuron activity and induction of depressive-like behavior by high-frequency stimulation of the subthalamic nucleus. Proc Natl Acad Sci U S A. 2007;104:17087–92.

[71] Toda H, Hamani C, Fawcett AP, Hutchison WD, Lozano AM. The regulation of adult rodent hippocampal neurogenesis by deep brain stimulation. J Neurosurg. 2008;108:132–8.

[72] Valenti O, Cifelli P, Gill KM, Grace AA. Antipsychotic drugs rapidly induce dopamine neuron depolarization block in a developmental rat model of schizophrenia. J Neurosci. 2011;31:12330–8.

[73] van Kuyck K, Demeulemeester H, Feys H, et al. Effects of electrical stimulation or lesion in nucleus accumbens on the behaviour of rats in a T-maze after administration of 8-OH-DPAT or vehicle. Behav Brain Res. 2003;140:165–73.

[74] Vitek JL. Mechanisms of deep brain stimulation: excitation or inhibition. Mov Disord. 2002;17 Suppl 3:S69–72.

[75] Welter ML, Houeto JL, Bonnet AM, et al. Effects of high-frequency stimulation on subthalamic neuronal activity in parkinsonian patients. Arch Neurol. 2004;61:89–96.

[76] Windels F, Bruet N, Poupard A, et al. Effects of high frequency stimulation of subthalamic nucleus on extracellular glutamate and GABA in substantia nigra and globus pallidus in the normal rat. Eur J Neurosci. 2000;12:4141–6.

[77] Windels F, Carcenac C, Poupard A, Savasta M. Pallidal origin of GABA release within the substantia nigra pars reticulata during high-frequency stimulation of the subthalamic nucleus. J Neurosci. 2005;25:5079–86.

[78] Winter C, Mundt A, Jalali R, et al. High frequency stimulation and temporary inactivation of the subthalamic nucleus reduce quinpirole-induced compulsive checking behavior in rats. Exp Neurol. 2008;210:217–28.

第 4 章 脑深部电刺激手术和技术
Surgical and Technical Aspects of Deep Brain Stimulation

Rick Schuurman　Stephan Chabardes　著
尹子霄　杨岸超　译　孟凡刚　张建国　校

> **摘要：** 立体定向手术技术的基础是通过将带有确定空间坐标的刚性框架置于颅骨上，或通过将颅骨固定于机器人系统中的内部空间参考系中，从而将三维空间坐标叠加在大脑上。MRI 扫描中确定的脑深部电刺激（deep brain stimulation，DBS）靶点的位置信息会被转换为空间坐标。之后通过附着在立体定向框架上的立体定向弧，或通过手术机器人的辅助机械臂，引导电极通过颅骨孔到达靶区。
> 　　此外，DBS 领域近来也有一些其他的技术创新。磁共振技术的进步让我们能够直视 DBS 的靶点结构，这使得电极植入更加精确。新的磁共振技术也有助于理解大脑神经元网络，从而进一步探究新靶点和新的 DBS 适应证。多数 DBS 植入术是在局部麻醉下进行的，目的在于术中评估症状缓解的程度及刺激靶区产生的不良反应。但这可能会在不久的将来被认为是多余的步骤，因为对于大多数适应证而言，术前 MRI 和术中电生理已经足以提供充分的信息来确定电极植入的最佳位置。最新的 DBS 系统能通过多方向的电极施加带有方向性的电流。这一进展可以进一步提高 DBS 的性能，且由于电流精度的增加，刺激带来的不良反应将减少。最后，闭环电刺激系统的发展将能使 DBS 根据患者的实时状况不断地调整电流释放。

一、概述

脑深部电刺激（DBS）是一种通过植入大脑的电极直接释放电流，从而影响或改变脑深部结构功能的一种治疗方式。这些颅内电极通过皮下延长导线连接到植入胸部或腹壁的刺激器。工程师可以对刺激器输出到颅内电极的电流释放方式进行编程，临床医生也可以通过外接程控设备调整刺激电流的参数。

二、DBS 电极的立体定向植入技术

DBS 的良好疗效要求高精度的电极植入。目前最常用的刺激靶点是：①丘脑的亚核，用于治疗震颤、任务相关性肌张力障碍、疼痛综合征和癫痫；②深部基底节核团，如底丘脑核用于治疗帕金森病，苍白球用于治疗伴或不伴结构性脑异常的全身性或局灶性肌张力障碍；③连接大脑各区域的深部白质束，用于治疗精神疾病（如强迫症）或震颤。

在精确 MRI 扫描使靶点结构可见后，可使用立体定向手术技术完成电极植入。

三、立体定向图谱

在立体定向手术中，会用到特殊的解剖图谱，这种图谱可以高度详细地描绘出大脑的解剖

结构。其使用一个虚拟的中心轴，用来连接前连合（AC）和后连合（PC），并在亚毫米级别精度上将大脑在轴向、冠状和矢状3个方向描绘出来，这使得所有图像的方向都与AC-PC轴平行或垂直。因此，大脑中每个结构都有一个相对于AC-PC轴的相对位置，且这个相对位置在大多数人是一致的。但是为了最终确定植入的确切位置，需要使用MRI扫描来纠正个体间微小的解剖差异。

通过使用特殊的软件，可以将立体定向解剖图谱投射到单个患者的MRI图像上。这样一来，我们就可以确定靶点在大脑中的精确位置，并且为这些靶区提供解剖坐标（图4-1）。

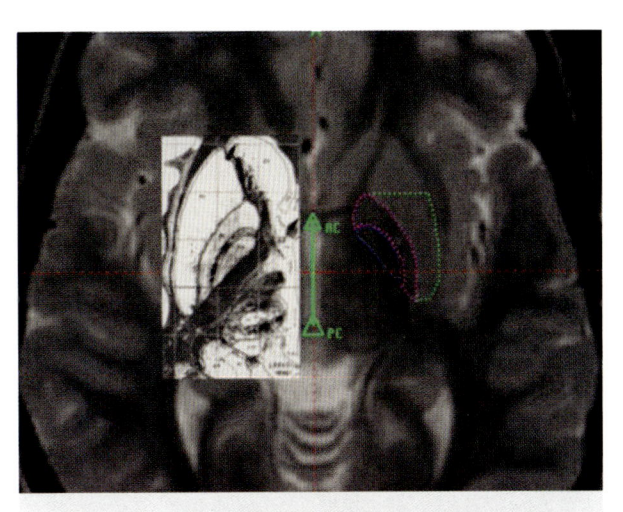

▲ 图 4-1 DBS 中用于确定靶点位置的轴向 MRI 影像示例，此例中靶点为苍白球

在图的中央，AC-PC 轴已画出。在图像的左侧，立体定向图谱作为示例已投射至大脑。在图像的右侧，通过利用手术计划软件画出苍白球的内部（蓝色）和外部（粉色）和壳核（绿色）的轮廓，从而调整图谱的位置以适应不同患者的个体解剖结构（根据该轴向图谱平面的延伸程度，壳核的前缘被切除）

四、基于立体定向框架的导航

在手术中颅骨会被固定在一个刚性框架上。这种所谓的立体定向框架（图4-2A）与颅骨和脑内结构都具有固定的位置关系。大多数立体定向框架由互成直角的直金属条构成，且在3个方向上都带有毫米尺度标记。这样，一个笛卡尔坐标系就投射到了大脑上，其中X轴表示左右，Y轴表示前后，Z轴表示上下。

将框架固定到头部后，就可以进行1.5T的MRI扫描，从而直接显示DBS靶点的空间位置，或者通过获得靶区邻近结构的位置信息，根据图谱间接获取靶点的位置。实际上，大多数团队都会进行术前3T（甚至7T）MRI扫描，以此使得靶点足够清晰可见。接着，通过手术计划软件，将术前影像与基于框架的1.5T MRI 或 CT 进行配准。

在对不同来源的图像进行配准的过程中，必须对不同MRI扫描序列图像所产生的不同程度的失真进行校正。然而，当今大多数MRI扫描仪都配备了足够精确的失真校正算法，同时计划软件也可以进行最终校正。

通过这种方式将MRI影像、图谱和立体定向框架结合，便能描绘出DBS靶点对于AC-PC轴的相对位置，并得到其相对于立体定向框架的空间坐标位置，这有助于术中的手术导航。

五、立体定向植入

在确定了靶点的空间坐标后，可将电极经过颅骨孔直线穿过大脑植入到靶区。使用MRI扫描建立的三维图像可以确定电极穿过大脑的轨迹路径。该路径由规划软件确定，其主要目的是避开所有可见的血管，从而最大程度减少出血的风险，进而减少大脑损伤。

患者接着被置于手术台上，头部被立体定向框架牢牢固定。之后在无菌环境下将手术打靶装置固定于框架上。该装置为一弧形设备（图4-2B），此弧形设备的虚拟圆心将与目标靶点的X、Y、Z轴空间坐标相重合。电极植入的角度在路径规划时已被算出。现在可以将电极沿着规划好的路径植入到大脑的靶区中。

六、术中测试

在确定DBS靶点的位置后，可以通过术中

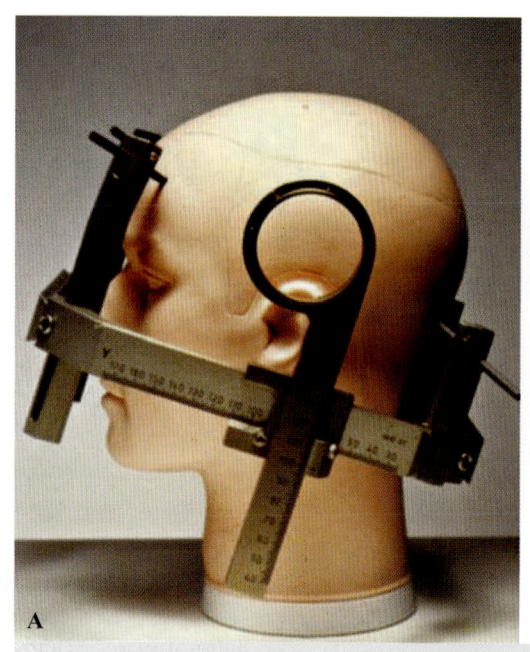

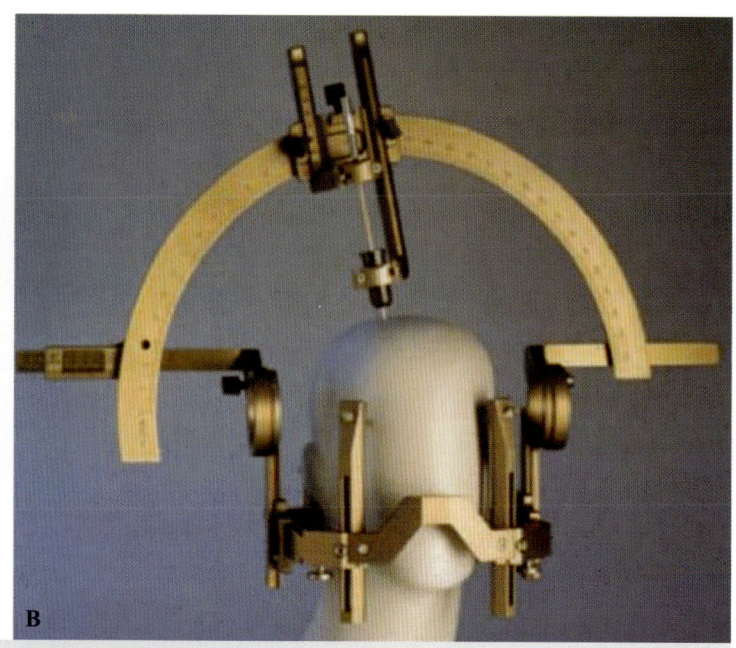

▲ 图 4-2　A. 立体定向框架固定于颅骨上，框架上的毫米标记提供了投射到大脑的笛卡尔坐标系；B. 立体定向弧固定于框架上，该弧所形成的虚拟圆心与靶点的坐标相重合。这样一来，电极（或其他任何手术器械）可以沿着预先确定好的路线植入靶点中

电生理和刺激测试验证该位置的优劣，但该方法仅适用于可以直接观察到改善的适应证（如在肌张力障碍或精神疾病中就不适用）。为使术中测试可以顺利进行，DBS 通常在局麻下植入，以便对靶区的病理生理脑活动进行最佳的记录，并使患者在清醒状态下提供对电刺激的临床反馈。

为使术中改善效果最大化，帕金森患者会在术前一晚停用抗帕金森药物，以保证在术中表现出最严重的临床症状。但是显然，停药状态下进行"清醒"颅内手术会给患者带来不小的负担，因此在手术中应特别注意患者的身体和情绪状态（另见第 7 章）。

为了对靶点进行神经生理学确认，可插入一个或几个平行于预定路径的微电极进行记录。信号可从靶区中的单个神经元获得，以此方式勾勒出各目标神经核团的边界，并将其用于计划的 MRI 扫描所确定的边界进行比较。

在通过影像和神经生理学方法确定靶区后，则开始进行测试刺激。术中刺激测试是术后真实刺激的模拟，其可以用来验证靶区刺激是否确实能够缓解疾病症状。例如，在帕金森患者中是否会减轻震颤和强直。此外，刺激测试可以帮助确定出现刺激相关不良反应的电流阈值，包括由于电流扩散至邻近结构而引起的眼球运动障碍、语言障碍或肌肉不自主收缩。

最后，根据影像学、神经生理学和临床相关信息，我们可以确定 DBS 电极的最佳位置。然后在 X 线的确认下将永久 DBS 电极植入于靶区，并将电极固定于颅骨上，这样电极不会在术后沿电极轴发生位移。

由于 DBS 通常双侧植入，对侧半球的术中测试和电极植入重复上述步骤。

接着，移除颅骨上的立体定向框架。在接下来的全麻手术中，将电极与延伸导线连接，延伸导线通过颈部皮下组织穿过锁骨下区域，并与神经刺激器相连接。刺激器被植于胸壁或腹壁皮下。

在 DBS 术中可以对处于清醒状态的运动障碍患者（如原发性震颤、肌张力障碍、帕金森病、疼痛综合征）进行术中测试，以获得患者的临床改善反馈用于指导最佳植入，从而增加有效电极植入的概率。对于因肌张力障碍而导致姿势严重异常的患者而言（特别是儿童），可以在全麻下进行 DBS 手术。在这些情况下，测试刺激仍然可以提供有关肌肉收缩等不良反应的电流阈值的反馈。对于癫痫和精神疾病等 DBS 适应证，由于无法观察到可靠的术中临时刺激效果，DBS 也可以在全麻下进行。

七、术中影像验证电极位置

尽管已经将电极放置到靶区，但是为避免临床效果不佳，仍需要检查是否有任何空间位置上的偏差。为达到该目的，有以下几种方法可供选择，包括最简单的 X 线，以及更加精确、复杂的技术，如术中 CT 或术中 MRI。

术中 CT 可以显示微电极（MER）和永久 DBS 电极的套管轨迹。图像以医学数字成像和通信（digital imaging and communications in medicine，DICOM）的格式获取，并且可以与在 3T MRI 上进行的术前计划相融合。这些影像使我们能够在术中发现任何电极位置上的偏差，并将之纠正（图 4-3）。

Zrinzo 和 Hariz（Aviles-Olmos 等，2014）描述了另一种方法，即通过术中 MRI 对电极位置进行验证。按照这种方法，仍然使用常规的立体定向框架植入电极，但在手术最后、取下立体定向框架之前必须对患者进行 MRI 扫描。

Larson 和 Starr（Starr 等，2009）提出了一种使用 clear point 系统的创新性方法，该方法强调在术中 MRI 实时引导下进行 DBS 电极植入。在这个概念下，患者被特定的工具固定于 MRI 装置中，并同时接受手术（图 4-4）。

八、其他植入方法

（一）Nexframe

没有立体定向框架也是可以进行 DBS 电极植入的。在这种情况下，较小的瞄准装置替代立体定向框架并被连接到颅骨上。同样通过 MRI 影像确定 DBS 靶点和植入轨迹。使用基准标记点代替框架透过皮肤固定到颅骨上，该基准标记点在 MRI 下可见。与一般神经外科手术导航的方式相同，该方法也应用了红外探测技术，并根据此来引导导航软件。

在颅骨的钻孔位置确定之后，瞄准装置（即所谓的 Nexframe）就被连接于颅骨上（Starr 等，2010）。在将套管固定于正确的植入方向后，即可计算植入深度并通过该套管将电极植入到靶区中。据报告，该系统的电极放置精确度与立体定

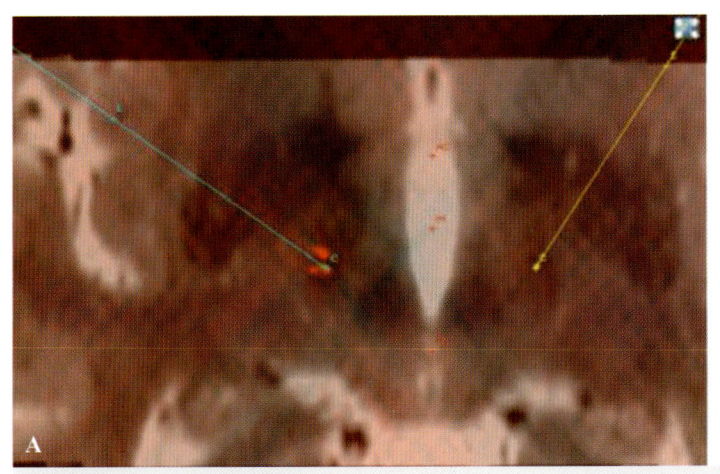

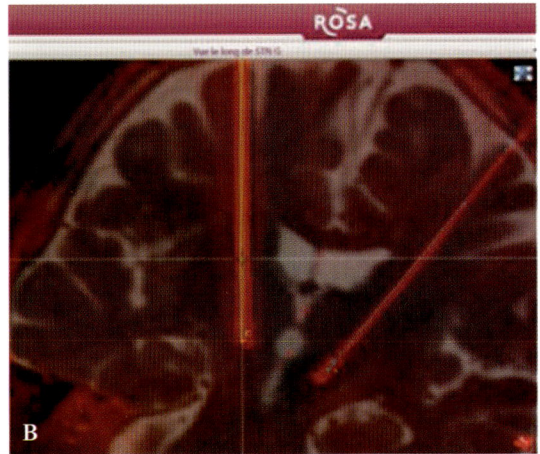

▲ 图 4-3　A. 显示红核、底丘脑核（STN）和 3 个微电极尖端进入 STN 的与术前 T_2 MRI 图像融合的术中影像；B. 显示红核、STN 和最终电极按照既定轨迹插入的与术前 T_2 MRI 图像融合的术中影像

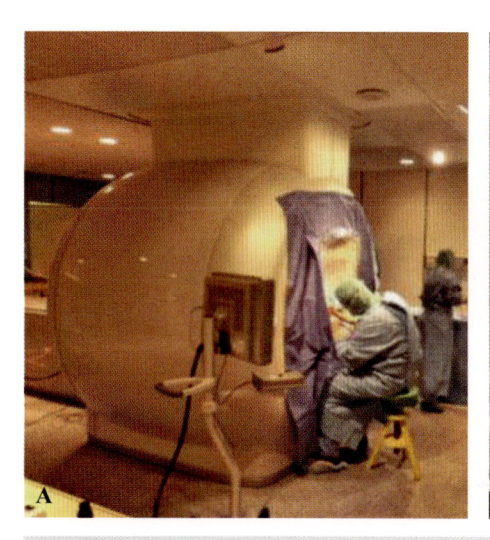

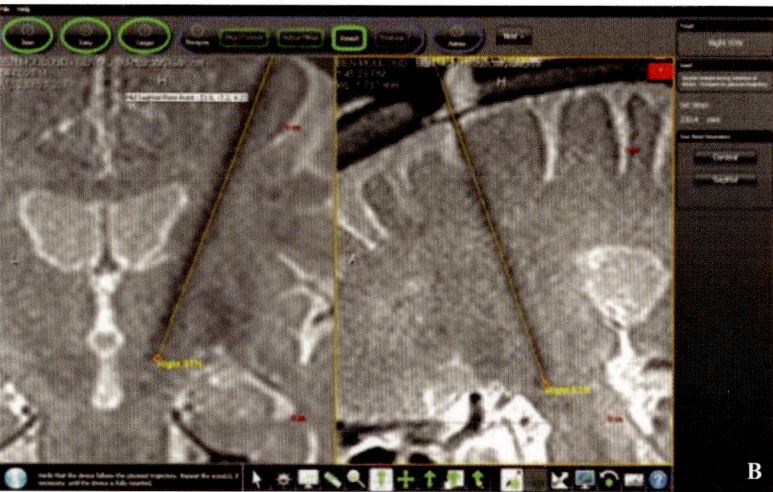

▲ 图 4-4　图示为在 Grenoble 大学使用 Clear Point 系统并借鉴由美国加利福尼亚大学旧金山分校（UCSF）的 Starr 和 Larson 提出的概念进行的 STN-DBS 电极植入的案例

向框架植入的精确度相当（Kelman 等，2010）。

（二）机器人引导的手术

机器人引导下的 DBS 电极植入已经被应用了 20 多年，然而最近的一些技术创新使得该技术得以被更加广泛地应用（有关综述，请参阅 Faria 等，2015）。机械臂可以代替立体定向弧来执行电极植入。借助机器人的导航软件，DBS 靶点的确定和路径的规划通过与框架手术相同的方式依据 MRI 影像实现。在手术过程中，将基准标记点透过皮肤固定至颅骨后，再次进行 CT 扫描三维成像，并将这些图像与进行手术计划的 MRI 进行融合。

这之后，通过刚性固定（使用框架作为头部固定器）将机械臂连接至颅骨框架，并且将机械臂的转向装置与术前计划系统建立共同参照系，这样该机械臂即可指向颅骨钻孔的位置。机械臂可以选择握持一个微型推动器（Microdrive），其能协助将多根套管植入大脑并指向靶区。接下来，插入深部电极并进行术中测试，最后完成永久 DBS 电极的植入（图 4-5）。

与常规框架手术相比，使用机械臂的优势在于精度更高（向量误差：机器人手术为 1~1.5mm，框架手术为 3mm）（Von Langdorff 等，2014），以及手术过程更快，尤其是在如立体脑电图（SEEG）这种需要多个植入路径的情况下。

九、近期和未来的技术发展

（一）影像学

MRI 早在 20 世纪 90 年代就被引入立体定向电极植入手术，最初它主要用于精准确定 AC-PC 轴的位置。与早年的脑室造影术相比，它可以更加精确地显示脑内解剖结构。此外，在路径规划中，MRI 的应用使得植入轨迹能够避开血管和脑室系统。

随着旨在显示基底节的新 MR 序列的发展，以及具有更高场强的 MR 的出现，DBS 的靶点结构将被更加清晰详细地显示出来（图 4-6）。这项技术使得术前对靶点的确定变得更加精确。

（二）DTI、连通性、fMRI

弥散张量成像（DTI）和示踪成像的使用为可视化大脑各种结构之间的白质连接提供了新的可能。该技术可能会为 DBS 治疗带来新的潜在靶点，也可能会优化现有的靶点。相关的例证包括齿状核-红核-丘脑束的可视化（可在大脑

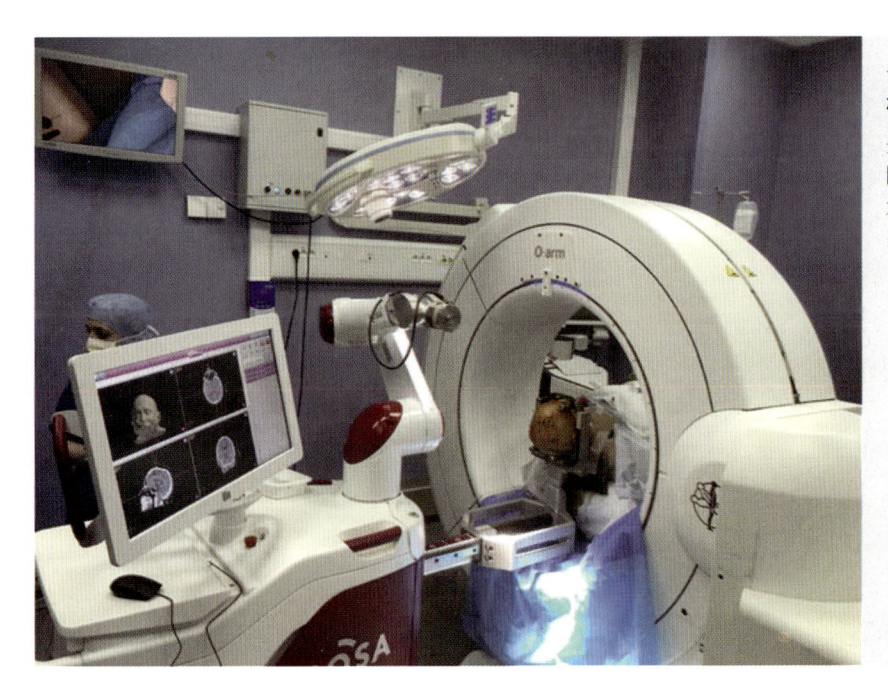

第 4 章 脑深部电刺激手术和技术
Surgical and Technical Aspects of Deep Brain Stimulation

◀ 图 4-5 在 Grenoble 大学进行的机器人引导的手术

头部固定器（此处为 Leksell 框架）被刚性固定于患者的头部。将患者置于术中扫描仪中（Oarm，Medtronic），以进行术中图像验证和导线放置

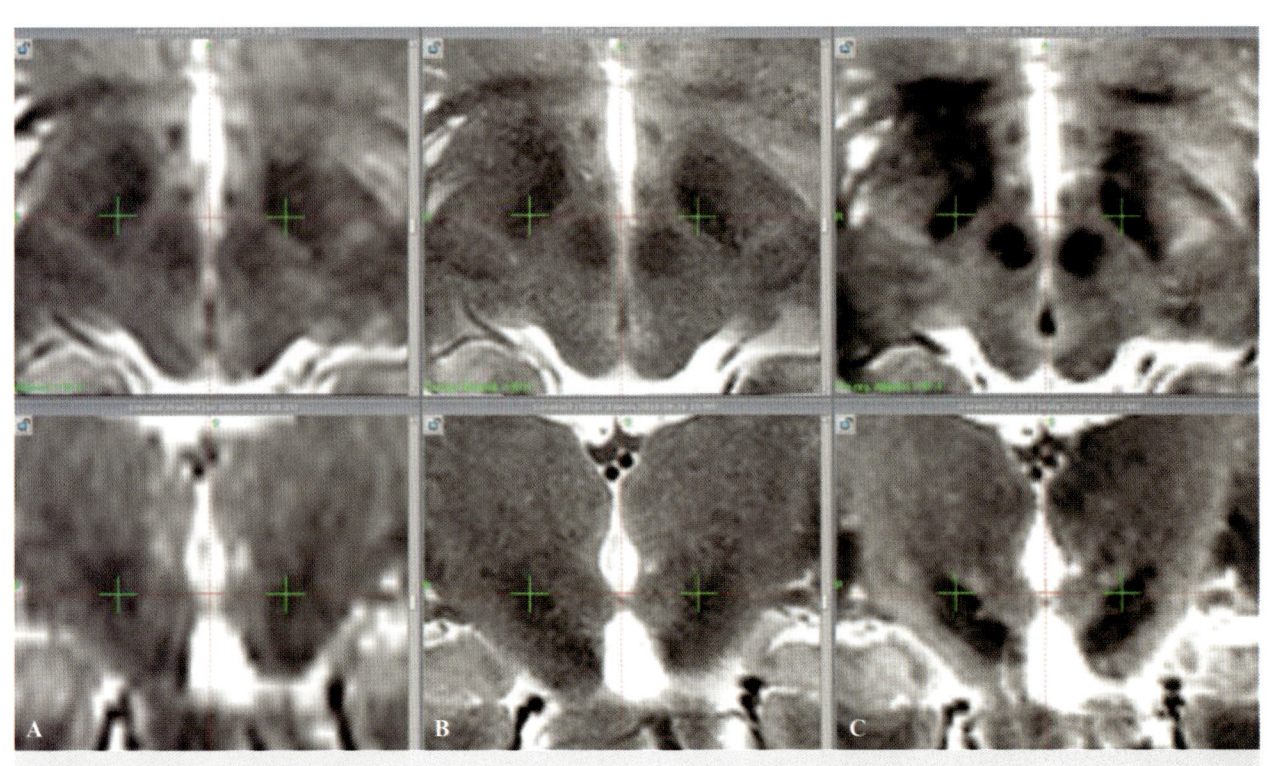

▲ 图 4-6 DBS 手术计划中帕金森病患者底丘脑核在 MRI 扫描中的详细投影

不同场强的 T_2 轴位（顶部）和冠位（底部）的 MR 扫描：A. 1.5T；B. 3T；C. 7T

不同平面刺激该结构以治疗震颤）（Coenen 等，2014），以及前脑内侧束的可视化（在焦虑症和情绪障碍的治疗中发挥重要作用）（Schlaepfer 等，2013）。连通性研究可以识别丘脑中的亚结构用以治疗疼痛（Kovanlikaya 等，2014）。

功能磁共振成像（fMRI）和连通性研究，除了可以直接描绘 DBS 靶点和加深关于现有靶点的理解之外（Lambert 等，2012），还有助于我们理解功能性大脑神经元网络，特别是当这些成像技术能在 DBS 植入时被同时使用（Figee 等，2013）。

（三）3D 影像计划平台

近来，利用可变图谱或解剖自动化分段技术，已经实现了对靶区及其周围结构的 3D 模型重建（图 4-7）。这些工具使我们能够在术前进行模拟或在术后重建电极的位置，还可以对电极周围的理论组织激活场（VTA）可视化。然而这些 3D 图像结果的精准度取决于原始图像的质量和"融合"过程，需要谨慎解释。

（四）全身麻醉下的 DBS 手术

目前帕金森病仍是 DBS 最常见的适应证，以上描述的手术策略是基于影像学、神经生理学和临床信息来共同确定最佳 DBS 电极位置的。目前大多数中心均在局麻下进行 DBS 手术。在过去，将这些技术结合起来并能够在术中判断 DBS 效果的优势大大超过了患者手术负担的劣势。但是，随着成像技术和全麻下神经生理学信号记录的进步（Pinkster 等，2009），术中进行临床测试的附加价值可能会减少。一项大中心的病例系列研究结果显示，在全麻下进行 DBS 植入与在同一中心在清醒状态下接受手术的患者（历史队列对照）的临床改善相当（Nakajima 等，2011）。

除减轻患者的负担外，全麻手术还可能带来较短的手术时间和较轻的术后意识障碍，从而缩短住院时间。未来研究需要进一步对局部麻醉和全身麻醉 DBS 进行比较，在减轻患者负担而又不降低干预质量的前提下，全麻手术是否应该被更广泛地应用以缩短治疗时间。

（五）方向性刺激

目前广泛使用的 DBS 电极有 4 个可激活触点，均可以被独立地开关。这些触点的长度为 1.5mm，间隔为 0.5 或 1.5mm。根据对刺激的临床反应，可以通过选择可激活触点的位置实现 DBS 放电位置沿 Z 轴垂直方向的上下移动。一般情况下，电流在每个有效触点向所有方向传递，不能在电极植入后选择 X 和 Y 轴的刺激方向。但由于电流在邻近结构（如内囊、内侧丘系或动眼神经纤维）中的播散可能会引起刺激相关不良反应，因此电流不能被无限制的增加以追求最优临床效果。

在新开发出的电极中，其触点不再是圆环状的，而是分成了 3 个部分。可以通过打开或

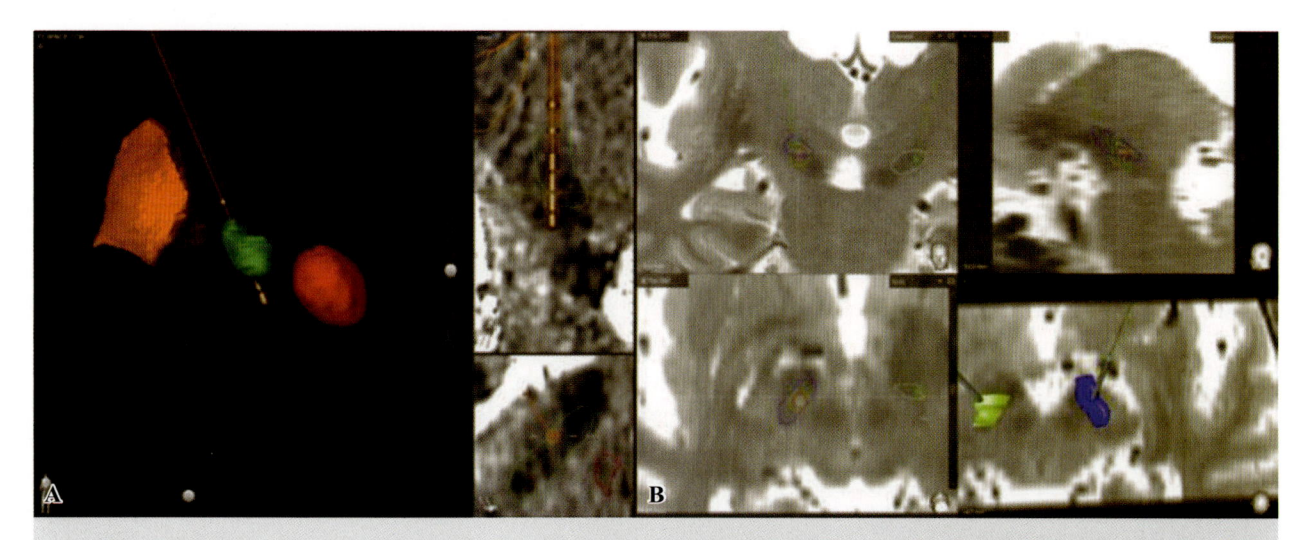

▲ 图 4-7 使用 Guide XT（Brain Lab）（A）和 Sure Tune（Medtronic）（B）将 DBS 电极植入 STN（绿色）中的 3D 图像

关闭其中的某一部分，从而创建一个不对称的刺激场，进而将刺激电流转向或偏离特定的方向（图4-8）。早期的研究表明，无论是在术中试验性植入的方向电极还是术后永久性植入的方向电极，均可通过控制电流方向来扩大治疗窗（临床疗效阈值和不良反应阈值之间的电压差值）。

（六）闭环式的自适应刺激

可以预见在不久的将来会出现闭环式的自适应刺激（详见第5章）。当前，DBS以固定的参数释放刺激，该参数会持续产生相同的电流，而与基于患者病情波动和疾病活动所需的实际刺激需求无关。根据病情的实时需求，输入系统的反馈可以使刺激参数实时发生变化。

在MTPT诱导的猴帕金森病模型中，运动皮质中的细胞活动为DBS系统提供了反馈。当帕金森症状加重时，DBS系统将会开启刺激，这一苍白球DBS显示出了闭环刺激的有效性（Rosin等，2011）。这种刺激形式的有效性也在人类中得到了证明。在帕金森病患者中，植入底丘脑核的DBS电极通过导线穿出皮肤接受外挂刺激，并测量脑细胞的局部场电位活动。与疾病严重程度相关的β活动增加可激活DBS，并带来与连续性DBS相当，甚至更优的临床改善（Little等，2013）。一旦永久性植入式闭环系统可以投入使用，我们可以更加深入地研究这种刺激方式带来的优势。

十、结论

自20世纪90年代以来，用于DBS的外科技术一直在不断发展，如今，高场强的新MRI序列的使用使绝大多数的解剖核团清晰可见。准确植入电极仍然是DBS手术的主要目标，通过在术中确认电极的准确放置，电极植入位置不佳的概率将被大大降低。方向性电极的使用能够在大多数情况下（尽管不是所有情况下）弥补电极放置位置的一些细微误差。然而，硬件技术和影像学的进步不代表能够忽视解剖学、生理学和临床神经病学或精神病学的基础理论知识，这些理论基础对于最优化DBS治疗是必不可少的。

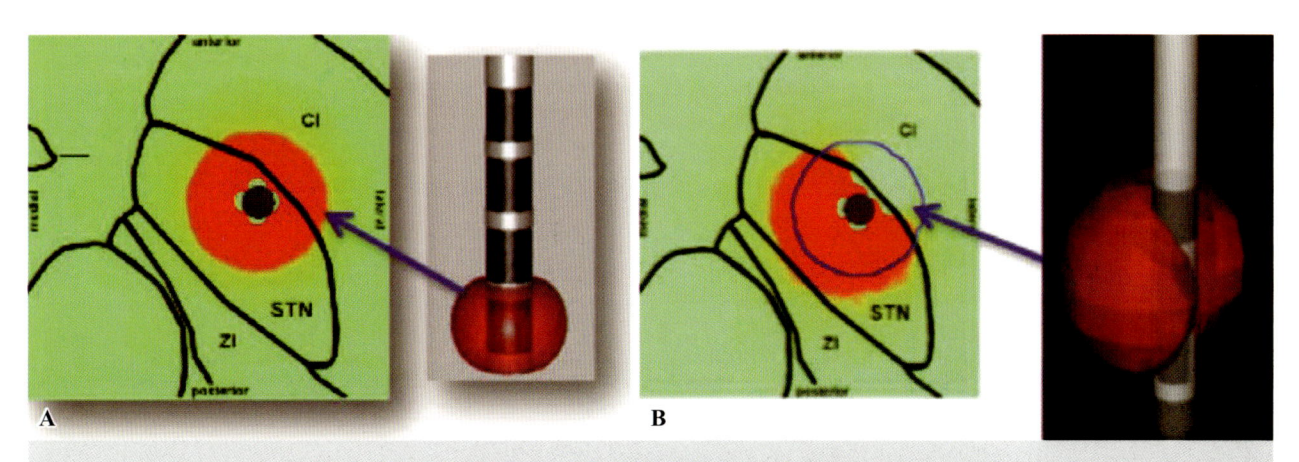

▲ 图4-8 在底丘脑核电流扩散的示意图

A. 从常规电极发出的电流会对邻近结构产生异常刺激，对底丘脑核（STN）刺激产生积极的临床作用而对内囊（CI）刺激产生不良反应；B. 通过方向电极来控制电流，可以对刺激场的形状进行调整，从而仅刺激靶点区

参考文献

[1] Aviles-Olmos I, Kefalopoulou Z, Tripoliti E, et al. Long-term outcome of subthalamic nucleus deep brain stimulation for Parkinson's disease using an MRI-guided and MRI-verified approach. J Neurol Neurosurg Psychiatry. 2014;85:1419–25.

[2] Coenen VA, Allert N, Paus S, et al. Modulation of the cerebello-thalamo-cortical network in thalamic deep brain stimulation for tremor. Neurosurgery. 2014;75:657–70.

[3] Contarino MF, Bour LJ, Verhagen R, et al. Directional steering: a novel approach to deep brain stimulation. Neurology. 2014;83:1163–9.

[4] Faria C, Erlhagen W, Rito M, De Momi E, Ferrigno G, Bicho E. Review of robotic technology for stereotactic neurosurgery. IEEE Rev Biomed Eng. 2015;8:125–37.

[5] Figee M, Luigjes J, Smolders R, et al. Deep brain stimulation restores frontostriatal network activity in obsessive-compulsive disorder. Nat Neurosci. 2013;16:386–7.

[6] Kelman C, Ramakrishnan V, Davies A, Holloway K. Analysis of stereotactic accuracy of the Cosman-Robert-wells frame and nexframe frameless systems in deep brain stimulation surgery. Stereotact Funct Neurosurg. 2010;88:288–95.

[7] Kovanlikaya I, Heier L, Kaplitt M. Treatment of chronic pain: diffusion tensor imaging identification of the ventroposterolateral nucleus confirmed with successful deep brain stimulation. Stereotact Funct Neurosurg. 2014;92:365–71.

[8] Lambert C, Zrinzo L, Nagy Z, et al. Confirmation of functional zones within the human subthalamic nucleus: patterns of connectivity and sub-parcellation using diffusion weighted imaging. NeuroImage. 2012;60:83–94.

[9] Little S, Pogosyan A, Neal S, et al. Adaptive deep brain stimulation in advanced Parkinson disease. Ann Neurol. 2013;74:449–57.

[10] Nakajima T, Zrinzo L, Foltynie T, et al. MRI-guided subthalamic nucleus deep brain stimulation without microelectrode recording: can we dispense with surgery under local anaesthesia? Stereotact Funct Neurosurg. 2011;89:318–25.

[11] Pinkster MO, Volkmann J, Falk D, et al. Deep brain stimulation of the internal globus pallidus in dystonia: target localisation under general anaesthesia. Acta Neurochir. 2009;151:751–8.

[12] Rosin B, Slovik M, Mitelman R, et al. Closed-loop deep brain stimulation is superior in ameliorating parkinsonism. Neuron. 2011;72:370–84.

[13] Schlaepfer TE, Bewernick BH, Kayser S, Madler B, Coenen VA. Rapid effects of deep brain stimulation for treatment-resistant major depression. Biol Psychiatry. 2013;73:1204–12.

[14] Starr PA, Martin AJ, Larson PS. Implantation of deep brain stimulator electrodes using interventional MRI. Neurosurg Clin N Am. 2009;20:193–203.

[15] Starr PA, Martin AJ, Ostrem JL, Talke P, Levesque N, Larson PS. Subthalamic nucleus deep brain stimulator placement using high-field interventional magnetic resonance imaging and a skull-mounted aiming device: technique and application accuracy. J Neurosurg. 2010;112:479–90.

[16] Steigerwald F, Muller L, Johannes S, Matthies C, Volkmann J. Directional deep brain stimulation of the subthalamic nucleus: a pilot study using a novel neurostimulation device. Mov Disord. 2016;31:1240–3.

[17] von Langsdorff D, Paquis P, Fontaine D. In vivo measurement of the frame-based application accuracy of the neuromate neurosurgical robot. J Neurosurg. 2014;31:1–4.

第 5 章 未来展望：自适应脑深部电刺激
Future Perspectives: Adaptive Deep Brain Stimulation

Martijn Beudel　Margot Heijmans　Jeroen G. V. Habets　Pieter L. Kubben　著
尹子霄　杨岸超　译　孟凡刚　张建国　校

> **摘要**：在过去的 10 年，神经调控，尤其是脑深部电刺激（deep brain stimulation，DBS），已经成为许多药物难治性神经精神疾病的一种重要治疗方式。然而 DBS 还存在很多缺陷，尤其在疗效、不良反应和效率上。这些缺陷的原因很大程度上可以归因于开环 DBS 的设计，其不考虑临床需求的变化，而持续地输出同等水平的刺激。规避这种缺陷的一种方法是使 DBS 能根据病理性神经活动或其他生物指标来进行反馈性的刺激。这种刺激模式称为自适应 DBS（adaptive DBS，aDBS）或闭环 DBS。目前临床上应用 aDBS 治疗的疾病只有癫痫。然而 aDBS 也开始应用于其他神经系统疾病研究中，主要是运动障碍性疾病，并取得了较好的结果。我们将在本章中深入探讨 aDBS 在神经和精神疾病中的运用和阻碍。本章将首先介绍 aDBS 的原理，之后介绍其适应证、可能的生物标志，以及 aDBS 运用于具体疾病的例证。最后，我们将讨论更多数据驱动的方法来使用 aDBS。

一、概述

脑深部电刺激（DBS）作为一种对难治性神经精神疾病的治疗方式，已经成功地在临床上使用了超过 30 年（见第 1 章）。尽管从最早用于临床以来 DBS 已经取得了许多技术进步，但总体而言其仍以大致相同的方式提供刺激；即仍以恒定的模式对深部核团进行高频刺激（开环刺激），若刺激不再有效和（或）引起不良反应，则手动调整刺激参数（图 5-1A）。尽管这些参数调整可能带来临床改善（Moro 等，2006），但目前形式的 DBS 潜力仍然有限。

帕金森病（Parkinson disease，PD）患者在多巴胺能药物关期，DBS 仅能使统一帕金森病评估量表（UPDRS）运动评分的改善率达到 45% 左右（Horn 等，2017）。其疗效有限的原因之一是 PD 症状的出现和严重程度均会随着时间的推移而改变，但传统的 DBS 只提供一种刺激模式，无法考虑症状的严重程度。癫痫作为一种典型的发作性疾病，其症状只在很短的时间内出现。但在 PD 中，症状不仅会因为多巴胺能系统的开关状态而出现短期波动，也会由于疾病进展在较长的时间间隔内发生波动。这种几乎可以在所有疾病中观察到，且在不同时间尺度上出现的波动性，已被证明是一种有用的调节 DBS 的生物标志。这种自适应形式的 DBS 被称作自适应 DBS（adaptive DBS，aDBS）、反应性 DBS 或闭环 DBS。为了表达上的一致性，本章将使用术语 aDBS 来进行统一的描述。

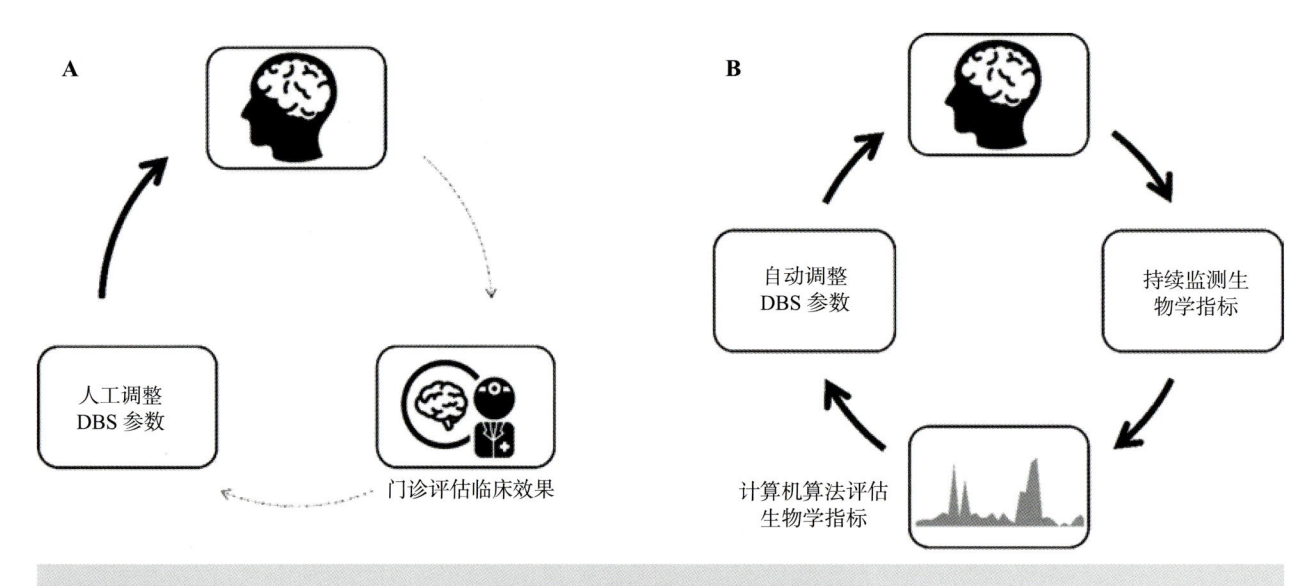

▲ 图 5-1 连续 DBS 和 aDBS 的比较

A. 在持续 DBS 中，临床医生在一段时间后评估治疗效果，并手动调整 DBS 参数；B. 在 aDBS 中，通过测量生物标志间接评估临床效果，并自动调整 DBS 参数。细虚箭表示偶发事件，粗实箭表示连续事件

二、aDBS 的一般概念

（一）aDBS 的原理

aDBS 系统基于一种闭环系统，该系统记录并分析一个或多个能反映患者临床状态（即症状严重程度）的变量，并确定刺激参数是否需要调整（图 5-1B）。由于 aDBS 以"按需"的方式提供刺激（即当症状出现时才给予刺激），aDBS 系统被认为是一种更有效的、刺激相关不良反应更少的、电池寿命更长的，以及更少习惯化的刺激系统。

开发 aDBS 系统的一个重要步骤是选择合适的生物标志。生物标志应该能够准确反映疾病的主要症状。为了实现这一点，有时需要额外的植入物或记录设备以获取基于生物标志的反馈信息。在选择生物标志时，应考虑额外植入物或设备的侵袭性，以及生物标志实时分析的计算要求（图 5-2）。本章将讨论可能的生物标志及其在 PD、原发性震颤、癫痫、肌张力障碍、强迫症（obsessive-compulsive disorder，OCD）和抽动秽语综合征中的优劣势。这并不意味着 aDBS 仅能适用于这些疾病，但目前尚缺乏实验和临床证据证明 aDBS 的其他适应证。

除 aDBS 系统的各种输入的选项外，aDBS 还有多种可能的输出选项，即刺激算法。根目前研究发现，应用于 aDBS 最常见的算法是调节 DBS 的刺激振幅（电压，图 5-3）。振幅的调节可分为二分类的开 / 关方式（Little 等，2013），即仅当输入信号超过某个阈值，以及标量方式时才开启刺激，即逐步调整刺激振幅（Rosa 等，2017）。除了振幅的调节外，还可能存在对临床症状（如震颤）或具有振荡性质的生物标志的相位依赖性刺激（Cagnan 等，2017）。通过这种相位依赖性刺激，DBS 的单次脉冲仅在特定的相位才被触发。目前尚没有研究系统地评估刺激参数对疗效的影响，刺激频率和刺激脉宽也可能在将来被用于改进 aDBS 系统（Fasano 和 Lozano，2014）。

（二）aDBS 的临床与技术实现

aDBS 在控制系统研究中有着长久的历史。尽管控制系统，即闭环系统，可以追溯到古代，麦克斯韦在 1868 年描述的一篇题为"论调控器"的论文划定了闭环系统的里程碑，其对闭环

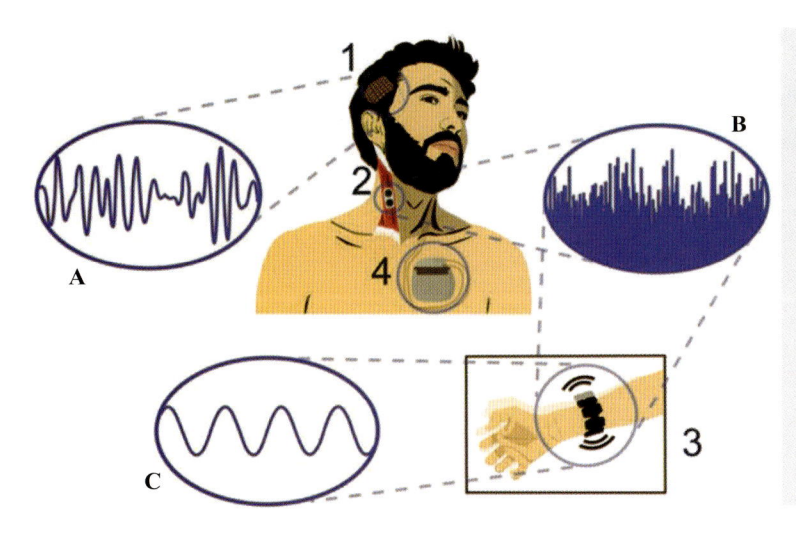

第 5 章　未来展望：自适应脑深部电刺激
Future Perspectives: Adaptive Deep Brain Stimulation

◀ 图 5-2　aDBS 的潜在记录位点（数字）和生物标志（字母）

1.颅内记录位点包括皮质和皮质下靶区；2.肌肉记录位点；3.外部记录位点；4.DBS 电池记录位点。A.局部场电位；B.肌电图；C.加速度信号（经许可转载，引自 Piña-Fuentes et al，*Neurosurgical Focus*，2018b）

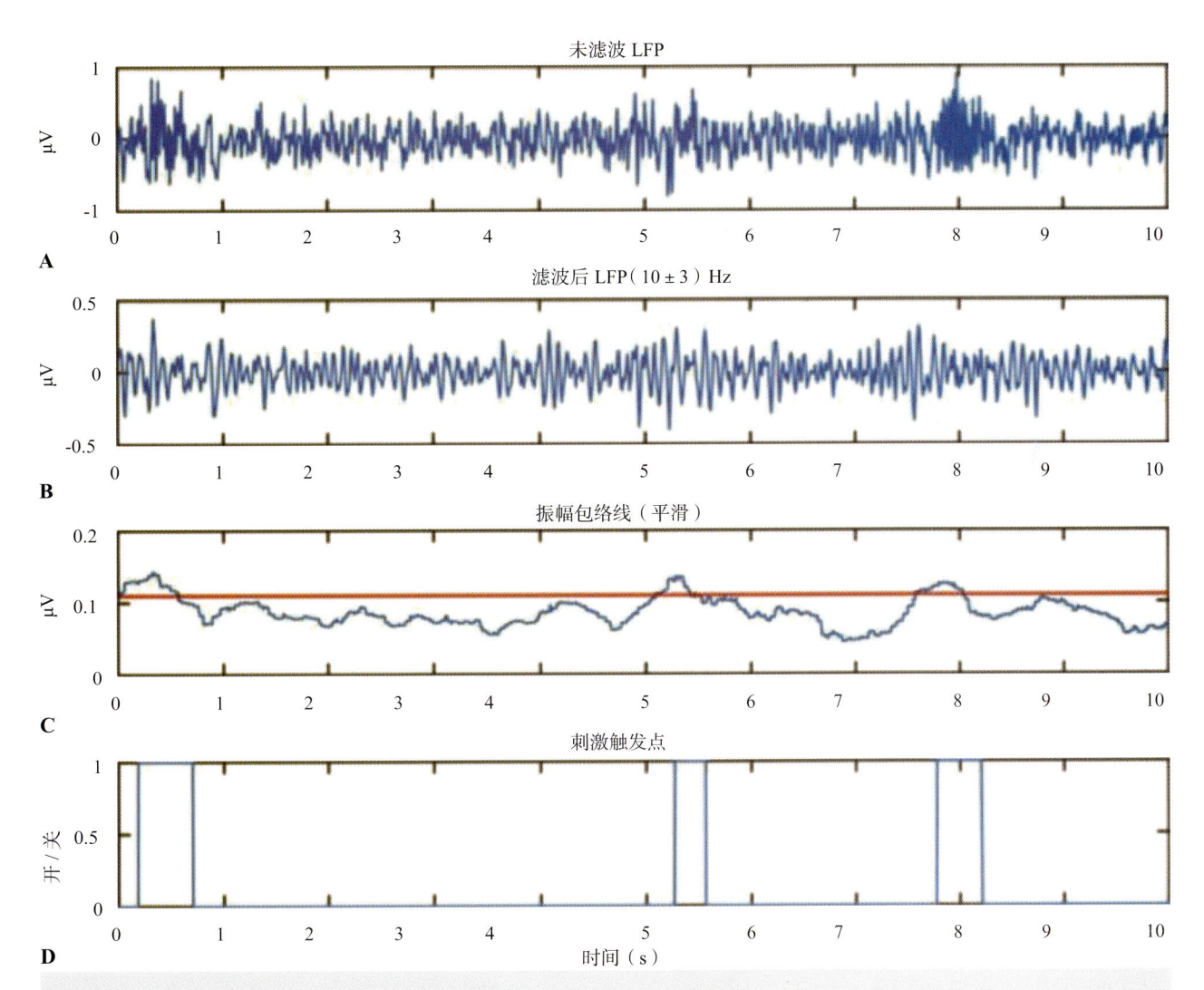

▲ 图 5-3　aDBS 算法的示例

A.肌张力障碍患者苍白球的未滤波的局部场电位（LFP）；B.低频范围中（4～12Hz）围绕峰值频率的滤波后 LFP；C.峰值频率的平滑振幅（振幅包络线），以及刺激阈值（红线）；D.刺激触发点，即开启 DBS 刺激的时刻。刺激触发点即振幅包络超过刺激阈值的时刻（经许可转载，引自 Piña-Fuentes et al，*Neurobiology of Disease*，2018a）

041

系统进行了较为正式的分析,包括自激振荡现象(Maxwell,1868)。aDBS 的第一个实验性证据可以追溯到 20 世纪 60—70 年代,在这期间,Delgado 用他的"刺激接收器"进行了实验。该"刺激接收器"能够基于黑猩猩杏仁核中的"纺锤波"活动(Horgan,2005)或运动检测器信号(Delgado 等,1976)来激发 aDBS。然而在医学领域,1980 年以前还没有在人类身上实现闭环技术的植入。直到 1980 年,Mirowski 等(1980)发表了第一篇描述植入式自动除颤器治疗恶性室性心律失常的论文。尽管在 1980 年心脏病学领域就取得了这一进展,但直到 2004 年闭环刺激才首次应用于癫痫(Kossoff 等,2004)。

有几个原因导致了心脏病学和神经病学中闭环刺激研发的延迟。首先,他们记录的病理信号的振幅不同(mV 与 μV),在神经病学中记录电信号需要更高的放大率和设备资源。其次,癫痫和心律失常的病理信号复杂程度不同,癫痫信号的记录需要更大的计算量及更多的设备资源。最后,中枢神经系统被头骨包围,其功能高度分化,这使得实现最佳空间定位更加困难。在非阵发性疾病如 PD 或震颤的 aDBS 治疗中这些问题则变得更加明显。以工程学的角度考虑从连续刺激转向自适应刺激时,首先应该考虑的是被检症状或生物标志物的采样率和频率,以及采集额外闭环特征所需要消耗的能量,这样才能确定需要哪些硬件设备。在 aDBS 刚刚起步的时期(Anderson 等,2008),电池的能量消耗是限制其发展的一个问题,但是今天由于可充电的起搏器(internalized pacemakers,IPG)已成为商业化产品并被常规植入,电池的能量消耗问题已不再是个棘手的问题。

三、aDBS 在运动障碍病中的应用

帕金森病

PD 是一种包括运动症状和非运动症状的进展性神经退行性疾病。除了长期随访中运动症状的性质和严重程度会随着时间而改变外,短期内运动症状也存在波动。其中最为人熟知的症状"开关"现象即为多巴胺能药物水平的波动引起的。在起病初期,服用低剂量的多巴胺能药物就可以相对容易地达到"开"状态,并维持一整天。然而,5 年之后大多数患者开始出现运动并发症(Hauser 等,2006)。这些运动并发症包括可预测或不可预测的运动改善波动(如"不起效""延迟起效"或"疗效减退")和不自主运动的出现(异动症)。该两种并发症都会使患者变得虚弱,是除难治性震颤和冲动控制障碍以外 DBS 最典型的手术指征。理论上,DBS 持续释放电流能够缓解 PD 运动症状。但事实上 DBS 术后的 PD 患者仍然需要多巴胺能药物治疗。其中一个重要的原因是 DBS 电极只刺激底丘脑核(subthalamic nucleus,STN)的运动区,而不刺激联络区和边缘区,这可能导致在缺乏多巴胺能药物的情况下出现如淡漠等非运动症状(Martinez-Fernandez 等,2016)。药物和 DBS 两种疗法的结合提示,即便"关"期症状很严重,运动症状波动仍然存在。然而,DBS 的上调潜力是有限的,因为大电流刺激更容易导致异动、其他刺激相关不良反应,甚至是运动迟缓(Chen 等,2006)。除了这些基于多巴胺能药物用量的症状波动之外,其他因素也会影响运动症状的严重程度。其中最重要的因素是疾病进展、压力、昼夜节律、并发疾病和疲劳。

总而言之,PD 的症状严重程度会随时间发生变化,但目前 DBS 仍以开环的方式提供刺激。若 DBS 能仅在需要时以闭环方式提供刺激,就能带来更好的疗效、减少刺激引起的不良反应、提高效率并减少(住院)参数调整的次数。为了实现 aDBS,症状的严重程度需要被持续规律地记录。目前有两种方法进行临床试验,一是直接记录中枢神经系统的神经活动,二是利用运动传感器记录运动。此外还有一种方法(即皮质下记录神经化学信号)仅在临床前研究中被探究过(Lee 等,2017)。由于目前这种方法存在局

限性，即需要额外的皮质下化学传感器，而且目前还没有相关的临床证据，我们将不再讨论这种方法（Graupe 等，2014）。在接下来的部分中，我们将更深入地讨论神经生理学记录和运动传感器记录的方法及其优缺点。未来必须考虑如何最好地对 aDBS 进行调整，如参数调整的频率（Habets 等，2018）。

四、神经电生理学方式

（一）皮质下神经电生理学方式

神经电生理记录在 DBS 中起重要作用（见第 6 章）。神经生理信号几乎可以从神经系统的任何位置被记录到。然而到目前为止，皮质下记录只在术中分辨皮质下结构时发挥作用（Verhagen 等，2015）。事实上，从不同皮质下核团的神经电生理记录中获得的神经"信号"不仅有助于确定 DBS 的最佳植入位点，还可以作为间接量化症状严重程度的生物标志物。由于 MRI 在 DBS 电极定位方面变得越来越重要（Brodsky 等，2017），因此在不久的将来，神经电生理记录可能会根据神经电生理信号与症状的存在或严重程度的相关性在调整 DBS 靶点位置方面发挥最重要的作用。在 PD 中，最为人们所知的神经活动异常是通过局部场电位记录到的 β（13～30Hz）频段内神经元活动同步性增强。

尽管增强的 β 振荡在 DBS 领域已被激烈讨论了近 20 年（Bronte-Stewart 等，2009；Brown 等，2001；Kuhn 等，2008），但其具体来源还尚不清楚。STN β 振荡的过度同步化与对侧肢体运动迟缓和僵直的严重程度显著相关（Beudel 等，2017）。相比于运动迟缓和僵直，静止性震颤和局部场电位（local field potential，LFP）间的相关性则不那么明显，或者说更复杂。从功率谱密度来看，震颤更与低 γ（30～45Hz）（Beudel 等，2015）和高频振荡（>200Hz）（Hirschmann 等，2016）有关。最近的一项研究通过将这些功率特征用于分类器算法，使得预测 PD 静止性震颤的准确率高达 84%（Hirschmann 等，2017）。目前这些 LFP 分析还不是"实时"的，且缺乏足够的准确度。基于这些原因，目前还无法实现在嵌入式 DBS 系统中应用此类分类器算法或将其用于 aDBS。

静止性震颤的临床表现被认为是一种代偿机制，以对抗与运动迟缓和强直相关的过度 β 同步（Helmich 等，2012）。STN β 活动和皮质 -STN 耦合的降低均与静止性震颤相关（Qasim 等，2016）。此外，β 频段可能包含 2 个独立的、与临床相关的 β 频段：低 β（11～15Hz）和高 β（19～27Hz）（Blumenfeld 等，2017；Priori 等，2004）。不同的 β 频段可能具有其独特的基底节 - 皮质运动区功能连接模式（Hirschmann 等，2011；Litvak 等，2011；Oswal 等，2016）。在最近的一项研究中，60Hz 和 140Hz 的 STN 刺激可导致相似的运动迟缓改善，但高 β 活动在 2 种刺激模式下均减弱，低 β 活动仅在 140Hz 刺激时减弱，而在 60Hz 刺激时增强（Blumenfeld 等，2017）。另一项研究表明，STN 内局部高 β 振荡同步性的抑制与连续 DBS（cDBS）带来的运动改善相关（Oswal 等，2016）。他们认为高 β 和低 βSTN 振荡分别通过超直接通路和间接通路耦合到不同的皮质运动区。尽管还未达成共识，但这些发现都有助于理解 cDBS 对 β 频段的调节。

aDBS 对 STN LFP 振幅的影响也尚不清楚。Tinkhauser 等（2017）发现与 cDBS 和无 DBS 相比，aDBS 会带来持续时间更短、振幅更低的 β "爆发"，这表明 aDBS 调节 STN 神经元同步化的方式与 cDBS 不同，而这导致了更短的同步化和更低的爆发幅度。此外，Giannicola 等发现 STN DBS 并不能像左旋多巴那样可以在所有患者中降低 β 振荡。此外，DBS 诱导的 LFP 衰减只有在伴随左旋多巴诱导的 β 振荡衰减时才能检测到（Giannicola 等，2010）。

目前大多数 LFP 研究的一个重要缺陷在于它们都是在术后即刻进行的。但由于术后植入电极周围的神经组织阻抗可逆性降低，结果可能存在偏差（Lempka 等，2009）。然而，一些证据表明，DBS 对 STN βLFP 的调控在 DBS 电极植入后 2 天和 30 天没有显著差异（Rosa 等，2010），甚至在 DBS 植入 7 年后仍然能被观察到（Giannicola 等，2012）。

Rosin 等（2011）首次在非人灵长类 PD 模型中描述了 aDBS 的概念。在这项具有里程碑意义的研究中，Rosin 使用皮质脑电图（electrocorticography，ECoG）记录非洲绿猴初级运动皮质（M_1）的放电活动，并发现基于此的 GPi aDBS 能较传统的连续 DBS 更好地缓解非洲绿猴的运动迟缓症状。然而生物标志物的记录和输出有效刺激之间存在延迟。Johnson 等（2016）在恒河猴 PD 模型中使用 STN aDBS，发现其能带来显著的僵直改善，但没有带来运动迟缓的改善。因此，他们对单独使用 STN LFP-β 功率作为生物标志提出质疑。他们认为，aDBS 系统可能需要多种 PD 表型特异的生物标志，并根据患者的症状特征进行调整。值得注意的是，该实验中的一个关键细节在于他们使用提示性运动来评估运动迟缓，而这种提示性运动对帕金森病的影响小于自发运动（Nieuwboer 等，2007）。

尽管非人灵长类动物 PD 模型中的 aDBS 研究对于生物标志的报道存在争议（Johnson 等，2016；Rosin 等，2011），目前 PD 中 aDBS 的临床研究仍主要以 STN β 振荡作为输入信号。Little 等（2013）首次描述了在 PD 患者身上进行 aDBS 的研究。通过盲法评估他们发现，与随机刺激和 cDBS 相比，单侧 STN aDBS 能带来更显著的震颤、运动迟缓和僵直的改善。但值得注意的是，纳入患者均有双侧症状而 aDBS 仅被单侧实施。在后续研究中，双侧 aDBS 相对于无刺激（Little 等，2016a）能够显著改善 UPDRS 运动评分，且没有引起在 cDBS 中所观察到的刺激诱发的构音障碍（Little 等，2016b）。此外，aDBS 与多巴胺能药物能够产生协同作用（Little 等，2016a）。最后，单侧和双侧 aDBS 均较 cDBS 能耗更低。Rosa 等（2017）在长期随访中发现 aDBS 相较于 cDBS 更不易引起左旋多巴诱导的异动症，但他们的评估也仅限于随机一天的评估结果而非一段时间内的结果（Arlotti 等，2018）。

如前所述，目前大部分 aDBS 实验都是在术后急性期内进行的。然而，Piña-Fuentes 等（2017）在 1 名长期植入 aDBS 的患者中记录到运动迟缓的改善，说明 aDBS 带来的改善并非由微损毁效应引起。但是 aDBS 的长期疗效仍应该在更大的样本中被证实。Velisar 等（2019）对此进行了首次尝试，但该研究并没有对 cDBS 和 aDBS 的疗效进行正式的比较。

（二）皮质神经电生理记录

由于纹状体多巴胺去神经化可导致皮质-基底节环路抑制功能的降低和振荡活动的增强（de Hemptinne 等，2013；Hammond 等，2007；Oswal 等，2016），研究人员基于该假说探索了 PD 患者皮质神经电生理活动作为 aDBS 生物标志的可能性。但目前为止，基于皮质振荡特征的 aDBS 研究均是在非人灵长类动物上开展的（见前述）。

近期的研究显示，PD 患者 ECoG 中能够记录到 M_1 区增强的相位振幅耦合（phase-amplitude-coupling，PAC）。PAC 是神经科学许多领域中一个新兴现象（Jensen 和 Colgin，2007），它描述了一个频段的振幅如何与另一个频段的相位相关。PAC 的一个常见例子是 PD 患者运动皮质的高频振荡（high-frequency oscillations，HFO）振幅与 STN 的 β 振荡相位之间存在相关性（van Wijk 等，2016；de Hemptinne 等，2013）。此外，STN DBS 能够降低这种 β-HFO 的 PAC，并且 PAC 降低的程度与临床评估的运动迟缓的改善程度一致（de Hemptinne 等，2015）。不仅如此，M_1 中窄带的 γ 振荡（60～90 Hz）与异动症的严重程度相关（Swann 等，2016）。这些 M_1 区的 ECoG 特征在长达 12 个月的时间内保持稳定（Swann 等，2018a）。

总而言之，这些研究表明 PD 患者的 ECoG 信号也可能是 aDBS 的潜在神经生理学生物标志。但仍要注意该方法存在一些明显的缺点，包括植入额外皮质电极带来的风险，计算 PAC 所需要的计算量，以及 PAC 与临床症状学之间的关系仍有待验证等（Van Wijk 等，2016）。基于皮质记录 aDBS 的长期植入安全性及临床疗效均有待验证。近期，通过使用窄带 $M_1\gamma$ 信号设计的 aDBS 在 2 名患者中被证明是可行且可耐受的（Swann 等，2018b）。

五、外部传感器方式

可穿戴传感器（即"可穿戴设备"）通过加速计和（或）陀螺仪客观检测运动（Grimaldi 和 Manto，2010）。加速计根据牛顿第二定律（力 = 质量 × 加速度）评估一个轴上的加速度和速度。陀螺仪评估角速度，除了单一的加速计以外，还能提供更多维度的信息。生理性运动和病理性运动之间的差异可以根据运动特征进行评估，如震颤（或运动）的平均振幅、2 个振幅之间的平均规律性、平均频率及峰值频率（Jeon 等，2017）。

基于可穿戴设备在检测 PD 患者运动症状方面的潜力，越来越多的研究将其作为 PD 患者 aDBS 的输入信号（Sanchez-Ferro 等，2016）。然而，由于大量不同类别商用传感器的出现，以及许多研究人员和公司没有公开提供他们的算法，这一研究领域正逐渐趋于异质化。

就震颤而言，加速计和陀螺仪可以相对容易地记录症状是否存在，以及症状的严重程度（Basu 等，2013；Khobragade 等，2015）。由于震颤是否出现很大程度上取决于患者的状态（例如 PD 震颤多发生于静止时，而原发性震颤多发生于活动时），因此较高的采样频率是必需的（至少和震颤频率达到一个数量级）。在首个基于 PD 患者震颤幅度的 aDBS 研究中（Malekmohammadi 等，2016），蓝牙手表作为传感器通过特定的接口（Nexus-D platform，by Medtronic，Minneapolis，MN，USA）被无线连接至反应性神经刺激器上（Activa PC + S by Medtronic）。在该项纳入 5 名患者的研究中，aDBS 仅需较低的电压就能有效抑制震颤，且刺激开启的时间仅为 cDBS 的一半。

尽管目前可穿戴设备最常被用于震颤的监测，但其也能用于监测 PD 患者的冻结步态（Rodriguez-Martin 等，2017）、运动迟缓和异动（Griffiths 等，2012；Hasan 等，2017）。通过手腕加速计评估的运动迟缓和异动与 UPDRS 运动评分（运动迟缓）和异常非自主运动量表（异动症）得分显著相关（Griffiths 等，2012）。但值得注意的是，这些研究都仅在被试静息态下记录，而不是在任务态下记录。因此，将这些范式转化到更符合实际应用场景（包括不同的运动）是非常重要的。

目前为止，基于可穿戴设备的 aDBS 还存在一些局限性。第一，可穿戴设备只能监测运动症状，不能提供非运动症状或 cDBS 不良反应的信息，这些症状也显著影响患者的生活质量；第二，由于自发性运动和病理性运动之间差异的复杂性，以及许多研究人员没有公开他们使用的算法，导致传感器算法的开发、验证及再实现的进展比较缓慢；第三，用于记录、传输和处理数据的硬件还不能满足所有必要的条件，如与 IPG 的无线通信。但是最近采用蓝牙接口的（实验性）平台为未来实现这些条件提供了可能（如 Medtronic 的 Nexus-e）。采用什么设备进行数据处理、电池寿命的限制，以及所有相关设备之间能否确保连通性是该领域未来需要解决的问题。

特发性震颤

丘脑 cDBS 是一种安全有效的治疗 ET 的手段，可带来长期的震颤缓解和功能改善（Baizabal-Carvallo 等，2014；Limousin 等，1999）。目前，沿齿状核 - 红核 - 丘脑束（DRT）的多个位点被用作 cDBS 的靶点（Holslag 等，2018），其中丘脑腹侧中间核（ventral intermediate nucleus，VIM）最常被使用。然而，该疗法存在一些缺陷，主要包括经常出现的语言和平衡障碍的不良反应，以及随时间推移出现的疗效减退（Baizabal-Carvallo 等，2014；Barbe 等，2011）。

基于类似于 PD 的原因，这些缺陷使人们开始关注 ET 中的 aDBS 疗法。

六、闭环方法

与 PD 相比，ET 中 aDBS 的生物标志只反映震颤而不反映其他运动症状。正如前文中关于 PD 中 aDBS 的章节所述，我们对震颤和皮质及皮质 LFP 之间关系的认识仍然有限。因此，大多数用于 ET 的实验性 aDBS 系统采用可穿戴设备作为信号输入，一些研究额外使用表面肌电图（surface electromyography, sEMG）作为附加输入。

Graupe 等（2010）在 1 名患者中证实，交替、非连续的 DBS 放电模式能有效抑制震颤且不会导致复发。通过直接检查 DBS-OFF 期未处理的 sEMG 信号，他们可使 DBS 在震颤再次出现之前被再次启动。同一个课题组之后提出了 aDBS 系统的原理证明，该系统基于腕部加速计和 sEMG 提供的数据，通过神经网络训练的计算算法预测震颤发生，预测特异性达到 86%、敏感性达到 100%（Basu 等，2013）。基于这些数据，他们认为可以减少 30% 的刺激时间，且不用担心震颤的复发。然而，对于严重震颤及震颤潜伏期短的患者而言，这种预测可能变得更加困难。

ET 中 aDBS 的最新实验设计采用了由三轴加速计构成的可穿戴设备。Cagnan 等的结果显示，就震颤抑制而言，不仅是 DBS 的频率非常重要，DBS 脉冲发放时间（相对于震颤相位）也非常重要（Cagnan 等，2014）。他们发现 ET 中的相位依赖性刺激对震颤幅度的调节与 PD 相比有显著不同，并提出了不同的潜在神经病理生理网络机制假说。潜在的震颤细胞的共振是造成这一现象的原因。后来，他们率先在 ET 和肌张力障碍性震颤中使用了相位特异性丘脑 aDBS，并证明其可以调节震颤幅度，具体根据 DBS 脉冲发放时间相对于持续性震颤相位的关系来调节振幅。相位特异性 aDBS 在入组的 ET 和肌张力障碍性震颤患者中达到了与高频 cDBS 相当的震颤抑制，且使用的总电能不足 cDBS 的一半（Cagnan 等，2017）。这一课题组还证实类似的相位依赖性刺激可被用于无创性皮质刺激（Brittain 等，2013）。

另一个课题组在同一名 ET 患者的单一病例研究中测试了两种 aDBS 方式（Herron 等，2017）。一个 aDBS 系统是通过装有加速计和陀螺仪的智能手表测得的震颤触发的，另一个是通过患者手臂上 4 个肌电电极的记录触发的。与 cDBS 相比，这两种 aDBS 策略分别导致 36% 的额外震颤和 85% 的电池节省，以及 7% 的额外震颤和 53% 的电池节省。作者认为，在震颤的发生和刺激阈值之间存在平衡，因此在开发 ET 中 aDBS 系统时需要确定电池损耗。此外他们还提出，未来的 aDBS 设备应达到多大程度的震颤减轻才能产生吸引力可能会决定患者的个人选择。总之，在为 ET 患者开发 aDBS 系统方面已经取得了不少有前景的进展。目前，包含加速计和陀螺仪的可穿戴设备，以及可能附加的肌电电极被用作监测震颤存在或出现的输入信号。合理地说，个体患者应在将来和他们的临床医生探讨预期震颤减少量与电池消耗量和可能的不良反应之间的权衡（另见"闭环方法"部分）。

肌张力障碍与 aDBS

肌张力障碍是一种由持续或间断肌肉收缩引起的、异常的、常常表现为重复性运动的运动障碍性疾病。药物难治性的肌张力障碍可通过 DBS 治疗（见第 14 章）。目前而言，DBS 对肌张力障碍的疗效个体差异较大，且疗效很难预测，因此为该疗法设计反馈环路非常困难。如果有一种能够可靠检测症状严重程度的生物标志出现，将无疑能推动该领域的进步。在活动性肌张力障碍中可以特异性地检测到低频振荡（4～12Hz）的增加（Barow 等，2014；Piña-Fuentes 等，2019）。此外，这种低频振荡功率谱密度（power spectral density, PSD）的波动性似乎与 PD 中 β 振荡的波动性相类似（Piña-Fuentes 等，2018a，b），低频振荡的振幅与肌张力障碍的严重程度显著相关（Neumann等，2017）。因此，苍白球低频振荡可能是肌张力障碍aDBS的一个合适的生物标志。然而，迄今为止，作为原理证明，低频振荡aDBS仅在1名患者身上进行了测试（Piña-Fuentes等，2018a, b），且仅作为次要结局指标。今后的研究需要进一步探索苍白球低频振荡作为肌张力障碍患者aDBS生物标志的潜力。此外，从肌电图和皮质脑电图中提取的其他生物标志也值得被探究（Piña-Fuentes等，2018b）。

七、癫痫与aDBS

癫痫是一种慢性神经系统疾病，其特征是反复、无法预料的发作。在大多数情况下癫痫可以通过抗癫痫药物治疗。然而，对于约30%的患者而言，抗癫痫药物不能充分控制癫痫发作（Kwan等，2010）。在这其中的一些患者中，手术切除癫痫病灶成了一种治疗选择。对于手术切除效果不理想或不适合手术的患者，神经调控疗法成了另一种选择。目前，癫痫有3种神经调控疗法，包括迷走神经电刺激（vagus nerve stimulation，VNS）、丘脑前核DBS和反应性皮质/皮质下神经刺激。临床上已经将闭环形式的神经调控应用于药物难治性癫痫（另见"概述"部分）。闭环设计对于癫痫而言是一种尤其合适的刺激方式，因为癫痫是一种典型的阵发性疾病，发作只在很短的时间内发生。

闭环VNS

人们在过去的几年中一直尝试开发闭环VNS系统，尽管VNS不是DBS的一种形式，但是闭环VNS的发展也与癫痫的aDBS有关，因为同样需要用到类似的生物标志。闭环VNS的概念起源于磁激活VNS。磁激活VNS使得看护者或患者自己在癫痫发作时能开启额外的刺激。2项研究测试了磁激活VNS在癫痫治疗中的可行性和有效性。其结果显示磁激活VNS能带来额外的积极效果，但由于大多数患者自身无法在发作时开启额外刺激，磁激活VNS需要额外的护理人员参与到刺激的手动激活中（Boon等，2001；Morris 3rd，2003）。这一缺陷为探索自动闭环VNS系统及合适的生物标志物提供了灵感。

由于在超过70%的癫痫发作中能观察到心率的增加，心率变化可以作为癫痫发作的其中一个潜在生物标志（Eggleston等，2014）。几个课题组均提出并验证了基于心率的闭环系统。这些概念验证性研究表明，以心率增加为生物标志的VNS是可行的，且在治疗癫痫患者方面具有潜力（Jeppesen等，2010；Osorio，2014；Shoeb等，2009；Van Elmpt等，2006）。这些积极的结果促成了心源性闭环VNS系统的开发，即AspireSR（Cyberonics，Houston，USA）。

2015年，AspireSR获得了FDA的批准。当由脉冲发生器中的ECG传感器测量的心率在癫痫开始时或发作中超过预先指定的阈值时，AspireSR会自动释放额外的刺激。一项前瞻性多中心研究评估了AspireSR在31例癫痫患者中的表现。这项研究表明AspireSR检测到超过80%的癫痫发作伴有心率改变。在癫痫发作后立刻甚至在癫痫发作前AspireSR就能判断到来的癫痫发作。因此该研究得出结论，AspireSR及其实现的基于心率的癫痫发作检测算法能够检测出伴随心率变化的癫痫发作（Boon等，2015）。最新的基于心率的癫痫检测算法进一步扩展了这些结果，该算法显示心率变异性可用于癫痫的早期检测，并可能可以被用于癫痫发作的预测，预测敏感性高达94.1%（Pavei等，2017）。SenTiva（LivaNova，London，UK）于2017年获得FDA批准。该闭环VNS系统也对心率的变化进行反应，并同时收集和记录体位信息，因为体位信息可能也与癫痫发作有关。由于该系统最近才获得批准，其性能仍需进一步评估。尽管基于心跳的闭环VNS对捕捉癫痫发作有很好的效果，但尚不清楚该刺激模式是否优于开环VNS系统。

八、闭环反应性皮质/皮质下刺

先前的研究表明，短暂的电刺激可以在癫痫发作时通过适当的方式诱发而终止后放电，该机制类似于自发的癫痫样脑电活动（Kros 等，2015；Lesser 等，1999；Motamedi 等，2002）。这类研究为利用癫痫样脑电活动（通过硬膜下电极记录）作为生物标志的闭环反应性电刺激提供发展的基础。

2004 年，闭环反应性皮质电刺激被首次应用于癫痫（Kossoff 等，2004）。在这项试验中，4 名患者使用了外挂的皮质栅格电极来记录并自动分析神经活动。当出现癫痫发作时给予皮质刺激。他们的主要发现是，在试验期内脑电图记录到的癫痫发作被抑制、临床癫痫发作次数显著减少，且没有观察到重大不良反应事件。1 年后，8 名进行颅内监测的癫痫患者（Osorio 等，2005）接受了集成的床旁闭环反应性电刺激系统（Peters 等，2001）的评估。这是通过将脑电图仪与恒流刺激器以闭环方式连接来完成的。通过这样做，可以在临床观察到或脑电图记录到癫痫发作时提供电刺激。这种反应性电刺激算法使得 8 名患者中的 4 名癫痫发作减少了 50% 以上（Osorio 等，2005）。这些概念验证性证据表明，闭环反应性神经电刺激是可行的、有效的。

2008 年，借助完全植入性装置让 1 名患者接受了同样的闭环神经电刺激（Anderson 等，2008），该设备被称为反应性神经电刺激系统（RNS，NeuroPace，Mountain View，USA）。该系统包括 1 个植入颅骨内的神经刺激器，以及 1~2 个放置在深部和或皮质致痫区用于记录和刺激的条状电极。RNS 的安全性和有效性已在可行性研究（n=65）、随机多中心双盲对照实验（n=191）和 7 年长期随访研究（n=230）中被证实（Bergey 等，2015；Heck 等，2014；Morrell 和 RNS System in Epilepsy Study Group，2011）。首先，研究表明与假刺激组患者相比，闭环反应性皮质刺激组患者的癫痫发作显著减少（Morrell and RNS System in Epilepsy Study Group，2011）。植入 5 个月后，所有受试者均接受闭环反应性电刺激，并完成 2 年的随访。结果显示，1 年后癫痫发作次数的中位数降低了 44%，2 年后降低了高达 53%（Heck 等，2014）。7 年的随访研究表明，植入后 3 年和 6 年癫痫发作降低率分别增加了 60% 和 66%（Bergey 等，2015）。

因此，这些研究得出结论，对癫痫病灶的闭环反应性神经刺激具有良好的耐受性和可接受的安全性，并且降低了癫痫发作的频率。从那以后，RNS 被成功地植入到许多难治性癫痫患者中，不仅使用了皮质栅格电极，而且还使用了 DBS 电极（Geller 等，2017；Jobst 等，2017）。未来的研究将有必要优化刺激算法，并在癫痫患者中进行闭环反应性神经刺激和非反应性神经刺激的对比。

九、抽动秽语综合征与 aDBS

抽动秽语综合征（Tourette syndrome，TS）是一种神经精神障碍性疾病，表现为运动性抽动和发声性抽动，常伴有精神病。对大多数患者来说，药物和（或）行为疗法是有效的，但有一部分 TS 患者对这些疗法不敏感。DBS 已成为治疗严重难治性 TS 的一种成熟的疗法。越来越多的证据显示，苍白球内侧核（globus pallidus internus，GPi）和丘脑中央中核－束旁核复合体 DBS 能为 TS 患者带来显著的抽动改善（Dowd 等，2017；Kefalopoulou 等，2015；Servello 等，2016）。尽管丘脑 DBS 在 TS 中的短期疗效比较显著，但在 12~78 个月后，丘脑 DBS 的不良反应（如乏力、视觉障碍或记忆问题）逐渐遮盖了其治疗作用（Smeets 等，2018）。由于 TS 是一种发作性疾病，抽动仅在很少的时间内发生，因此 aDBS 也可应用于抽动抑制效果较好、刺激相关不良反应较少的 TS 患者。

最近的研究表明，在 GPi、GPe 及丘脑中记录到的神经电生理信号（如 LFP）在抽动时具有特定的放电模式（Bour 等，2015；Israelashvili 等，2017；Jimenez-Shahed 等，2016；Maling 等，

2012）。有研究发现抽动与 GPi 中高频振荡和 γ 带活动的增加相关（Jimenez-Shahed 等，2016），且抽动前会出现反复的丘脑 – 皮质同步放电（Bour 等，2015）。此外，DBS 治疗后丘脑 γ 带活动的增强与抽动改善的程度显著相关（Maling 等，2012），且在单个 GP 神经元内能够观察到与抽动相关的瞬时频率的变化（Israelashvili 等，2017）。除了这些抽动特异性的神经生理学特征外，还可以从 DBS 电极记录和分析 LFP。因此，LFP 可能有助于识别抽动发作，而基于 LFP 的 aDBS 系统可能可以在 TS 中发挥作用。

Shute 等（2016）使用长期植入的丘脑和硬膜下皮质电极来识别抽动的神经生理学特征，并将其用于开发抽动检测器。该研究还检验了抽动相关神经生理特征的一致性和可重复性。在 2 名 TS 患者中，通过丘脑 – 皮质低频（1～10Hz）相干的增强检测到抽动。在 6 个月的随访期内，识别持续复杂性抽动的平均敏感性为 88.6%，特异性为 96.3%。如前所述，本研究除使用 DBS 电极外还使用了硬膜下皮质电极来优化抽动监测。但缺点是该监测方法需要额外的植入设备。Marceglia 等在自己和既往对抽动发作时丘脑 LFP 特征研究的基础上，提出了一种识别抽动的 aDBS 系统。他们认为每个患者都有其最优的 DBS 刺激参数。如果丘脑 α 频段（8～12Hz）能量下降至少 20%，且 α 频段及低频振荡（2～7Hz）能量在 α 频段能量最初下降后的 250ms 内随后增加 150%，则提示应调整 DBS 参数。而当低频振荡能量下降超过峰值能量的 50% 时，aDBS 系统应再次将参数更改为基线状态时的设置（Marceglia 等，2017）。

虽然用于 TS 的 aDBS 系统较早就被提出，但目前为止仅有 1 项 aDBS 的概念验证性研究在 TS 患者中被开展（Molina 等，2018），该研究纳入了 1 名 TS 患者，对其进行了长期 aDBS 的观察，双侧 DBS 植入于丘脑中央中核 – 束旁核复合体。DBS 的植入设备是 RNS，其最初设计用于治疗癫痫（见"神经生理学方式"一节）。通过个体化的抽动识别检测器监测抽动。本例患者抽动时可见 5～15Hz 功率谱密度的提高。该研究的主要发现是，aDBS 是安全、可耐受的，能带来与传统 DBS 无差异的抽动改善，同时增加 36% 的预期电池寿命（Molina 等，2018）。

综上所述，TS 中的 aDBS 仍处于研发阶段。这也是因为 TS 的 cDBS 还尚未十分成熟。研究者应开展更大规模、随机和双盲随访的研究，并尝试其他可能有效的 DBS 靶点如 GPi，同时监测 aDBS 对刺激相关不良反应及精神并发症的影响。

十、强迫症

强迫症（obsessive compulsive disorder, OCD）是一种神经精神障碍性疾病，其特征表现为重复出现的、无法控制的强迫想法和（或）强迫行为。腹侧纹状体/腹侧内囊 DBS 可用于治疗严重的慢性药物难治性 OCD（Provenza 等，2019）。强迫症或许是 aDBS 的潜在适应证，因为其在刺激不足（可能导致 OCD 症状改善不佳）和过度刺激（可能导致躁狂症）之间存在微妙的平衡（Widge 等，2016）。DBS 对伏隔核异常活动的校正作用可能能作为 aDBS 的一个生物标志（Figee 等，2013）。然而，OCD 的异质性特征，以及其数天、数周或数月的动态变化状态使得寻找适合的 aDBS 输入信号非常困难。心理学监测或电生理可能是首先需要研究的方向。

十一、未来的发展方向

目前，aDBS 仅在癫痫患者中得到临床应用。尽管越来越多的证据表明 aDBS 也能够被用于运动障碍性疾病（Meidahl 等，2017）和神经精神性疾病（Marceglia 等，2017），其真实价值仍有待于在临床和实际应用中被证实，包括其对非运动症状方面的影响。但这主要取决于具有闭环特性的 DBS 硬件的开发。现有的 aDBS 系统主要是将 DBS 电极与体外的具有闭环特征的 IPG 相连接（Malekmohammadi 等，2016），下一步我们应开发并检验一体化植入的具有闭环特征的 IPG 系统。这可以是装载了 LFP/ECoG 计算分析功能的系统，可以是能够无线接收加速计或（表面）肌电信号的设备，也可以是在 IPG 中直接嵌入加速计或陀螺仪的系统。能耗是此类硬件开发的关键限制，其开发还受到采样率的影响。目前大部分 aDBS 中的采样率较高（>100 个采样点/秒）。由于 PD 的 LFP 存在波动性大和爆发放电等特征，因此对于 PD 中"基于爆发放电（burst-based）"的 aDBS，高（且连续）的采样率是必需的。然而，还需要探索其他策略（例如每半小时短暂地检测一次 β 能量）是否同样有益处。总之，闭环特性与其他新兴刺激模式的整合，如"协同复位"（Adamchic 等，2014），以及发展更精细、同步化更高的自适应调节模式必将改变 aDBS 的未来。

参考文献

[1] Adamchic I, Hauptmann C, Barnikol UB, et al. Coordinated reset neuromodulation for Parkinson's disease: proof-of- concept study. Mov Disord. 2014;29(13):1679–84.

[2] Anderson WS, Kossoff EH, Bergey GK, Jallo GI. Implantation of a responsive neurostimulator device in patients with refractory epilepsy. Neurosurg Focus. 2008;25(3):E12.

[3] Arlotti M, Marceglia S, Foffani G, Volkmann J, Lozano AM, Moro E, et al. Eight-hours adaptive deep brain stimulation in patients with Parkinson disease. Neurology. 2018;90:e971–6.

[4] Baizabal-Carvallo JF, Kagnoff MN, Jimenez-Shahed J, et al. The safety and efficacy of thalamic deep brain stimulation in essential tremor: 10 years and beyond. J Neurol Neurosurg Psychiatry. 2014;85(5):567–72.

[5] Barbe MT, Liebhart L, Runge M, et al. Deep brain stimulation in the nucleus ventralis intermedius in patients with essential tremor: habituation of tremor suppression. J Neurol. 2011;258(3):434–9.

[6] Barow E, Neumann W-J, Brücke C, Huebl J, Horn A, Brown P, et al. Deep brain stimulation suppresses pallidal low frequency activity in patients with phasic dystonic movements. Brain. 2014;137:3012–24.

[7] Basu I, Graupe D, Tuninetti D, et al. Pathological tremor prediction using surface electromyogram and acceleration: potential use in 'ON-OFF' demand driven deep brain stimulator design. J Neural Eng. 2013;10(3):036019.

[8] Bergey GK, Morrell MJ, Mizrahi EM, et al. Long-term treatment with responsive brain stimulation in adults with refractory partial seizures. Neurology. 2015;84(8):810–7.

[9] Beudel M, Little S, Pogosyan A, et al. Tremor reduction by deep brain stimulation is associated with gamma power suppression in Parkinson's disease. Neuromodulation. 2015;18(5):349–54.

[10] Beudel M, Oswal A, Jha A, et al. Oscillatory beta power correlates with Akinesia-rigidity in the Parkinsonian subthalamic nucleus. Mov Disord. 2017;32(1):174–5.

[11] Blumenfeld Z, Koop MM, Prieto TE, et al. Sixty-hertz stimulation improves bradykinesia and amplifies subthalamic low-frequency oscillations. Mov Disord. 2017;32(1):80–8.

[12] Bogdan DI, van Laar T, Oterdoom DLM, Drost G, van Dijk JMC, Beudel M. Optimal parameters of deep brain stimulation in essential tremor: a meta-analysis and novel programming strategy. Abstract # 1395, Movement disorders conference. 2019.

[13] Boon P, Vonck K, Van Walleghem P, et al. Programmed and magnet-induced vagus nerve stimulation for refractory epilepsy. J Clin Neurophysiol. 2001;18(5):402–7.

[14] Boon P, Vonck K, van Rijckevorsel K, et al. A prospective, multicenter study of cardiac-based seizure detection to activate vagus nerve stimulation. Seizure. 2015;32:52–61.

[15] Bour LJ, Ackermans L, Foncke EM, et al. Tic related local field potentials in the thalamus and the effect of deep brain stimulation in Tourette syndrome: report of three cases. Clin Neurophysiol. 2015;126(8):1578–88.

[16] Brittain JS, Probert-Smith P, Aziz TZ, Brown P. Tremor suppression by rhythmic transcranial current stimulation. Curr Biol. 2013;23(5):436–40.

[17] Brodsky MA, Anderson S, Murchison C, et al. Clinical outcomes of asleep vs awake deep brain stimulation for Parkinson disease. Neurology. 2017;89(19):1944–50.

[18] Bronte-Stewart H, Barberini C, Koop MM, et al. The STN beta-band profile in Parkinson's disease is stationary and shows prolonged attenuation after deep brain stimulation. Exp Neurol. 2009;215(1):20–8.

[19] Brown P, Oliviero A, Mazzone P, et al. Dopamine dependency of oscillations between subthalamic nucleus and pallidum in Parkinson's disease. J Neurosci. 2001;21(3):1033–8.

[20] Cagnan H, Little S, Foltynie T, et al. The nature of tremor circuits in parkinsonian and essential tremor. Brain. 2014;137(Pt 12):3223–34.

[21] Cagnan H, Pedrosa D, Little S, et al. Stimulating at the right time: phase-specific deep brain stimulation. Brain. 2017;140(1):132–45.

[22] Chen CC, Brucke C, Kempf F, et al. Deep brain stimulation of the subthalamic nucleus: a two-edged sword. Curr Biol. 2006;16(22):R952–3.

[23] de Hemptinne C, Ryapolova-Webb ES, Air EL, et al. Exaggerated phase-amplitude coupling in the primary motor cortex in Parkinson disease. Proc Natl Acad Sci U S A. 2013;110(12):4780–5.

[24] de Hemptinne C, Swann NC, Ostrem JL, et al. Therapeutic deep brain stimulation reduces cortical phase-amplitude coupling in Parkinson's disease. Nat Neurosci. 2015;18(5):779–86.

[25] Delgado JM, Delgado-García JM, Grau C. Mobility controlled by feedback cerebral stimulation in monkeys. Physiol Behav. 1976;16:43–9.

[26] Dowd RS, Pourfar M, Mogilner AY. Deep brain stimulation for Tourette syndrome: a single-center series. J Neurosurg. 2017:1–9.

[27] Eggleston KS, Olin BD, Fisher RS. Ictal tachycardia: the head-heart connection. Seizure. 2014;23(7):496–505.

[28] Fasano A, Lozano AM. The FM/AM world is shaping the future of deep brain stimulation. Mov Disord. 2014;29(2):161–3.

[29] Figee M, Luigjes J, Smolders R, et al. Deep brain stimulation restores frontostriatal network activity in obsessive-compulsive disorder. Nat Neurosci. 2013;16:386–7.

[30] Geller EB, Skarpaas TL, Gross RE, et al. Brain-responsive neurostimulation in patients with medically intractable mesial temporal lobe epilepsy. Epilepsia. 2017;58(6):994–1004.

[31] Giannicola G, Marceglia S, Rossi L, et al. The effects of levodopa and ongoing deep brain stimulation on subthalamic beta oscillations in Parkinson's disease. Exp Neurol. 2010;226(1):120–7.

[32] Giannicola G, Rosa M, Servello D, et al. Subthalamic local field potentials after seven-year deep brain stimulation in Parkinson's disease. Exp Neurol. 2012;237(2):312–7.

[33] Graupe D, Basu I, Tuninetti D, et al. Adaptively controlling deep brain stimulation in essential tremor patient via surface electromyography. Neurol Res. 2010;32(9):899–904.

[34] Graupe D, Tuninetti D, Slavin KV, Basu I. Closed-loop electrochemical feedback system for DBS. J Neurosurg. 2014;121(3):762–3.

[35] Griffiths RI, Kotschet K, Arfon S, et al. Automated assessment of bradykinesia and dyskinesia in Parkinson's disease. J Parkinsons Dis. 2012;2(1):47–55.

[36] Grimaldi G, Manto M. Neurological tremor: sensors, signal processing and emerging applications. Sensors (Basel). 2010;10(2):1399–422.
[37] Habets JG, Heijmans M, Kuijf ML, et al. An update on adaptive deep brain stimulation in Parkinson's disease. Mov Disord. 2018;33(12):1834–43.
[38] Hammond C, Bergman H, Brown P. Pathological synchronization in Parkinson's disease: networks, models and treatments. Trends Neurosci. 2007;30(7):357–64.
[39] Hasan H, Athauda DS, Foltynie T, Noyce AJ. Technologies assessing limb bradykinesia in Parkinson's disease. J Parkinsons Dis. 2017;7(1):65–77.
[40] Hauser RA, McDermott MP, Messing S. Factors associated with the development of motor fluctuations and dyskinesias in Parkinson disease. Arch Neurol. 2006;63(12):1756–60.
[41] Heck CN, King-Stephens D, Massey AD, et al. Two-year seizure reduction in adults with medically intractable partial onset epilepsy treated with responsive neurostimulation: final results of the RNS system pivotal trial. Epilepsia. 2014;55(3):432–41.
[42] Helmich RC, Hallett M, Deuschl G, et al. Cerebral causes and consequences of parkinsonian resting tremor: a tale of two circuits? Brain. 2012;135(Pt 11):3206–26.
[43] Herron JA, Thompson MC, Brown T, et al. Chronic electrocorticography for sensing movement intention and closed-loop deep brain stimulation with wearable sensors in an essential tremor patient. J Neurosurg. 2017;127(3):580–7.
[44] Hirschmann J, Ozkurt TE, Butz M, et al. Distinct oscillatory STN-cortical loops revealed by simultaneous MEG and local field potential recordings in patients with Parkinson's disease. Neuroimage. 2011;55(3):1159–68.
[45] Hirschmann J, Butz M, Hartmann CJ, et al. Parkinsonian rest tremor is associated with modulations of subthalamic high-frequency oscillations. Mov Disord. 2016;31(10):1551–9.
[46] Hirschmann J, Schoffelen JM, Schnitzler A, van Gerven MAJ. Parkinsonian rest tremor can be detected accurately based on neuronal oscillations recorded from the subthalamic nucleus. Clin Neurophysiol. 2017;128(10):2029–36.
[47] Holslag JAH, Neef N, Beudel M, et al. Deep brain stimulation for essential tremor: a comparison of targets. World Neurosurg. 2018;110:e580–4.
[48] Horgan J. The Forgotten Era of Brain Chips. Scientific American. 2005;293(4):66–73.
[49] Horn A, Reich M, Vorwerk J, et al. Connectivity predicts deep brain stimulation outcome in Parkinson disease. Ann Neurol. 2017;82(1):67–78.
[50] Israelashvili M, Smeets AY, Bronfeld M, et al. Tonic and phasic changes in anteromedial globus pallidus activity in Tourette syndrome. Mov Disord. 2017;32(7):1091–6.
[51] Jensen O, Colgin LL. Cross-frequency coupling between neuronal oscillations. Trends Cogn Sci. 2007;11(7):267–9.
[52] Jeon H, Lee W, Park H, et al. Automatic classification of tremor severity in Parkinson's disease using a wearable device. Sensors (Basel). 2017;17(9)
[53] Jeppesen J, Beniczky S, Fuglsang-Frederiksen A, et al. Detection of epileptic-seizures by means of power spectrum analysis of heart rate variability: a pilot study. Technol Health Care. 2010;18(6):417–26.
[54] Jimenez-Shahed J, Telkes I, Viswanathan A, Ince NF. GPi oscillatory activity differentiates tics from the resting state, voluntary movements, and the unmedicated parkinsonian state. Front Neurosci. 2016;10:436.
[55] Jobst BC, Kapur R, Barkley GL, et al. Brain-responsive neurostimulation in patients with medically intractable seizures arising from eloquent and other neocortical areas. Epilepsia. 2017;58(6):1005–14.
[56] Johnson LA, Nebeck SD, Muralidharan A, et al. Closed-loop deep brain stimulation effects on parkinsonian motor symptoms in a non-human primate—is beta enough? Brain Stimul. 2016;9(6):892–6.
[57] Kefalopoulou Z, Zrinzo L, Jahanshahi M, et al. Bilateral globus pallidus stimulation for severe Tourette's syn-drome: a double-blind, randomised crossover trial. Lancet Neurol. 2015;14(6):595–605.
[58] Khobragade N, Graupe D, Tuninetti D. Towards fully automated closed-loop deep brain stimulation in Parkinson's disease patients: a LAMSTAR-based tremor predictor. Conf Proc IEEE Eng Med Biol Soc. 2015;2015:2616–9.
[59] Kossoff EH, Ritzl EK, Politsky JM, et al. Effect of an external responsive neurostimulator on seizures and electrographic discharges during subdural electrode monitoring. Epilepsia. 2004;45(12):1560–7.
[60] Kros L, Rooda OH, De Zeeuw CI, Hoebeek FE. Controlling cerebellar output to treat refractory epilepsy. Trends Neurosci. 2015;38(12):787–99.
[61] Kuhn AA, Kempf F, Brucke C, et al. High-frequency stimulation of the subthalamic nucleus suppresses oscillatory beta activity in patients with Parkinson's disease in parallel with improvement in motor performance. J Neurosci. 2008;28(24):6165–73.
[62] Kwan P, Arzimanoglou A, Berg AT, et al. Definition of drug resistant epilepsy: consensus proposal by the ad hoc task force of the ILAE commission on therapeutic strategies. Epilepsia. 2010;51(6):1069–77.
[63] Lee KH, Lujan JL, Trevathan JK, et al. WINCS harmoni: closed-loop dynamic neurochemical control of therapeutic interventions. Sci Rep. 2017;7:46675.
[64] Lempka SF, Miocinovic S, Johnson MD, et al. In vivo impedance spectroscopy of deep brain stimulation electrodes. J Neural Eng. 2009;6(4):046001.
[65] Lesser RP, Kim SH, Beyderman L, et al. Brief bursts of pulse stimulation terminate afterdischarges caused by cortical stimulation. Neurology. 1999;53(9):2073–81.
[66] Limousin P, Speelman JD, Gielen F, Janssens M. Multicentre European study of thalamic stimulation in parkinsonian and essential tremor. J Neurol Neurosurg Psychiatry. 1999;66(3):289–96.
[67] Little S, Pogosyan A, Neal S, et al. Adaptive deep brain stimulation in advanced Parkinson disease. Ann Neurol. 2013;74(3):449–57.
[68] Little S, Beudel M, Zrinzo L, et al. Bilateral adaptive deep brain stimulation is effective in Parkinson's disease. J Neurol Neurosurg Psychiatry. 2016a;87(7):717–21.
[69] Little S, Tripoliti E, Beudel M, et al. Adaptive deep brain stimulation for Parkinson's disease demonstrates reduced speech side effects compared to conventional stimulation in the acute setting. J Neurol Neurosurg Psychiatry. 2016b;87(12):1388–9.
[70] Litvak V, Jha A, Eusebio A, et al. Resting oscillatory cortico-subthalamic connectivity in patients with Parkinson's disease. Brain. 2011;134(Pt 2):359–74.
[71] Malekmohammadi M, Herron J, Velisar A, et al. Kinematic adaptive deep brain stimulation for resting tremor in Parkinson's disease. Mov Disord. 2016;31(3):426–8.
[72] Maling N, Hashemiyoon R, Foote KD, et al. Increased thalamic gamma band activity correlates with symptom relief following deep brain stimulation in humans with Tourette's syndrome. PLoS One. 2012;7(9):e44215.
[73] Marceglia S, Rosa M, Servello D, et al. Adaptive deep brain stimulation (aDBS) for Tourette syndrome. Brain Sci. 2017;8(1)
[74] Martinez-Fernandez R, Pelissier P, Quesada JL, et al. Postoperative apathy can neutralise benefits in quality of life after subthalamic stimulation for Parkinson's disease. J Neurol Neurosurg Psychiatry. 2016;87(3):311–8.
[75] Maxwell JC. I. On governors. Proc R Soc Lond. 1868;(16):270–283.
[76] Meidahl AC, Tinkhauser G, Herz DM, et al. Adaptive deep brain stimulation for movement disorders: the long road to clinical therapy. Mov Disord. 2017;32(6):810–9.
[77] Mirowski M, Reid PR, Mower MM, et al. Termination of malignant ventricular arrhythmias with an implanted automatic defibrillator in human beings. N Engl J Med. 1980;303(6):322–4.
[78] Molina R, Okun MS, Shute JB, et al. Report of a patient undergoing chronic responsive deep brain stimulation for Tourette syndrome: proof of concept. J Neurosurg. 2018;129(2):308–14.
[79] Moro E, Poon YY, Lozano AM, et al. Subthalamic nucleus stimulation: improvements in outcome with reprogramming. Arch Neurol. 2006;63(9):1266–72.
[80] Morrell MJ, RNS System in Epilepsy Study Group. Responsive cortical stimulation for the treatment of medically intractable

partial epilepsy. Neurology. 2011;77(13):1295–304.
[81] Morris GL 3rd. A retrospective analysis of the effects of magnet-activated stimulation in conjunction with vagus nerve stimulation therapy. Epilepsy Behav. 2003;4(6):740–5.
[82] Motamedi GK, Lesser RP, Miglioretti DL, et al. Optimizing parameters for terminating cortical afterdischarges with pulse stimulation. Epilepsia. 2002;43(8):836–46.
[83] Neumann W-J, Horn A, Ewert S, Huebl J, Brücke C, Slentz C, et al. A localized pallidal physiomarker in cervical dystonia. Ann Neurol. 2017;82:912–24.
[84] Nieuwboer A, Kwakkel G, Rochester L, Jones D, van Wegen E, Willems AM, et al. Cueing training in the home improves gait-related mobility in Parkinson's disease: the RESCUE trial. J Neurol Neurosurg Psychiatry. 2007;78:134–40.
[85] Osorio I. Automated seizure detection using EKG. Int J Neural Syst. 2014;24(2):1450001.
[86] Osorio I, Frei MG, Sunderam S, et al. Automated seizure abatement in humans using electrical stimulation. Ann Neurol. 2005;57(2):258–68.
[87] Oswal A, Beudel M, Zrinzo L, et al. Deep brain stimulation modulates synchrony within spatially and spectrally distinct resting state networks in Parkinson's disease. Brain. 2016;139(Pt 5):1482–96.
[88] Pavei J, Heinzen RG, Novakova B, et al. Early seizure detection based on cardiac autonomic regulation dynamics. Front Physiol. 2017;8:765.
[89] Peters TE, Bhavaraju NC, Frei MG, Osorio I. Network system for automated seizure detection and contingent delivery of therapy. J Clin Neurophysiol. 2001;18(6):545–9.
[90] Piña-Fuentes D, Little S, Oterdoom M, et al. Adaptive DBS in a Parkinson's patient with chronically implanted DBS: a proof of principle. Mov Disord. 2017;32(8):1253–4.
[91] Piña-Fuentes D, van Zijl JC, van Dijk JMC, Little S, Tinkhauser G, Oterdoom DLM, et al. The characteristics of pallidal low-frequency and beta bursts could help implementing adaptive brain stimulation in the parkinsonian and dystonic internal globus pallidus. Neurobiol Dis. 2018a;121:47–57.
[92] Piña-Fuentes D, Beudel M, Little S, van Zijl J, Elting JW, Oterdoom DLM, et al. Toward adaptive deep brain stimulation for dystonia. Neurosurg Focus. 2018b;45:E3–8.
[93] Piña-Fuentes D, van Dijk JMC, Drost G, van Zijl JC, van Laar T, Tijssen MAJ, et al. Direct comparison of oscillatory activity in the motor system of Parkinson's disease and dystonia: a review of the literature and meta-analysis. Clin Neurophysiol. 2019;130:917–24.
[94] Popovych OV, Lysyansky B, Tass PA. Closed-loop deep brain stimulation by pulsatile delayed feedback with increased gap between pulse phases. Sci Rep. 2017;7(1):1033.
[95] Priori A, Foffani G, Pesenti A, et al. Rhythm-specific pharmacological modulation of subthalamic activity in Parkinson's disease. Exp Neurol. 2004;189(2):369–79.
[96] Provenza NR, Matteson ER, Allawala AB, et al. The case for adaptive neuromodulation to treat severe intractable mental disorders. Front Neurosci. 2019;13:152.
[97] Qasim SE, de Hemptinne C, Swann NC, et al. Electrocorticography reveals beta desynchronization in the basal ganglia-cortical loop during rest tremor in Parkinson's disease. Neurobiol Dis. 2016;86:177–86.
[98] Rodriguez-Martin D, Sama A, Perez-Lopez C, et al. Home detection of freezing of gait using support vector machines through a single waist-worn triaxial accelerometer. PLoS One. 2017;12(2):e0171764.
[99] Rosa M, Marceglia S, Servello D, et al. Time dependent subthalamic local field potential changes after DBS surgery in Parkinson's disease. Exp Neurol. 2010;222(2):184–90.
[100] Rosa M, Arlotti M, Marceglia S, et al. Adaptive deep brain stimulation controls levodopa-induced side effects in Parkinsonian patients. Mov Disord. 2017;32(4):628–9.
[101] Rosin B, Slovik M, Mitelman R, et al. Closed-loop deep brain stimulation is superior in ameliorating parkinsonism. Neuron. 2011;72(2):370–84.
[102] Sanchez-Ferro A, Elshehabi M, Godinho C, et al. New methods for the assessment of Parkinson's disease (2005 to 2015): a systematic review. Mov Disord. 2016;31(9):1283–92.
[103] Servello D, Zekaj E, Saleh C, et al. Sixteen years of deep brain stimulation in Tourette's syndrome: a critical review. J Neurosurg Sci. 2016;60(2):218–29.
[104] Shoeb A, Pang T, Guttag J, Schachter S. Non-invasive computerized system for automatically initiating vagus nerve stimulation following patient-specific detection of seizures or epileptiform discharges. Int J Neural Syst. 2009;19(3):157–72.
[105] Shute JB, Okun MS, Opri E, et al. Thalamocortical network activity enables chronic tic detection in humans with Tourette syndrome. Neuroimage Clin. 2016;12:165–72.
[106] Smeets AY, Duits AA, Leentjens AF, et al. Thalamic deep brain stimulation for refractory Tourette syndrome: clinical evidence for increasing disbalance of therapeutic effects and side effects at long-term follow-up. Neuromodulation. 2018;21(2):197–202.
[107] Swann NC, de Hemptinne C, Miocinovic S, et al. Gamma oscillations in the hyperkinetic state detected with chronic human brain recordings in Parkinson's disease. J Neurosci. 2016;36(24):6445–58.
[108] Swann NC, de Hemptinne C, Miocinovic S, et al. Chronic multisite brain recordings from a totally implantable bidirectional neural interface: experience in 5 patients with Parkinson's disease. J Neurosurg. 2018a;128(2):605–16.
[109] Swann NC, de Hemptinne C, Thompson MC, Miocinovic S, Miller AM, Gilron R, et al. Adaptive deep brain stimulation for Parkinson's disease using motor cortex sensing. J Neural Eng. 2018b;15(4):046006.
[110] Tinkhauser G, Pogosyan A, Little S, et al. The modulatory effect of adaptive deep brain stimulation on beta bursts in Parkinson's disease. Brain. 2017;140(4):1053–67.
[111] van Elmpt WJ, Nijsen TM, Griep PA, Arends JB. A model of heart rate changes to detect seizures in severe epilepsy. Seizure. 2006;15(6):366–75.
[112] van Wijk BC, Beudel M, Jha A, et al. Subthalamic nucleus phase-amplitude coupling correlates with motor impairment in Parkinson's disease. Clin Neurophysiol. 2016;127(4):2010–9.
[113] Velisar A, Syrkin-Nikolau J, Blumenfeld Z, Trager MH, Afzal MF, Prabhakar V, et al. Dual threshold neural closed loop deep brain stimulation in Parkinson disease patients. Brain Stimul. 2019;12:868.
[114] Verhagen R, Zwartjes DG, Heida T, et al. Advanced target identification in STN-DBS with beta power of combined local field potentials and spiking activity. J Neurosci Methods. 2015;253:116–25.
[115] Widge AS, Licon E, Zorowitz S, et al. Predictors of hypomania during ventral capsule/ventral striatum deep brain stimulation. J Neuropsychiatry Clin Neurosci. 2016;28(1):38–44.

第6章 基底节的神经生理学与脑深部电刺激
Neurophysiology of the Basal Ganglia and Deep Brain Stimulation

Boran Urfalı　Yasin Temel　Hagai Bergman　著
刘钰晔　王 秀　译　韩春雷　杨岸超　张建国　校

摘要：我们对基底节生理学和脑深部电刺激（DBS）的理解，来源于数十年来对实验动物模型和患者基底节的研究。

经典的基底节模型描述了连接皮质与纹状体，以及基底节输出结构的直接、间接和超直接通路。基底节的输出核团调节运动皮质的兴奋性。在帕金森病中，多巴胺耗竭会导致运动皮质兴奋性降低和运动迟缓。该模型预测多巴胺耗竭后底丘脑核（STN）活动增加，提示 DBS 的治疗机制可能是通过恢复 STN 正常的放电模式来实现。

较新的基底节计算模型将它们描绘成一个执行/评价（actor/critic）强化学习网络。actor 即基底节的主轴，负责连接编码实时状态的所有皮质区域和大脑运动中枢。critic，或称为教师，即中脑多巴胺能神经元，负责对预测与现实不匹配的信息进行编码。在该模型中，多巴胺的主要作用是调节皮质-纹状体间的突触连接效力。皮质-纹状体突触连接效力决定了行为策略，即状态与动作的耦合。

最近新基底节计算模型结合了经典的直接/间接通路和现代强化学习模型的主要特点。基底节 critics（神经递质，包括投射至纹状体的多巴胺能、胆碱能、5-羟色胺能和组胺能神经递质）可以调节纹状体神经元和皮质-纹状体突触连接效力。该模型进一步表明，基底节网络是编码状态和动作的大脑结构之间的默认连接。

基底节神经递质的变性或异常活动可导致基底节主轴神经元的活动异常。由于基底节网络是状态和动作之间的默认连接，其他神经网络（如皮质-皮质网络）不能代偿基底节的异常活动。因此，基底节相关神经和精神疾病的治疗可以通过抑制基底节主轴来实现。通过损毁或 DBS 调控，使基底节网络的功能失活（信息损伤），然后功能被其他神经元网络代偿，从而恢复正常的行为。

一、概述

本章以帕金森病（Parkinson disease, PD）为例说明基底节的神经生理学。PD 是最常见的基底节疾病，而且目前对 PD 动物模型有着深入的研究。如今 DBS 术中电生理监测导航定位刺激靶点的过程也为我们提供更多的基底节生理信息。

二、基底节的神经生理模型

（一）经典的直接或间接 D_1/D_2 基底节网络模型

如今，多数神经病学教科书认为基底节是大脑闭环连接的一部分，其通过直接和间接通路连接运动皮质和其他所有皮质（Albin 等，1989；Bergman 等，1990）。运动皮质通过皮质-脊髓（或锥体）通路投射到脊髓水平，控制肌肉的激活和运动（图 6-1）。

该基底节模型强调了两条分离的通路结构。两条通路起始于纹状体的投射神经元 [中型多棘神经元（medium spiny neurons，MSN）]，汇聚于基底节的输出结构苍白球内侧部（internal segment of the globus pallidus，GPi）和黑质网状部（substantia nigra pars reticulata，SNr）。纹状体投射神经元表达两种类型的 G 蛋白偶联的多巴胺受体。"直接通路"始于表达多巴胺 D_1 受体的 MSN，并（直接）通过单突触 GABA 抑制 GPi/SNr。起始于 D_2 受体 MSN 的"间接通路"投射是多突触和去抑制性的，通过苍白球外侧部（external globus pallidus，GPe）和底丘脑核（STN）谷氨酸能神经元兴奋 GPi/SNr。多巴胺对这两条基底节通路有不同的作用。多巴胺可以兴奋 D_1-MSN，促进直接途径的传递，抑制 D_2-MSN，阻碍间接途径的传递。

这一经典的直接/间接 D_1/D_2 基底节模型改变了临床生理学和神经科学的历史。它为 MPTP 处理的 PD 猴模型的生理研究提供了一个总体框架（图 6-2）。研究报告指出，在多巴胺耗竭后，GPe 神经元的平均放电频率降低。另一方面，有报告称 GPi（Miller 和 DeLong，1987；Filion 和 Tremblay，1991）和 STN（Bergman 等，1994）的放电频率增加。灵长类动物模型（Filion 等，1991；Papa 等，1999；Heimer 等，2006）和患者（Hutchinson 等，1997；Merello 等，1999；Lee 等，2007）接受多巴胺替代疗法后，苍白球放电频率均有逆转趋势。

经典的 D_1/D_2 直接/间接模型也可以解释多巴胺替代治疗 PD 的生理机制。多巴胺前体和突触后激动药可以使纹状体恢复正常的多巴胺基础水平，从而提高运动皮质的兴奋性水平，改善帕金森病的运动障碍。同样，通过其他方法使 STN 和 GPi 失活也可以减少基底节对运动相关丘脑皮质网络的抑制性输出的过度激活，例如 γ-氨基丁酸（gamma aminobutyric acid，GABA）激动药（Wichmann 等，1994）、损毁（Bergman 等，1990；Wichmann 等，1994）或 DBS（基于 DBS 模拟失活假说，见后述）。

最近的解剖学研究表明，基底节之间的连接比经典的直接或间接 D_1/D_2 模型所描述的要复杂得多。图 6-2 描绘了我们当前的基底节网络模型（Deffains 等，2016）。此外，方框和箭模型（图 6-1 和图 6-2）在解释基底节活动和 PD 的动态模式方面存在不足。研究通过记录 MPTP 干预猴模

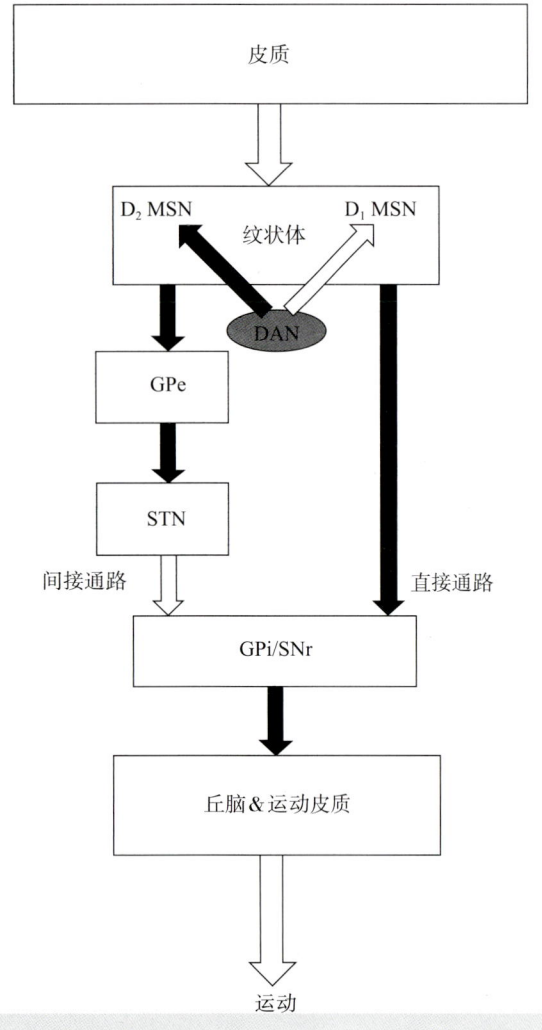

▲ 图 6-1　经典的直接/间接 D_1/D_2 基底节模型
白箭代表兴奋作用，即谷氨酸能、多巴胺能影响 D_1-MSN 连接；黑箭代表抑制作用，即 GABA 能、多巴胺能影响 D_2-MSN 连接
DAN. 中脑多巴胺能神经元；GPe. 苍白球外侧部；GPi. 苍白球内侧部；MSN. 纹状体中型多棘（投射）神经元；SNr. 黑质网状部；STN. 底丘脑核

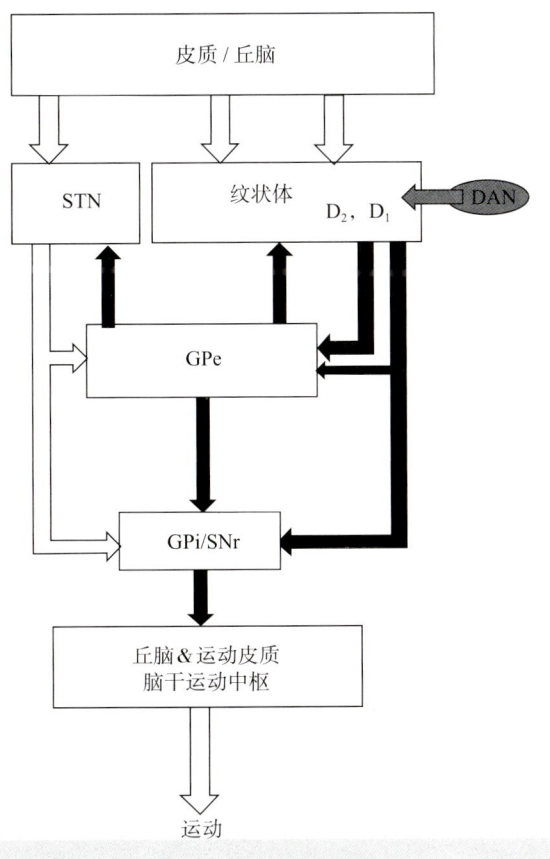

▲ 图 6-2 最新的基底节模型

白箭和黑箭分别代表兴奋性（谷氨酸）、抑制性（GABA）和多巴胺能（作用方式取决于突触后多巴胺受体）连接

DAN. 中脑多巴胺能神经元；GPe. 苍白球外侧部；GPi. 苍白球内侧部；D_1、D_2. 纹状体中型多棘（投射）神经元；SNr. 黑质网状部；STN. 底丘脑核

型（Miller 和 DeLong，1987；Filion 和 Tremblay，1991；Bergman 等，1994）和接受 DBS 手术的 PD 患者（Levy 等，2002a，b；Weinberger 等，2009；Zaidel 等，2010）的棘波和场电位活动发现，在震颤或 θ 频率（3～7Hz）和 β 频率范围（人类为 13～30Hz，MPTP 处理的猴模型为 8～20Hz），周期性爆发放电的基底节神经元比例增加。最后，这些方框和箭模型忽略了基底节在强化学习（见后述）和行为环境适应中的角色。

（二）基底节的强化学习模型

更现代的计算机模型将基底节视为执行/评价（actor/critic）强化学习网络（Schultz 等，1997）。主轴或 actor 部分连接编码当前状态的皮质区域，如看到、听到和记住的内容。主轴负责实现状态和动作之间的评估，如行为策略。中脑多巴胺能神经元扮演着评价方或教师（teacher）的角色。他们计算预测与现实之间的差异，即预测误差。预测误差用于更新对未来的预测，如果现实比预测更好则加强动作的关联，比预测更差则进行削弱，来优化行为策略。

在基底节解剖学方面（图 6-3），基底节主轴（actor）的神经网络将编码状态的皮质和丘脑神经元与皮质和脑干运动中枢连接起来。中脑多巴胺能神经元是基底节网络的评价方。它们正常的背景活动（4～5 个棘波/秒）编码了预测和现实之间的预测误差。积极的预测误差（现实比预测好）是由多巴胺神经元的爆发性放电编码的。另外，预期奖励缺失、厌恶事件，以及其他的负性预测错误（现实比预测更差）通过抑制棘波活动来编码（Schultz，2001；Tobler 等，2005）。多巴胺能活性变化及皮质和纹状体的协同放电，导致皮质 - 纹状体突触效率的可塑性变化（如长时程增强），从而调节由皮质活动编码的状态与动作之间的联系。

这种基底节的执行/评价（actor/critic）强化学习模型彻底改变了目前对无模型或程序式、盲从式学习的生理机制的理解。该模型还为某些与基底节相关的疾病提供了理论观点，例如解释缓慢进展的左旋多巴诱导运动障碍。但对于经典的直接或间接 D_1/D_2 模型，该模型有其自身的缺陷。例如，以基底节为基础的强化学习模型未能为多巴胺激动药和拮抗药（如阿扑吗啡或氟哌啶醇）的超快作用提供机制解释。此外，该模型假设一种单一的模式——快感或惩罚，来控制行为，可能没有完全描述人类和动物的多维情感。

（三）基底节的多目标优化模型

中脑多巴胺能神经元并不是基底节的唯一调节器。纹状体胆碱能中间神经元、中缝背侧 5- 羟色胺能（5-HT）神经元和灰结节 - 乳头体的组胺能神经元也可以调节基底节的活动，因此被认为是基底节评价系统的一部分（图 6-4）。在

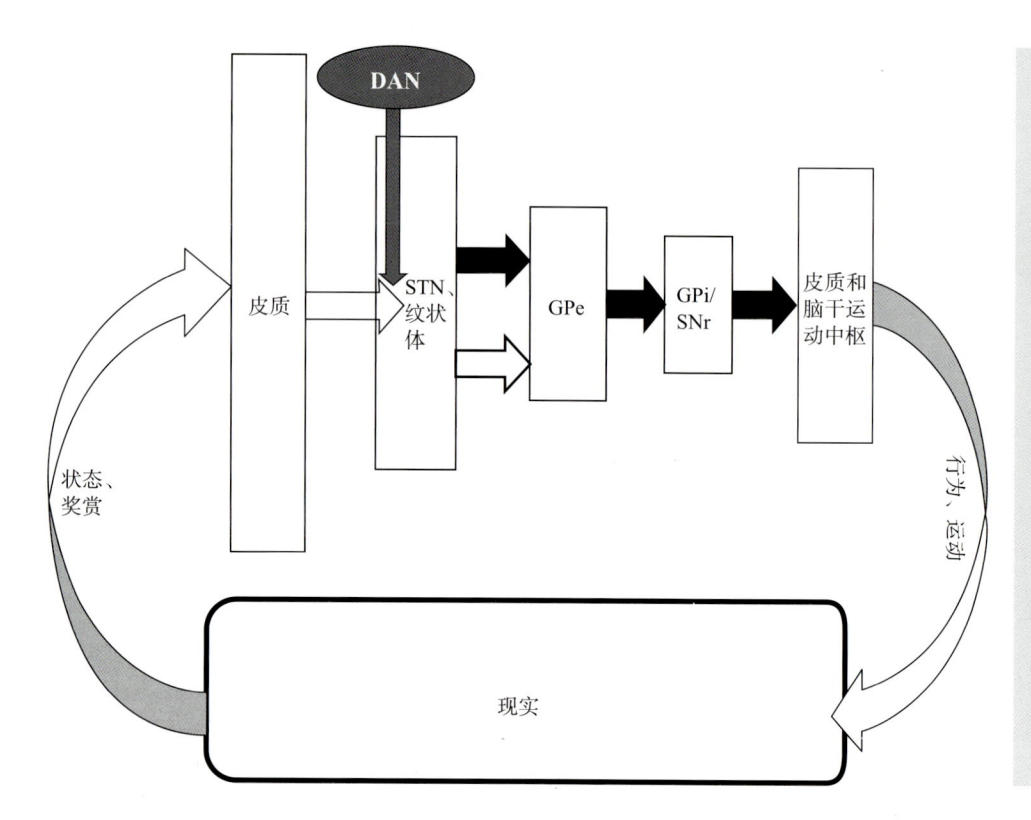

图6-3 基底节的执行/评价(actor/critic)强化模型的解剖学描述

执行（actor）是连接编码当前状态的皮质区域和大脑运动中枢的基底节主轴；评价方（critic）教师代表是中脑多巴胺能神经元。评价方（critic）对愉悦预测误差进行了编码，并调节了状态和动作之间的耦合DAN. 中脑多巴胺能神经元；GPe. 苍白球外侧部；GPi. 苍白球内侧部；SNr. 黑质网状部；STN. 底丘脑核

这个多元模型中，基底节计算目标是在未来累积收益最大化和行为成本或信息成本最小化之间进行评价，提供了多个目标优化（Parush等，2011）。在这个多目标优化模型中，每个基底节的评价方（critic）都扮演着双重角色。与上述强化模型相似，基底节区评价方（critic）影响皮质-纹状体突触的功能，还影响纹状体投射神经元的兴奋性，从而在收益和成本之间权衡。

多评价方（critic）、多目标优化模型（图6-4）更好地展示了基底节执行/评价（actor/critic）网络的复杂性。评价方（critic）对纹状体兴奋性和皮质-纹状体突触功能的综合影响，可以解释超快效应（如阿扑吗啡）和缓慢的程序性学习。此外，该模型还解释了对非多巴胺能评价方（critic）在基底节生理学和病理生理学中的作用，包括PD患者的多巴胺-乙酰胆碱调控的运动功能和5-羟色胺相关的抑郁。

三、脑深部电刺激的神经生理学

治疗PD的第一步是用左旋多巴或突触后多巴胺激动药进行多巴胺替代治疗（dopamine replacement therapy, DRT）。DRT的目标是恢复多巴胺生理功能的全部动态范围，包括阶段性爆发释放和持续基线水平。然而，多巴胺能轴突的出芽增加、多巴胺受体的过度敏感，以及在DRT多年后发生的其他病理生理变化，会导致纹状体中多巴胺的异常动态变化。经过数年的DRT治疗后，诸如左旋多巴引起的运动障碍等不良反应将显著影响生活质量。

经典的直接/间接D_1/D_2模型和MPTP灵长类动物模型中的生理记录提示治疗的重点从评价方（DRT）转移到基底节的执行方（STN或GPi的DBS）。生理学研究表明，MPTP处理猴模型的基底节主轴神经元的放电速率、放电模式和同步化发生了变化。在猴和人类中，这些过度活跃的基底节核团的失活可以改善帕金森病的症状并提示在DRT治疗失败后仍有新的治疗手段。DBS的机制仍然存在争议，但大多数人同意信息损伤假说，即DBS的快速效应与失活的效应类似。这与基底节网络是编码当前状态和行动的

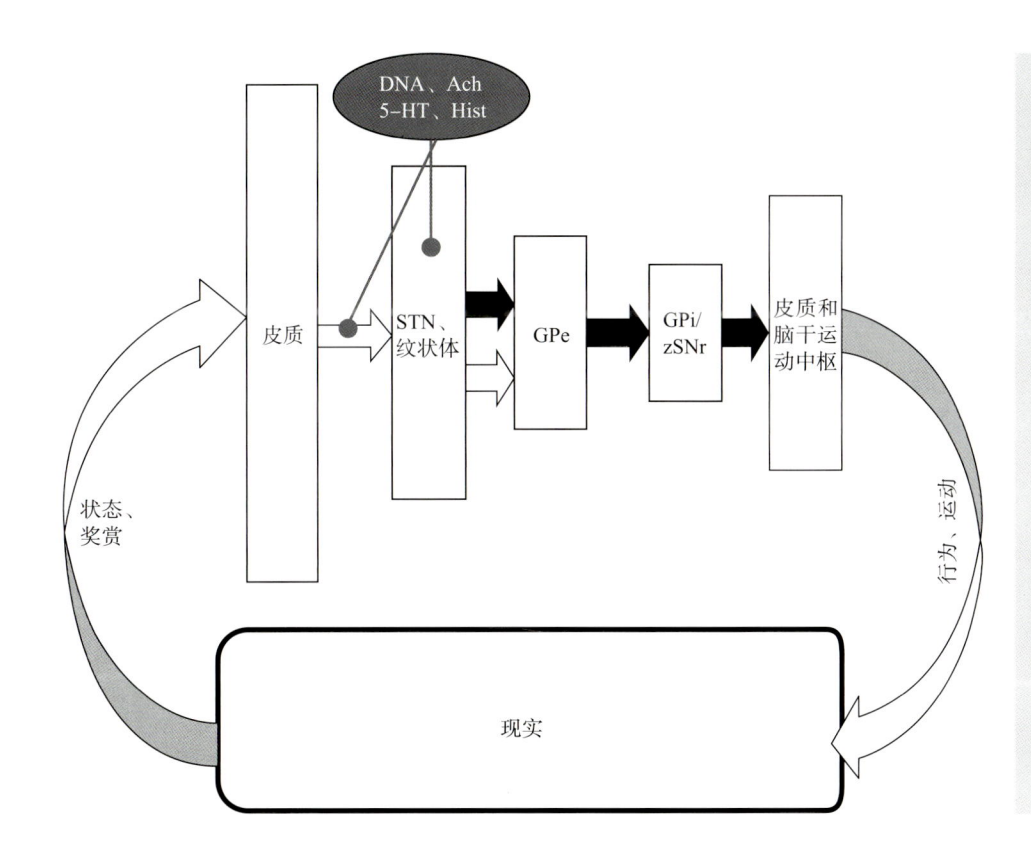

图 6-4 基底节多目标优化模型的解剖学描述

基底节评价方（critic）通过调节纹状体投射神经元的兴奋性、状态 - 动作耦合，以及通过调节皮质 - 纹状体突触的作用，对基底节主轴的兴奋性产生多重和不同的影响
5-HT.5- 羟色胺；Ach. 胆碱能中间神经元；DAN. 中脑多巴胺能神经元；GPe. 苍白球外侧部；GPi. 苍白球内侧部；Hist. 组胺；SNr. 黑质网状部；STN. 底丘脑核

神经结构之间的默认、快速和无意识联系的概念是一致的，例如 Kahneman 所著《思维的快与慢》（*Thinking Fast and Slow*，2011）中的默认系统。还有许多其他的网络，例如以皮质和小脑为中心的网络。这些网络在状态和动作之间也同时提供平行连接（图 6-5）；但由于基底节是状态和动作之间的默认连接，其他网络并不能补偿异常的基底节活动。抑制基底节的异常活动可以用其他网络进行补偿，并重新建立接近正常状态 - 动作的耦合。

沿主轴进行信息汇聚的独特特征决定了基底节失活带来的严重效应（Bar-Gad 等，2003）。这种漏斗式（信息流）结构能够使正常的基底节提取当前状态的特征（可能与运动行为有关），这些特征对于正在进行的和下一步将要进行的运动很重要。另外，当基底节"表现不佳"时，医生可以基于这种漏斗式结构，通过基底节局部微小结构的失活而对皮质和脑干产生重大影响。最近的证据表明，STN 是基底节生理和病理生理活动的"驱动力"，这为 STN 作为最佳的 DBS 靶点提供了另一种支持，至少对于 PD 而言是这样（Deffains 等，2016）。

但是基底节靶点的永久失活仅能通过毁损实现，因此并不被推荐作为治疗选择。DBS 是一个可逆和可调节的过程，因此更适合当前对治疗有效性和伦理的要求。PD 和其他基底节疾病的现代治疗已经从在基底节评价方神经递质水平上的化学操作，转移到对基底节执行方放电活动的干预。DBS 治疗对其他与基底节相关的运动障碍也有效，如肌张力障碍和特发性震颤，目前正在尝试用于基底节参与发病的精神障碍，如强迫症和重度抑郁症。

四、总结

我们对基底节网络和相关疾病（如 PD）的理解，是由基底节的计算模型决定的。经典的直接或间接 D_1/D_2 模型假定多巴胺和基底节的作用在于调节运动皮质的兴奋性；执行 / 评价（actor/critic）强化模型假设多巴胺的作用是调节皮质 -

▲ 图 6-5 基底节网络是神经系统中连接"状态和行为"的众多神经网络之一

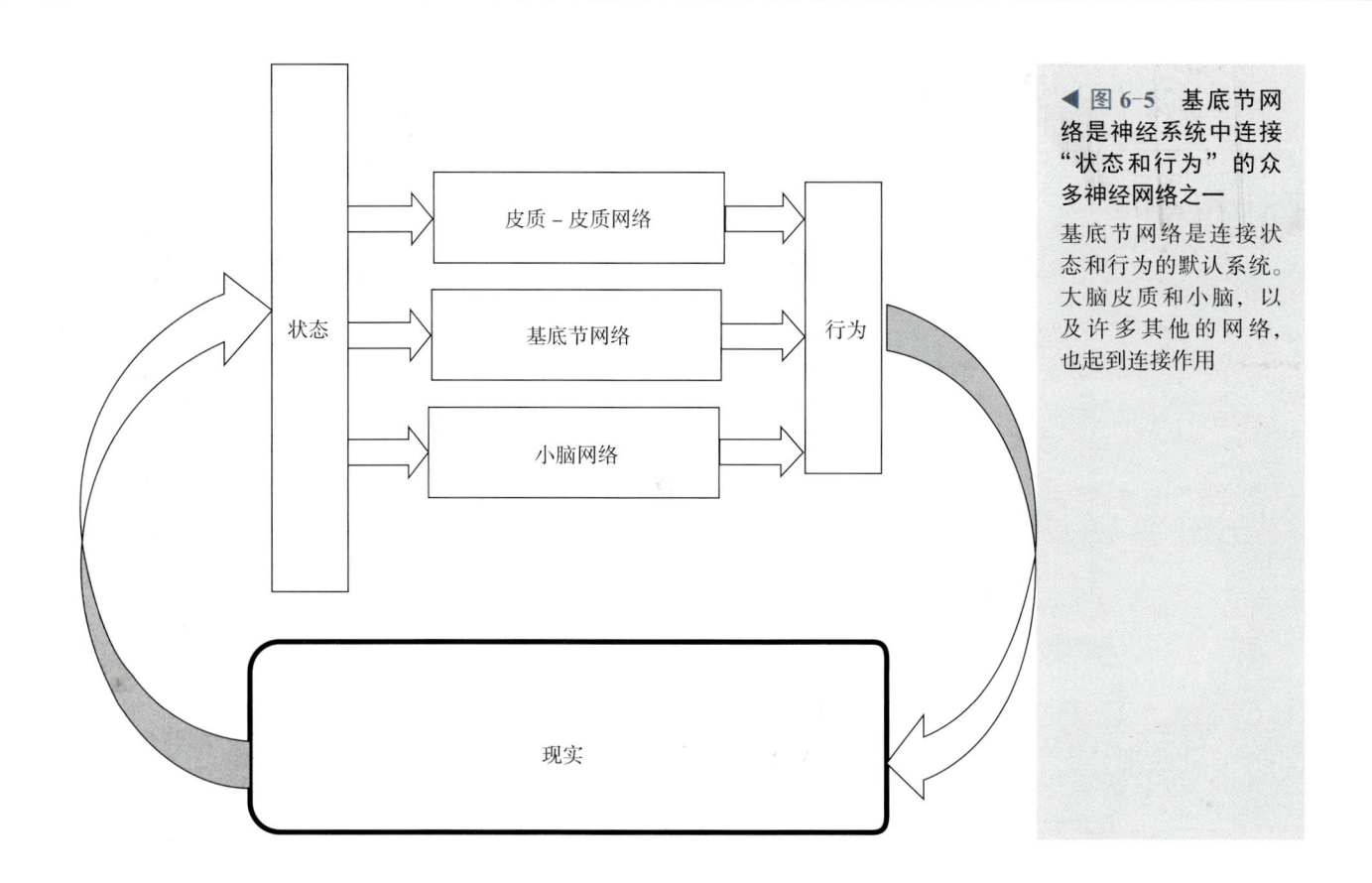

基底节网络是连接状态和行为的默认系统。大脑皮质和小脑，以及许多其他的网络，也起到连接作用

纹状体的突触效应和行为策略；第三代模型，多评价、多目标优化模型，假定在基底节中存在不止一个多巴胺能评价或老师（teacher）。基底节评价方通过调节纹状体的兴奋性和突触效率，并实现正在进行和未来行为的多目标优化。

基底节执行/评价多目标优化模型可用于改进新一代 DBS 设备，将为患者提供更好的治疗。如今 DBS 必须由医生每 2～10 周进行一次调整，但 PD 的动态性和复杂性要求对参数的调整更频繁、更复杂。这可以通过闭环 DBS 方法来实现（Rosin 等，2011；另见第 5 章）。未来的闭环 DBS 设备将致力于实现患者运动和非运动症状的多目标优化，同时将 DBS 治疗的不良反应降至最低。

参考文献

[1] Albin RL, Young AB, Penney JB. The functional anatomy of basal ganglia disorders. Trends Neurosci. 1989;12:366–75.
[2] Bar-Gad I, Morris G, Bergman H. Information processing, dimensionality reduction and reinforcement learning in the basal ganglia. Prog Neurobiol. 2003;71:439–73.
[3] Bergman H, Wichmann T, DeLong MR. Reversal of experimental parkinsonism by lesions of the subthalamic nucleus. Science. 1990;249:1436–8.
[4] Bergman H, Wichmann T, Karmon B, DeLong MR. The primate subthalamic nucleus. II. Neuronal activity in the MPTP model of parkinsonism. J Neurophysiol. 1994;72:507–20.
[5] Deffains M, Iskhakova L, Katabi S, Israel Z, Bergman H. Subthalamic, not striatal, activity correlates to basal ganglia downstream activity in normal and parkinsonian monkeys. Elife. 2016;5. pii: e16443. https://doi.org/10.7554/eLife.16443.
[6] Filion M, Tremblay L. Abnormal spontaneous activity of globus pallidus neurons in monkeys with MPTP-induced parkinsonism. Brain Res. 1991;547:142–51.
[7] Filion M, Tremblay L, Bedard PJ. Effects of dopamine agonists on the spontaneous activity of globus pallidus neurons in monkeys with MPTP-induced parkinsonism. Brain Res. 1991;547:152–61.
[8] Heimer G, Rivlin-Etzion M, Bar-Gad I, Goldberg JA, Haber SN, Bergman H. Dopamine replacement therapy does not restore the full spectrum of normal pallidal activity in the 1-methyl-4-phenyl-1,2,3,6-tetra-hydropyridine primate model of parkinsonism. J Neurosci. 2006;26:8101–14.
[9] Hutchinson WD, Levy R, Dostrovsky JO, Lozano AM, Lang AE. Effects of apomorphine on globus pallidus neurons in parkinsonian patients. Ann Neurol. 1997;42:767–75.
[10] Lee JI, Verhagen ML, Ohara S, Dougherty PM, Kim JH, Lenz FA. Internal pallidal neuronal activity during mild drug-related dyskinesias in Parkinson's disease: decreased firing rates and altered firing patterns. J Neurophysiol. 2007;97:2627–41.
[11] Levy R, Hutchison WD, Lozano AM, Dostrovsky JO. Synchronized neuronal discharge in the basal ganglia of parkinsonian patients is limited to oscillatory activity. J Neurosci. 2002a;22:2855–61.
[12] Levy R, Ashby P, Hutchison WD, Lang AE, Lozano AM, Dostrovsky JO. Dependence of subthalamic nucleus oscillations on movement and dopamine in Parkinson's disease. Brain. 2002b;125:1196–209.

[13] Merello M, Balej J, Delfino M, Cammarota A, Betti O, Leiguarda R. Apomorphine induces changes in GPi spontaneous outflow in patients with Parkinson's disease. Mov Disord. 1999;14:45–9.

[14] Miller WC, DeLong MR. Altered tonic activity of neurons in the globus pallidus and subthalamic nucleus in the primate MPTP model of parkinsonism. In: Carpenter MB, Jayaraman A, editors. The basal ganglia II. New York: Plenum Press; 1987. p. 415–27.

[15] Papa SM, DeSimone R, Fiorani M, Oldfield EH. Internal globus pallidus discharge is nearly suppressed during levodopa-induced dyskinesias. Ann Neurol. 1999;46:732–8.

[16] Parush N, Tishby N, Bergman H. Dopaminergic balance between reward maximization and policy complexity. Front Syst Neurosci. 2011;5:22.

[17] Rosin B, Slovik M, Mitelman R, Rivlin-Etzion M, Haber SN, Israel Z, Vaadia E, Bergman H. Closed-loop deep brain stimulation is superior in ameliorating parkinsonism. Neuron. 2011;72:370–84.

[18] Schultz W. Reward signaling by dopamine neurons. Neuroscientist. 2001;7:293–302.

[19] Schultz W, Dayan P, Montague PR. A neural substrate of prediction and reward. Science. 1997;275:1593–9.

[20] Tobler PN, Fiorillo CD, Schultz W. Adaptive coding of reward value by dopamine neurons. Science. 2005;307:1642–5.

[21] Weinberger M, Hutchison WD, Lozano AM, Hodaie M, Dostrovsky JO. Increased gamma oscillatory activity in the subthalamic nucleus during tremor in Parkinson's disease patients. J Neurophysiol. 2009;101:789–802.

[22] Wichmann T, Soares J. Neuronal firing before and after burst discharges in the monkey Basal Ganglia is predictably patterned in the normal state and altered in parkinsonism. J Neurophysiol. 2016;95:2120–33.

[23] Wichmann T, Bergman H, DeLong MR. The primate subthalamic nucleus. III. Changes in motor behavior and neuronal activity in the internal pallidum induced by subthalamic inactivation in the MPTP model of parkinsonism. J Neurophysiol. 1994;72:521–30.

[24] Zaidel A, Spivak A, Grieb B, Bergman H, Israel Z. Subthalamic span of beta oscillations predicts deep brain stimulation efficacy for patients with Parkinson's disease. Brain. 2010;133:2007–21.

第7章 脑深部电刺激手术麻醉
Anaesthesia for Deep Brain Stimulation Surgery

Michaël J. Bos　Boukje J. E. Hermans　Wolfgang F. Buhre　著
刘钰晔　王秀　译　韩春雷　杨岸超　张建国　校

> **摘要**：在药物难治性运动障碍（帕金森病、特发性震颤和肌张力障碍）、癫痫，以及精神疾病如强迫症等的外科治疗方面，脑深部电刺激（deep brain stimulation, DBS）已被广为接受。DBS手术可以在不同的麻醉方式下进行，但是为满足神经外科医生的治疗需求和个人偏好，多数中心选择局部麻醉。然而目前尚未证实哪一种麻醉手段更适合DBS手术。麻醉医生在围术期面临的挑战取决于所治疗的神经精神疾病的种类。麻醉的目的旨在提供理想的手术条件、保证患者舒适并有利于定位靶点。另外麻醉医师需意识到围术期的并发症及相应处理手段。本章节将针对DBS手术患者的麻醉管理进行系统、前沿性的综述。

一、概述

在药物难治性运动障碍疾病，如帕金森病（PD）、特发性震颤和肌张力障碍及其他神经系统疾病，如癫痫和精神疾病［如强迫症（obsessive-compulsive disorder, OCD）、抽动秽语综合征（Tourette syndrome，TS）］等的外科治疗方面，脑深部电刺激（DBS）已被广为接受（Benabid 等，2009；Miocinovic 等，2013）。传统DBS手术多在清醒、局部麻醉和（或）镇静状态下进行以利于神经电生理监测和临床评估。清醒手术中，麻醉医生需要面临的任务，包括为患者创造舒适、安全的环境以减少突发的运动行为、最大限度减少麻醉对微电极记录（microelectrode recording, MER）的影响并能保证患者术中配合临床评估。从这方面来讲，成功的DBS手术需要神经外科、神经内科、神经电生理和麻醉医生的密切配合（Poon 和 Irwin，2009）。除了清醒DBS手术外，另一种麻醉方式即全身麻醉。随着近期立体定向技术和术中影像技术的发展，全麻DBS手术也逐渐被推广，但是高剂量全麻药物对MER的影响目前尚未明了且不能行术中测试。尽管存在这些不足，目前报道显示，全身麻醉DBS手术同样有较好的运动功能改善预后（Ho 等，2018）。

除与手术相关的问题外，由于DBS患者术中需要头架固定，术中如何对患者进行气道管理是麻醉医生面临的重要问题，尤其在应用低剂量麻醉药物时。呼吸道并发症仍然是麻醉相关并发症和死亡的主要原因（Venkatraghavan 等，2006）。

在这篇综述中，我们列举了DBS术中麻醉医生需要关注的问题。本章节将简单介绍DBS手术过程，拟手术患者术前进行的专科疾病评估，随后介绍不同的麻醉技术、麻醉对MER的影响，以及常见的麻醉并发症。

二、手术过程简要介绍

DBS 手术分 2 步进行，首先是脑内电极植入，随后是神经刺激器植入。部分中心是在同一次手术先后完成 2 步，而部分中心是分 2 次手术完成，在第二次手术中进行刺激器植入。

患者头颅固定好立体定向框架后完成影像扫描（CT 或磁共振影像），随后设计电极路径获得合适的靶点坐标。患者被转运到手术室并将框架固定于手术床上。皮肤切开后，颅骨钻孔并切开硬膜。微电极按照设计路径进行置入，邻近靶点区域在不同的位置进行 MER 记录。随后进行临床症状测试以确定刺激治疗效果并最大可能减少刺激相关不良反应。基于信号记录和术中测试，明确最佳电极位置后按照原有路径植入永久电极。电极的颅外部分置于皮下并缝合关闭切口。

患者全身麻醉进行 DBS 手术的第二步。刺激器被埋置于胸部锁骨下区域或腹部右下象限区域皮下组织内，并通过延长导线与电极相连。

三、术前注意事项

多学科术前评估的重要内容是评估患者是否适合手术治疗，麻醉医生需要考虑患者的一般身体状况、精神疾病史和认知功能。全面的气道评估对于 DBS 手术是有非常重要的，尤其对于全程或部分过程需要清醒局麻的患者。所有进行 DBS 电极植入的患者均应被认为是困难气道，因为固定于头部的框架限制了颈部活动，且多数立体定向头架鼻前有一横杆，也限制了术中气道的管理。因此对于术中所有阶段的气道保护均应该提前做好计划，并且需要在术前与整个手术团队一起讨论完成。理想情况下，科室应该联合整个手术团队对此类情况进行培训以提高对于术中紧急情况的处理能力（Chakrabarti 等，2014）。

除了常规术前评估外，患者还需要进行麻醉相关评估，因为患者可能存在与治疗疾病相关的并发症。

（一）帕金森病

PD 患者可能存在多个生理系统的功能受损，如呼吸、心血管、胃肠道和骨骼肌系统的功能紊乱。通常情况下，呼吸系统功能紊乱是由于运动迟缓、僵直和呼吸机的不协调运动所致，受损程度与 PD 疾病的严重程度密切相关。临床发现多达 1/3 患者存在阻塞性通气障碍（Hovestadt 等，1989；Nicholson 等，2002），因此 PD 患者易合并呼吸系统感染。另外，上呼吸道功能紊乱合并咳嗽反射减弱、吞咽困难时可能出现分泌物潴留、肺不张和通气障碍。PD 患者术后坠积性肺炎的发生率显著高于非 PD 患者（Pepper 和 Goldstein，1999）。除了上述潜在的呼吸系统相关危险因素外，PD 患者以下并发症的发生率还可能增加，包括喉痉挛、阻塞型睡眠呼吸暂停综合征和术后呼吸衰竭等（Nicholson 等，2002）。

心血管功能紊乱在 PD 患者中同样常见，最常见的致残症状是直立性低血压与自主神经功能紊乱（Ziemssen 和 Reichmann，2010）。多种多巴胺能药物如左旋多巴和三环类抗抑郁药通过抑制交感神经系统或阻滞 α 肾上腺素能活动可能会导致或者加重低血压的情况（John 等，1984）。若围术期需应用升压药，建议应用快速起效药物。其他常见的心脏并发症包括高血压、心律失常和血容量不足。术前应妥善处理高血压，以减少 DBS 术中颅内出血的风险。若术前收缩压和舒张压分别＞160mmHg 和 110mmHg，手术应该延期进行（Hartle 等，2016）。对于合并有慢性高血压的患者，抗高血压药物应规律坚持服用，突然停用抗高血压药物可能引起交感神经的过度兴奋而引起严重高血压、心动过速、焦虑、头痛和烦乱等情况（Aronow，2017）。

消化系统的功能紊乱在 PD 患者也较为常见并可累及胃肠道的各个水平。导致胃肠道功能紊乱的可能原因，包括黑质-纹状体破坏引起的多巴胺缺乏、迷走神经背核受累，以及肠道固有神经系统的神经病理改变等情况（Del Tredici 等，2002；Halliday 等，1990）。PD 早期或进展期均可能出现胃轻瘫症状，可表现为恶心、呕吐、饱腹感和腹部舒张不良等情况。为了降低胃轻瘫的症状，手术前可以考虑应用促动力药和抗呕吐药如昂丹司琼或抗组胺药（Pfeiffer，2011）。

过度流涎是疾病的晚期症状，其本身不是由于唾液分泌过多，而是因为吞咽动作的频率和功能下降引起。应用抗毒蕈碱类药物如莨菪碱或格隆铵类药物将增加唾液黏稠度并进一步损伤吞咽功能。

吞咽困难在PD患者中被频繁报道，是发生呼吸道并发症的潜在危险因素，尤其是在患者镇静状态下。目前尚不能明确吞咽困难是否是疾病进展的表现，其可发生在疾病的早期，偶尔也会作为患者的主诉就诊。口咽部和食管的功能障碍都可能造成患者的吞咽困难（Fasano等，2015；Noyce等，2012）。

接近50%患者存在营养不良的情况，具体机制目前尚不明确，但是年龄、运动症状、疾病严重程度和抑郁等可能是营养不良的相关原因。术前需要对患者的营养水平进行评估。因为营养不良，患者可存在贫血、低蛋白血症和电解质紊乱等情况。葡萄糖利用水平通常被破坏，术前需要检测患者的血糖水平。

认知损害是PD患者常见的非运动症状。认知损害患者围术期易出现谵妄，因此术前应评估患者的认知功能状态。超过20%的患者DBS术后可出现谵妄表现。术中配合程度高的患者，在清醒手术部分能够回答问题或配合完成任务是非常重要的。从这个角度来说，术前向患者全面解释手术的整个过程，并对手术的每一步骤有一个较好的精神心理准备对降低焦虑情绪是有必要的。术前或围术期焦虑情绪可导致血压升高，从而增加了颅内出血的风险（Aarsland等，2017；Carlson等，2014；Venkatraghavan等，2010）。

在与神经外科医生讨论后，合理指导患者停用专科治疗药物，因为所有患者需停药以利于术中进行电刺激和临床评估。这样会对围术期护理进一步增加挑战，因为停药状态可能会加重患者的疾病症状（Burton等，2004）。

（二）特发性震颤

特发性震颤是一种累及双侧上肢的动作性震颤综合征，病史在3年以上，伴或不伴有其他肢体的震颤，多无其他神经系统体征，如肌张力障碍或帕金森综合征。特发性震颤症状多因应激或劳累时加重。治疗药物包括β受体拮抗药，如普萘洛尔和托吡酯（Bhatia等，2018）。除了与年龄和认知下降等相关的麻醉注意事项外，特发性震颤无疾病特异性的心肺相关麻醉风险。部分患者服用β肾上腺素能受体阻滞药（普萘洛尔）可能导致患者术中易出现心动过缓或低血压；服用抗惊厥药物（扑痫酮）可能存在肝脏细胞色素P_{450}同工酶的诱导作用（Bloor等，2017；Louis，2016）。特发性震颤DBS手术多采用清醒麻醉方式。

（三）肌张力障碍

肌张力障碍患者术前评估重点，包括肌张力障碍运动和痉挛的严重程度、已知的触发因素和麻醉药物与左旋多巴、抗胆碱能治疗药物的相互作用。全面的气道评估是术前必需的，尤其在手术清醒麻醉或镇静阶段。颈部或口咽部肌张力障碍患者的气道管理更为复杂，部分病情严重患者需要在清醒和纤维支气管镜直视下进行气管插管。除了运动症状，肌张力障碍患者可能存在体重下降、营养不良、精神心理障碍（如焦虑和重度抑郁症）（Smit等，2016；Venkatraghavan等，2016）。

（四）癫痫

癫痫患者的DBS手术通常在全身麻醉下进行。癫痫患者DBS手术相关的心肺并发症与年龄对照组相似。癫痫术前需要进行包括精神心理并发症在内的全面健康评估。围术期患者维持抗癫痫药物治疗是必需的，麻醉医生需要了解常见抗癫痫药物的药理特征、药代动力学特征，以及与麻醉药物的动态相互作用（Perks等，2012）。

(五)强迫症

强迫症(obsessive-compulsive disorder, OCD)是以强迫行为为特征的慢性精神疾病。患者可能经历较长时间后才得以诊断并通常具有严重的致残性。术前评估重点包括强迫行为的范围和严重程度,以及对并发症的评估,比如情绪障碍、焦虑和人格障碍等情况。OCD 的药物治疗通常包括 5- 羟色胺能抗抑郁药,如 5- 羟色胺再摄取抑制药(serotonin reuptake inhibitors, SSRI)或三环类抗抑郁药(tricyclic antidepressant, TCA)氯米帕明。5- 羟色胺再摄取抑制药对麻醉管理无明显干预,需密切注意联合用药,以及药物经过 CYP450 系统代谢后的效应,尤其对于服用苯二氮䓬类药物的患者。突然停用 SSRI 容易出现撤药症状(如流感症状、疲倦和肌肉疼痛)。对于服用 TCA 的患者,麻醉管理需要密切注意不良反应和药物相互作用。TCA 的作用机制是加强 5- 羟色胺能和去甲肾上腺素能的活动,TCA 对组胺能、胆碱能和 α₁ 肾上腺素能的抑制作用是产生不良反应的机制。需要谨慎关注 TCA 对心血管的影响和与特殊神经递质的相互作用,如去甲肾上腺素。TCA 可以增加去甲肾上腺素能神经末梢神经递质的储存。当应用间接作用的血管收缩药时,可能会引起肾上腺素的过渡释放,所以对拟交感作用药物的应用需要谨慎。抗胆碱能药物同样可引起临床问题,因为术中多种麻醉药物同样存在抗胆碱效应。突然停用 TCA 可能会引起生理性撤药反应,表现为与药物作用相反的表现,如流涕、寒战和精神萎靡等(Fleisher, 2006)。服用 SSRI 和 TCA 的患者因存在血小板水平的 5- 羟色胺能减少而存在出血风险。这些效应会被非甾体抗炎药加强。血小板释放的 5- 羟色胺对血小板聚集和血凝块形成中发挥重要作用(Saraghi 等, 2018)。因此,这些药物术前建议停用,但是停药可能会加重临床症状。

(六)抽动秽语综合征

抽动秽语综合征(Tourette syndrome)是儿童期起病的神经精神功能障碍,临床以运动性和发声性冲动为特征。大多数抽动秽语综合征患者合并神经行为障碍,如注意力缺乏多动症、抑郁和强迫症。术前评估需要涵盖这些功能紊乱及运动性冲动的严重程度,尤其对于清醒阶段的 DBS 手术。手术室紧张的氛围可能会加重临床症状。抽动秽语综合征的药物治疗,包括 α 受体拮抗药(可乐定和胍法辛)、神经松弛药(氟哌啶醇、匹莫齐特、利培酮、奥氮平)和苯甲酰胺类药物(舒必利和硫必利)。麻醉医生术前了解这些药物的药理特征和与麻醉药物的相互作用至关重要。

四、术前检查

常规实验室检查应该包括全血细胞计数、血型和交叉配血试验、血清尿素、肌酐和电解质水平。PD 患者多存在血糖利用障碍,因此术前应检测患者血糖水平。除非患者既往存在凝血功能障碍、肝肾衰竭等病史,凝血功能(PTTK 和 INR)检查不是必需的。术前建议对 PD 患者或存在已知心血管风险因素的患者进行 12 导联心电图检查(标准和实践规范委员会;美国麻醉医师协会麻醉术前评估工作组等, 2012)。

五、DBS 术中抗凝血药和抗血小板治疗

目前针对 DBS 手术抗凝血药和抗血小板药物应用管理的文献较少且仅有几篇病例报道,尚无长期随访研究和指南文件。因此建议 DBS 术前在合适时间停用所有抗凝血药物和抗血小板药物(Ashkan 等, 2015;Lazio 和 Simard, 1999)。

六、麻醉技术

多种麻醉技术被报道应用于 DBS 手术,包括局部或区域麻醉联合麻醉监测管理、清醒镇静、睡眠 – 清醒 – 睡眠或全身麻醉技术。尽管

部分文献报道清醒麻醉技术在减少麻醉药物对MER监测的影响存在优势，但是目前尚未证实哪一种麻醉方式对DBS手术更好（Harries等，2012；Maltête等，2004；Poon和Irwin，2009；Venkatraghavan和Manninen，2011）。所有麻醉技术将在下文进行简要介绍。

（一）麻醉前用药

通常来说，麻醉前用药的目的是进行麻醉准备、降低患者焦虑、疼痛和减少分泌物以辅助手术，以及减少术后恶心和呕吐等情况的发生。麻醉术前用药不是术前管理的常规操作，需要在个体水平针对性考虑。麻醉前用药需要谨慎应用，尤其是苯二氮䓬类和γ-氨基丁酸（gamma-aminobutyric acid，GABA）受体的拮抗药，因为这些药物可能会对手术及MER造成干扰。患者术前常规服用的心血管和呼吸系统用药应该坚持服用，这些专科疾病治疗的药物停用是需要与手术团队进行首要讨论的内容。

（二）监测麻醉管理联合局部或区域麻醉

对于安装立体定向头架患者进行的清醒麻醉技术中，局部或区域麻醉可以使镇静药和镇痛药物的剂量减少到最小。固定杆穿刺点应用短效和长效麻醉药混合进行局部浸润麻醉。每个患者的麻醉药物总剂量需要谨慎计算（包括镇痛效果不理想时的补充药物剂量）。常用的局部麻醉药物包括布比卡因、左布比卡因、罗哌卡因或利多卡因。另外可以额外添加肾上腺素以延迟麻醉药物吸收、延长并增强麻醉效果并降低切口的出血（Kirksey等，2015）。药物的生化特征，如局麻药的脂溶性、药物容积和浓度，将会影响药物的作用时间。麻醉效应可维持6～8h，部分原因是与额外应用的血管升压药或可乐定等有关。应用罗派卡因或左布比卡因的优势在于其心血管和神经毒性不良反应较经典的布比卡因小，但是该不同点与临床的相关性在多篇述评中被质疑（El-Boghdadly和Chin，2016；Kirksey等，2015）。

除了局部麻醉外，头皮麻醉也可以采用区域麻醉技术。每一侧头皮可以通过阻滞7根皮神经来完成。前额皮肤是由三叉神经分支（V₁支）眶上神经和滑车上神经来支配。颧颞神经，即三叉神经分支（V₂分支），支配小部分前额和颞区皮肤。耳颞神经同样是三叉神经分支（V₃分支），支配颞区皮肤、下嘴唇、下面部、耳郭和耳上皮肤。枕小神经，C₂或C₃脊神经的分支，支配后头部耳郭后皮肤区域。枕大神经，C₂脊神经的分支，支配后头部其余部分的头皮感觉。耳大神经，C₂或C₃脊神经分支，支配腮腺、乳突和耳郭部位的皮肤感觉。需要注意的是头皮神经阻滞仅仅是表面麻醉，像深部结构如硬膜，则需要额外麻醉或静脉镇痛药物（Costello和Cormack，2004；Burnand和Sebastian，2014）。

DBS手术需要应用标准的术中监测，包括心电图、非侵入性动脉压监测、血氧和呼气末CO_2监测。对于术中血压波动管理存在挑战的患者，可以考虑应用瞬时动脉压监测。由于运动伪差的影响，非侵入性血压测量可能不准确。应用侵入性血压监测的原因是清醒患者术中反复进行血压测量会带来不适感（Moore等，2008；Venkatraghavan等，2010）。考虑到DBS手术时长的原因，必须要进行导尿。

手术台上维持合适的姿势对保证患者的舒适和配合至关重要。患者头颈部在低位颈椎水平保持适当角度的屈曲、寰枕关节伸展位。颈部和双肩下垫一个枕头减少患者不适。髋关节和膝关节屈曲10°～15°且腰椎需要保持生理且舒适的姿势。双腿屈曲且膝下垫有毛毯或者软垫用以保持稳定和舒适。应用保温毛毯可以帮助患者保温。面前的清洁的塑料手术帘可以使得患者有清晰视野且有助于麻醉医生与患者进行交流。麻醉医生在帮助患者和手术医生术中交流中起到核心作用并鼓励患者保持良好心态参与手术配合（Erickson和Cole，2007；Rozet和Vavilala，2007；Venkatraghavan等，2010）。

（三）清醒镇静

麻醉技术中除了局部或区域麻醉联合MAC

外，清醒镇静技术也可以考虑应用。这项技术的目的是在保持患者自主呼吸通气的同时根据不同手术阶段或者患者需要（如焦虑、疼痛或者严重的不自主运动）来调整相应的镇静水平。在安置固定杆、皮肤切开和颅骨钻孔时加深镇静水平，而当MER和临床评估时降低或者停止镇静药物水平，在所有神经电生理监测完成后再次增加镇静药物水平。清醒镇静麻醉的优势在于避免气道操作及相关并发症（Khatib等，2008）。

目前清醒镇静最常用的药物与全身麻醉药物一样：丙泊酚和瑞芬太尼。丙泊酚因本身有较好的脂溶性而起效快，由于其初始分布半衰期短暂，患者即很快清醒。对老龄患者（尤其PD多属老龄患者），推荐低剂量应用以保证低容量分布。丙泊酚可以抑制呼吸，甚至在镇静剂量水平即可抑制缺氧诱导的呼吸驱动和高碳酸血症引起的生理反应。上述作用机制与GABA介导的抑制性神经递质传递易化有关。由于基底节对GABA存在较好的敏感性，GABA受体机制相关的麻醉药物对MER可能存在影响。尽管文献报道应用丙泊酚会使得神经元电活动模式发生变化，但是多项研究证实在应用丙泊酚情况下进行MER监测是可能的（Grant等，2015；Hutchison等，2003；Maltête等，2004；Raz等，2010）。除了对MER的影响，丙泊酚同样可引起运动障碍并能抑制震颤，这些效应可能会干扰术中临床测试。

瑞芬太尼是一种合成的超短效阿片类物质，其本身多个特点使得该药物较为适合应用于DBS手术。瑞芬太尼存在短时清除半衰期和时量相关半衰期，其通过非特异性的血浆或组织脂酶成分进行代谢且对肝肾功能没有太多的依赖。瑞芬太尼可以提供快速镇痛作用并对中枢神经系统存在较小的抑制作用。瑞芬太尼对MER的影响尚不完全明了，因此建议在开始MER之前1～2min停用瑞芬太尼（Grant等，2015；Kisilewicz等，2017；Lamperti，2015）。其他药物如可乐定和短效阿片类物质如阿芬太尼或芬太尼也可能在DBS手术中应用。对于DBS手术常用镇静药物综述已在表7-1中列出（Burnand和Sebastian，2014；Erickson和Cole，2007；Raz等，2010）。

清醒DBS手术新的麻醉方向即α$_2$受体激动药右美托咪定的应用。作为一种镇静药物，右美托咪定存在较多的优势。右美托咪定药物效果包括了镇静、镇痛和抗焦虑效应，患者接受语言刺激时很容易被叫醒。另外在镇静剂量下的右美托咪定不会抑制PD患者的震颤症状，是保证术中临床测试的理想药物。右美托咪定对呼吸系统和高碳酸血症反射性生理反应等方面无明显抑制作用，其另一优势在于抑制应激反应以减少血压波动。右美托咪定对GABA受体并无影响，后者是基底节主要抑制性神经递质。GABA受体激活可影响MER甚至使得MER无法进行。部分报道提示右美托咪定在低剂量［<0.5μg/（kg·h）］应用条件下安全且对MER质量无明显影响。对右美托咪定不良反应的关注较为重要，包括低血压、心动过缓、恶心、呕吐等。部分文献报道在高剂量应用时患者反而表现为烦乱激惹行为，这种情况对固定在头架状态下的患者较为危险（Rozet等，2006；Rozet，2008）。

许多麻醉医生在临床测试时倾向于停用所用镇静药物以减少药物干扰因素的可能。丙泊酚和瑞芬太尼需在临床测试前10～15min停用。尽管瑞芬太尼低剂量持续应用对MER影响很小，也建议在MER前数分钟停用。一旦所有测试完成，需要加深镇静水平或开始启动全身麻醉（Grant等，2015；Sarang和Dinsmore，2003）。

（四）睡眠-清醒-睡眠麻醉技术

在睡眠-清醒-睡眠麻醉过程中，患者接受全身麻醉并在MER和临床测试阶段保持清醒状态。在这种麻醉过程中，麻醉医生面临多项挑战，包括适宜的镇静状态、镇痛深度、保持稳定的血流动力学及气道安全。在第一阶段，应用丙泊酚进行诱导。在维持阶段，静脉用和吸入用麻醉药物同时应用，多推荐短效阿片药物如瑞芬太尼。在第二阶段，麻醉状态应该顺利转换，避

表 7-1 DBS 术中常用镇静药物

药物名称	药物作用	不良反应
α₂ 受体激动药		
右旋美托咪啶	• 镇静、镇痛和抗焦虑作用 • 类似自然睡眠状态而无呼吸抑制 • 对 GABA 受体无影响 • 短效	• 剂量依赖的低血压 • 心动过缓 • 高剂量对 MER 存在影响 • 高剂量可能出现烦躁激惹行为
GABA 受体激动药		
丙泊酚	• 短效，快速起效 • 缓慢给药至预期效果	• 影响 MER，不同的组织器官或不同疾病状态疗效存在差异 • 抑制震颤 • 存在运动障碍诱导效应 • 镇静/呼吸抑制和低血压等效应与药物剂量相关
咪达唑仑	• 抗焦虑作用	• 过度镇静和呼吸抑制 • 烦乱激惹行为 • 存在运动障碍诱导效应 • 干扰 MER
阿片类药物		
舒芬太尼/芬太尼	• 强阵痛效应 • 对 MER 影响最小	• 抑制震颤 • 引起肢体强直 • 长效 • 呼吸抑制
瑞芬太尼	• 超短效，缓慢滴定给药 • 强镇痛效应	• 引起肢体强直 • 高剂量抑制震颤 • 呼吸抑制

免咳嗽或其他不良反应。在第二阶段，患者因进行 MER 和临床测试，需要保持清醒状态。在某些情况下，低剂量丙泊酚单独或联合瑞芬太尼应用以减少患者术中不适。部分文献证实低剂量丙泊酚或瑞芬太尼应用期间进行的神经监测是可靠的。除丙泊酚外，阿片类药物应用频率可适时调整以改善患者的舒适程度。在第三阶段，即 MER 和宏刺激结束后，患者可再次进行全身麻醉。在该阶段，麻醉药物不会再干扰术中记录或测试，理论上讲本阶段麻醉药物的应用已无特殊限制（Erickson and Cole，2007；Hans 等，2000；Manninen 等，2006）。

喉罩是 PD 患者术中麻醉常用的气道设备，因为喉罩较容易插入、拔出或重复插入而对患者的头位不需要过多的要求。喉罩的另一重要优势就是在轻度麻醉阶段患者更容易接受，因此保证手术的顺利进行。麻醉医生必须认识到喉罩首次置入成功率＞90%，但是在正常人群中仍有 1.1% 的失败率。在固定立体定向头架的特殊患者置入失败率可能更高（Ramachandran 等，2012）。

如果在睡眠-清醒-睡眠麻醉技术第三阶段出现喉罩位置不良则需要紧急处理。通过面罩通气适当预吸氧对于头架固定患者较为困难，因此氧饱和度很快因此而下降。在这种紧急情况下，可以考虑再次尝试喉罩复位或面对面插管；另外一种选择是及时尽快移除固定头架。此时面罩通气需要立即启用并保持气道通畅姿势（下颌上抬和头后仰），随后应用直视喉镜或视频喉内镜辅助下进行气管插管（Frerk 等，2015）。

（五）全身麻醉

在 DBS 手术中，若患者因过度恐惧而不能耐受清醒手术、配合程度差、严重的药物关期症状及儿童患者，全身麻醉是有必要的。另外，全身麻醉也适合于不需要术中临床测试的 DBS 手术（如 OCD 和癫痫）。

运动障碍疾病 DBS 手术全身麻醉的重要不足之处在于其对 MER 的干扰，但是部分小样本回顾性研究报道全身麻醉条件下的 MER，可以在 PD 患者和肌张力障碍患者底丘脑核、苍白球和黑质记录到电信号。这些研究并未发现全麻 DBS 术中与清醒手术存在差异，在这些研究中挥发性（七氟烷和地氟烷）和静脉性（丙泊酚联合鸦片类药物）麻醉药物均有报道应用。重要的是，在高剂量麻醉药物条件下神经元典型爆发式电活动消失。既往研究结论也是值得质疑的，因为这部分研究多属小样本研究而且使用的麻醉药物也存在差异，目前仍然需要前瞻性、双盲、高质量研究对比不同麻醉药物在全麻手术中对 MER 质量的影响（Castrioto 等，2016；Moll 等，2013；Sanghera 等，2003；Tsai 等，2015；Yamada 等，2007）。

临床刺激测试的目的是测试临床疗效和不良反应，然而在全身麻醉手术，由于对震颤和僵直等症状的抑制作用而无法完成相关的刺激测试，而且像感觉异常和异常运动等刺激不良反应同样也不能进行评估。对接受苍白球电刺激手术患者，另一种可能完成的测试即通过闪光刺激诱发电位来检测视束功能（Lozano 等，1997）。

随着影像技术的发展，靶点定位和 DBS 电极手术置入可以在术中磁共振或 CT 引导下完成，而不需要进行 MER 监测或术中临床测试。近年来几篇报道显示应用先进术中影像学进行 DBS 手术与传统清醒手术相比，术后疗效无明显差异。然而这些研究多数是回顾性研究、样本量较少并且应用的麻醉和手术技术存在明显的异质性。更进一步讲，这些研究多是在高水平专业机构完成，这些机构对术中影像技术的应用有丰富的经验，所以这样的研究结论难以在所有 DBS 中心进行推广（Burchiel 等，2013；Chen 等，2017；Ho 等，2018；Matias 等，2018；Sheshadri 等，2017）。尽管如此，目前的研究结论表明 DBS 手术全身麻醉有较好的应用前景。

七、麻醉药物对微电极记录的影响

清醒 DBS 手术的目的即是进行 MER 记录和术中测试，有近 20 年多项研究旨在探讨不同麻醉药物对 MER 的影响。总览所有的研究，目前尚不能明确麻醉药物能在多大程度上影响 MER。大多数研究属于回顾性研究，且不同研究间麻醉药物应用方案和患者选择（年龄、适应证和疾病严重程度）异质性大，因此不能形成确定的结论（Grant 等，2015）。

目前我们的大多理解都是来源于病例报道或小样本病例研究。MER 期间，神经元的背景电活动和棘波放电模式对准确定位核团位置非常重要。麻醉药物主要是通过 γ- 氨基丁酸（GABA）受体影响神经元背景电活动和棘波放电，而且多成剂量依赖型。另外麻醉药物在不同核团对神经元电活动的影响是不一样的，核团 GABA 能纤维输入起到主要作用，因为多数麻醉药物可以增强 GABA 的抑制作用（Galvan and Wichmann，2007；Raz 等，2010）。

（低剂量）麻醉状态下 PD 患者 STN MER 可以成功完成，在记录过程中应用的各种麻醉技术均有报道，包括清醒镇静状态（应用丙泊酚和右美托咪啶，无气道操作）和全身麻醉（静脉或吸入麻醉药物）。尽管麻醉药物会降低棘波活动，多数研究证实仍可以用以定位靶点，但是这些研究没有准确说明药物对神经元背景活动的影响、对棘波电活动的抑制程度，以及定位针道的次数等结论（Elias 等，2008；Lin 等，2008；Maltete 等，2004；Moll 等，2013）。

预料中的是，麻醉药物对苍白球内侧部和外侧部电活动的影响比较明显，因为苍白球本身存在丰富的 GABA 能纤维支配（Kita 等，2006）。在肌张力障碍患者和动物模型上获得的数据均发现全身麻醉对苍白球神经元的放电频率有明显的抑制作用。挥发性麻醉药物可以明显降低 PD 患者苍白球放电频率，但是同等剂量的麻醉药物对全身麻醉下进行 DBS 手术的肌张力障碍患者的放电频率却没有影响。PD 患者内侧苍白球神经元活动对挥发性麻醉药物的敏感性较肌张力患者高（Hutchison 等，2003；Peduto 等，1991；Sanghera 等，2003）。

苯二氮䓬类药物是直接的 GABA 受体激动药，可以完全抑制 MER 且可以诱导运动障碍。术中抗焦虑用药时，可考虑应用右美托咪啶。尽管既往研究显示 GABA 能神经元的调控是影响 MER 的关键机制，短效鸦片受体激动药如瑞芬太尼也可以影响 MER，其具体机制尚不明确（Erickson 和 Cole，2007；Grant 等，2015；Kouvaras 等，2008）。

瑞芬太尼是通过非 GABA 介导机制发作用，但其对神经元活动的影响机制尚不明确，对于 DBS 手术可能是较好的麻醉选择。到目前为止，多个研究已经显示低剂量右美托咪啶对底丘脑核和苍白球内侧部 MER 的影响是最小的（Lee 等，2007；Morace 等，2016；Rozet，2008；Sassi 等，2013）。

八、并发症

（一）围术期并发症

DBS 电极置入术中和术后均有可能出现与手术或麻醉相关的严重并发症。不同研究报道的不良反应的发生率存在差异，术中并发症的发生率整体为 12%～16%。最常见的并发症包括围术期气道梗阻、严重高血压和癫痫（Fenoy 和 Simpson，2014；Khatib 等，2008；Venkatraghavan 等，2006）。

（二）呼吸系统并发症

1.6%～2.2% 患者术中出现呼吸系统相关并发症，发生原因包括过度镇静，因为出血或癫痫发作等颅内事件引起的意识水平下降。术前应该准备好相应的开通气道和通气设备，因为对安装立体定向头架患者的相关气道管理是一个很大的挑战（Khatib 等，2008；Venkatraghavan 等，2010）。

（三）心血管系统并发症

对运动障碍或严重痉挛患者术中进行血流动力学监测较为困难，但是早期识别高血压或者低血压事件非常重要。高血压是术中常见事件，可能原因包括焦虑、疼痛、不适或术前高血压治疗不充分。高血压将增加颅内出血的风险，因此在术中置入电极前应严格控制动脉压以避免颅内出血。尽管术中理想血压水平尚无明确结论，多数推荐收缩压需控制在 140mmHg 以下（Binder 等，2005；Gorgulho 等，2005；Zrinzo 等，2012）。如果术中出现高血压事件，需要依据病因应用短效药物对症治疗，常用抗高血压药物包括拉贝洛尔、艾司洛尔或肼苯哒嗪；针对应激反应，可以应用短效镇静或镇痛药物，如右美托咪啶或瑞芬太尼。低血压的出现较为少见，但若出现需要谨慎关注，因为低血压可能影响脑灌注和加深镇静状态。低血压的原因包括过度镇静、过量抗高血压药物应用，也有可能是因为低血容量或者自主神经功能障碍（Osborn 等，2015；Sanchez-Ferro 等，2013）。

静脉空气栓塞是一种少见、但是威胁生命的心血管并发症。静脉空气栓塞是因为开放的静脉腔内压力低于大气压造成，这种情况可发生于患者处在头部高于心脏的姿势体位。患者处于半坐位且存在低血容量时将增加静脉气体栓塞的风险。静脉气体栓塞的后果取决于气体体积和气体进入的频率。临床上当大量气体进入血管时才表现有症状。在清醒患者进行钻孔过程中，患者突然的剧烈咳嗽可能是静脉气体栓塞的症状。静脉栓塞患者在低氧血症出现之前，可存在明显的血流动力学表现，如突然的低血压。大量气体快速进入心脏可导致三尖瓣和肺动脉瓣功能障碍进而造成右心室流出道梗阻，随后导致突然循环停滞。若患者同时存在卵圆孔未闭，突然空气栓塞可能出现脑卒中或者心肌梗死。心脏多普勒超声或者经食管超声可能能够早期识别空气栓塞（Palmon 等，1997）。静脉气体栓塞的发生率为 1.3%～4.5%。静脉气体栓塞的治疗多数是支持性的，应集中于如何避免空气进一步进入静脉系统，如生理盐水填充术区或者骨蜡封闭骨缘，并且降低头颅水平至心脏水平以下（Chang 等，2011；Hooper 等，2009）。

（四）神经系统并发症

术中或术后神经系统并发症的发生率为 0.3%～4.5%，包括肢体力弱、谵妄和癫痫发作等。癫痫发作多发生在刺激测试阶段且多为局灶起源，发生率为 0.8%～4.5%。多数癫痫发作可自发缓解，不过有时需要低剂量苯二氮䓬类或丙泊酚治疗。在 0.3%～3.8% 的患者可发生意识丧失，对这类情况的发病原因的即刻判断较为困难。疲劳、镇静、颅内出血、癫痫发作或气颅均可能是相关原因。因颅内出血或神经损伤引起的意识障碍需要临床迅速、积极地治疗（Kenney 等，2007；Umemura 等，2003；Venkatraghavan 等，2006；Voges 等，2006）。

九、术后管理

患者 DBS 术后早期主诉多为疲劳，主要是与 DBS 手术中患者的紧张和情绪反应相关。但是在部分病例中，疲劳和困倦是由于气颅或谵妄状态的表现。术后头痛也较为常见，可以应用对乙酰氨基酚联合阿片类或 α_2 受体激动药如可乐定治疗。若患者头痛症状对多种药物治疗均无效，可以考虑应用艾司氯胺酮。推荐所有 DBS 术后患者进行 24h 神经监护，包括身体条件比较好且手术时间短、无并发症的年轻患者，随后可以考虑早期转入普通病区。对 PD 患者术后尽早恢复 PD 药物治疗，这样有助于患者尽快恢复和缓解紧张压力。术后延迟药物治疗或者改变用药方案可加重临床症状并诱发严重运动障碍或肌张力障碍（Blanshard 等，2001；Osborn 等，2015；Urasaki 等，2013）。

十、DBS 刺激器置入手术麻醉

DBS 手术第二步是植入神经刺激器。DBS 电极连接延长导线，通过皮下隧道延伸至锁骨下区域或腹部右下 1/4 象限并与刺激器相连接。通常刺激器是在电极植入术后 1～4 周后植入，但是也有部分中心将刺激器和电极同期植入。植入过程可以在应用喉罩或气管插管全身麻醉下进行，相关风险与心脏起搏器植入手术相类似。术中对麻醉药物的选择无特殊限制。

十一、结论

随着手术适应证和人口老龄化的增加，DBS 手术需求也将持续增加，对于擅长功能神经外科手术麻醉的专家需求也会逐渐增加。各医学中心也会依据神经外科医生的手术需求和患者状态建立自己的 DBS 手术相关麻醉技术。到目前尚未证实哪一种麻醉技术更适合 DBS 手术。最重要的是，DBS 手术成功有赖于合理患者选择、专注的手术团队和标准的手术和麻醉流程。

参考文献

[1] Aarsland D, Creese B, Politis M, et al. Cognitive decline in Parkinson disease. Nat Rev Neurol. 2017;13:217–31.

[2] Aronow WS. Management of hypertension in patients undergoing surgery. Ann Transl Med. 2017;5:227.

[3] Ashkan K, Alamri A, Ughratdar I. Anti-coagulation and deep brain stimulation: never the twain shall meet? Stereotact Funct Neurosurg. 2015;93:373–7.

[4] Benabid AL, Chabardes S, Mitrofanis J, Pollak P. Deep brain stimulation of the subthalamic nucleus for the treatment of Parkinson's disease. Lancet Neurol. 2009;8:67–81.

[5] Bhatia KP, Bain P, Bajaj N, et al. Consensus statement on the classification of tremors. From the task force on tremor of the International Parkinson and Movement Disorder Society. Mov Disord. 2018;33:75–87.

[6] Binder DK, Rau GM, Starr PA. Risk factors for hemorrhage during microelectrode-guided deep brain stimulator implantation for movement disorders. Neurosurgery. 2005;56:722–32.

[7] Blanshard HJ, Chung F, Manninen PH, et al. Awake craniotomy for removal of intracranial tumor: considerations for early discharge. Anesth Analg. 2001;92:89–94.

[8] Bloor M, Nandi R, Thomas M. Antiepileptic drugs and anesthesia. Paediatr Anaesth. 2017;27:248–50.

[9] Burchiel KJ, McCartney S, Lee A, Raslan AM. Accuracy of deep brain stimulation electrode placement using intraoperative computed tomography without microelectrode recording. J Neurosurg. 2013;119:301–6.

[10] Burnand C, Sebastian J. Anaesthesia for awake craniotomy. Contin Educ Anaesth Crit Care Pain. 2014;14:6–11.

[11] Burton DA, Nicholson G, Hall GM. Anaesthesia in elderly patients with neurodegenerative disorders: special considerations. Drugs Aging. 2004;21:229–42.

[12] Carlson JD, Neumiller JJ, Swain LD, et al. Postoperative delirium

in Parkinson's disease patients following deep brain stimulation surgery. J Clin Neurosci. 2014;21:1192–5.
[13] Castrioto A, Marmor O, Deffains M, et al. Anesthesia reduces discharge rates in the human pallidum without changing the discharge rate ratio between pallidal segments. Eur J Neurosci. 2016;44:2909–13.
[14] Chakrabarti R, Ghazanwy M, Tewari A. Anesthetic challenges for deep brain stimulation: a systematic approach. N Am J Med Sci. 2014;6:359–69.
[15] Chang EF, Cheng JS, Richardson RM, et al. Incidence and management of venous air embolisms during awake deep brain stimulation surgery in a large clinical series. Stereotact Funct Neurosurg. 2011;89:76–82.
[16] Chen T, Mirzadeh Z, Ponce FA. "Asleep" deep brain stimulation surgery: a critical review of the literature. World Neurosurg. 2017;105:191–8.
[17] Committee on Standards and Practice Parameters; American Society of Anesthesiologists Task Force on Preanesthesia Evaluation, Apfelbaum JL, Connis RT, et al. Practice advisory for preanesthesia evaluation an updated report by the American Society of Anesthesiologists Task Force on Preanesthesia Evaluation. Anesthesiology. 2012;116:522–38.
[18] Costello TG, Cormack JR. Anaesthesia for awake craniotomy: a modern approach. J Clin Neurosci. 2004;11:16–9.
[19] Cravedi E, Deniau E, Giannitelli M, et al. Tourette syndrome and other neurodevelopmental disorders: a comprehensive review. Child Adolesc Psychiatry Ment Health. 2017;11:59.
[20] Del Tredici K, Rüb U, De Vos RA, et al. Where does parkinson disease pathology begin in the brain? J Neuropathol Exp Neurol. 2002;61:413–26.
[21] El-Boghdadly K, Chin KJ. Local anesthetic systemic toxicity: continuing professional development. Can J Anaesth. 2016;63:330–49.
[22] Elias WJ, Durieux ME, Huss D, Frysinger RC. Dexmedetomidine and arousal affect subthalamic neurons. Mov Disord. 2008;23:1317–20.
[23] Erickson KM, Cole DJ. Anesthetic considerations for awake craniotomy for epilepsy. Anesthesiol Clin. 2007;25:535–55.
[24] Fasano A, Visanji NP, Liu LW, et al. Gastrointestinal dysfunction in Parkinson's disease. Lancet Neurol. 2015;14:625–39.
[25] Fenoy AJ, Simpson RK Jr. Risks of common complications in deep brain stimulation surgery: management and avoidance. J Neurosurg. 2014;120:132–9.
[26] Fleisher LA. Anesthesia and uncommon diseases. 6th ed. Philadelphia, PA: Elsevier/Saunders, 2006
[27] Frerk C, Mitchell VS, McNarry AF, et al. Difficult airway society 2015 guidelines for management of unanticipated difficult intubation in adults. Br J Anaesth. 2015;115:827–48.
[28] Galvan A, Wichmann T. GABAergic circuits in the basal ganglia and movement disorders. Prog Brain Res. 2007;160:287–312.
[29] Gorgulho A, De Salles AA, Frighetto L, Behnke E. Incidence of hemorrhage associated with electrophysiological studies performed using macroelectrodes and microelectrodes in functional neurosurgery. J Neurosurg. 2005;102:888–96.
[30] Grant R, Gruenbaum SE, Gerrard J. Anaesthesia for deep brain stimulation: a review. Curr Opin Anaesthesiol. 2015;28:505–10.
[31] Halliday GM, Li YW, Blumbergs PC, Joh TH, et al. Neuropathology of immunohistochemically identified brainstem neurons in Parkinson's disease. Ann Neurol. 1990;27:373–85.
[32] Hans P, Bonhomme V, Born JD, et al. Target-controlled infusion of propofol and remifentanil combined with bispectral index monitoring for awake craniotomy. Anaesthesia. 2000;55:255–9.
[33] Harries AM, Kausar J, Roberts SA, et al. Deep brain stimulation of the subthalamic nucleus for advanced Parkinson disease using general anesthesia: long-term results. J Neurosurg. 2012;116:107–13.
[34] Hartle A, McCormack T, Carlisle J, et al. The measurement of adult blood pressure and management of hypertension before elective surgery. Anaesthesia. 2016;71:326–37.
[35] Ho AL, Ali R, Connolly ID, et al. Awake versus asleep deep brain stimulation for Parkinson's disease: a critical comparison and meta-analysis. J Neurol Neurosurg Psychiatry. 2018;89:687–91.
[36] Hooper AK, Okun MS, Foote KD, et al. Venous air embolism in deep brain stimulation. Stereotact Funct Neurosurg. 2009;87:25–30.
[37] Hovestadt A, Bogaard JM, Meerwaldt JD, et al. Pulmonary function in Parkinson's disease. J Neurol Neurosurg Psychiatry. 1989;52:329–33.
[38] Hutchison WD, Lang AE, Dostrovsky JO, Lozano AM. Pallidal neuronal activity: implications for models of dystonia. Ann Neurol. 2003;53:480–8.
[39] Johns DW, Ayers CR, Carey RM. The dopamine agonist bromocriptine induces hypotension by venous and arteriolar dilation. J Cardiovasc Pharmacol. 1984;6:582–7.
[40] Kenney C, Simpson R, Hunter C, et al. Short-term and long-term safety of deep brain stimulation in the treatment of movement disorders. J Neurosurg. 2007;106:621–5.
[41] Khatib R, Ebrahim Z, Rezai A, et al. Perioperative events during deep brain stimulation: the experience at Cleveland Clinic. J Neurosurg Anesthesiol. 2008;20:36–40.
[42] Kirksey MA, Haskins SC, Cheng J, Liu SS. Local anesthetic peripheral nerve block adjuvants for prolongation of analgesia: a systematic qualitative review. PLoS One. 2015;10:e0137312.
[43] Kisilewicz M, Rosenberg H, Vaillancourt C. Remifentanil for procedural sedation: a systematic review of the literature. Emerg Med J. 2017;34:294–301.
[44] Kita H, Chiken S, Tachibana Y, Nambu A. Origins of GABA(A) and GABA(B) receptor-mediated responses of globus pallidus induced after stimulation of the putamen in the monkey. J Neurosci. 2006;26:6554–662.
[45] Kouvaras E, Asprodini EK, Asouchidou E, et al. Fentanyl treatment reduces GABAergic inhibition in the CA1 area of the hippocampus 24 h after acute exposure to the drug. Neuropharmacology. 2008;55:1172–82.
[46] Lamperti M. Adult procedural sedation: an update. Curr Opin Anaesthesiol. 2015;28:662–7.
[47] Lazio BE, Simard JM. Anticoagulation in neurosurgical patients. Neurosurgery. 1999;45:838–47.
[48] Lee JY, Deogaonkar M, Rezai A. Deep brain stimulation of globus pallidus internus for dystonia. Parkinsonism Relat Disord. 2007;13:261–5.
[49] Lin SH, Chen TY, Lin SZ, et al. Subthalamic deep brain stimulation after anesthetic inhalation in Parkinson disease: a preliminary study. J Neurosurg. 2008;109:238–44.
[50] Louis ED. Non-motor symptoms in essential tremor: a review of the current data and state of the field. Parkinsonism Relat Disord. 2016;22:S115–8.
[51] Lozano AM, Kumar R, Gross RE, et al. Globus pallidus internus pallidotomy for generalized dystonia. Mov Disord. 1997;12:865–70.
[52] Maltête D, Navarro S, Welter M, et al. Subthalamic stimulation in Parkinson disease: with or without anesthesia? Arch Neurol. 2004;61:390–2.
[53] Manninen PH, Balki M, Lukitto K, Bernstein M. Patient satisfaction with awake craniotomy for tumor surgery: a comparison of remifentanil and fentanyl in conjunction with propofol. Anesth Analg. 2006;102:237–42.
[54] Matias CM, Frizon LA, Nagel SJ, et al. Deep brain stimulation outcomes in patients implanted under general anesthesia with frame-based stereotaxy and intraoperative MRI. J Neurosurg. 2018;129:1572–8.
[55] Miocinovic S, Somayajula S, Chitnis S, Vitek JL. History, applications, and mechanisms of deep brain stimulation. JAMA Neurol. 2013;70:163–71.
[56] Moll CK, Payer S, Gulberti A, et al. STN stimulation in general anaesthesia: evidence beyond 'evidence-based medicine'. Acta Neurochir Suppl. 2013;117:19–25.
[57] Moore C, Dobson A, Kinagi M, Dillon B. Comparison of blood pressure measured at the arm, ankle and calf. Anaesthesia. 2008;63:1327–31.
[58] Morace R, De Angelis M, Aglialoro E, et al. Sedation with α2 agonist dexmedetomidine during unilateral subthalamic nucleus deep brain stimulation: a preliminary report. World Neurosurg. 2016;89:320–8.
[59] Nicholson G, Pereira AC, Hall GM. Parkinson's disease and anaesthesia. Br J Anaesth. 2002;89:904–16.

[60] Noyce AJ, Silveira-Moriyama L, Gilpin P, et al. Severe dysphagia as a presentation of Parkinson's disease. Mov Disord. 2012;27:457–8.

[61] Osborn IP, Kurtis SD, Alterman RL. Functional neurosurgery: anesthetic considerations. Int Anesthesiol Clin. 2015;53:39–52.

[62] Palmon SC, Moore LE, Lundberg J, Toung T. Venous air embolism: a review. J Clin Anesth. 1997;9:251–7.

[63] Peduto A, Concas A, Santoro G, et al. Biochemical and electrophysiologic evidence that propofol enhances GABAergic transmission in the rat brain. Anesthesiology. 1991;75:1000–9.

[64] Pepper PV, Goldstein MK. Postoperative complications in Parkinson's disease. J Am Geriatr Soc. 1999;47:967–72.

[65] Perks A, Cheema S, Mohanraj R. Anaesthesia and epilepsy. Br J Anaesth. 2012;108:562–71.

[66] Pfeiffer RF. Gastrointestinal dysfunction in Parkinson's disease. Parkinsonism Relat Disord. 2011;17:10–5.

[67] Poon CC, Irwin MG. Anaesthesia for deep brain stimulation and in patients with implanted neurostimulator devices. Br J Anaesth. 2009;103:152–65.

[68] Ramachandran SK, Mathis MR, Tremper KK, et al. Predictors and clinical outcomes from failed Laryngeal Mask Airway Unique™: a study of 15,795 patients. Anesthesiology. 2012;116:1217–26.

[69] Raz A, Eimerl D, Zaidel A, et al. Propofol decreases neuronal population spiking activity in the subthalamic nucleus of Parkinsonian patients. Anesth Analg. 2010;111:1285–9.

[70] Rezai AR, Kopell BH, Gross RE, et al. Deep brain stimulation for Parkinson's disease: surgical issues. Mov Disord. 2006;21:S197–218.

[71] Roessner V, Plessen KJ, Rothenberger A, et al. European clinical guidelines for Tourette syndrome and other tic disorders. Part II: pharmacological treatment. Eur Child Adolesc Psychiatry. 2011;20:173–96.

[72] Rozet I. Anesthesia for functional neurosurgery: the role of dexmedetomidine. Curr Opin Anaesthesiol. 2008;21:537–43.

[73] Rozet I, Vavilala MS. Risks and benefits of patient positioning during neurosurgical care. Anesthesiol Clin. 2007;25:631–53.

[74] Rozet I, Muangman S, Vavilala MS, et al. Clinical experience with dexmedetomidine for implantation of deep brain stimulators in Parkinson's disease. Anesth Analg. 2006;103:1224–8.

[75] Sánchez-Ferro A, Benito-León J, Gómez-Esteban JC. The management of orthostatic hypotension in Parkinson's disease. Front Neurol. 2013;4:64.

[76] Sanghera MK, Grossman RG, Kalhorn CG, et al. Basal ganglia neuronal discharge in primary and secondary dystonia in patients undergoing pallidotomy. Neurosurgery. 2003;52:1358–70.

[77] Saraghi M, Golden L, Hersh EV. Anesthetic considerations for patients on antidepressant therapy – Part II. Anesth Prog. 2018;65:60–5.

[78] Sarang A, Dinsmore J. Anaesthesia for awake craniotomy—evolution of a technique that facilitates awake neurological testing. Br J Anaesth. 2003;90:161–5.

[79] Sassi M, Zekaj E, Grotta A, et al. Safety in the use of dexmedetomidine (Precedex) for deep brain stimulation surgery: our experience in 23 randomized patients. Neuromodulation. 2013;16:401–6.

[80] Sheshadri V, Rowland NC, Mehta J, et al. Comparison of general and local anesthesia for deep brain stimulator insertion: a systematic review. Can J Neurol Sci. 2017;44:697–704.

[81] Smit M, Kuiper A, Han V, et al. Psychiatric co-morbidity is highly prevalent in idiopathic cervical dystonia and significantly influences health-related quality of life: results of a controlled study. Parkinsonism Relat Disord. 2016;30:7–12.

[82] Tomic S, Pekic V, Popijac Z, et al. What increases the risk of malnutrition in Parkinson's disease? J Neurol Sci. 2017;375:235–8.

[83] Tsai ST, Chuang WY, Kuo CC, et al. Dorsolateral subthalamic neuronal activity enhanced by median nerve stimulation characterizes Parkinson's disease during deep brain stimulation with general anesthesia. J Neurosurg. 2015;123:1394–400.

[84] Umemura A, Jaggi JL, Hurtig HI, et al. Deep brain stimulation for movement disorders: morbidity and mortality in 109 patients. J Neurosurg. 2003;98:779–84.

[85] Urasaki E, Fukudome T, Hirose M, et al. Neuroleptic malignant syndrome (parkinsonism–hyperpyrexia syndrome) after deep brain stimulation of the subthalamic nucleus. J Clin Neurosci. 2013;20:740–1.

[86] Venkatraghavan L, Manninen P. Anesthesia for deep brain stimulation. Curr Opin Anaesthesiol. 2011;24:495–9.

[87] Venkatraghavan L, Manninen P, Mak P, et al. Anesthesia for functional neurosurgery: a review of complications. J Neurosurg Anesthesiol. 2006;18:64–70.

[88] Venkatraghavan L, Luciano M, Manninen P. Review article: anesthetic management of patients undergoing deep brain stimulator insertion. Anesth Analg. 2010;110:1138–45.

[89] Venkatraghavan L, Rakhman E, Krishna V, et al. The effect of general anesthesia on the microelectrode recordings from pallidal neurons in patients with dystonia. J Neurosurg Anesthesiol. 2016;28:256–61.

[90] Voges J, Waerzeggers Y, Maarouf M, et al. Deep-brain stimulation: long-term analysis of complications caused by hardware and surgery—experiences from a single centre. J Neurol Neurosurg Psychiatry. 2006;77:868–72.

[91] Yamada K, Goto S, Kuratsu J, et al. Stereotactic surgery for subthalamic nucleus stimulation under general anesthesia: a retrospective evaluation of Japanese patients with Parkinson's disease. Parkinsonism Relat Disord. 2007;13:101–7.

[92] Ziemssen T, Reichmann H. Cardiovascular autonomic dysfunction in Parkinson's disease. J Neurol Sci. 2010;289:74–80.

[93] Zrinzo L, Foltynie T, Limousin P, Hariz MI. Reducing hemorrhagic complications in functional neurosurgery: a large case series and systematic literature review. J Neurosurg. 2012;116:84–94.

第8章 程控：通用特性
Programming: General Aspects

Clecio de Oliveira Godeiro Jr.　Elena Moro　Erwin B. Montgomery Jr.　著
王慧敏　胡文瀚　译　王　秀　杨岸超　张建国　校

> **摘要**：过去20年来，虽然对脑深部电刺激（DBS）治疗的一些潜在获益或不良反应尚不明确，但对于大脑如何对个体化DBS脉冲做出反应还是有一定程度的了解。众所周知，DBS是通过电极触点作负极向周围轴突产生动作电位而作用。DBS脉冲通过神经元轴突的细胞膜去极化启动电压门控通道进而在轴突发挥作用。
>
> DBS设备可设定电流（恒压刺激模式下的电压）、脉冲宽度并结合神经生物物理学特性以达到DBS程控的最佳治疗。DBS原始效应的启动是通过整个系统滴定效应来实现的，包括反滴效应和正滴效应。而DBS的次级效应对临床疗效也至关重要。振荡活动及其相互作用导致临床效应的周期性现象。因此虽然DBS的电流和脉冲宽度对原始效应极为重要，但DBS的频率对次级效应也至关重要。所以在程控时相对独立的电流和脉冲宽度，频率也须作为一个独立的控制参数。由此总电能输出（TEED）不能作为一个全面的概括。
>
> DBS程控治疗的有效性和高效率涉及广泛。程控不仅仅是调整电流、脉冲宽度、频率和触点参数。在运动障碍病如帕金森病等治疗中，需要将DBS治疗与其他治疗方法综合应用。治疗所需工具不仅包括DBS程控设备，还需要评估DBS疗效的工具，特别是在DBS程控中存在多重复杂因素影响时。然而，有相当多的证据表明，适当的DBS编程可以极大地改变患者的生活质量。

一、概述

脑深部电刺激治疗（DBS）比最佳药物治疗更有效、更安全。帕金森病（PD）的前瞻性对照试验证实了这一点（Weaver等，2012）。还有证据来自于前瞻性非对照试验，在这些试验中，药物疗效减弱的患者仍然可以通过DBS得到改善。对于这些患者而言，DBS比最佳药物治疗更有效。同样地，当其他替代疗法失效时，DBS通常会有其治疗优势。DBS挑战了生理学和病理生理学的基本概念（Montgomery，2012），是神经病学的一项重大进展，可能会取代运动障碍疾病如PD治疗中已有的神经递质替代疗法。

（一）伦理

DBS治疗需要开启刺激器并设置最佳刺激参数。开机前DBS没有获益。所以DBS的最优效果取决于程控人员的技能、知识、经验和奉献精神。医生和卫生专业人员较其他人员更加权威（Montgomery，2018）。通常，患者依赖于程控人员的专业性和医德，而程控人员在工作中则本着负责的工作态度。此外，程控人员有义务完成自己的工作，所有程控人员需要在条件允许的情况下为患者提供最佳的照护，并尽可能改善护理的条件及环境。程控人员通过承担集体责任以回报社会。我们期望程控这个职业能够产生有价值的东西，这也是绝大多数程控人员对自己的期望。问责制是一种价值判断。我们不应该耻于以"好"或"不好"来描述境况，也许这是最诚实的做法。

目前的问题是程控人员不足和如何解决这一不足。指出那些不好的情况、环境和行为是一种责任。这种评价是针对整体的情境和行动的，而不是针对某个程控人员。回顾分析2个运动障碍病中心41例DBS术后疗效不满意患者，其中37%的患者术后程控方案不理想，重新程控后得到显著改善（Okun等，2005）。很难说程控人员为何没有确认患者不佳状态。通过调整刺激参数和药物，甚至可以改善DBS治疗PD的固有疗效（Moro等，2006）。当然这并不意味着程控的目标可以是不切实际的完美状态。完美可以是期望，却不一定是必然。在本章中，反复指出了现实中的限制及其对DBS程控的影响。

（二）程控的多种方法及发展史

粗略回顾有关DBS程控相关描述发现了程控治疗方案的多样性。该多样性值得深思。如果每种方案在每种情境下都能实现合理预期结果，这是否意味着用哪种方法并不重要？然而，之前的研究发现，有一定比例的患者没有达到合理的预期结果，而是重新程控后得以改善。如果不是每种方式都能达到合理的预期结果，那么哪种方法是最好的呢？如果有更好的模式，如何说服程控员使用该模式？最后一个问题很关键，如果只知道一种特定的模式，程控人员就不太可能对这种方法提出质疑。Abraham Maslow 在1966年曾说，"如果你唯一的工具是一把锤子，把所有东西都当成钉子的想法很诱人。"本章的主题是为程控人员提供神经生理学理论和实践工具，而不是现象学、模式识别或基础的默认方式。

正如将讨论的那样，有3种通用的DBS程控方式。这些方式已经在医学中根深蒂固地存在了几个世纪。临床医生已经潜意识地适应了特定的治疗方式，很难选择其他的治疗方式。这样的描述并非贬损，而是历史的遗留问题。值得注意的是，这些方法不是随意的，而是临床医生认知的直接结果（Montgomery，2018）。更大的问题是当默认一种立场会阻碍对其他观点的判断分析。这种情况对临床术后DBS照护预期的改善并无好处。

（三）程控方法

根据疾病及治疗将程控方法分为3种。一种方法是设置每根电极及刺激参数直到患者达到合理的预期值，或者患者和程控人员出现疲劳效应，即"猎枪法"。该方法源于古希腊以来的经验主义，即个体现象都是新生或独特的。其假设最佳治疗是根据患者个体的情况来定而非按一般原则推断。从过去经验或他人经验中归纳是没有意义的。DBS程控的另一种方法是复制平常或典型的电极设置［例如激活的阴极（负极）和阳极（正极）的组合］和刺激参数［电压或电流幅度、脉冲宽度（PW）和频率］。这种方法类似于教条主义，他们认为诊断和治疗可以直接参考已有知识，如专家共识。举个生动例子，使用组织激活体积（VTA）的工程建模来指导编程。一项研究称建模与否在减少资源要求方面没有显著性差异（Pourfar等，2015）。但是因研究者未使用合适的非劣效性研究设计，其研究结果是无法得到解释。如前所述，将VTA作为典型是使用不当的。相反，应该是静电场的体积（VES）。DBS程控的第三种方法是基于电学、电子学、生理学、解剖学和逻辑学的基本原理的。理性主义者或对症治疗医师例证该法，他们试图将各种现象与基本原理相结合加以理解（Montgomery，2018）。这些方法是源于对广泛临床表现多样化的理论认识，而非实践证实（Montgomery，2018）。

073

目前没有任何理论或经验证实哪种方法优于其他。事实上，大多数程控人员是将这些方法进行组合使用，虽然也会强调某一方法。尚无对照试验来比较这些方法，部分原因是这些方法还没有充分系统化，不能对参与这些试验的程控人员进行分类。每种方法需要不同的假设和不同的含义。例如，采用第二种方法即教条法可以最大限度地提高效率，但需要最佳电极设置和刺激参数的个体化差异最小化。换而言之，教条法是假定所有患者相关的因素都是平均而典型的，而这在现实中是不可能的。第三种方法即理性法，假设DBS患者的临床多样性可分解为数个基本理论和实践单元，这在实际中可能发生，也可能无法实现。第一种方法即经验法，则侧重于个体化，该方法无预定方案，需面对较多的电极设置与刺激参数的组合。无论何种方法至少要实现疗效最大化且不良反应最小化。

本章通过讨论DBS基础理论指导程控的观点来支持理性DBS程控方法。涉及电学、电子学、生理学和生理解剖学学科。教条法不灵活，经验法又因电极和刺激参数的多重组合而过分灵活。理性法在完成原理的初步理解后就会节省成本，同时能够随着进展进行适时整合。整合所依据的电学、电子学、生理学和生理解剖学原理虽大相径庭，但其本身不会有太大改变。DBS的电极是分段独立的，划分的触点都能够分配电流，并设置多种刺激模式以便能够更大程度的改善患者症状。这也造成了DBS程控治疗更加复杂化。

有趣的是从DBS首次用于运动障碍病（Cooper等，1980）到发展为公认的临床疗法（Benabid等，1987），关于DBS治疗的作用机制，并没有多少理论和时间依据。因此，教条法和经验法的普遍使用就不足为奇了。如今即便已经了解大量关于神经元如何反馈DBS脉冲的理论，但对于其作用机制仍不清楚。这也反映出生理学和病理生理学知识的不足。事实上，最初的观点认为高频DBS是抑制作用而低频刺激则激活靶点核团，这一理论指导了DBS程控的设置，尽管该理论在当时被认为可能是错误的（Montgomery和Baker，2000）。

这并不是说神经元放电频率没有降低，在某些情况下，通过刺激突触前末端释放神经递质，从而导致突触后神经元超极化。这种细胞的超极化可能导致突触前神经元动作电位的减少。与此同时，却发现轴突丘的动作电位起始节或近端轴突的节间（Ranvier节点）处可诱发动作电位（Coombs等，1957；Llinas和Terzuolo，1964；Steriade等，1974；McIntyre和Grill，1999）。因此深入理解神经元对DBS刺激的反应，虽然复杂，却是掌握理性程控法的重要工具。

二、DBS近似效应和电压门控离子通道

（一）DBS的近似效应

脑深部电刺激的原始或近似效应引起可兴奋细胞周围电场的变化，这些可兴奋细胞在大脑中可以移动电荷（离子）。这种生理效应必须由那些对静电场变化敏感的可兴奋细胞来调节。主要的敏感元素是电压门控离子通道。这些通道通常位于轴突上，因此，DBS刺激的直接作用可能是由轴突介导的。静电场的变化导致轴突细胞膜上的电压发生超极化或去极化。当去极化超过阈值时，产生动作电位。除非产生动作电位，否则很大比例的神经元不会产生生理效应，尤其是那些最终被DBS激活的生理网络下游的神经元。还需要关注神经树突上的其他受体，例如，N-甲基-D-天冬氨酸（NMDA）受体会受到周围静电场变化的影响。但具体效应尚不明确。

神经元效应是由静电场变化的方向决定的。例如，阴极（负极）DBS刺激可能会在周围的轴突产生去极化，达到阈值时就会产生动作电位。阳极（正极）电刺激通常产生轴突的超极化，减少动作电位产生的可能性。但是超极化可以导致电压门控离子通道的激活，当超极化完成时，神经元就会反弹激活（Montgomery，2006）。反弹性兴奋普遍存在于基底神经节-丘脑-皮质系

统的神经元中。

DBS 刺激的效果取决于轴突表面的静电场产生的电荷量，电荷量则由电荷施加的速度（电流）和脉冲宽度（PW）的持续时间决定。电荷量用微库仑（μC）计量。电流是由电荷被施加在轴突上的强度（电压）和电荷流动的阻力（电阻）决定的。电压（V）、电流（I）、电阻（R）通过欧姆定律联系起来，V=I·R。这些因素为 DBS 程控人员优化 DBS 治疗提供机制支持。

DBS 刺激的频率也可以用来优化治疗。然而，DBS 的频率效应更为复杂。DBS 刺激的常规频率下，轴突上单个神经元动作电位的发生概率是微不足道的。要产生直接的效果，就必须有 DBS 脉冲刺激（时间总和）的重叠效应，至少需要达到每秒 300 个脉冲的刺激。若 DBS 频率的影响只是简单的时间叠加，频率增加的生理效应应该是单调递增的，但事实并非如此（Huang 等，2014）。与之相反，DBS 可能通过阴极（触点为负极）周围大量轴突产生的同步动作电位的空间总和而产生临床效应。

生理效应也取决于 DBS 电极触点周围的生理解剖。刺激预期轴突是获益的必要条件，而刺激非预期轴突可能会产生不良反应。不同患者的局部解剖可能存在很大差异，同一个患者由于神经元迁徙亦导致解剖不同，进而使得 DBS 程控更加复杂。尽管如此，生理解剖的知识仍可以帮助程控操作人解释脑深部电刺激的临床疗效。结合对神经电生理机制的理解，可以指导优化 DBS 的最佳治疗。例如，可以重建图 8-1 中假设所示的 VES（区别于 VTA）的区域解剖结构。

然而，更重要的是要意识到指导 DBS 程控的 VES 假设并非解剖学上的最佳靶点，实际上是生理学上的靶点。底丘脑核（STN）作为靶点的观点是错误的。事实上真正的靶点是指 STN 的感觉运动区，而其边缘区和认知区域是需要避开的。迄今为止，尚无解剖学成像来划分 STN 的分区；仅推断感觉 - 运动区的位置在某种程度上与解剖相关。该相关的强弱决定了基于影像学方法的稳定性。而基于电生理特性的方法则并不

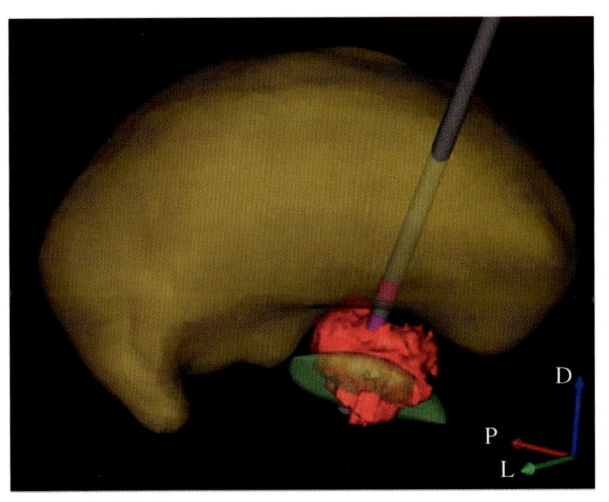

基于 DTI 的组织介质，电极封装

▲ 图 8-1 显示了作者在研究中称之为组织激活体积（VTA），实际上是静电场的体积

该模型基于患者的磁共振成像（MRI）创建的。扩散张量成像（DTI）用以计算影响 DBS 相关静电场的体积和形状的组织阻抗。黄色较大的结构是丘脑，绿色的是底丘脑核。红色体积为静电场的体积（引自 Butson 等，2007）

依赖于此假设。同样，DBS 的靶点也并非特指丘脑腹侧中间核（Vim）或苍白球内侧部（GPi）。而是指与患者主要功能障碍相应的亚区。

必须考虑的局部生理解剖还包括轴突通路。事实上，考虑到 DBS 脉冲信号在产生轴突动作电位方面的近似效应，DBS 作用很可能是由靶点附近的轴突通路介导的。图 8-2 显示了 STN 周围的一些相关通路。有相当多的证据表明，DBS 作用的一种治疗机制是在从皮质到 STN 的超直接通路中产生动作电位（图 8-2C 中的紫色部分）。不良反应可能是由于刺激皮质脊髓通路导致强直性肌肉收缩（图 8-2B 中的白色通路），以及刺激小脑丘脑束引起共济失调（图 8-2D 中橙色部分）。

（二）DBS 和药物治疗

除影响 DBS 治疗的生理因素外，还存在一些实际问题。以 PD 的 DBS 治疗为例，需要 DBS 与药物协同作用。事实上，DBS 的程控需要结合药物动力学(临床反应随药物周期的变化)

的时间变化。我们在优化 DBS 时不能忽略药物治疗，尤其是当 DBS 治疗药物引起的并发症时。至少对于 PD 治疗，DBS 程控人员不仅要有神经电生理和解剖学的专业知识，还要有药理相关的专业知识。由此，我们需要程控人员在所有方面都有相应的能力。

（三）综合性决策

除教条法，DBS 程控通常需要综合性决定。了解如何综合制定 DBS 程控方案与其他决策相比获益更多。实际上，每项决策都源于诊断，例如，判断特定患者的疗效或不良反应是什么？每项决策都需要兼顾所用工具正面和负面预期值。例如，程控者要评判某个 DBS 方案有用（阳性预测值，PPV）或无用（阴性预测值，NPV）。高 PPV 和 NPV 的方法或工具使得 DBS 程控更高效且有效。注意评判工具可能只是患者和程控人员之间的沟通交流，程控人员是否准确取得重要数据（假阴性）或是否误判患者陈述（假阳性）？答案取决于医生沟通中的敏感性，比如医生是否询问潜在数据和特异性资料。假设医生询问了此类问题，其取得准确信息的能力（概率）又如何？单独看敏感性或特异性对诊断而言并非有效指标。相反，必须将特异性和敏感性与贝叶斯定理中的先验概率结合起来，以便表明与该问题有关的问题属于什么可能性。结合特异性，敏感性和先验概率可以确定 PPV 和 NPV。

三、DBS 程控的生态学

DBS 的目的是改善患者的生活质量，伦理要求对患者的特殊问题进行滴定治疗。因为没有两名患者的疾病影响方式或优先顺序完全相同，所以最佳的 DBS / 药物联合治疗方案可能也不完全相同。个性化的术后 DBS 程控需要大量的精力和资源，而程控员常作为"守门员"。脑深部电刺激的程控员须在特定的医疗环境中进行操作，这可能会极大地影响可用来进行治疗的资源和物流。因此，很可能没有两个诊所是完全相同

的。通常，DBS 程控的选择涉及相互竞争的利益之间的道德权衡，如资源和精力的支出。在患者药物最少状态下进行程控是最好的方式，如在药物治疗后禁食一夜。如此便需要医生清晨查看患者，这样会增加程控员日程安排的压力。同样地，在患者恢复药效时，需要观察 DBS 和药物的协同效应，尤其是不良反应。DBS 程控的推荐方案需要认识到资源需求和限制。鉴于这种多样性，本章唯一实用的方法是总结理想目标，以及影响实现该目标的因素，DBS 程控员能够以最佳的操作流程实现其患者的利益最大化。

不同的制造商有不同的 DBS 系统，讨论不同 DBS 设备所特有的程控方法是不切实际的。神经电生理理论可以指导程控员使用相应的 DBS 系统，而这些电生理理论基础又受到不同设计方案和工作原理的影响。可充电刺激器的出现大大改变了优化策略。在过去，电池使用寿命是固定的，电极配置和刺激参数的选择要保护电池寿命。程控人员尽量将刺激振幅、PW 和频率最小化。甚至有人提议使用 ≤ 60 微秒（μs）的 PW。但如后所述，从神经电生理的角度来看，这并不是最佳的选择，而且很可能对可充电刺激器的患者来说已不相关。

四、初始 DBS 程控的神经生理学内容

（一）轴突动作电位的生成是 DBS 的主要机制

脑深部电刺激通过在激活触点周围产生静电场来发挥作用。电场将带电离子移动到细胞膜的表面，以影响可兴奋细胞细胞膜上的电势。因此，DBS 首先作用于神经元中的电压敏感结构。最可能涉及的结构是细胞膜上的电压门控离子通道，这些通道主要位于轴突的细胞膜上。一般来说，这些通道是根据通过该通道的离子来定义的，包括钠离子（Na^+）、钾离子（K^+）、钙离子（Ca^{2+}）、氯离子（Cl^-），以及改变细胞膜电势的

第 8 章 程控：通用特性
Programming: General Aspects

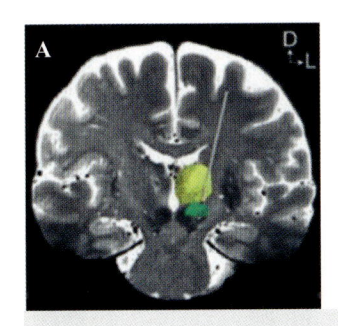

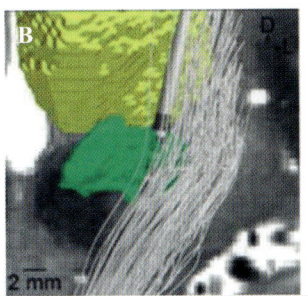

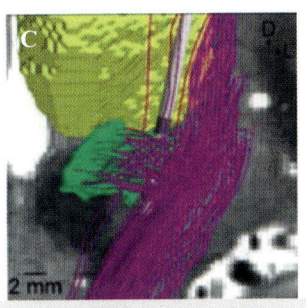

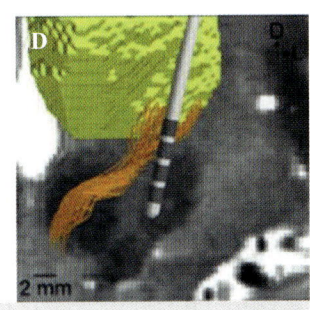

▲ 图 8-2 患者特异性轴突通路
A. 7T T₂ 加权磁共振图像的冠状面，以及 DBS 电极（Medtronic model 3389）、丘脑（黄色）和底丘脑核（绿色）；100 例人群纤维：B. 内囊纤维（白色流线）；C. 超直接通路（粉红色流线）；D. 小脑丘脑束（橙色流线）

离子电导。例如，要改变 Na^+ 电导，必须将细胞膜去极化［开放（译者注：超极化应该是开放的细胞膜电压，原著此处错误）细胞膜上的电压］到一定的阈值，而超极化（降低细胞膜上的电压）可能会影响 K^+ 通道。值得注意的是，细胞膜上存在许多不同的离子通道，虽然一些通道有着相同的离子，如 Na^+、K^+、Ca^{2+}，但其反应则存在很大差异（Ranck，1975）。

电压门控离子通道受 DBS 感应的静电场变化的影响。电压门控离子通道的变化使得细胞膜上电势发生改变，这种变化导致 DBS 脉冲产生的初始变化正反馈放大，如增加细胞膜 Na^+ 内流。随之而来的则是负反馈，降低效果，如 Na^+ 电压门控的离子通道失活并导致全或无动作电位。

当 DBS 脉冲为阴极（负极）时，在轴突表面会沉积负电荷，降低细胞膜外表面的净正性。当去极化超过阈值时，Na^+ 通道打开（初始反应），正电荷从电池的外部流向内部。该变化导致细胞膜外的正电荷进一步流失，并进一步去极化（二次反应正反馈）。去极化达到一定水平，就会打开其他的离子通道，比如 K^+ 通道，而 Na^+ 通道失活（负反馈）。K^+ 通道的激活导致正离子从细胞内流向细胞外，从而增加了细胞外的正极，称为超极化（图 8-3）。净响应是一个动作电位，它是 DBS 脉冲的直接作用。此外，动作电位导致其他离子通道的后期变化。例如，可能 Na^+ 通道失活，致使该结构变得难以接受随后的 DBS 脉冲。同样，随之可能会激活 Ca^{2+} 通道，造成

超极化之后的去极化，从而导致反弹或重复性动作电位。因此，在细胞膜的水平存在前馈和后馈机制，是高度非线性的。这意味着，在神经元上沉积负电荷以激发反应之间的关系不是简单增加电流（DBS 脉冲的振幅）和 PW 的问题。换言之，输出的总电能 = 刺激电流（安培、电压 ÷ 电阻）× PW × DBS 脉冲的频率（Brocker 和 Grill，2013），而不是控制变量。

（二）恒流恒压

DBS 神经生理反应依赖于改变神经系统靶点可兴奋细胞细胞膜上的电位。电位的变化取决于移动到细胞膜上的电荷数量［以微库仑（μC）计］。因此，决定神经元反应的关键因素是电流和脉冲宽度，而不是电压和脉冲宽度（Montgomery，2017）。电流乘以脉冲宽度可确定沉积在神经元膜上电荷的微库仑。只知道电压和脉冲宽度，并不能知道沉积了多少微库仑，除非知道前面所述欧姆定律所讨论的电阻值。在相同的电压和脉冲宽度下，如果电阻不同，则产生不同的微库仑。恒流（CC）刺激通过改变电压来补偿电阻的变化，而恒压（CV）刺激则不能进行代偿。因此，CC 比 CV 刺激更可取。随着时间的推移，阻抗可能会发生变化，特别是 DBS 植入的最初几个月变化最为明显。因此，CV 刺激的有效参数下，反应良好的患者发现，即使刺激参数没有任何变化，但其对 DBS 的反应会发生变化。此外，由于每个患者的阻抗可能

077

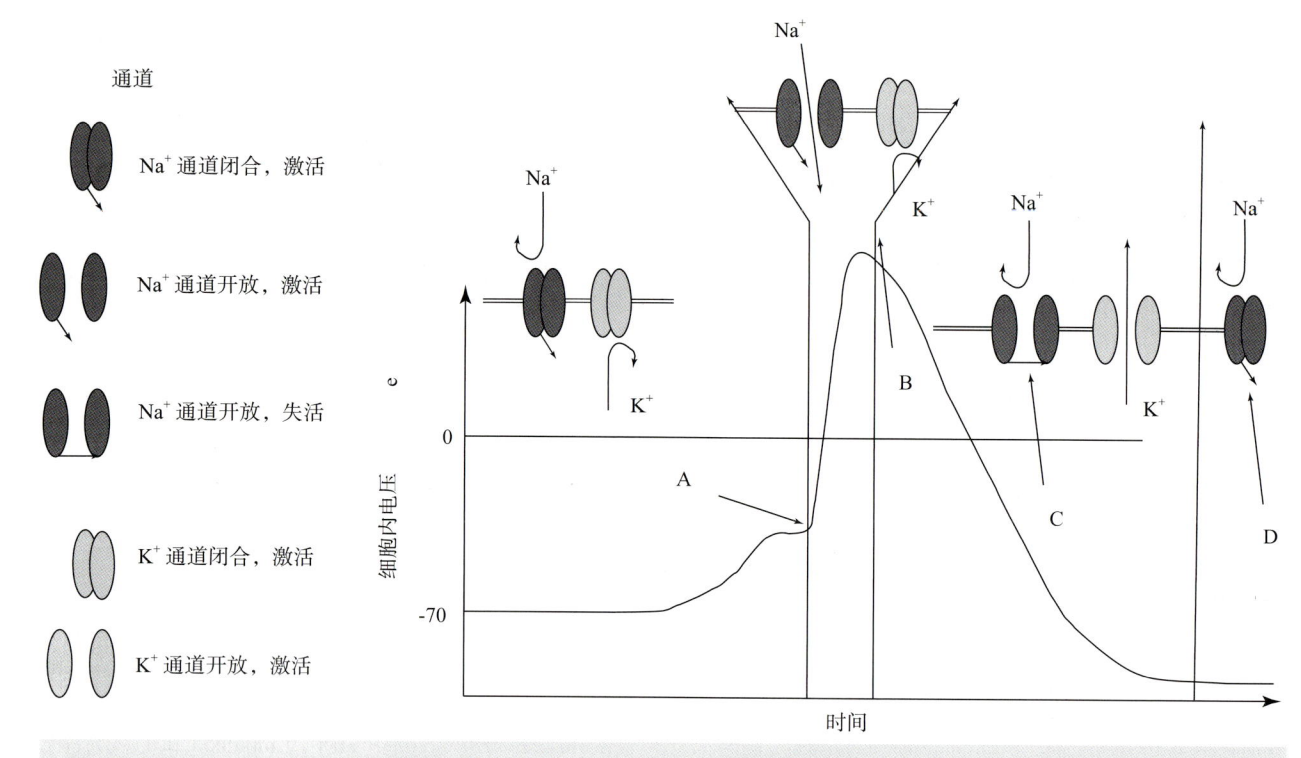

▲ 图 8-3 动作电位分布示意图

当神经元达到其静息膜电位或电压时，离子进入或离开神经元的离子通道就会关闭。因此，钠离子（Na⁺）不能进入神经元，钾离子（K⁺）不能离开。静息电压或电位（A）随后增加到 Na⁺ 通道阈值，打开 Na⁺ 通道，Na⁺ 进入神经元。Na⁺ 的流入进一步降低了膜电压，这种现象称为去极化。随着去极化，附加的 Na⁺ 通道打开，连锁反应产生动作电位。进一步的去极化到达阈值，K⁺ 通道打开，K⁺ 外流（B）。K⁺ 的这种流出将膜电压推向负值。极化还可以使 Na⁺ 通道（C）失活，从而阻止 Na⁺ 进一步内流。K⁺ 持续流出产生的负电压大于静止膜的负电压。此时的神经元已实现超极化。此时，Na⁺ 通道关闭并重新激活（D）（经许可转载，引自 Montgomery，2010）

不同，而且阻抗可能随着电极设置的不同而改变，因此很难从一个患者的经验总结为另一个患者的期望效果（Lempka 等，2009；Wei 和 Grill，2009；Sillay 等，2010，2013）。

除了阻抗对电荷传递有影响外，电极与脑组织间的电容也影响波形（DBS 刺激时间内电压或电流的变化）（Miocinovic 等，2009）。对于 CV 刺激，电荷积聚在大脑/电极界面上，导致电压累积以抵抗额外电荷的流动。最终的结果是 DBS 脉冲每一阶段所沉积的电荷减少，从而降低了 DBS 刺激的效果。DBS 的 CC 无此现象，有利于该模式的应用。

可以肯定的是，CV 和 CC 刺激都能提供电压和电流。按照欧姆定律，刺激期间的电压通过电阻与电流相关，E（电压）=I（电流）×R（电阻）。这并不是说 CC 刺激具有不同的生理作用。而是关于如何控制微库仑的传递的问题。在 CC 刺激中，电流是直接调控的，在设置了脉冲宽度的情况下，CC 刺激将在每个脉冲相位上产生恒定的微库仑电荷。在 CV 刺激中，电压是直接调控的，电流（进而是微库仑）取决于电阻。使用 CC 刺激可简化对动作电位生成的控制，能够对同一患者不同时间，以及不同患者之间的 DBS 进行比较。对患者个体而言，问题不在于 CC 或 CV 刺激是否更有效或更安全（Okun 等，2012；Ramirez de Noriega 等，2015；York 和 Moro，2017），因为无论哪种方式，都可以对两者进行设置，以获得相同的神经电生理反应，且在每个脉冲相位上传递相同数量的微库仑电荷。消除阻抗变化的潜在混淆，一定程度上有助于理解个体患者因时间而发生变化的现象，且能更方便与其他患者进行比较，以便于普及知识和方法。

(三) 动作电位产生的选择性

动作电位产生的关键决定因素是轴突细胞膜的去极化程度。而去极化的程度又取决于DBS脉冲每个节段传输的静电荷数［以微库仑（μC）计量］和激活的电压门控离子通道数（图8-4）。决定动作电位发生阈值的首要因素是暴露于细胞膜上的阴极（负极）电压门控离子通道和沉积的电荷量。轴突膜电压门控离子通道密度最高的区域一般为突触前末端。在该区域中，有大量的电压门控钙离子（Ca^{2+}）通道参与突触前末端去极化进而释放神经递质。因此，突触前末端可能具有最低的动作电位产生阈值。需要注意的是电刺激产生的动作电位可以是逆行电位，因为靠近刺激点的轴突节段会发起异常向下传递的顺行电位。有髓鞘轴突中动作电位起始区段或第一节间也分布有高密度的电压门控离子通道，通常为钠（Na^+）离子通道。大直径和小直径的无髓鞘轴突可能具有类似的电压门控离子通道密度。直径较大的轴突具有较大的表面积，可通过电容的电学特性积聚更多电荷。

在CC刺激模式下，微库仑数是电流（mA）和PW（μs）的乘积，其中1mA × 1000μs=1μC。轴突产生动作电位的灵敏度也取决于电压门控离子通道的密度，即轴突细胞膜单位表面面积上的通道数。同时，静电力的方向会引起静电荷的流动［从阴极（负）接触开始，流向阳极（正）接触］。因此我们关注的是从阴极到阳极的电流矢量正交的表面积（90°）。

髓鞘轴突通常具有激活动作电位的最低阈值，其次是大的无髓鞘轴突，而小的无髓鞘轴突具有最高阈值。不幸的是，我们很难知道哪种类型的神经轴突具有疗效，哪种类型的神经轴突具有不良反应。就STN-DBS而言，大量证据表明，投射到STN或经过STN的皮质神经元有髓神经轴突中动作电位的产生可能介导了这种益处（而强直性肌肉收缩可能是一种不良反应）。脑电图（EEG）中诱发电位集中反向动作电位的现象证明了以上观点（Walker等，2012）。此外，一项针对STN-DBS的啮齿动物模型的光遗传研究表明，激活STN的皮质投射会带来益处，直接增加或减少STN神经元活性则没有任何益处（Gradinaru等，2009）。

需要补充说明的是，安全限制是30μC/（cm^2·PW），cm^2指的表面积，PW是刺激相位，是当电流在一个方向上，阴极或阳极的应用。使用安全限制是为了避免实际组织损伤，而不是为了避免因刺激非计划轴突产生不良反应。微库仑数由PW和刺激电流（mA）决定；后者由电压和阻抗决定。大多数情况下，通过了解刺激电流幅度可以解决此安全问题。然而，这可能会被CV刺激所误导，因为电压和PW不能精确地确定在每个刺激阶段注入的微库仑数。

(四) 振幅

刺激脉冲的振幅是微库仑所传递的电荷数。微库仑传输可以来自设定的电流（CC刺激模式），也可以来自电压驱动（在CV刺激模式）。从神经电生理学的角度来看，认为刺激电流与PW的影响是独立的，这是不合逻辑的。通常使用的刺激振幅是指施加到DBS电极触点的电流或电压。刺激振幅可以独立于PW进行调控，该现象在一定程度向程控员传递除其神经电生理学不同的讯息。在正文的其余部分，刺激幅度可以理解为电流或电压，除非需要对电流和电压进行特定的区分。

DBS疗效取决于在最佳频率下每个DBS脉冲产生足够数量的动作电位。每一次DBS脉冲产生动作电位的轴突数量取决于DBS脉冲每个相位注入轴突表面的电荷微库仑总数。电荷的数量取决于将负电荷推到神经元上的力、静电场或电压场，以及电荷流动的电阻（欧姆定律）。静电场从阴极（负极触点）扩散，就像一块石头被扔进池塘表面所产生的涟漪。当波纹扩散时，波纹的周长增加。从动量守恒（能量守恒）来看，波纹的振幅必然随着周长的增加而减小。这个类比可以扩展到三维表面，如球体，在这种情况

高阈值 ⟶ 低阈值

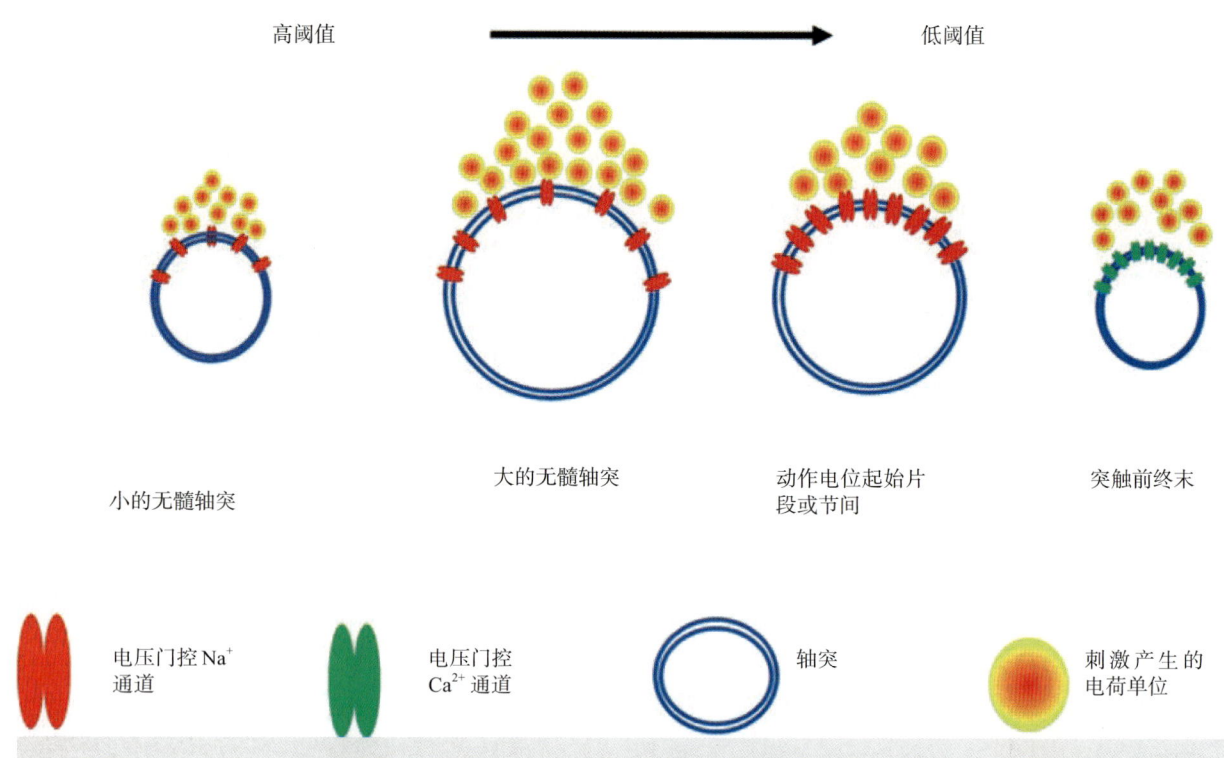

小的无髓轴突　　　大的无髓轴突　　　动作电位起始片段或节间　　　突触前终末

电压门控 Na⁺ 通道　　　电压门控 Ca²⁺ 通道　　　轴突　　　刺激产生的电荷单位

▲ 图 8-4　导致动作电位产生阈值差异的各种因素的示意图
包括受电荷沉积影响的电压门控离子通道的数量。这是由细胞膜中通道的密度和暴露于静电场的细胞膜面积决定的

下，能随着半径的平方下降。因此，静电场的强度将随着距阴极的距离增加而降低。此外，当静电场扩散时，电荷或电压会穿过更多的脑组织。由于脑组织具有阻抗，当静电场远离阴极移动时，与静电场驱动的电荷流相反将导致电荷沉积减少。

电极的结构使静电场的形状变得复杂。在均匀介质中，单极刺激模式，以植入的刺激器作阳极，静电场是球形的，静电场的梯度相对较低。换言之，静电场的强度从中心向外逐渐减小。双极刺激是在 DBS 电极上设置阳极和阴极，宽距双极即两极之间有多个触点间隔，与单极刺激相比，双极刺激约束更强，其静电场是椭圆形。在某种程度上，因为双极刺激中，静电场的强度随着阴极和阳极之间的距离而增加。较窄的双极刺激会产生相对较低的静电场。电场强度与阴极和阳极之间的距离有关，宽间距的双极组合更具显著优势。然而，大脑不是均匀的，因此对电荷流动的电阻率也不是均匀的。因此，在实际应用中，静电场的形状可能会很复杂。

（五）静电场的体积与组织激活的体积

有种误解认为通过了解 DBS 电极线周围脑组织的电阻率和刺激参数，就可以确定产生动作电位的轴突的体积。该体积被称之为组织激活体积（VTA），有人提出以此方式确定的 VTA 可以有效指导 DBS 程控。但实际上确定的是静电场（VES）的体积。根据轴突的性质和分布，实际的 VTA 可能与 VES 有很大的不同（图 8-5）。根据 VES 中实际的神经元成分，VTA 可能会有很大的不同（图 8-6）。

（六）脉冲宽度

脉冲宽度（PW）是指电脉冲的每个相位被传送到目标的持续时间。出于安全考虑，DBS 脉冲包含两相或两组分。第一相在一个方向上注入电流，然后在第二相中在相反方向上注入电流，例如阴极（负极）相接阳极（正极）相或阴

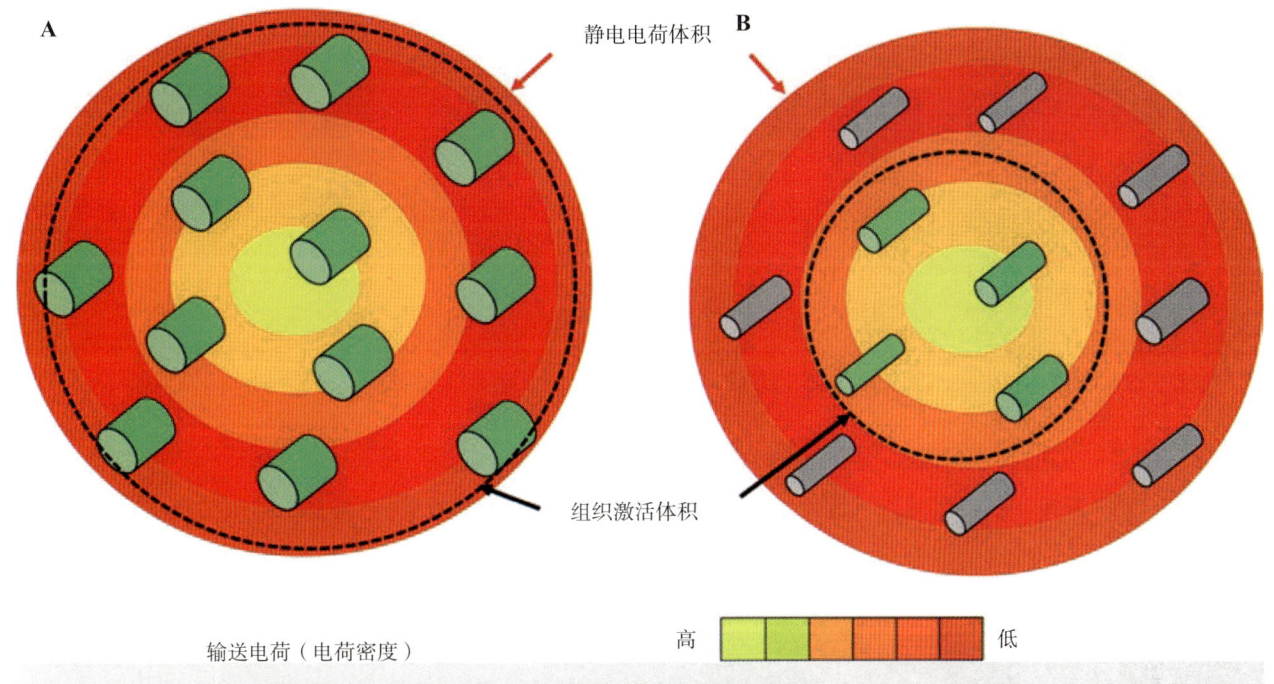

▲ 图 8-5 静电电荷密度体积（VES）与组织激活体积（VTA）的示意图

VES 的体积是从刺激电流源（无论是 CC 还是 CV）辐射出来的梯度。空间范围是由施加在刺激部位的电压和周围组织的电阻率决定的。在这种情况下，假定组织电阻率是均匀的，以 VES 为球形。此外，不考虑电极与脑界面的电容。这 2 个 VES 是一样的。圆柱体代表轴突。从（A）中可以看出，与（B）中所示的小直径轴突相比，轴突的直径更大，并且在较低的电荷密度下会产生动作电位（显示为绿色物体）。如图（B）所示，即使 VES 相同（B）中具有较大直径轴突的 VTA 远远大于具有小直径轴突的 VTA

极（负极）相接阳极（正极）相。通常，PW 指的是 DBS 脉冲的初始相位。

PW 影响神经元轴突产生动作电位的阈值，例如，有髓轴突与较大的无髓轴突相比，在 PW 较小的时候产生轴突电位，而较大的无髓轴突与较小的无髓轴突相比，可以产生更短的 PW 动作电位。该效应被称为"时间轴"，且对此效应的分析在技术上很复杂。有兴趣者可参阅 Ranck 及其同事的论文（1975）。一些关于 PW 对临床现象学影响的研究（Holsheimer 等，2000；Groppa 等，2014）表明，随着 PW 的增加，其对临床现象学的影响逐渐增强。每个试验都表明，在一定的 PW 下，临床效果与 PW 之间的关系渐近，此后脉冲宽度的增加并不会显著增加临床反应（图 8-7）。

PW 的程控设置与文献中推荐的 PW 有相当大的差异（Volkmann，2006；Steigerwald，2018）。然而，如图 8-7 所示，情况并不是那么明确。可以肯定的是，如果一个人愿意充分增加刺激幅度，神经生理反应几乎可以在任何 PW 达到，而组织安全是唯一的限制。此外，在一定脉冲宽度时，临床反应的阈值与 PW 之间的关系似乎渐近，因此 PW 的进一步增加不太可能显著增加临床效果。这一现象在 Moro 等（2002）的研究中得到了证明（图 8-8）。

鉴于以上对脉冲宽度的讨论，问题出现了，为什么在某些研究中，特别是在肌张力障碍患者，需要更大的脉冲宽度。之前关于时间轴的讨论主要涉及单个动作电位的产生。非常大的脉冲宽度可能在刺激脉冲持续期间产生多个动作电位（图 8-9）。脉冲宽度持续时间内的多个动作电位可以通过时间求和的方式放大 DBS 效应。每个动作电位在前一个动作电位的效应消散之前发生，因此具有累加效果（时间总和）。然而，对于单个动作电位的产生，无论刺激振幅加倍还是

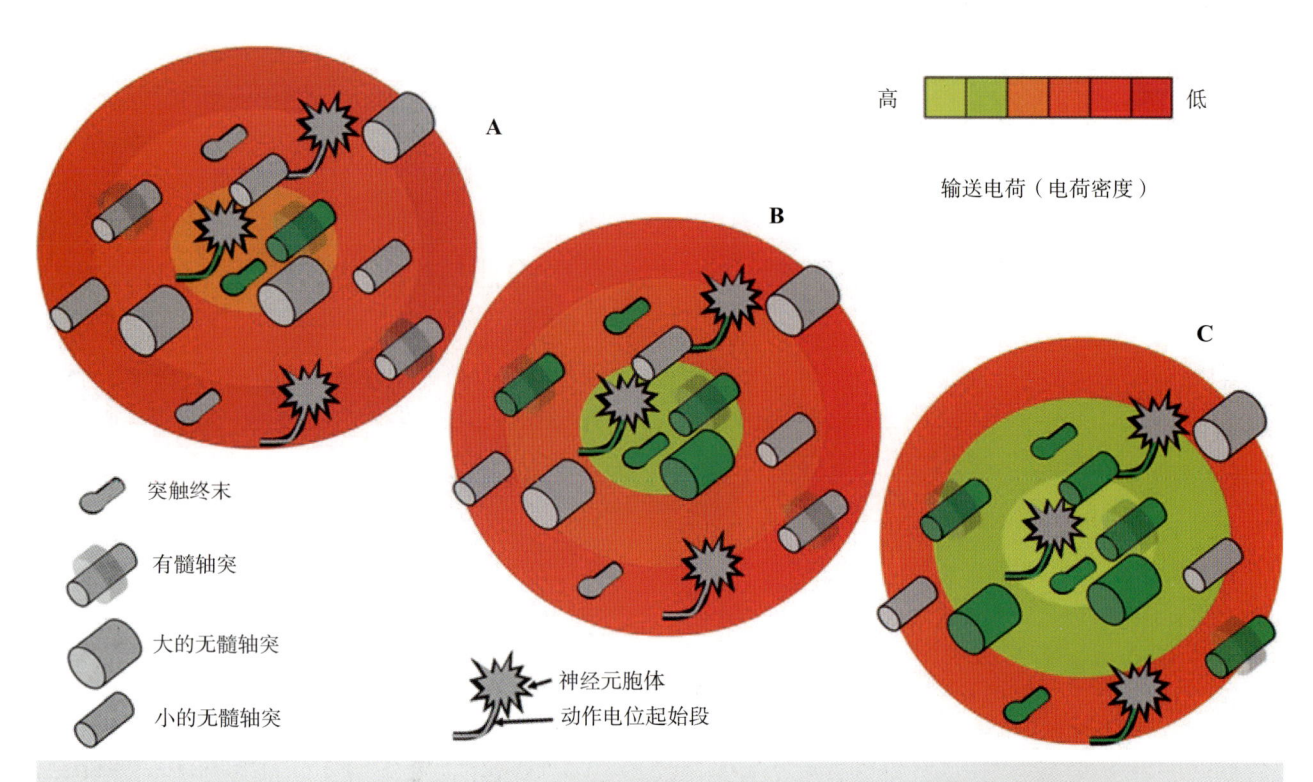

▲ 图 8-6 静电电荷密度（VES）体积与图 8-3 中所描述的组织激活体积的示意图表示

3 种体积的静电电荷密度强度均呈递增趋势。还示意性地表示了各种神经元元件，如突触末端，髓鞘轴突，大的无髓鞘轴突，小的无髓鞘轴突，以及当轴突从体中出现时的动作电位起始区段。这些元素中的每个元素都有不同的产生动作电位的静电电荷密度阈值。突触末端具有最低阈值，其次是动作电位起始区段，然后是髓鞘轴突，其后是具有最高阈值的大直径无髓鞘轴突与小的无髓鞘轴突。可以看出，增加静电电荷密度会激活不同的神经元元素（绿色）和激活元素的数量

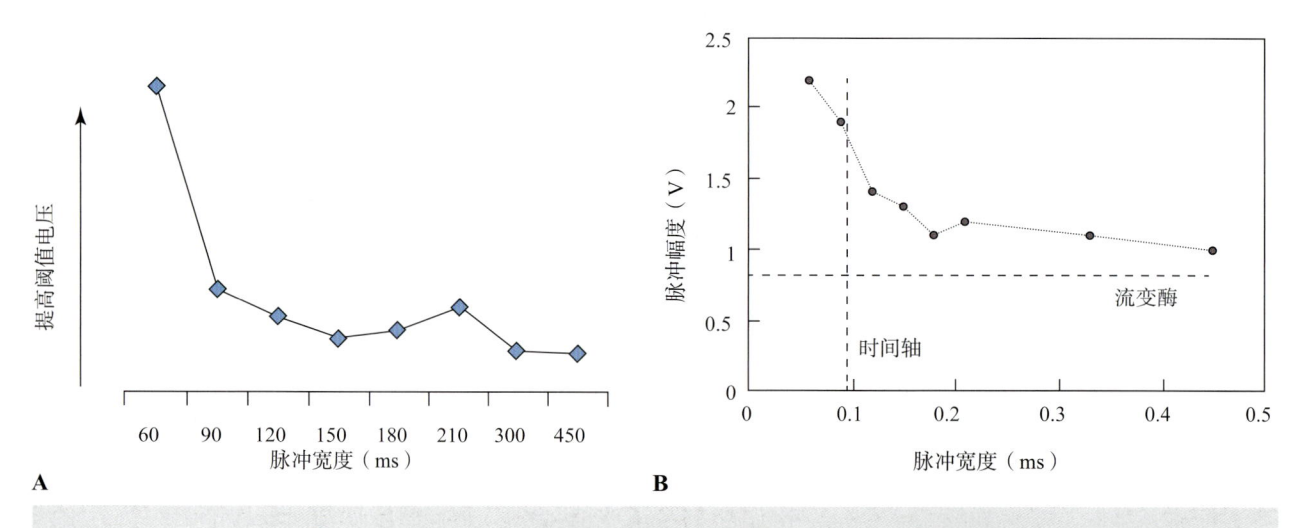

▲ 图 8-7 随着脉冲宽度的增加，阈值（刺激幅度）转变为神经生理反应

A. 根据 Groppa 等（2014）发表的原始数据重建；B. 来自于 Holsheimer 等（2000）原创。值得注意的是，即使最短的 PW 也会有神经生理反应，尽管将需要最大的刺激振幅。此外，两个图都表明该关系在某些 PW 处渐近，并且 PW 的进一步增加可能无效，因为响应阈值不太可能显著降低（经许可转载，引自 Montgomery，2017）

▲ 图 8-8　不同 PW 对运动迟缓和僵直的有效性研究

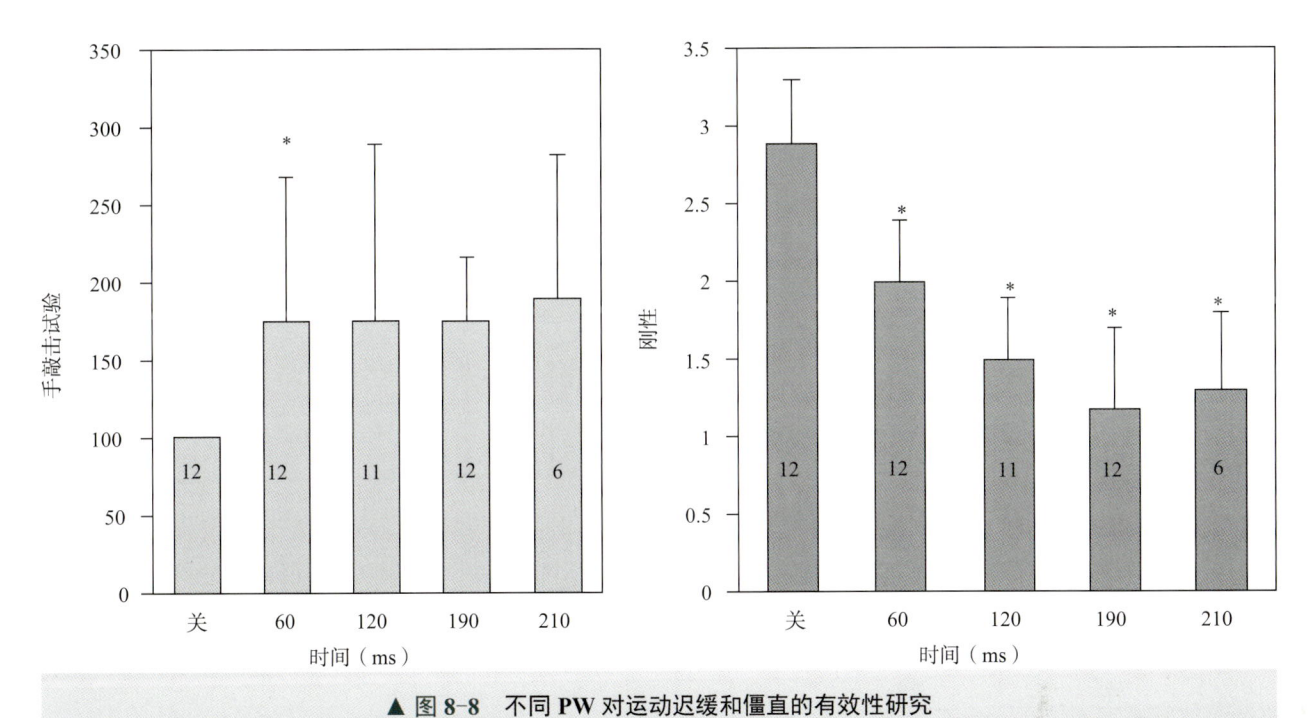

可以看出，经过一定的 PW 后，临床反应渐近，这表明更大 PW 刺激不可能增加反应性（经许可转载，引自 Moro 等，2002）

PW 加倍，传递到大脑和从电池中获取的净电荷都是一样的。

在大多数情况下，选择 PW 的一种方法是，在临床效果渐近于增加 PW 时，只设置 PW，而不显著降低阈值（图 8-7）。例如，人们可以将 PW 设置为 150μs，这是因为认识到更高的 PW 不可能独自增加临床效果，而较短的 PW 可能需要更高的刺激幅度。就基本的生理学而言，这种方法不太可能产生太大的影响，然而简化 DBS 程控可以转化为提高 DBS 程控的效率和降低成本。

（七）频率

脑深部电刺激频率是指每秒脉冲数（pps）。文献经常将 DBS 频率与赫兹（Hz）混淆，可能是因为混淆了连续的谐波振荡机制。DBS 是周期性的，意味着重复，但这并不意味着其是一种振荡现象，因此，DBS 的作用机制可能不像相互作用的连续谐波振荡（Montgomery，2017）。

许多研究用以检验 DBS 频率对各种神经系统疾病及刺激部位的临床作用（Benabid 等，1991；Moro 等，2002）。遗憾的是大多数只研究了少量的 DBS 频率。假设 DBS 频率与临床疗效之间的关系很复杂，为准确地表达这种关系就必须对关系中变化最快部分的频率进行至少 2 倍频率的采样。以此类推，如果要获得每秒 100 次波动信号的表达，就必须每秒至少采样 200 次。如果降低采样率，结果会有噪声干扰，测试也会慢得多。因此，大多数研究不太可能充分采样不同的可用 DBS 频率，导致 DBS 频率和临床反应的实际关系存在错误陈述。Huang 等（2014）研究植入刺激器（IPG）的 PD 患者手运动迟缓在不同频率下的疗效（图 8-10）仅对手运动迟缓而言，几乎每位受试者在相对低频（<25pps）时和在高频刺激时都有同样的改善。

Huang 等（2014））的研究也证明了个体间的差异性。然而多数其他研究因将受试者的反应进行平均化（Benabid 等，1991；Limousin 等，1995），类似低通滤波器的作用，其得出的 DBS

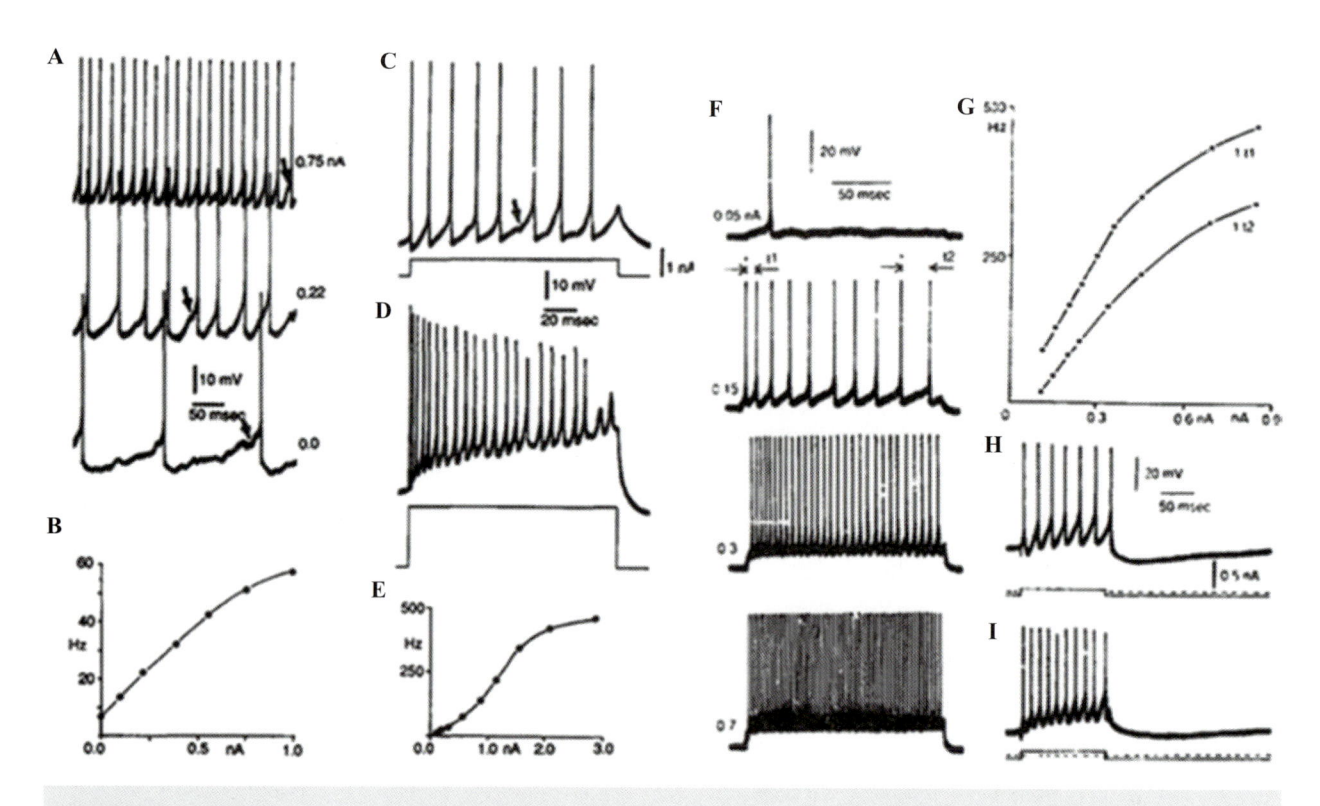

▲ 图 8-9 研究细胞内去极化注入电流的影响，A 至 E 是（Kita 和 Kitai，1991）啮齿类动物的苍白球神经元［人的苍白球外侧部（GPe）的同源物］，F 至 I 则是（Nakanishi 等，1987）啮齿动物底丘脑核神经元。在 A 至 E，持续注入电流会产生重复的动作电位（C、D 和 I）。正如可以理解的那样，电荷注入非常长，可能类似于 DBS 中非常长的 PW，从而产生了多重动作电位

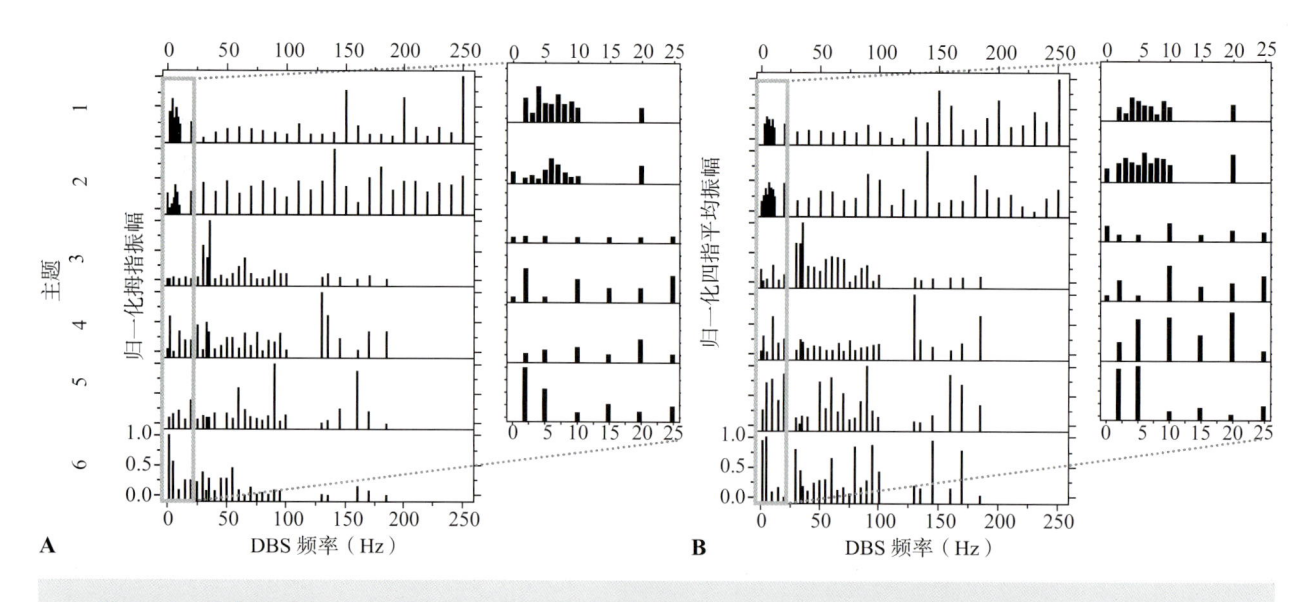

▲ 图 8-10 每个受试者（A）拇指和（B）手指（各指集合）均值标准化的运动幅度。脱落处表示在受试者的 IPG 中无法获得相应频率。峰值与大幅运动有关，出现于多个频率。小图显示的是低频时的幅度

频率与临床疗效之间缓慢变化的结论是错误的。在文献中经常看到当对多个受试者进行平均后其频率和临床疗效之间呈单调递增的关系。不幸的是这些可能的错误陈述已被视为证明高频DBS有效、低频无效的证据，进而导致对其潜在生理机制的推断无效。

患者个体化最佳DBS频率是无法预测的。肌张力障碍患者可能会对低频刺激产生反应（Alterman等，2007）。低频（60～80pps）可能对PD患者的步态障碍更有益（Moreau等，2008；Ricchi等，2012）。与较高频率（60～80pps）相比，低频率（10～25pps）脚桥核DBS对PD患者的药物难治性冻结步态改善更好（Ferraye等，2010；Moro等，2010；Thevathasan等，2018）在大多数患者中，较高的频率甚至会加重症状（Nosko等，2015）。但是在可充电IPG的设置时，DBS的起始频率设置为130pps是非常合理的，尤其这个范围内DBS频率的使用有长足的经验（Moro等，2002）。如图8-10所示，DBS程控者应该愿意探索更宽范围的DBS频率。

过去认为高频DBS抑制刺激靶点产生治疗作用，而低频则激活靶点加重症状（Montgomery和Baker，2000）。在其他众多的合理可能性中，系统振荡学说是一种潜在的解释。根据该理论，基底神经节 - 丘脑 - 皮质系统组织为一组相互连接、可折返的非线性振荡器，呈现不同的电路长度和频率（Montgomery，2016）。该系统包含一个较长的闭环反馈回路，该回路显示了从运动皮质到壳核到GPe到GPi到丘脑到运动皮质的投影。因此，该闭环的重入活动将花费更长的时间来穿过环路，产生更低频率的振荡。与此同时，在腹外侧丘脑和运动皮质之间也存在闭环反馈回路，其产生短回路长度和高频通路（Montgomery，2000）。不同的症状和体征可能取决于不同的环路，从而受到不同的频率影响（Santaniello等，2015）。对临床疗效不理想，增加刺激幅度或脉冲宽度无改善且无不良反应时，可以调节频率（Volkmann等，2006）。

（八）电极配置

将电极配置与刺激参数区分开来是有所裨益的。前者包括用于刺激的正负电极触点的组合。电极的配置能决定VES的大小，形状，位置及密度，而刺激参数则决定与VTA相关的动作电位的产生。电极配置的项目，包括双相DBS脉冲初始相位的极向（负或是正），正负电极触点之间的距离，以及激活的触点的数目。对电刺激场的目标化和精准配置使局部神经元产生反应，类似于"雕刻"VES和VTA，从而与局部生理解剖相吻合。

这里面有一些潜在的混淆会导致错误。每一个电极触点上将通过所有的正负电流，包括单极刺激中的仅能作为正极的IPG盒子，因此，命名将参考双相DBS脉冲初始相位的极向，尽管正极触点在第二相位的时候将通过负性电流，但这与负性电极触点在初始相位中流经的负性电流所产生的临床效应有所不同，因为在这两个相位中的双相脉冲是不对称的。相比于第二相位来说，初始相位较高的刺激电压决定了VES中较大的刺激体积，从而激活了较多的轴突。然而，基于安全的考虑，所有相位都通过了相同数量微库仑的放电。不幸的是，目前没有标准的电极触点命名法则，当在不同系统间进行切换时，这就会产生混淆。尽管存在这些差别，只有较少量的工作来描述个体系统且本章中出现的类似的尝试即将过时。然而，DBS的程控人员在面对植入不同系统的患者群体时需要清楚这些差别。

五、特别功能

我们将在整体层面讨论一些特别功能，而不是针对市面上特定的型号。这些特别功能包括交叉和方向特性，后者通过分布于垂直在DBS电极长轴平面的分段电极触点刺激VES的某些区段。同样，某些系统能够对同一DBS电极的不同触点施加不同的电流从而使刺激电流分段化。随着技术的进展及对与疾病病理生理的深化认识，人们对 DBS 作用机制认识的进一步加深，DBS 将继续演化进步。举例而言，光遗传学技术促使特定外源基因表达，改变离子通透性，从而影响基因启动子。这些分子技术以激活或抑制神经元的方式为未来的神经调节疗法提供了令人难以置信的精确度。

（一）交叉

这包括快速而交替地刺激电极触点，通常在不同的触点组上使用 2 组不同的电流或电压和脉冲宽度进行刺激。例如，可以将 2V 或 mA（取决于特定 IPG 可用的模式）和 90μs PW 施加到触点 A 和 C，而将 4V 或 mA（取决于特定 IPG 可用的模式）和 120μs PW 施加到触点 B 和 D。这样就建立了独特而复杂的 VES（Wojtecki 等，2011；Miocinovic 等，2014）。但是，2 组脉冲的精确管理可能会受到限制。例如，交叉的 DBS 的频率可能会受到限制。此外，一组脉冲相对于第二组脉冲的时相是固定的，并且默认参数不一定是最佳的。

（二）方向性刺激

最初，DBS 电极触点分布于垂直于电极长轴的平面上，组成了围绕电极圆周完整的环。因此，电流完全投射在 DBS 电极触点周围。最新的进展包括分段电极，其中电极周围的空间被分为扇区或区段。因此，这样就可以投射成围绕电极周围的扇区性 VES。例如，如果 DBS 电极在 STN 后方附近（刺激会引起持续的感觉异常），则可以使用朝前的分段触点。这些电极使 VES 更好地适应局部生理解剖结构（Pollo 等，2014；Schüpbach 等，2017）。但是，分段的电极可能会产生"边缘效应"，其中静电场沿边缘的强度更大，而不是从触点中心向外突出（有异于直觉）。这就使 DBS 电极的定位和程控更加复杂（Montgomery，2017）。

（三）电流的分段化

某些 IPG 仅允许将相同的电流或电压传递到所有刺激触点。新的 IPG 可以在所有刺激触点间差异性地分配总电流，这样就能在 DBS 电极附近的局部生理解剖结构周围形成复杂的静电场，而且处于这些静电场中的轴突种类又能决定刺激体积的大小。

六、新增特征与功能的社会危害

尽管增加了复杂性和资源需求，但是日益增长的 DBS 程控特性和功能可能会帮助更多的患者。自动程控系统正在开发中，例如，通过特殊的磁共振成像（MRI）扫描对 VES 建模。然后确定电极配置和刺激参数，从而将建好的 VES 放置在假想的最佳目标位置。但是，实际目标是生理标和解剖定位，可能只会使 DBS 程控人员"靠近"。其他可能的方法包括对患者进行一系列特定的电极配置和刺激参数调查，以记录临床反应，而不一定达到最终所需的配置和参数。模型是基于电张力维度上创建的，而不是基于解剖学或空间上的。

具有众多程控算法选项的 DBS 系统可能已经太复杂而无法有效利用。对自动程控的依赖引发了严重的道德和潜在法律问题，例如医疗责任与产品责任。从产品责任的其他示例推断，这个问题可能需要程控人员了解自动计算机系统的性质，以及如何修改该系统。在美国，枪支制造商通常不对个人使用枪支的行为负责，因此，对因使用枪支而造成的任何伤害不承担责任。法院认为，合理的人很容易理解枪支的风险，因此，枪支使用者会知道枪支是危险的，因此使用者应承担全部责任。

在其他情况下，医疗专业人员把问题集中在医疗器械的缺陷是否为"专利"，因此应可识别并防止该缺陷带来的损害。尚不清楚 DBS 程控人员如何识别自动计算机化 DBS 程控设备中的缺陷，尤其是在使用某种形式机器学习（人工智能）的情况下，而实际的算法或解决程控问题的确切方法在原则上则无法知晓（Hutson，2018）。从历史上看，医院或其他机构要比医疗专业人员持有更严格或更高的标准。至少在某些情况下，即便使用自动 DBS 程控设备软件，DBS 程控人员也应该认识到偏离标准的结果。

七、DBS 脉冲的远端效应

大多数讨论集中在对单个 DBS 脉冲的电神经生理反应。但是，DBS 的效用要复杂得多，因为每个脉冲的影响会在整个相关网络中传播，例如基底神经节－丘脑－皮质－小脑系统。单个脉冲的影响可能会重新进入相同的递归网络，从而延长单个脉冲的作用，然后单个脉冲与后续脉冲相互作用。例如，皮质脑电图显示单个 DBS 脉冲诱发的电位不同于一系列脉冲所诱发的电位（Baker 等，2002）。此过程可能有助于解释（尽管可能有其他解释）DBS 频率的复杂影响。此外，随着时间的推移，重入过程使整个相关网络中发展出复杂的变化（Montgomery，2017），而必要的反应演变可能解释了 DBS 启动时临床现象不同程度的滞后（以及 DBS 停止后的延迟）。对于这些问题的探索才刚刚开始，由于它们是 DBS 效应的基础，因此必须对这些效应有更深入的了解。神经元轴突"远端"对单个 DBS 脉冲的反应，可能使 DBS 有效的治疗更广泛范围的神经和心理疾病。

有一种趋势将 DBS 机制解释为"区域性"的。然而，这样的假设很少考虑到非区域性的效应。正如之前讨论过的，DBS 脉冲的近端效应是来自于轴突中动作电位的产生。通常，人们更多地考虑动作电位的正向传导，很少考虑其逆向传导的影响。这样的逆向作用传导到神经元体中，因此可能影响神经元随后的兴奋性。但是，许多神经元具有轴突侧支，因此，逆向动作电位会进入轴突侧支的分支，并以正向方向进入下一个神经元。因此，作用广泛传导到整个相关网络。

爱因斯坦曾说过"一切都应该尽可能地简单，但不要过于简单"。任何比实际生理学简单的理论都必须视为近似值，因此值得怀疑。相对于实际生理学更大程度简化的理论应该引起更大的怀疑。神经生理学是非常复杂的，这并不是一个空洞的事实，经常被认为是可以免除怀疑论的。此外，除了阈值电位产生动作电位以外，神经元间的相互作用是高度非线性的。非线性说明刚好在阈值以下的相对较大的电位变化与跨阈值的小变化具有非常不同的影响。因此，参与 DBS 效应的生理功能可能是"混沌"和"复杂"的。

对混沌和复杂系统有足够的了解，可以深入了解 DBS 的作用机制。更全面的讨论超出了本章的范围，但是存在一些有趣的关于混沌和复杂的特征性现象。首先，许多这样的系统可以自组织成临时稳定的状态（亚稳态），它们之间可以进行快速转换（分叉）。亚稳态可能是一种极限循环振荡器，它可能与 DBS 又相互作用，而 DBS 本身被认为是非线性离散振荡器（Montgomery，2017，参阅 17 章：离散神经振荡器）。其次，混沌和复杂系统显示的对初始条件的依赖性在开始时稍有变化就会产生非常不同的结果。因此，在精准的正确时间施加的单个或少量 DBS 脉冲可能会引起初始条件的微小变化，从而导致截然不同的结果，这并不意外。此属性可能是"协调复位"概念的解释，其中短暂的脉冲串会持续改善 PD 的症状和体征（Tyulmankov 等，2018；Wang 等，2016；Adamchic 等，2014）。但是，用"协调复位"理论很难解释如上所述的 DBS 频率与临床效果或反应延迟之间的复杂关系。此外，"协调复位"的概念是基于基底神经节－丘脑－皮质系统内病理性同步化神经元活动为病因的理论上，而其余的活动则使网络去同步化。虽然在病理情况下确实增加了同步，但有大量证据表明 DBS 实际上会提高同步，但在某种程度上是一种"嘈杂的同步"（Montgomery，2017）。"协调复位"可能是正确的，但其原因是错误的。至少，这种"协调复位"是 DBS 反应为非线性的一个例子，并且是神经生理学涉及混乱和复杂性的可能指标。

八、脑深部电刺激程控的主要原则

当前，最佳的 DBS 程控并不直接遵循电学、电子学、生物物理学、神经生理学、病理生理学和生理解剖学原则。换言之，如果仅基于上述原则，则无法先验性地预测最佳的电极配置和刺激参数。但是，一旦完成了单极测试，则这些原则有助于决定下一步的工作。尽管 DBS 诱导的神经反应的种类正在增加，但是尚未清楚这些反应中的哪一种产生了治疗作用（如果有的话），抑或是导致了不良影响（Montgomery，2017）。基于个体的 DBS 程控在很大程度上仍然是一个经验性的过程—首先进行尝试，然后根据响应做出了修改。对原则的了解确实有助于决策，尤其是从何处开始，以及接下来要进行哪些修改。

（一）经验原则：了解 DBS 程控人员面临的挑战

程控人员的基本任务是为患者提供最佳的生活质量。先验不可能把电极配置和刺激参数等同于生活质量。则需要使用替代物或生物标记物来衡量生活质量，而且，这些指标在 DBS 程控生态系统内必须可行。值得注意的是这些指标只是工具。与谚语"一个可怜的工匠责备他的工具"的相反的是"一个好工匠了解他的工具"。日益进步的 DBS 相关电子产品只是可用工具的一部分。需要其他工具来优化利用先进的 DBS 电子设备，例如"认知"工具。下一节将重点介绍这些工具，阐述它们的性质和局限性，使得这些工具也能不断发展。

一旦选好了衡量生活质量的度量指标，就可以构建其与电极配置和刺激参数之间的相关性，从而对电极配置和刺激参数进行预测，尽可能获得最佳收益和最小刺激相关不良事件的风险。影响这些相关性的因素包括：①指标的性质及其发生变动后该指标的滞后时间；②电极配置和刺激参数可调整的参数空间巨大；③ DBS 系统的多样性和多重性；④患者个体对 DBS 反应的异质性；⑤ DBS 程控阶段的组织和管理。因此，我们将对一般原则进行讨论，并利用示例讨论这些原则在操作层面上如何发挥作用，DBS 程控人员有望从这些原则中构建出最佳方法。

DBS 的适应证和刺激靶点数目正在迅速扩大。讨论每种适应证的每个靶点超出了本章的范围。我们将通过描述一定数量的病例来说明原理和概念。内容将集中在帕金森病和肌张力障碍 DBS 的典型病例。理想的指标应包含以下特点：①预测最佳生活质量（类似于阳性预测值）；②预测无不良反应（类似于阴性预测值）；③指示 DBS 响应；④相对于观察时间而言，对任何刺激变化的反应迅速；⑤快速消散反应；⑥评估者之间和评估者内部的可靠性高；⑦在 DBS 程控环境中毫无问题地使用。

（二）帕金森病

量化 DBS 的度量标准

DBS 程控的有效性取决于在程控过程中测量 DBS 效应的工具。对 DBS 效应的评估不准会增加疗效不佳的风险。通常使用运动障碍学会统一帕金森病评定量表（MDS-UPDRS）评估 DBS 的疗效（Goetz 等，2008）。事实上，通常将 MDS-UPDRS 第Ⅲ部分（运动检查）的一些子量表作为量化 DBS 程控的指标。理想情况下，MDS-UPDRS 第Ⅲ部分应该是生活质量的可靠预测因素，而生活质量是术后 DBS 治疗的最终目标。其中Ⅰ、Ⅱ部分相关性最强，而第Ⅲ部分和第Ⅳ部分之间仅有中度相关性，且预测能力较低，如生活质量指标［如 PD 问卷 -39（PDQ-39）］对应的 R^2 所示。如果 PDQ-39 是可靠的指标，程控的最佳度量标准则是第Ⅱ部分（He 等，2016）。在另一项研究中，第Ⅲ部分与 PDQ-39 之间的相关性 $r = 0.193$，可见其对生活质量的预测能力较差（Daniels 等，2011）。UPDRS 的第Ⅱ部分虽然是生活质量的更好预测因素，但并不适用，因为这个子量表需要在更长的时间范围内进行评估和判断。问题可能在于 PDQ-39，而不是 UPDRS。因此，目前除了在术后随访时使用

MDS-UPDRS 第Ⅲ部分作为 DBS 程控的度量标准外，很少有其他选择。然而，人们在使用它时仍应该谨慎。

基于上述考虑决定应用 UPDRS 第Ⅲ部分，那么该如何使用？忽略左右侧时，其中包含了 19 个（考虑侧别时为 26）项目。如果对每一组电极配置和刺激参数组合均进行 19 个项目的评估，所需时间导致它在 DBS 程控生态下内并不可行。是否可以减少评估的项目数量？因子分析表明，可以将 19 个项目依据 7 个因素进行分组（若不考虑侧别则为 6 个；Goetz 等，2008）。

其他一些问题也需要考虑，例如响应刺激变化而改变度量标准所需的时间。震颤、手指轻敲和手打开 / 关闭的潜伏期为数秒；然而，步态和平衡的变化需要数十分钟。考虑到存在响应潜伏期和 DBS 程控门诊的条件，将步态评估作为度量标准并不可行。尽管如此，在程控过程中的某个时间点评估步态至关重要（Temperli 等，2003）。完成电极配置和刺激参数的设置后，也应该在潜伏期后注意观察声音和言语表现，以及其他不良反应。例如，感觉异常和强直性肌肉收缩可能在数秒后出现，而步态或平衡异常加重可能需要数十分钟才能表现出来。一些不良反应，如情绪、冲动和认知的改变可能需要数天或数周才能被识别。

不良反应有可能与所治疗疾病的症状或体征相混淆，因此要对此有所预判并保持谨慎。皮质脊髓束受累可降低运动灵活性，这一改变可与运动迟缓恶化相混淆。对于底丘脑核的 DBS，可能会将初始肌肉收缩误判为感觉异常，程控者可能难以分辨内侧丘系与皮质脊髓束的刺激。

何时开始 DBS 程控及 DBS 电极植入，取决于生物物理、神经和社会学因素。患者从 DBS 程控的手术中恢复，是指在刚刚植入 DBS 电极时的"损毁效应"，或类似于微丘脑切开、微苍白球切开或微丘脑下部切开的短暂改善效应消失后（这些术语错误地暗示了假定的作用机制），患者已可以进行配合。水肿、急性和慢性胶质增生等生物物理因素影响着电荷的传导，关键在于这些因素随时间的变化。CC 系统的情况则不同，可在患者神经功能稳定时启动。另外还要考虑社会学因素，如医疗费用的覆盖范围和报销政策。

九、辅助治疗的潜在混杂效应

有时多种原因会引起同一现象，当 DBS 和其他治疗（如药物）之间的协同效应成为混杂因素时，DBS 与辅助治疗的同时存在会产生负面影响。因此，必须控制辅助治疗的作用，而这取决于它们在 DBS 程控期间的动态变化。在 DBS 程控期间，辅助治疗作用的出现并非是有序的。如果辅助药物的作用在 DBS 程控过程中不断变化，则无法从 DBS 的疗效中区分出辅助治疗的作用。如果辅助治疗的半衰期非常长，不需要直接控制辅助治疗。例如，肌肉肉毒毒素在 DBS 程控过程中的作用可能不变，因此不容易混淆 DBS 程控。还有一些其他的半衰期很长的药物。左旋多巴的血浆半衰期很短，约为 90min，在 DBS 程控期间肯定会波动。因此，应根据预期在 DBS 程控期间控制左旋多巴的使用。当辅助治疗效应处于最低状态时（例如，对于半衰期相当短的药物，经过一夜禁食后），执行 DBS 程控可能是最佳的。但是，程控者必须考虑到关机期间的残疾程度，因为他们可能会遇到组织和安全问题。

如果处在辅助治疗的疗效最小化状态，应在疗效最大化状态下对患者的辅助治疗进行重新评价。由于在疗效最小化时辅助治疗与 DBS 的协同效应很弱，最大化状态下这种显著协同作用可能会引起不良反应。应在患者结束程控之前评估这种情况。

我们在削弱辅助治疗的作用方面，应该采取多大的力度？这个问题至少有 2 个方面需要考虑。第一，收益递减的拐点何时出现？第二，削弱总体治疗是否有价值？一种重要的情况是，在尚未出现不良反应而又未能达到预期收益时，收益递减的拐点始终不出现。通常假定患者能够达到预期结局，同前述的 PD 患者，UPDRS 指标改善 50%~60%。然而，即使是预期目标也是可以调整的，因为许多患者可以达到更好效果。如果没有达到合理的预期收益水平，则可以考虑 DBS 系统故障、电极错位、程控工作不充分或已知对 DBS 相对耐受的疾病的回顾性记录，如多系统萎缩。

在一定成本下提高患者或护理者的满意度是我们的目标，那么 DBS 和辅助治疗的组合就显得相对次要。然而，成本的概念是复杂的。最大化 DBS 和最小化辅助治疗可降低总成本。请注意，手术中多数情况下 DBS 的成本是"已支付"的；因此，进一步提高临床疗效的成本主要在于 DBS 程控的时间。而药物成本的降低可能抵消一部分成本。

将治疗、DBS 和辅助治疗量化以使患者或护理者满意的过程是复杂的，特别是考虑到患者和护理者的期望，因而程控者可能会采用家长式管理。DBS 程控者可能会否认强烈的家长式主义，即主动而直接地反对患者的利益；然而相对柔和的家长式主义却更加普遍。柔和的家长式颠覆了患者的自主权，并剥夺了患者有权接受的利益，仅由自己武断地决定患者已经达到令人满意的控制水平。通过充分的咨询可以减少患者或护理者不切实际期望。之后，可以建设性地消除异见，并就收益递减方面的进一步积极管理进行讨论。

有效的 DBS 程控可以更快解决残疾和相关风险。无效的脑深部电刺激程控对患者、程控者和社会的成本 - 收益比都会造成损害。因此，缩小电极配置和刺激参数的范围非常重要。选取单个固定的脉冲宽度将减少参数可调控空间。使用最差状态的刺激参数进行单极测试至少可在最初排除不可用的电极配置，从而减少参数可调控空间（Volkmann 等，2006）。

肌张力障碍

临床反应的出现明显延迟增加了肌张力障碍程控的困难，因而这里对于肌张力障碍进行了分析。任何临床检查的改善可能都要经过长时间的连续刺激（数小时或数天）后才可显现（Coubes 等，2000）。在许多方面，这与 PD 和特发性震颤的 DBS 程控有所不同。与在强迫症中观察到的情况相似，肌张力障碍患者获益的潜伏期较长，对于 DBS 现有的和未发现的多种适应证可能都存在此现象。

理想情况下，可以使用有临床意义的量化的 DBS 度量标准。对于颈部肌张力障碍，最常用的是多伦多西部痉挛性斜颈评定量表（TWSTRS）（Kupsch 等，2011）。在一项肉毒杆菌毒素治疗的研究中，TWSTRS 唯一有意义的变化是降低 3 分；然而，实际临界值似乎随着初期疾病的严重程度而变化，因此，对于受累更严重的患者，可能需要更大幅度的降低才有意义（Espay 等，2018）。Espay 等（2018）建议取降低 12 分作为有临床意义的合理估计值。程控者依据既往临床试验推断个体患者的需求并不合理。或许最重要的是，TWSTRS 与具有临床意义的指标之间存在合理的相关性。

更多情况下，多数研究使用 Burke–Fahn–Marsden 肌张力障碍量表（BFMDRS）评价非局灶性肌张力障碍治疗效果（Vidailh 等，2005；Kupsch 等，2006；Volkmann 等，2012；Meoni 等，2017）。对 BFMDRS 的临床分析指出了其局限性（Albanese 等，2013）。除运动检查外，还有针对残疾的子量表。然而，这些指标均未针对有临床意义的差异进行分析。当然，残疾子量表不适用于程控中 DBS 的量化。

建议在后期随访时将改善 > 25% 作为 BFMDRS 运动评分的最低标准（Volkmann 等，2012；Meoni 等，2017）。在一项的纳入 24 项研究 Meta 分析中，包含了 523 例患者，末次随访（平均 32.5 个月；24 项研究）时 BFMDRS 运动评分的平均绝对改善率和百分比分别为 26.6 分（95%CI 22.4~30.8 分）和 65.2%（95%CI 59.6%~70.7%）（Moro 等，2017）。但是，接受平均改善率意味着如果程控者在此时停止，相当数量的患者将无法获得超出预期的改善。

肌张力障碍可能具有时相性（运动性肌张力障碍和肌张力障碍震颤）和强直性成分（Liu 等，2006；Yokochi 等，2018）。这些不同的动力学形式可能对 DBS 有不同的反应（Chung 和 Huh，2016）。一些人认为，相位性肌张力障碍症状的临床获益潜伏期更短，这可能使程控更容易；但相位成分的改善是否足以预测有临床意义的强直性症状改善尚不清楚。然而，程控对强直性肌张力障碍的影响随着时间不断变化增加了程控的难度。

肌张力障碍改善的长潜伏期背后的神经生理学机制尚不明晰。一种可能是神经生理系统适应性的主动学习形式。虽然仅为推测，一个有趣的概念可能是在联合突触输入处彼此间相互加强从而形成了 Hebbian 学习模式。DBS 在轴突中产生顺向和逆向传导的动作电位。逆向电位可侵入树突引起大量去极化。因此，当树突去极化形成 Hebbian 学习时，正常突触输入到达的概率大大提高。

由于在肌张力障碍中刺激的疗效通常会延迟，难以根据临床反应逐渐量化刺激的度量标准。因此，一些研究团队建议以调整后（10%～15%）的强度开始刺激，该强度应低于诱导不可逆不良反应发生的阈值。一旦获得稳定的临床获益，可逐渐降低刺激强度，直至肌张力障碍症状再次出现，以避免高刺激强度导致更快速的电池耗竭（Kupsch 等，2011）。然而，使用可充电脉冲发生器时，这种方法可能是不必要的。

十、神经影像对 DBS 程控者的重要性

通常 DBS 程控相对简单，但 DBS 手术失败并不少见，原因还包括程控之外的其他方面（Okun 等，2005；Moro 等，2006）。当患者获益不明显时，在调整电极前要先考虑接下来需要花费多少。制定决策时，程控人员对电极位置的准确性有多大把握也十分重要。若 DBS 程控人员同时参与了 DBS 电极植入手术，尤其是作为术中神经生理学专家，具有一定优势。如果对电极位置的准确性信心不足，则用神经影像定位到电极实际位置后调整电极。当 DBS 电极置入比较满意时，则不必调整电极，即可继续投入，以期达到最佳疗效。

DBS 的程控是一个积累经验的过程。对于程控的临床疗效不佳的患者，寻找原因的过程是一个良好的学习机会。张力性气颅引起脑组织移位可能是电极移位的常见原因，进而会导致 DBS 程控失败（Montgomery，2017）。因此，在 DBS 电极植入手术后立即进行神经影像学检查非常有帮助，如 MRI（可安全地兼容 DBS 系统的），因为颅内气体将在几天内被吸收。推迟影像学检查的时间，可能会无法识别张力性气颅。

可以通过临床症状的明显改善确定最佳的 DBS 电极位置。如果无法实现，可以通过神经影像确定电极位置。但必须强调的是，神经影像与解剖学靶点相关，却无法验证临床上有重要价值的生理学靶点位置。但是，如果术后影像显示电极位置明显偏离了常用的 DBS 有效靶点，则很可能是电极位置存在问题。放射学方面，可以通过 MRI 或计算机断层扫描（CT）定位电极位置。两种治疗方式各有优缺点，其安全性、准确性和可靠性各不相同（Castro 等，2006；Guo 等，2007）。

关于识别电极位置的最佳神经影像技术尚未达成共识。虽然 MRI 能对靶点部位实现良好的解剖学可视化，但是它可能产生伪影并影响最终的坐标。CT 扫描也是如此，CT 扫描是依据大脑中典型的放射强度设计的。然而，CT 中使用符合骨密度的设置可以减少 DBS 电极造成的散射伪影。不良事件的病例报告增强了人们对植入设备患者 MRI 检查安全性的担忧（由于磁场中电极和邻近组织的发热，以及设备的功能紊乱），尽管大规模队列研究报道的不良事件较为罕见（Larson 等，2008）。相比之下，CT 提供了良好的电极定位准确性，但缺乏足够的软组织对比度，难以实

现解剖学靶点的可视化。例如，CT 并不总能可靠地识别黑质或 STN（Pinsker 等，2008）。一种方法是将术后 CT 扫描与术前 MRI 相结合，在消除电极伪影的同时还保留了 MRI 的高分辨率和组织对比度（Geevarghese 等，2016）。

只考虑影像学检查的风险而忽略其收益（根据临床需求定义）是不合理的。缺乏影像学检查可能会对患者的治疗产生严重影响。医学上的每一个决定都是风险和潜在获益之间的权衡。虽然有不良反应的病例报告，但这些不良反应比较少见，如果因噎废食，则无异于因青霉素过敏史不详而为咽喉部链球菌感染患者直接开出红霉素治疗。

十一、初始程控和随访

DBS 程控时，通常首先评估 DBS 系统的物理和电生理特性。例如，需要检查植入硬件上的皮肤表面是否存在感染或糜烂。可通过测量阻抗检查电生理特性。此外，之前的测量值可用作排除故障的参考。高阻抗提示开路，这可能意味着 DBS 导线损坏、受到牵拉或脉冲发生器（脉冲发生器）受损。低阻抗可能表示系统中存在短路。有多种方法可以用于检查阻抗。通常，阻抗代表 1000 Hz 正弦交流电的电阻。也可使用 DBS 脉冲波形和脉冲序列测量阻抗，这种模式具有特定的电极配置和刺激参数。

DBS 引起的生理效应和临床效应有较大的个体差异，造成了初始电极配置和刺激方面的问题。如前所述，如果使用不可充电的 DBS 系统，也必须注意脉冲发生器电池放电的导电问题。一种方法是使用最小化的刺激振幅、脉冲宽度和频率，并使用单个阴极（负极触点）。这种情况下，对慢性 DBS，选择能诱发出疗效的最低阈值和最宽治疗窗（定义为刚出现疗效的阈值和出现不良反应的阈值之间的差异）的电极触点（Krack 等，2002）。使用可充电系统时，这一标准相对宽松。

DBS 电极周围的局部生理解剖特征是不良反应的强预测因素。首先进行单极测试，对每个触点施加刺激，直至出现不良反应或达到刺激振幅上限。通常，不良反应由相关轴突中直接产生的动作电位引起，如强直性肌肉收缩、感觉异常和强直性眼球偏斜。此时临床疗效并不是主要的观察目标，因为临床疗效背后的机制复杂，使得不同 DBS 频率下的效应难以预测。根据图 8-8，假设该研究结果具有普适性，那么初始 DBS 频率设置为 150pps 比较理想。脉冲宽度是值得考虑的问题；然而，考虑到过去的讨论和单极测试，最佳的初始脉冲宽度可能为 150μs。请注意，这并不代表治疗的 DBS 脉冲宽度应该如此之高，尽管根据之前的讨论，保持该脉冲宽度值能够降低 DBS 程控的难度。程控仪也可以使用较短的脉冲宽度，即使这可能需要更大的绝对刺激振幅。单极测试时，刺激振幅方面重要的是相对关系或差异。

完成单极测量和电极配置后，下一步是调试一系列的频率，比如保持固定脉冲宽度，测量 130～180pps 的最大受益，由于一些证据指出了高度特异的最佳 DBS 频率（图 8-8），因此不能直接使用预测、假定或者默认值。确定最佳 DBS 频率后，下一步应该实现临床疗效的优化和不良反应的最小化。然而，考虑到个体差异，以及 DBS 靶点、电极和脉冲发生器的多样化，更具体的建议远远超出了我们探讨的范围，感兴趣的读者可参考其他资料（Hariz 等，2013；Amon 和 Alesch，2017；Montgomery，2017；Wagle, Shukla 等，2017）。

十二、患者参与

可充电系统中电池维护非常关键，这依靠患者或护理者的共同努力。DBS 系统故障可能导致严重不良反应，例如 PD 患者的神经阻滞药恶性综合征。通常，患者教育应该通俗易懂，例如，在没有遥控器和充电器的情况下患者不得旅行（不得将这些设备放在检查过的、可能被错放的航空行李中）。即使在不需要脉冲发生器的开机早期，也要养成对脉冲发生器例行检查的习惯，以便在需要时形成稳定的习惯。患者应定期检查自己是否有感染或皮肤糜烂。此外，患者和护理人员应警惕可能对 DBS 产生不利影响的电场环境。此外，患者和护理人员应该注意，并非每个医生或护理人员都足够了解 DBS 的复杂性。事实上，患者应随身携带遥控器，以免因紧急情况将其送至急诊室，而急诊室人员既不了解 DBS 也没有处理 DBS 的工具。患者还应了解，如心电图、肌电图或某些类型的 MRI 等医学检查，需要暂时关闭 DBS，急诊室工作人员必须在这时关闭遥控器。

DBS 程控的实践过程中，应该注意到患者的具体情况。然而，程控者可能会建议患者（如特发性震颤患者）在夜间关闭 DBS，以节省电池电量并降低耐受风险（Deuschl 等，2006），而患者很少依从。此外，许多脉冲发生器允许患者在程控仪设定的限值范围内更改各种刺激参数。在这种情况下，程控者必须确保患者掌握了调整方法，并设置限值，将患者或护理者程控的上限限制在安全范围内。

有时很容易忽视一个事实，即 DBS 电极的另一端是一个普通的人，与常人一样有缺点、恐惧、优雅和勇气。John Donne 对患者的观点进行了准确描述，至今仍然适用："我像医生对待疾病那样，一丝不苟地观察医生，我看到了他的害怕；我与他分享内心的恐惧，而我的害怕比他的走地更快；他极力将自己的恐惧掩盖，我却以对此更加敏感"（Donne，2012）。

程控依赖于患者的配合与反馈，因此患者是帮助医生实现 DBS 疗效的重要环节。如果程控者能够与其他关心患者的人一样，认识到自身的缺点和恐惧，然后尽力提供最好的照料，将会给患者带来多么大的福音？DBS 治疗也可能会造成程控者的焦虑，掌握相应的处理方法能够帮助其消除焦虑。

十三、DBS 程控的未来展望

闭环 DBS 或自适应 DBS（aDBS）可对潜在生理信号做出响应，从而实时地调整 DBS 参数。aDBS 设备可对反映患者临床状态变化的特定变量进行测量和分析。基于对控制变量的分析，aDBS 系统计算出一组新的刺激参数并将其发送给植入式刺激器，这些参数能更有效地控制患者的症状（Arlotti 等，2016）。运动障碍疾病中 aDBS 的生物标志物可能与病理生理学直接相关，可通过 DBS 刺激器检测到它们，通常是神经电生理信号，如局部场电位（LFP）。生物标志物也可能是与病理生理学相关但无因果关系的其他指标，如肌电图或加速计这样的惯性传感器（Beudel 等，2018）。随着技术的发展，神经递质的电化学指标可能被用作生物标志物。

最终，每个 aDBS 都面临着和其他诊断方法同样的问题，判断是否需要应用或调整 DBS，即阳性和阴性预测值。首先，生物标志物通常是一个持续波动的信号，如 β 频率的功率。然而，该决策涉及一个二分类变量，即是改变或不改变 DBS 参数。因此，可能存在触发 DBS 改变的功率阈值。但请注意，这可能不是单一的阈值，能使其在跨过阈值时实现快速切换（类似将一个旧白炽灯泡接通插座后灯光闪烁，是由于这里有一个点存在断续接触）。我们不希望 aDBS 出现这种情况。为避免上述闪烁现象，可使用滞后效应，设置较高的阈值用于调整 aDBS，然后降低阈值以逆转 aDBS 的变化。

每种诊断方法都有其特异性和敏感性。敏感性的定义为生物标志物超过阈值，且根据目前的生理状态需要将 aDBS 调整至状态 X 的概率。特异性的定义为生物标志物未超过阈值，且考虑到目前生理状态无须将 aDBS 调整至状态 X 的概率。此外，对于判断 aDBS 中某一特定生物标志物的应用价值，特异性和敏感性并非有效的预测因素。此外，考虑先验概率也很重要。生物标志物存在的概率是多少？例如，当 15%～20% 的 PD 患者中不存在 β 频段 LFP 振荡功率的增加时，即使有较高的特异性和灵敏度，该指标仍不可靠。到目前为止，很少有研究证明 aDBS 在临床方面的价值优于恒定的常规 DBS；请注意，这个概念不同于统计假设检验中接受或拒绝无效假设。

过去有一种假设，即 DBS 的起效为全或无的单一机制，可立即开启、立即关闭。大量证据表明该假设是错误的。STN 记录的神经元活动与对侧 STN 附近的短序列 DBS 刺激相关，证实了复杂的、渐变的响应过程（Montgomery，2017）。同样，许多临床疗效需要较长的 DBS 才能起效。例如，运动迟缓的改善可能需要几分钟的 DBS 才能出现，而步态可能需要 20min。同样，许多临床疗效的消除，也需要等到 DBS 中止后相当长的时间。

DBS 出现效应的潜伏期类似于药理学研究中的洗入效应。同样重要的是洗脱效应的概念。对于 aDBS，如果单个 DBS 刺激序列（individual trains of DBS）的延迟比洗脱效应更短，则可以将 aDBS 视为连续 DBS。事实上，许多 aDBS 研究的本质可能更像是连续 DBS。然而，关于洗脱持续时间的数据非常少，并且不同临床效应和靶点之间可能存在差异。一项相关研究对 PD 患者施加了 STN 附近的循环模式 DBS（Montgomery，2005）。在该研究中，与 0.1s 开和 0.1s 关的 DBS 相比，连续 DBS 对运动症状的改善更明显。然而，而 0.5s 开和 0.5s 关的 DBS 和连续 DBS 之间在运动速度上没有显著统计学差异，尽管可能存在某种趋势。假如连续 DBS 和 0.5s 开和 0.5s 关的 DBS 之间没有差异，洗脱效应需要的时间可能＞0.1s 但≤0.5s。另外一种情况是，洗脱期＞0.5s，此时脉冲序列≥0.5s 且无＜0.5s 间隙的 aDBS 可能与连续 DBS 效应相同。

尽管存在上述问题，但 aDBS 在未来仍具备取得重要突破的潜力。上述概念比较复杂，因而思考和处理这些问题显得至关重要。

十四、结论

DBS 程控有许多不同的方法，这里提倡的方法是基于电学、电子学、生物物理学和局部生理解剖原理的方法。然而，治疗作用的确切机制尚不清楚。研究已经证实了神经组织对 DBS 脉冲的多种响应方式。这些知识在当下可以用于 DBS 的选择，同时也能够指导 DBS 技术未来的发展。

DBS 产生静电场，驱动电荷（离子）移动到神经元表面，产生去极化和超极化。电压门控离子通道对充分的去极做出反应，在轴突产生动作电位。这些动作电位在神经系统中进行广泛的顺向和逆向传播。了解特定轴突如何对活动性电极触点（电极配置）和刺激参数（电流、脉冲宽度和频率）做出响应，有助于我们优化 DBS 的疗效。

DBS 具有一套复杂的生态背景，需要考虑的因素并不局限于调整电极配置和刺激参数，还应该结合当地医疗资源，应用"认知"的或概念性的方法更好地完成 DBS 程控。

参考文献

[1] Adamchic I, Hauptmann C, Barnikol UB, Pawelczyk N, Popovych O, Barnikol TT, Silchenko A, Volkmann J, Deuschl G, Meissner WG, Maarouf M, Sturm V, Freund HJ, Tass PA. Coordinated reset neuromodulation for Parkinson's disease: proof-of-concept study. Mov Disord. 2014;29(13):1679–84. https://doi.org/10.1002/mds.25923. Epub 2014 Jun 28. PubMed PMID: 24976001; PubMed Central PMCID: PMC4282372).

[2] Albanese A, Sorbo FD, Comella C, et al. Dystonia rating scales: critique and recommendations. Mov Disord. 2013;28(7):874–83.

[3] Alterman RL, Miravite J, Weisz D, Shils JL, Bressman SB, Tagliati M. Sixty Hertz pallidal deep brain stimulation for primary torsion dystonia. Neurology. 2007;69(7):681–8.

[4] Amon A, Alesch F. Systems for deep brain stimulation: review of technical features. J Neural Transm (Vienna). 2017;124(9):1083–91.

[5] Arlotti M, Rosa M, Marceglia S, Barbieri S, Priori A. The adaptive deep brain stimulation challenge. Parkinsonism Relat Disord. 2016;28:12–7.

[6] Baker KB, Montgomery EB Jr, Rezai AR, Burgess R, Lüders HO. Subthalamic nucleus deep brain stimulus evoked potentials: physiological and therapeutic implications. Mov Disord. 2002;17(5):969–83. PubMed PMID: 12360546

[7] Benabid AL, Pollak P, Louveau A, Henry S, de Rougemont J. Combined (thalamotomy and stimulation) stereotactic surgery of the VIM thalamic nucleus for bilateral Parkinson disease. Appl Neurophysiol. 1987;50(1–6):344–6.

[8] Benabid AL, Pollak P, Gervason C, Hoffmann D, Gao DM, Hommel M, Perret JE, de Rougemont J. Long-term suppression of tremor by chronic stimulation of the ventral intermediate thalamic nucleus. Lancet. 1991;337(8738):403–6.

[9] Beudel M, Cagnan H, Little S. Adaptive brain stimulation for movement disorders. Prog Neurol Surg. 2018;33:230–42.

[10] Brocker DT, Grill WM. Principles of electrical stimulation of neural tissue. Handb Clin Neurol. 2013;116:3–18.

[11] Bronstein JM, Tagliati M, McIntyre C, Chen R, Cheung T, Hargreaves EL, Israel Z, et al. The rationale driving the evolution of deep brain stimulation to constant-current devices. Neuromodulation. 2015;18(2):85–8; discussion 88–9

[12] Butson CR, Cooper SE, Henderson JM, McIntyre CC. Patient-specific analysis of the volume of tissue activated during deep brain stimulation. NeuroImage. 2007;34(2):661–70. Epub 2006 Nov 17. PubMed PMID: 17113789; PubMed Central PMCID: PMC1794656

[13] Castro FJ, Pollo C, Meuli R, Maeder P, Cuisenaire O, Cuadra MB, Villemure JG, et al. A cross validation study of deep brain stimulation targeting: from experts to atlas-based, segmentation-based and automatic registration algorithms. IEEE Trans Med Imaging. 2006;25:1440–50.

[14] Chung M, Huh R. Different clinical course of pallidal deep brain stimulation for phasic- and tonic-type cervical dystonia. Acta Neurochir. 2016;158(1):171–80; discussion 180

[15] Coombs SJ, Curtis DR, Eccles JC. The interpretation of spike potentials of motoneurons. J Physiol. 1957;39:198–231.

[16] Cooper IS, Upton AR, Amin I. Reversibility of chronic neurologic deficits. Some effects of electrical stimulation of the thalamus and internal capsule in man. Appl Neurophysiol. 1980;43(3–5):244–58.

[17] Coubes P, Roubertie A, Vayssiere N, Hemm S, Echenne B. Treatment of DYT1-generalised dystonia by stimulation of the internal globus pallidus. Lancet. 2000;355(9222):2220–1.

[18] Daniels C, Krack P, Volkmann J, Raethjen J, Pinsker MO, Kloss M, Tronnier V, et al. Is improvement in the quality of life after subthalamic nucleus stimulation in Parkinson's disease predictable? Mov Disord. 2011;26(14):2516–21.

[19] Dayal V, Grover T, Limousin P, et al. The effect of short pulse width settings on the therapeutic window in subthalamic nucleus deep brain stimulation for Parkinson's disease. J Parkinsons Dis. 2018;8(2):273–9

[20] Deuschl G, Herzog J, Kleiner-Fisman G, Kubu C, Lozano AM, Lyons KE, Rodriguez-Oroz MC, et al. Deep brain stimulation: postoperative issues. Mov Disord. 2006;21 Suppl 14:S219–37.

[21] Donne J. Devotions upon emergent occasions: together with death's duel. Scotts Valley, CA: Createspace Independent Publishing Platform; 2012.

[22] Espay AJ, Trosch R, Suarez G, Johnson J, Marchese D, Comella C. Minimal clinically important change in the Toronto Western Spasmodic Torticollis Rating Scale. Parkinsonism Relat Disord. 2018;52:94–7.

[23] Ferraye MU, Debû B, Fraix V, Goetz L, Ardouin C, Yelnik J, Henry-Lagrange C, et al. Effects of pedunculopontine nucleus area stimulation on gait disorders in Parkinson's disease. Brain. 2010;133:205–14.

[24] Geevarghese R, O'Gorman Tuura R, Lumsden DE, Samuel M, Ashkan K. Registration accuracy of CT/MRI fusion for localisation of deep brain stimulation electrode position: an imaging study and systematic review. Stereotact Funct Neurosurg. 2016;94(3):159–63.

[25] Goetz CG, Tilley BC, Shaftman SR, Stebbins GT, Fahn S, Martinez-Martin P, Poewe W, et al.; Movement Disorder Society UPDRS Revision Task Force. Movement Disorder Society-sponsored revision of the Unified Parkinson's Disease Rating Scale (MDS-UPDRS): scale presentation and clinimetric testing results. Mov Disord. 2008;23(15):2129–70.

[26] Gradinaru V, Mogri M, Thompson KR, Henderson JM, Deisseroth K. Optical deconstruction of parkinsonian neural circuitry. Science. 2009;324(5925):354–9.

[27] Groppa S, Herzog J, Falk D, Riedel C, Deuschl G, Volkmann J. Physiological and anatomical decomposition of subthalamic neurostimulation effects in essential tremor. Brain. 2014;137(Pt 1):109–21.

[28] Guo T, Parrent AG, Peters TM. Surgical targeting accuracy analysis of six methods for subthalamic nucleus deep brain stimulation. Comput Aided Surg. 2007;12(6):325–34.

[29] Hariz M, Blomstedt P, Zrinzo L. Future of brain stimulation: new targets, new indications, new technology. Mov Disord. 2013;28(13):1784–92.

[30] He L, Lee EY, Sterling NW, Kong L, Lewis MM, Du G, Eslinger PJ, et al. The key determinants to quality of life in Parkinson's disease patients: results from the Parkinson's Disease Biomarker Program (PDBP). J Parkinsons Dis. 2016;6(3):523–32.

[31] Holsheimer J, Dijkstra E, Demeulemeester H, Nuttin B. Chronaxie calculated from current-duration and voltage-duration data. J Neurosci Methods. 2000;97:45–50.

[32] Huang H, Watts RL, Montgomery EB Jr. Effects of deep brain stimulation frequency on bradykinesia of Parkinson's disease. Mov Disord. 2014;29(2): 203–6.

[33] Hutson M. Has artificial intelligence become alchemy? Science. 2018;360(6388):478. PubMed PMID: 29724937. https://doi.org/10.1126/science.360.6388.478.

[34] Kita H, Kitai ST. Intracellular study of rat globus pallidus neurons: membrane properties and responses to neostriatal, subthalamic and nigral stimulation. Brain Res. 1991;564(2):296–305.

[35] Krack P, Fraix V, Mendes A, Benabid AL, Pollak P. Postoperative management of subthalamic nucleus stimulation for Parkinson's disease. Mov Disord. 2002;17(Suppl 3):S188–97.

[36] Kupsch A, Benecke R, Müller J, Trottenberg T, Schneider GH, Poewe W, Eisner W, et al.; Deep-Brain Stimulation for Dystonia Study Group. Pallidal deep-brain stimulation in primary generalized or segmental dystonia. N Engl J Med. 2006;355(19):1978–90.

[37] Kupsch A, Tagliati M, Vidailhet M, Aziz T, Krack P, Moro E, Krauss JK. Early postoperative management of DBS in dystonia: programming, response to stimulation, adverse events, medication changes, evaluations, and troubleshooting. Mov Disord. 2011;26 Suppl 1:S37–53.

[38] Larson PS, Richardson RM, Starr PA, Martin AJ. Magnetic resonance imaging of implanted deep brain stimulators: experience in a large series. Stereotact Funct Neurosurg. 2008;86(2):92–100.

[39] Lempka SF, Miocinovic S, Johnson MD, Vitek JL, McIntyre CC. In vivo impedance spectroscopy of deep brain stimulation electrodes. J Neural Eng. 2009;6:046001.

[40] Limousin P, Pollak P, Benazzouz A, Hoffmann D, Broussolle E, Perret JE, Benabid AL. Bilateral subthalamic nucleus stimulation for severe Parkinson's disease. Mov Disord. 1995;10(5):672–4.

[41] Liu X, Yianni J, Wang S, Bain PG, Stein JF, Aziz TZ. Different mechanisms may generate sustained hypertonic and rhythmic bursting muscle activity in idiopathic dystonia. Exp Neurol. 2006;198(1):204–13.

[42] Llinas RR, Terzuolo CA. Mechanisms of supraspinal actions upon spinal cord activities. Reticular inhibitory mechanisms on alpha extensor motoneurons. J Neurophysiol. 1964;27:579–91.

[43] Maslow AH. The psychology of science. Manhattan: Harper & Row; 1966.

[44] McIntyre CC, Grill WM. Excitation of central nervous system neurons by non-uniform electric fields. Biophys J. 1999;76:878–88.

[45] Meoni S, Fraix V, Castrioto A, Benabid AL, Seigneuret E, Vercueil L, Pollak P, et al. Pallidal deep brain stimulation for dystonia: a long term study. J Neurol Neurosurg Psychiatry. 2017;88(11):960–7.

[46] Miocinovic S, Lempka SF, Russo GS, Maks CB, Butson CR, Sakaie KE, Vitek JL, et al. Experimental and theoretical characterization of the voltage distribution generated by deep brain stimulation. Exp Neurol. 2009;216(1):166–76.

[47] Miocinovic S, Khemani P, Whiddon R, Zeilman P, Martinez-Ramirez D, Okun MS, Chitnis S. Outcomes, management, and potential mechanisms of interleaving deep brain stimulation settings. Parkinsonism Relat Disord. 2014;20(12):1434–7.

[48] Montgomery EB Jr. Effect of subthalamic nucleus stimulation patterns on motor performance in Parkinson's disease. Parkinsonism Relat Disord. 2005;11(3):167–71.

[49] Montgomery EB Jr. Effects of GPi stimulation on human thalamic neuronal activity. Clin Neurophysiol. 2006;117(12):2691–702.

[50] Montgomery EB Jr. Basal ganglia physiology and pathophysiology: a reappraisal. Parkinsonism Relat Disord. 2007;13(8):455–65.

[51] Montgomery EB Jr. Deep brain stimulation programming: principles and practice. 1st ed. Oxford: Oxford University Press; 2010. ISBN 978-0-19-973852-6.

[52] Montgomery EB Jr. The epistemology of deep brain stimulation and neuronal pathophysiology. Front Integr Neurosci. 2012;6:78.

[53] Montgomery EB Jr. Modeling and theories of pathophysiology and physiology of the basal ganglia–thalamic–cortical system: critical

analysis. Front Hum Neurosci. 2016;10:469.
[54] Montgomery EB Jr. Deep brain stimulation programming: mechanisms, principles and practice. 2nd ed. Oxford: Oxford University Press; 2017.
[55] Montgomery EB Jr. Medical reasoning: the nature and use of medical knowledge. Oxford: Oxford University Press; 2018.
[56] Montgomery EB Jr., Baker KB. Mechanisms of deep brain stimulation and future technical developments. Neurol Res. 2000;22(3):259–66.
[57] Moreau C, Defebvre L, Destée A, Bleuse S, Clement F, Blatt JL, Krystkowiak P, et al. STN-DBS frequency effects on freezing of gait in advanced Parkinson disease. Neurology. 2008;71(2):80–4.
[58] Moro E, Esselink RJ, Xie J, Hommel M, Benabid AL, Pollak P. The impact on Parkinson's disease of electrical parameter settings in STN stimulation. Neurology. 2002;59:706–13.
[59] Moro E, Poon YY, Lozano AM, Saint-Cyr JA, Lang AE. Subthalamic nucleus stimulation: improvements in outcome with reprogramming. Arch Neurol. 2006;63(9):1266. -72-36
[60] Moro E, Piboolnurak P, Arenovich T, Hung SW, Poon YY, Lozano AM. Pallidal stimulation in cervical dystonia: clinical implications of acute changes in stimulation parameters. Eur J Neurol. 2009;16(4):506–12.
[61] Moro E, Hamani C, Poon YY, Al-Khairallah T, Dostrovsky JO, Hutchison WD, Lozano AM. Unilateral pedunculopontine stimulation improves falls in Parkinson's disease. Brain. 2010;133(pt 1):215–24.
[62] Moro E, LeReun C, Krauss JK, Albanese A, Lin JP, Walleser Autiero S, Brionne TC, et al. Efficacy of pallidal stimulation in isolated dystonia: a systematic review and meta-analysis. Eur J Neurol. 2017;24(4):552–60.
[63] Nakanishi H, Kita H, Kitai ST. Intracellular study of rat substantia nigra pars reticulata neurons in an in vitro slice preparation: electrical membrane properties and response characteristics to subthalamic stimulation. Brain Res. 1987;437(1):45–55.
[64] Nosko D, Ferraye MU, Fraix V, Goetz L, Chabardès S, Pollak P, Debû B. Low-frequency versus high-frequency stimulation of the pedunculopontine nucleus area in Parkinson's disease: a randomised controlled trial. J Neurol Neurosurg Psychiatry. 2015;86(6):674–9.
[65] Okun MS, Tagliati M, Pourfar M, Fernandez HH, Rodriguez RL, Alterman RL, Foote KD. Management of referred deep brain stimulation failures: a retrospective analysis from 2 movement disorders centers. Arch Neurol. 2005;62(8):1250–5.
[66] Okun MS, Gallo BV, Mandybur G, Jagid J, Foote KD, Revilla FJ, Alterman R, et al; SJM DBS Study Group. Subthalamic deep brain stimulation with a constant-current device in Parkinson's disease: an open-label randomised controlled trial. Lancet Neurol. 2012;11(2):140–9.
[67] Pinsker MO, Herzog J, Falk D, Volkmann J, Deuschl G, Mehdorn M. Accuracy and distortion of deep brain stimulation electrodes on postoperative MRI and CT. Zentralbl Neurochir. 2008;69(3):144–7.
[68] Pollo C, Kaelin-Lang A, Oertel MF, Stieglitz L, Taub E, Fuhr P, Lozano AM, et al. Directional deep brain stimulation: an intraoperative double-blind pilot study. Brain. 2014;137(Pt 7):2015–26.
[69] Pourfar MH, Mogilner AY, Farris S, Giroux M, Gillego M, Zhao Y, Blum D, Bokil H, Pierre MC. Model-based deep brain stimulation programming for Parkinson's disease: the GUIDE pilot study. Stereotact Funct Neurosurg. 2015;93(4):231–9. https://doi. org/10.1159/000375172. Epub 2015 May 14. PubMed PMID: 25998447
[70] Ramirez de Noriega F, Eitan R, Marmor O, Lavi A, Linetzky E, Bergman H, Israel Z. Constant current versus constant voltage subthalamic nucleus deep brain stimulation in Parkinson's disease. Stereotact Funct Neurosurg. 2015;93:114–21.
[71] Ranck JB. Which elements are excited in electrical stimulation of mammalian central nervous system: a review. Brain Res. 1975;98:417–40.
[72] Ricchi V, Zibetti M, Angrisano S, Merola A, Arduino N, Artusi CA, Rizzone M, et al. Transient effects of 80 Hz stimulation on gait in STN DBS treated PD patients: a 15 months follow-up study. Brain Stimul. 2012;5:388–92.

[73] Santaniello S, McCarthy MM, Montgomery EB Jr, Gale JT, Kopell N, Sarma SV. Therapeutic mechanisms of high-frequency stimulation in Parkinson's disease and neural restoration via loop-based reinforcement. Proc Natl Acad Sci U S A. 2015;112(6):E586–95.
[74] Schüpbach WMM, Chabardes S, Matthies C, Pollo C, Steigerwald F, Timmermann L, Visser Vandewalle V, et al. Directional leads for deep brain stimulation: opportunities and challenges. Mov Disord. 2017;32(10):1371–5.
[75] Sillay KA, Chen JC, Montgomery EB. Long-term measurement of therapeutic electrode impedance in deep brain stimulation. Neuromodulation. 2010;13(3):195–200.
[76] Sillay KA, Rutecki P, Cicora K, Worrell G, Drazkowski J, Shih JJ, Sharan AD, et al. Long-term measurement of impedance in chronically implanted depth and subdural electrodes during responsive neurostimulation in humans. Brain Stimul. 2013;6(5):718–26.
[77] Steigerwald F, Timmermann L, Kühn A, Schnitzler A, Reich MM, Kirsch AD, Barbe MT, et al. Pulse duration settings in subthalamic stimulation for Parkinson's disease. Mov Disord. 2018;33(1):165–9.
[78] Steriade M, Deschenes M, Oakson G. Background firing and responsiveness of pyramidal tract neurons and interneurons. J Neurophysiol. 1974;37:1065–92.
[79] Temperli P, Ghika J, Villemure JG, Burkhard PR, Bogousslavsky J, Vingerhoets FJ. How do parkinsonian signs return after discontinuation of subthalamic DBS? Neurology. 2003;60(1):78–81.
[80] Thevathasan W, Debu B, Aziz T, Bloem BR, Blahak C, Butson C, Czernecki V, et al.; Movement Disorders Society PPN DBS Working Group in collaboration with the World Society for Stereotactic and Functional Neurosurgery. Pedunculopontine nucleus deep brain stimulation in Parkinson's disease: a clinical review. Mov Disord. 2018;33(1):10–20.
[81] Tyulmankov D, Tass PA, Bokil H. Periodic flashing coordinated reset stimulation paradigm reduces sensitivity to ON and OFF period durations. PLoS One. 2018;13(9):e0203782. https://doi. org/10.1371/journal. pone.0203782. eCollection 2018. PubMed PMID: 30192855; PubMed Central PMCID: PMC6128645
[82] Urasaki E, Fukudome T, Hirose M, Nakane S, Matsuo H, Yamakawa Y. Neuroleptic malignant syndrome (parkinsonism-hyperpyrexia syndrome) after deep brain stimulation of the subthalamic nucleus. J Clin Neurosci. 2013;20(5):740–1. https:// doi.org/10.1016/j. jocn.2012.04.024. Epub 2013 Mar 5. PubMed PMID: 23465352
[83] Vidailhet M, Vercueil L, Houeto JL, Krystkowiak P, Benabid AL, Cornu P, Lagrange C, et al.; French Stimulation du Pallidum Interne dans la Dystonie (SPIDY) Study Group. Bilateral deep-brain stimulation of the globus pallidus in primary generalized dystonia. N Engl J Med. 2005;352(5):459–67.
[84] Volkmann J, Herzog J, Kopper F, Deuschl G. Introduction to the programming of deep brain stimulators. Mov Disord. 2002;17(Suppl 3):S181–7.
[85] Volkmann J, Moro E, Pahwa R. Basic algorithms for the programming of deep brain stimulation in Parkinson's disease. Mov Disord. 2006;21(Suppl 14):S284–9.
[86] Volkmann J, Wolters A, Kupsch A, Müller J, Kühn AA, Schneider GH, Poewe W, et al. DBS Study Group for Dystonia. Pallidal deep brain stimulation in patients with primary generalised or segmental dystonia: 5-year follow-up of a randomised trial. Lancet Neurol. 2012;11(12):1029–38.
[87] Wagle Shukla A, Zeilman P, Fernandez H, Bajwa JA, Mehanna R. DBS programming: an evolving approach for patients with Parkinson's disease. Parkinsons Dis. 2017;2017:1–11.
[88] Walker HC, Huang H, Gonzalez CL, Bryant JE, Killen J, Cutter GR, Knowlton RC, Montgomery EB, Guthrie BL, Watts RL. Short latency activation of cortex during clinically effective subthalamic deep brain stimulation for Parkinson's disease. Mov Disord. 2012;27(7):864–73.
[89] Wang J, Nebeck S, Muralidharan A, Johnson MD, Vitek JL, Baker KB. Coordinated reset deep brain stimulation of subthalamic nucleus produces long-lasting, dose-dependent motor improvements in the 1-Methyl-4-phenyl-1,2,3,6-tetrahydropyridine

non-human primate model of parkinsonism. Brain Stimul. 2016;9(4):609–17. https://doi.org/10.1016/j. brs.2016.03.014. Epub 2016 Mar 22. PubMed PMID: 27151601

[90] Weaver FM, Follett KA, Stern M, Luo P, Harris CL, Hur K, Marks WJ Jr, et al.; CSP 468 Study Group. Randomized trial of deep brain stimulation for Parkinson disease: thirty-six-month outcomes. Neurology. 2012;79(1):55–65.

[91] Wei XF, Grill WM. Impedance characteristics of deep brain stimulation electrodes in vitro and in vivo. J Neural Eng. 2009;6:046008.

[92] Wojtecki L, Vesper J, Schnitzler A. Interleaving programming of subthalamic deep brain stimulation to reduce side effects with good motor outcome in a patient with Parkinson's disease. Parkinsonism Relat Disord. 2011;17(4):293–4.

[93] Yokochi F, Kato K, Iwamuro H, Kamiyama T, Kimura K, Yugeta A, Okiyama R, et al. Resting-state pallidal-cortical oscillatory couplings in patients with predominant phasic and tonic dystonia. Front Neurol. 2018;9:375.

[94] York MK, Moro E. No differences in neuropsychological outcomes between constant current and voltage current subthalamic deep brain stimulation for Parkinson's disease. Ann Transl Med. 2017;5(7):177.

第 9 章 神经心理学评估
Neuropsychological Assessment

Marjan Jahanshahi **著**
袁天硕 石 林 **译** 赵宝田 杨岸超 张建国 **校**

> **摘要：** 脑深部电刺激（DBS）旨在通过控制目标症状来改善其功能，进而最终提高患者的生活质量（QoL）。一些可通过 DBS 治疗的疾病（如帕金森病）存在认知障碍或严重的精神症状，这些症状与运动症状无关，但会影响患者生活质量和术后疗效，因此进行术前筛查从而排除这些影响 DBS 效果的严重认知障碍或精神症状是很有必要的。由于任何脑部手术都有着使认知功能降低的潜在风险，所以即便是术前认知功能基本完好的疾病（如特发性肌张力障碍）也需要进行术前和术后认知功能评估。此外，由于电极位置、邻近脑区的扩散激活、刺激对于所涉及网络远隔部位的影响等多种机制的作用，患者很可能出现行为或情绪的变化，这也需要进行严格的术前和术后评估。综上所述，DBS 是一个能改变患者生活的外科手术，它可以在相对较短的时间内对患者的症状和体征产生巨大影响，并改变他们的日常生活、心理，以及与他人的交往。虽然 DBS 所导致的变化很大程度上都是积极的，但就算是积极的改变也需要患者及家属去适应和调整。神经心理学评估可在术前筛查和排除患有严重认知障碍或精神疾病的患者，并建立认知、情绪、行为、社会心理功能，以及生活质量的术前基线，以便与术后变化进行比较，这对于量化 DBS 的疗效及记录任何可能的不良反应都非常有意义。临床神经心理学家作为多学科团队的一部分，应在患者的术前教育和术前准备中发挥作用，以应对 DBS 带来的生活改变，以及术后社会心理失调。

一、概述

脑深部电刺激（DBS）是治疗帕金森病（PD）、特发性震颤和肌张力障碍的公认疗法，并已扩展到治疗其他疾病，如 Tourette 综合征、强迫症（OCD）、抑郁症，最近还成为治疗痴呆的潜在疗法。

神经心理学重点关注认知障碍。但情绪和行为的改变也可能会对认知功能产生影响，在解释认知功能障碍时也要考虑到这些因素。因此神经心理学评估不仅涉及认知方面，如智力、注意力、记忆力和学习能力、执行功能、感觉语言等标准化测试，还包括情绪行为方面的标准化访谈和有效的问卷调查等。

二、脑深部电刺激治疗运动障碍性疾病

本书广泛涵盖了 DBS 治疗帕金森病和肌张力障碍的各种靶点及其对患者运动症状和生活质

量（QoL）的影响（见第 12 章和第 14 章）。考虑到 DBS 手术在认知、心理和社会心理方面的影响，本章的重点将放在 PD 和肌张力障碍方面，因为已有大量文献报道了 DBS 对这两种运动障碍性疾病在认知、情绪和行为方面的影响，并且 DBS 用于这两种疾病的历史也是最长的。对于其他疾病［如特发性震颤（Tröster 等，1999）、癫痫（Fisher 等，2010）、抑郁症（McNeely 等，2008）和 OCD（Mallet 等，2008；Tyagi 等，2019）］而言，虽然目前已有的经验性证据较少，但针对多种脑部不同靶点进行 DBS 治疗，从认知角度看通常也是安全的，术后也能够改善情绪和生活质量。

三、帕金森病

（一）DBS 对于认知的影响

轻度认知障碍（MCI），尤其是执行功能障碍是 PD 的早期征象之一（Muslimovic 等，2005；Litvan 等，2011，2012；综述见 Dirnberger 和 Jahanshahi，2013）。一部分 PD 患者随着疾病的进展而继发痴呆，据估计在患病 20 年后痴呆症的发生率为 80%（Emre 等，2007；Hely 等，2008；Gratwicke 等，2015）。

PD 患者 DBS 术前的神经心理学情况已有所概述（Voon 等，2006；Tröster 2017）。这种神经心理学评估包括认知方面的评估和筛查，以排除痴呆和严重的难治性精神疾病。已发表的关于 DBS 对认知影响的大多数研究都是针对 PD 患者的，而且这些患者在术前都经过了神经心理学筛查，并选择排除了痴呆和严重认知功能障碍。一项德国的 DBS 研究结果强调了这种术前认知筛查的重要性（Witt 等，2011）。术前在 Mattis 痴呆评分量表中得到临界分数的患者（n=12）在帕金森问卷 39（PDQ-39；其中一部分改善主要是由于 3 例患者，其余 9 例患者术后 PDQ-39 得分均下降）的生活质量方面改善最差，这与未手术的"最佳药物治疗"对照组没有区别，并且明显不如 Mattis 术前认知评估显示"完好"的 3 组。

几项 Meta 分析检验了底丘脑核脑深部电刺激（STN-DBS）和苍白球内侧部脑深部电刺激（GPi-DBS）对 PD 认知的影响（表 9-1）。这些结果均表明 STN-DBS 和 GPi-DBS 不会导致任何严重的认知功能变化，然而语言流利性和执行功能（如 Stroop 色字干扰任务测试）的进一步恶化是在 STN-DBS 和 GPi-DBS 治疗 PD 后经常出现的主要认知功能减退。在比较 STN-DBS 和 GPi-DBS 对认知影响的 3 项 Meta 分析中，2 项（Wang 等，2016；Combs 等，2015）表明 STN-DBS 与更严重的认知不良反应有关，而另一项 Meta 分析（Elgebaly 等，2017）认为在对认知影响方面 2 个靶点都没有证据支持。美国的一项 STN-DBS 和 GPi-DBS 的双盲随机试验表明 2 个靶点对认知的影响大致相同，但 STN-DBS 组的认知处理速度下降更快（Follett 等，2010），并且 STN-DBS 术后 36 个月的 Mattis 痴呆评分量表得分下降更快（Weaver 等，2012）。一项荷兰的随机对照试验 NSTAPS 得出结论，在认知、情绪和行为的不良反应方面，STN 和 GPi 靶点是相同的，但 STN 靶点在药物"关"期运动症状的控制、日常活动、药物减量方面具有优势（Odekerken 等，2013）。

表 9-2 中列出的数个病例或分组研究中，研究了脚桥核（PPN）DBS 对 PD 认知功能的影响。其结果并不一致，有些研究认为在接受了短期低频 PPN-DBS 后 PD 患者认知的一些方面得到了改善，如语言语法（Zanini 等，2009）、延迟语义记忆和回溯（Ceravolo 等，2011）、工作记忆（Costa 等，2010），以及与注意力改善有关的整体认知方面（Ricciardi 等，2015），也有一些研究表明患者术后语言功能下降（Pinto 等，2014），但认知功能没有变化（Leimbach 等，2019）。

这些都是基于 1～11 例患者的小样本研究，并且 8 项研究中有 5 项研究的患者同时接受了 STN 或未定带 DBS 和 PPN-DBS。因此单纯由 PPN-DBS 导致的认知功能改变仍不清楚。除了

表 9-1 关于 STN-DBS 或 GPi-DBS 对 PD 认知方面影响的神经心理学证据的 8 个 Meta 分析的详细信息

研究者（出版年份）	研究数量	样本数量	DBS 靶点	方法学	主要发现
Parsons 等（2006）	28	612	STN	• 包括个案或组间研究，DBS 开机 vs. 关机，术前 vs. 术后的研究，认知方面的随机效应值	• 语义语音方面的口语流利度显著下降。此外，执行功能、语言学习和记忆的下降是显著的，尽管效应量较小
Combs 等（2015）	38	1622	STN GPi	• 包括单侧和双侧 DBS，随机效应值	• STN-DBS 导致精神运动速度、记忆力、注意力、执行功能和整体认知的小幅下降，语义和语音口语流利度中度下降。与 STN-DBS 相比，GPi-DBS 导致的认知下降较少，即注意力小幅下降，语言流利性小幅/中等下降
Xie（2016）	10	797	STN	• 包括 3 项 RCT 研究，7 项对照研究。固定和随机测试效应值	• 与对照组相比，STN-DBS 导致整体认知、记忆、言语流利性和执行功能下降。在其他认知领域无明显差异
Wang 等（2016）	7	521	STN vs. GPi	• 仅包括 4 项 RCT，均为单侧和双侧 DBS，认知领域的固定和随机效应值	• 与 GPi-DBS 相比，STN-DBS 与注意力下降、工作记忆、语音流利性、学习记忆和术后整体认知的下降有关。2 个靶点在生活质量和精神类作用方面没有差异
Martinez-Martinez 等（2017）	50	69~246 每次测试	STN vs. GPi	• 仅关注了执行功能的测试，包括固定和随机测试效应值	• 发现了认知语言流利性、抑制性功能有下降的趋势。其他功能的评估中术前后无差异
Elgebaly 等（2017）	4	345	STN vs. GPi	• RCT，固定和随机测试效应值	• STN DBS 与 GPi DBS 相比，大多数神经心理学结果均无统计学差异。在神经心理学方面，现有证据不支持任何一个靶点更具优势
Jahanshahi 和 Leimbach（submitted）[a]	12	DBS n=410 PD 对照 n=440	STN	• 神经心理学对照研究，认知方面随机效应值	• 语义和语音口语流利程度的中等效应值表明，手术组下降幅度更大。其他认知方面的效应值很小

RCT. 随机对照试验

a. 引自 Jahanshahi M and Leimbach. The short and long-term cognitive effects of subthalamic deep brain stimulation in Parkinson disease（submitted）

第9章 神经心理学评估
Neuropsychological Assessment

表9-2 关于PPN-DBS对帕金森病（PD）或帕金森病痴呆（PD-D）或进行性核上性麻痹（PSP）患者认知功能影响的个案或组水平研究

研究者	数量	DBS靶点和侧别	随访时间	神经心理学测试	运动症状相关的发现	认知方面的发现
Zanini等（2009）	5PD	• 双侧PPN • 双侧STN	6、12个月	• 故事生成任务	• UPDRS-Ⅲ提高	• 低频刺激改善了语言的语法方面
Costa等（2010）	5PD	• 双侧PPN • 双侧STN	3个月	• 卡片分类测试、语音VF、RPM、RAVLT、Rey的复杂图形测试、记忆广度测试、Corsi方块敲击测试、TMT	• UPDRS-Ⅲ提高	• 工作记忆显著提升
Thevathasan等（2010）	11PD	• 双侧PPN • 单侧PPN • 双侧ZI	2~38个月	• 简单反应时任务、数字警戒任务、选择性反应时任务	• 步态和平衡能力提高	• 在注意力测试中，反应速度提高但反应准确性没有提高
Ceravolo等（2011）	6PD	• 双侧PPN • 双侧STN	12个月	• CVLT、记忆广度、TMT、语音VF、BNT	• UPDRS-Ⅲ提高	• 执行功能和延迟语言回忆得到改善
Pinto等（2014）	7PD	• 双侧PPN • 双侧STN	12个月	• 言语任务	• 未评估	• 语言功能下降
Ricciardi等（2015）	1PD-D	• 单侧PPN	6、48个月	• MMSE、RPM47、RAVLT、记忆广度、WASI、NART、WAIS Ⅲ词命名、MFTC、Stroop	• UPDRS-Ⅲ轻度提高	• 全面性的改善
Leimbach等（2019）	5PD 2PSP	• 双侧PPN	12个月	• MMSE、DRS-2、WASI、NART、WAIS Ⅲ WMI & PSI、CVLT、Stroop、TMT、VF、VCALT	• UPDRS-Ⅲ提高	• 在大多数测试中没有变化

STN.底丘脑核；ZI.未定带；UPDRS.统一帕金森评估量表；CVLT.California语言学习测试；RPM.Rey渐进矩阵；RAVLT.Rey听觉语言学习测试；BNT.Boston命名测试；MMSE.简易精神状态检查表；MFTC.多特征目标消除；WASI.韦氏成人智力测验；WAIS Ⅲ WMI & PSI.Wechsler成人智力量表工作记忆指数和处理速度指数；NART.全国成人阅读测验；VCALT.视觉联想学习测试

少数研究（Costa 等，2010；Ricciardi 等，2015；Leimbach 等，2019），大部分研究仅涉及了有限的神经心理学评估项目，表9-2列举的研究只对短期 PPN 刺激的作用进行了研究，没有比较 PPN-DBS 手术前后的认知变化。少数有着手术前后数据的研究（Pinto 等，2014；Ricciardi 等，2015；Zanini 等，2009；Leimbach 等，2019）表明认知方面仅有微小的改变。

很多研究还探索了丘脑腹侧中间核（Vim）DBS 治疗 PD 后认知方面的变化。两项早期研究（Caparros-Lefebvre 等，1992；Tröster 等，1997）表明了 Vim-DBS 的对于认知功能的安全性，但其中第一项研究中也发现 9 名患者中有 5 名出现了轻微的语言流利性减退。随后 Tröster 等（1998）发表了一个 42 岁的男性 PD 病例的详细神经心理学评估，包括在 Vim-DBS 手术前后，以及开、关机的评估结果。术后，患者的语言流利性（下降 2 个标准差）和加州语言学习测试中的情景记忆（下降 1.3 个标准差）显著减退，但却在 Mattis 痴呆评分量表（主要是造句类题目）和威斯康星卡片分类测验中的表现更好。刺激时语言流利性会有轻微改善但情景记忆在开机时会减退。随后同一个研究小组报道了 6 例接受 Vim-DBS 的 PD 患者在认知、情绪、生活质量方面的结果（Woods 等，2001）。术后 1 年，患者在 Mattis 痴呆评分量表的概念化子测验中得分提高（相对于基线），还在即时情景回忆、远期延迟回忆、Beck 抑郁评估表、Beck 焦虑评估表、PDQ-39 生活质量评估中的自述抑郁和焦虑方面得到了改善。通过一系列的认知测试，对 9 例患者（包括 5 例 PD 患者）Vim 刺激的短期作用进行研究发现，除了刺激左侧 Vim 时出现情景记忆回忆的轻微下降外，单侧 Vim-DBS 没有造成认知方面的其他改变（Loher 等，2003）。通常人们认为，Vim-DBS 几乎不会出现认知方面的不良反应。

（二）DBS 的精神类不良反应

精神类症状包括抑郁、焦虑、淡漠、幻觉、妄想和药物引起的冲动控制障碍（ICD），这些都是 PD 的非运动症状（Jahanshahi 和 Marsden，1998）。术前筛查严重精神疾病非常重要，因为有证据表明术前的精神症状术后仍会存在，还会影响到术后运动症状改善带来的生活质量提高。Houeto 等（2006）报道一部分病例在 STN-DBS 术后出现重度抑郁症、自杀、广场恐惧症或一般性焦虑等精神症状，这些问题在术前就已存在，有时会持续到术后。

目前有大量关于 DBS 在 PD 患者中的精神类不良反应的文献，其中包括单个或多病例报道以及队列研究。也有一些关于 DBS 术后精神症状的综述（Voon 等，2006；Volkmann 等，2010；Castrioto 等，2014）。一些对照试验（Deuschl 等，2006；Follett 等，2010；Weaver 等，2012；Williams 等，2010；Schuepbach 等，2013；Witt 等，2008）表明很多精神类不良反应是短期，并且可控的。术后 STN-DBS 的自评量表抑郁和焦虑也有所改善或没有变化，但相比最佳药物治疗，DBS 术后的抑郁发作频率更高（Castrioto 等，2014；Witt 等，2008；Schuepbach 等，2013）。一项回顾性多中心研究显示 STN-DBS 术后自杀风险会增加（Voon 等，2008），但在之后并未得到来自随机对照试验的前瞻性证据的证实（Weintraub 等，2013）。此外在早期的研究中（Voon 等，2008），很多患者术后没有逐渐减少多巴胺类药物的剂量，而在现在这是标准治疗操作并可能有助于预防此类精神症状。从精神类疾病的角度看，通常认为 Vim-DBS 是更安全的。但近期却有报道 1 名 56 岁的男性患者在接受了卡比多巴和左侧 Vim-DBS 后自杀未遂的案例（Ayobello 等，2019）。

L'hommee 等（2012）应用 Ardouin 量表评估了 63 名 STN-DBS 术前和术后 1 年的 PD 患者（Ardouin 等，2009；Rieu 等，2015）。术后患者的认知方面没有变化，统一帕金森评分量表（UPDRS）的运动症状方面改善 45%，多巴胺类药物剂量减少 73%。他们研究显示术前 ICD、多巴胺失调综合征和"关"期烦躁在手术后得到了明显改善，存在1例术后新发多巴胺药物滥用的病例，还有2例患者自杀未遂。淡漠是PD常见的精神症状，其发病率在20%~60%（Pagonabarraga等，2015），对生活质量有着负面影响（Benito-Leo等，2012）。有报道表明STN-DBS术后淡漠可出现恶化或进展（Czernecki等，2008；L'hommee等，2012；Thobois等，2010；Martinez-Fernandez等，2016）。例如，在L'hommee等的研究中（2012），术前没有患者存在淡漠，但这一数字在术后1年增加到21%。术后淡漠加重一部分原因可能是由于STN-DBS术后可能出现的多巴胺药物减量，使中脑边缘系统多巴胺能神经元突触前退化的作用显现（Thobois等，2010）。在一个包含88例接受STN-DBS的PD患者队列研究中，术后1年27%的患者出现淡漠。虽然淡漠组和非淡漠组在运动症状方面均得到改善，但淡漠组在生活质量（PDQ-39）、抑郁和焦虑方面没有改善，而非淡漠组在这些方面均得到改善（Martinez-Fernandez等，2016）。因此，术后淡漠似乎抵消了STN-DBS提高生活质量和改善情绪的效果。

在一项针对接受STN-DBS的PD患者的关于精神症状的长期随访研究中，Abbes等（2018）应用Ardouin行为量表从术前到术后3~10年随访了69例PD患者。平均随访时间为6年，除进食行为和性欲亢进外，所有的ICD和多巴胺失调综合征的发生均减少。兴奋或关期烦躁等神经精神类波动也得到显著改善。但与之相反的是随访时有25%的患者出现淡漠，而手术前这一数字仅为3%。数据的回顾性分析表明存在几例抑郁、焦虑、淡漠和ICD的短暂发作。

病理性赌博和购物及性欲亢进等ICD是多巴胺药物治疗PD后的特征表现，发生在15%~25%的患者（Lim等，2008；Weintraub 2008）。单或多病例研究表明DBS可以改善术前已有的ICD（Ardouin等，2006；Lim等，2009）。但也有研究表明STN-DBS可使已有的ICD症状加重或在术后诱发新的ICD（Smeding等，2007；Halbig等，2009；Lim等，2009；for review see Broen等，2011）。术后ICD症状是否较术前加重或者新发，可能取决于每个患者术后多巴胺药物的适量减少或DBS参数调整。有学者提出STN是一种"临时制动器"以阻止人们的冲动行为，并在做出决定之前留出时间去积累动机，但是STN-DBS会干扰STN的这种临时制动功能从而可能导致冲动（Frank等，2007）。现在有一些关于接受STN-DBS或单侧底丘脑核毁损术的PD患者冲动行为的报道，在范式测验中的试验性研究也显示出类似结果（Jahanshahi 2013；Jahanshahi等，2015a），如Stroop颜色干扰任务（Jahanshahi等，2000）、有奖赏的概率决策任务（Frank等，2007）、关于运动抑制的停止信号任务（Obeso等，2013；Obeso等，2014）、需要运动克制的"继续或停止任务"的反应时间（Georgiev等，2016）、涉及速度和准确性指令下感知决策的移动点任务（Pote等，2016）。抑制不当、习惯性、强势的反应也是执行控制的重要组成和自我控制的基础。很多研究认为额叶-纹状体-底丘脑核-苍白球环路构成了无意/习惯性和目标导向性抑制网络，从而允许适应性行为（Jahanshahi等，2015b）。

有研究报道，4例患者在DBS术后出现了新的功能性运动障碍（如坐位时右腿功能性踢腿或右腿功能性震颤），其中2例PD患者接受的双侧DBS-STN，这种术后可能出现的并发症可以通过就诊咨询和术后调控来缓解（Breen等，2018）。

（三）术后社会心理功能

PD对患者的影响，尤其是抑郁、认知障碍等方面，都已被广泛报道（Schrag等，2000；Rahman等，2008）。大部分接受DBS的PD患者术后运动症状和生活质量会得到显著改善（Deuschl等，2006；Weaver等，2012；Follett等，2010；Williams等，2010）。虽然手术改善了患者运动症状，但在一些治疗中心的部分手术病例出现了STN-DBS术后的社会心理适应性变差（Agid等，2006；Houeto等，2002；Schupbach等，

2006；Gisquet 2008；Haahr 等，2010；Haahr 等，2011；Bell 等，2011）。Shahmoon 和 Jahanshahi（2017）回顾了 PD 患者在接受 STN-DBS 后的社会心理适应性相关研究，总结出关于术后社会心理适应性的 6 个共同的问题：①术后伴侣和家人对患者的期望过高；②由于术后运动症状的改善，患者才真正认识到帕金森病对他们生活"损害"的程度；③由于术后调控刺激器主要由临床团队负责，所以患者术后失去了对疾病的管理和控制；④患者经过自身调整并学会了与 PD 共存后，变得对生活失去了激情或有些淡漠；⑤术后症状的改善使得患者和家人需要重新适应，重新回到正常生活也是很困难的；⑥与体内设备和脑内电极有关的自我形象方面的困扰。虽然 DBS 术后社会心理失调的患者仅占少数，但仍应在手术前后均采取适当的措施，以防止出现此类情况从而抵消了 DBS 对患者运动症状的改善和生活质量的提高。

四、肌张力障碍

（一）DBS 对于认知的影响

原发性肌张力障碍或 DYT1 基因相关的肌张力障碍患者没有表现出任何严重的认知功能缺陷，在神经心理学研究中将这些肌张力障碍患者与年龄匹配的健康对照组（Jahanshahi 等，2003；Balas 等，2006；Allam 等，2007；Bugalho 等，2008；Aleman 等，2009；Romano 等，2014；Foley 等，2017）或相较于标准数据（Scott 等，2003；Jahanshahi 和 Torkamani 2017；Jahanshahi 2017）进行比较，也仅发现了独立的执行功能障碍。但继发性肌张力障碍患者可能伴有从轻度认知损害至痴呆不同程度的认知功能障碍（Torkamani 和 Jahanshahi，2014）。

运动障碍协会工作组制订了肌张力障碍患者 DBS 术前和术后神经心理和神经精神病学评估的指南，还回顾了有关 DBS 治疗肌张力障碍对认知、情绪、行为，以及生活质量方面影响的文献（Jahanshahi 等，2011）。少数神经心理学研究（表 9-3）表明 GPi/STN-DBS 不会对肌张力障碍患者的认知功能产生任何不良反应（Halbig 等，2005；Pillon 等，2006；Kleiner-Fisman 等，2007；Jahanshahi 等，2014；Owen 等，2015；Dinkelbach 等，2015），但也有研究发现个别患者出现认知下降或在术后的持续注意力或语言流利性的测试中得分降低（Halbig 等，2005；Kiss 2007；Kleiner-Fisman 等，2007；Jahanshahi 等，2013；Owen 等，2015）。在没有设置对照组或未能采用类似版本的认知测试的情况下，范式的练习效应、术后抗胆碱能药物剂量的减少和运动症状的改善都是潜在的混淆因素，在研究术前和术后认知变化时需要弄清这些因素的影响。对于继发性肌张力障碍 DBS 方面的研究也发现了类似的情况，研究中包括了一些认知方面的测试（Jahanshahi 等，2011）。尽管肌张力障碍患者 DBS 术后出现认知障碍的情况并不常见，但任何形式的脑部手术均具有这种潜在风险，因此我们建议在治疗肌张力障碍患者时应该谨慎操作并在手术前后进行简要的认知评估（Jahanshahi 等，2011）。

（二）DBS 的精神类不良反应

抑郁、焦虑、OCD 都是原发性或继发性肌张力障碍常见的精神类不良反应（Jahanshahi 2005；Torkamani 和 Jahanshahi 2014，Jahanshahi 2017）。但我们还尚不清楚肌张力障碍的精神类并发症是疾病的主要特征，还是致残、不雅的运动障碍所导致的继发症状，也尚无证据能够支持这两种猜测（Jahanshahi 2017；Torkamani and Jahanshahi 2014）。现有的大部分关于 DBS 对肌张力障碍影响的研究都已筛查并排除了那些存在药物治疗无效的难治性严重精神疾病的病例。伴有轻至中度抑郁的原发性肌张力患者通常会从 GPi-DBS 中得到改善（Halbig 等，2005；Kupsch 等，2006；Kiss 2007；Valldeoriola 等，2010）。但可能是由于术后减少了用于控制术前肌张力障碍运动症状苯二氮䓬类药物剂量，术

第9章 神经心理学评估
Neuropsychological Assessment

表 9-3 脑深部电刺激对肌张力障碍认知功能的影响的神经心理学研究

研究者	样本数量和类型	年龄	排除标准	方法学	双侧DBS靶点	随访时间	主要发现
Halbig 等 (2005)	n=15, 13例特发性, 2例迟发性	13—68	临床访谈, 无排除标准	Mattis 痴呆评分量表、Stroop 测试、TMT、语言流利性（语音和语义）、记忆广度、简易预提示任务的反应时间、RAVLT、BDI、BAI、Montgomery Asberg 抑郁量表、Snaith-Hamilton 娱乐量表、简易精神评定量表、Bech-Rafaelsen 躁狂评分量表、PDQ-39	GPi	平均：6.5个月，范围 3~12个月	• 手术组认知功能水平没有变化，部分患者 TMT A 有所改善
Pillon 等 (2006)	n=22	14—54	MMSE<24	Raven 渐进矩阵、WAIS-R（相似性、计算）、Grober 和 Buschke 测验、WCST、语言流利性、语义和语音）、TMT、BDI	GPi	12个月	• 组水平的认知方面没有变化，但在 Raven 渐进矩阵、WAIS-R（相似性）、WCST（非持久性错误）、自由语言回忆中的表现有轻微提高，但统计学显著
Kleiner-Fisman 等 (2007)	n=4, 主要是CD，但有2例患者有其他类型肌张力障碍	41—56	MMSE<24	WAIS Ⅲ 子测试（记忆广度、符号搜索、字母-数字顺序、计算、相似性、符号搜索、数字符号）、Wisconsin 卡片分类测试、Stroop 测试、试行测试、语音和语义语言流利性、Boston 命名测试、BDAE、复杂概念材料测试、Hopkins 语言学习测试-修订版、简易视空间记忆测试-修订版、敲击测试、简易绘画测试、时钟绘画测试、STAI、SF-36	STN	3个月，12个月	• 术前：语言和视觉记忆方差未报告。所有4名患者的执行功能均出现轻度但不显著下降。1名患者的语言记忆显著下降，另外2名患者的视觉记忆下降但最后的结论是 STN-DBS 并没有显著改变患者的认知功能
Jahanshahi 等 (2014)	n=14, 7例 DYT1 基因阳性	18—64	无	MMSE、全国成人阅读测试、WAIS-R、语言 IQ（词汇、相似度、记忆广度、语义）、WCST、语言流利性（语音、语义、交替语义）、PASAT、RAVLT、Stroop、自定顺序指示、Boston 命名测试、简要 RMF、分级命名测试、BDI、BAI、AES	GPi	12个月	• GPi-DBS 不影响 IQ、记忆、语言和执行功能。术后唯一可靠的变化是在 PASAT 中的表现较差。DYT1 基因对术后认知方面没有影响
Owen 等 (2015)	13名儿童, 4例 DYT1 基因阳性, 3例患有原发性肌张力障碍叠加综合征	6—18	无	儿童记忆量表子测试和 WMS 语言和非语言记忆（记忆广度、字母-数字顺序）、工作记忆指数（编码、符号搜索和删除）、WISC-Ⅳ、WASI 的感知推理指数（词汇、相似度、理解力）	GPi	11名患者随访12个月，2名随访36个月	• 术后认知功能基本保持稳定并有10名患者得到改善。改善主要表现在语言理解和感知推理方面。3名患者在一些方面表现变差（处理速度、语言或视觉记忆、感知推理）
Dinkelbach 等 (2015)	n=13CD	39—69	无	RAVLT、记忆广度、WMS-块距前进、图形记忆的非语言学习测验、数字顺序测试、语言流利性（语音、语义、交互语音、交互语义）、Stroop、Benton 线条方向判断、每日注意对象和空间感知测试组、心算、多选题词汇测试以获取得分 IQ 评估、CDQ-24	GPi	12个月	• 除了交替语义的语言流利性下降外，其他任何认知方面测量均无改变

BAI.Beck 焦虑量表；BDI.Beck 抑郁量表；AES. 淡漠评估量表；EQ 5D EuroQoL. 生活质量量表；MMSE. 简易智力状态检查量表；RAVLT.Rey 听觉语言学习测试；SF-36. 健康调查量表 36；TMT. 连线测试；WCST.Wisconsin 卡片分类测试；PASAT. 同步听觉系列加法测试；RMF. 人脸识别记忆；BDAE.Boston 诊断失语症检查；CDQ-24. 颈部肌张力障碍问卷 24；WAIS. 韦氏成人智力测验；WMS. 韦氏记忆量表；WISC-Ⅳ. 韦氏儿童智力量表第 4 版；CD. 认知功能衰退

后患者的焦虑症状仍会存在（Jahanshahi 等，2011）。GPi-DBS 与"肌张力障碍叠加综合征"精神类疗效的相关性尚不明确（Contarino 等，2011；Kemmotsu 等，2011；Torkamani 和 Jahanshahi 2014）。虽然 OCD 是肌张力障碍中另一种常见的精神症状，但迄今为止尚无研究报道过 DBS 手术对肌张力障碍强迫症状的影响。有一个病例报道了植入的电极偏了杏仁核区，导致了伴有妄想的抑郁和严重的淡漠（Piacentini 等，2008）。自杀是 DBS 手术治疗原发性肌张力障碍最严重的精神类不良反应。在 Foncke 等（2006）的研究样本中，16 名肌张力障碍病例中有 2 名（12.5%）自杀。自杀是个多因素决定的行为，目前仍不清楚 DBS 后的自杀行为是刺激扩散至边缘系统环路的结果，还是反映了术后对于改变的再适应问题。自杀是 DBS 术后一种可以预防的不良反应，详细的术前精神类筛查和定期的术后随访对此是很重要的（Jahanshahi 等，2011）。

（三）术后社会心理功能

肌张力障碍会使生活质量（QoL）降低（Ben-Shlomo 等，2002；Page 等，2007）。相较于 PD 或多发性硬化等其他疾病，肌张力障碍尤其影响 QoL 的情绪部分（Camfield 等，2002）。已有的研究表明 DBS 术后肌张力障碍患者的 QoL 会有所改善（Jahanshahi 等，2011）。所有的 DBS 研究都使用了通用的 QoL 量表，例如 EuroQoL 和 Short Form 36（SF-36），这有利于其与一般人群或其他神经系统疾病的规范数据进行比较。但也有例外，如头-颈肌张力障碍这种特殊疾病的 QoL 评估[Cervical Dystonia Questionnaire 24（CDQ-24）；Muller 等，2004]，此类针对特殊疾病的 QoL 量表的缺失可能会使得 DBS 对于疾病的特异性作用被忽视（Maier 等，2016）。此外有研究表明，肌张力障碍患者对自身疾病的反应的主要特征，是与姿态异常和耻辱感有关的畸形、病态的外在形象，以及自我贬低（Jahanshahi 和 Marsden, 1988,，1990a，b；Lewis 等，2008；Page 等，2007；Papathanasiou 等，1997；Papathanasiou 等，2001），所以如果仅用普通的 QoL 评估方法将会忽略掉 DBS 对于这些社会心理学维度的影响。除了需要针对肌张力障碍的 QoL 量表外，还需要评估 DBS 手术对于心理健康其他方面的影响，比如自尊、外在形象、就业、婚姻关系、社交活动、肌张力障碍羞耻感等社会功能。

Hariz 等（2011）使用半结构化访谈和定性分析的方式，对 13 名接受了 GPi-DBS 的各类肌张力障碍的患者进行了研究，并描述了患者术后的共同经历。其中的主题有"与致残和毁容的疾病作斗争""接受 DBS 是对人生转折点的探寻""品味自己的真实潜能""在指导下转变"。有很多患者提出需要术后支持。1 名受试者在一段关于 DBS 的陈述中，强调了对术后心理治疗和支持的需要："即使我得到了新的身体，但却没有得到新的想法。就像做整容手术，你可能会改变自己鼻子，但你对自己的感觉仍然是一样的。"

五、影响 DBS 在认知和精神方面效果的因素

为了能够预防和控制 DBS 术后出现的任何认知或精神类问题，确定与之相关的因素是尤为重要的。年龄更大、术前应用更多剂量左旋多巴、术前存在明显的认知缺陷、中线症状严重是与增加 PD 患者术后出现认知缺陷的可能性的相关因素（Saint-Cyr 等，2000；Daniels 等，2010；Smeding 等，2011；Hariz 等，2000）。电极未准确放置在 STN 背外侧或手术针道通过脑室或尾状核，这些可能与认知下降有关（Cakmakli 等，2009；Tsai 等，2007；York 等，2009；Witt 等，2013）。此外也有学者认为刺激参数（如振幅和频率）也与注意力和语义记忆测试的下降有关（Francel 等，2004）。

关于 STN-DBS 对行为和情绪影响的相关因素的证据较少。一些关键因素可能与手术操作有关，例如微电极通过的次数或电极的位置，这些

都可能会涉及 STN 的边缘部。由于 STN 的体积较小，所以电流可能会扩散到边缘部从而导致精神类不良反应。Houeto 等（2006 年）认为，一些 DBS 术后的精神症状可能反映了与手术无关的原有情绪问题的重现或加剧。术后左旋多巴剂量的减少可能是导致淡漠进展的关键因素，已有研究证实这种淡漠可通过重新应用或增加左旋多巴药物剂量而得到缓解（Castrioto 等，2014）。能够影响 DBS 治疗肌张力障碍在认知和精神方面作用的因素目前还尚不清楚。

多种社会心理因素同样重要。患者及家属对手术结果的过高期望，也会影响到患者术后的调整（Maier 等，2016）。DBS 对运动症状的改善是显著并立即产生的，这可能意味着在术前严重残疾的患者在 1~2 周就可以完全恢复健康和活动能力。患者和家属也需要时间来适应这种急剧而快速的功能改变（Shahmoon 和 Jahanshahi 2017）。进行脑部手术是一件重要的"人生大事"，无论对于患者还是家人都是充满不确定、焦虑、压力的一段时期（Shahmoon 和 Jahanshahi 2017）。事实证明，来自社会的支持具有缓冲作用，可以帮助患者减轻压力。缺乏足够的社会支持可能与术后并发症有关。患者功能状态的改善可能会使他们的角色发生改变。患者可能将不再依赖伴侣或子女的照顾，伴侣护理的角色也发生了改变。这种家庭动态和人际关系的变化需要时间进行调整，如果解决不当则可能引发精神或行为问题（Shahmoon 和 Jahanshahi 2017）。即使运动功能得到了改善，但仍可能有一些患者并不愿放弃"患病角色"，不想恢复到就业、分担家务、照顾家庭这些正常角色当中。

六、预防/减少 DBS 手术的认知和精神类不良反应

通过认真的筛选患者可以避免许多 DBS 手术的认知和精神类不良反应。术前的神经心理学评估不仅应侧重于评估认知功能和鉴别严重的精神类疾病，还应记录患者所处的社会环境。如下文所述，应该对患者和家属进行术前教育，使其了解在术后 6~12 个月他们可能在生活、角色、互动方面发生的变化，这也可能会预防 DBS 手术所致的快速改变，以及在社会心理方面的不良反应。术后刺激触点的精准选择和刺激参数的设置或调整，对于缓解运动症状和避免不良反应来说也是至关重要的。逐渐减少多巴胺类药物剂量可以避免出现淡漠。在术后 6~12 个月，DBS 治疗团队可以通过电话或接诊来与患者沟通，以便能及早发现和治疗精神类并发症和社会适应问题。其中有些问题可能需要直接的医学或心理学治疗。

七、神经心理学家在患者术后心理调节中的作用

有学者认为 DBS 手术具备重大压力性人生事件的几个特点，一生经历一次的稀有性，对于手术结果及不良反应风险的不确定性，最重要的是它能给患者的运动症状、日常活动、独立性、个人身份、情绪、计划/期望和角色带来巨大的改变，而这一切都需要社会心理调整（Shahmoon 和 Jahanshahi 2017）。因此，Shahmoon 和 Jahanshahi（2017）提出了一些建议，以优化手术患者的术后社会心理适应性调整，其中包括增加患者选择标准，应考虑到患者的婚姻关系和社会环境，使患者对于手术结果的期望更加明确，针对 DBS 术后患者及其家属可能发生的身体、心理、社会方面的改变进行更全面、细致的准备工作，并为需要进行心理治疗的患者提供如认知行为治疗等心理疗法，以改善术后适应性。

这项关于 PD 或肌张力障碍患者术后社会心理调整的研究主要采用定期访谈的方式，也强调了我们目前的结果衡量指标，如 UPDRS 和 PDQ-39 更适用于记录运动特征和 QoL 方面的改善，而不能完全反映患者术后的全部经历。所以，制定并验证一种更为敏感的评估方法，以量化 DBS 术后患者面临的社会心理挑战将是非常有价值的。

八、结论

神经心理学家作为多学科 DBS 团队中的一员，在术前评估、手术患者的选择、术前准备并教育患者及家属以应对 DBS 所带来的改变、处理术后出现的任何社会心理失调等方面发挥着重要作用。

参考文献

[1] Abbes M, Lhommée E, Thobois S, et al. Subthalamic stimulation and neuropsychiatric symptoms in Parkinson's disease: results from a long-term follow-up cohort study. J Neurol Neurosurg Psychiatry. 2018;89:836–43.

[2] Agid Y, Schupbach M, Gargiulo M, et al. Neurosurgery in Parkinson's disease: the doctor is happy, the patient less so? J Neural Transm Suppl. 2006;70:409–14.

[3] Aleman GG, de Erausquin GA, Micheli F. Cognitive disturbances in primary blepharospasm. Mov Disord. 2009;24:2112–20.

[4] Allam N, Frank JE, Pereira C, Tomaz C. Sustained attention in cranial dystonia patients treated with botulinum toxin. Acta Neurol Scand. 2007;116:196–200.

[5] Ardouin C, Voon V, Worbe Y, et al. Pathological gambling in Parkinson's disease improves on chronic subthalamic nucleus stimulation. Mov Disord. 2006;21:1941–6.

[6] Ardouin C, Chereau I, Llorca PM, Lhomme E, et al. Assessment of hyper- and hypo-dopaminergic behaviours in Parkinson's disease. Rev Neurol (Paris). 2009;165:845–56.

[7] Ayobello A, Saway B, Greenage M. Attempted suicide in a Parkinsonian patient treated with DBS of the VIM and high dose carbidopa-levodopa. Case Rep Psychiatry. 2019;2019:2903762.

[8] Balas M, Peretz C, Badarny S, et al. Neuropsychological profile of DYT1 dystonia. Mov Disord. 2006;21:2073–7.

[9] Bell E, Maxwell B, McAndrews MP, et al. A review of social and relational aspects of deep brain stimulation in Parkinson's disease informed by healthcare provider experiences. Parkinsons Dis. 2011;2011:871874.

[10] Benito-Leo NJ, Cubo E, Coronell C. Impact of apathy on health-related quality of life in recently diagnosed Parkinson's disease: the ANIMO study. Mov Disord. 2012;27:211–8.

[11] Ben-Shlomo Y, Camfield L, Warner T, the Epidemiological Study of Dystonia in Europe (ESDE) Collaborative Group. What are the determinants of quality of life in people with cervical dystonia. J Neurol Neurosurg Psychiatry. 2002;72:608–14.

[12] Breen DP, Rohani M, Moro E, et al. Functional movement disorders arising after successful deep brain stimulation. Neurology. 2018;90:931–2.

[13] Broen M, Duits A, Visser-Vandewalle V, et al. Impulse control and related disorders in Parkinson's disease patients treated with bilateral subthalamic nucleus stimulation: a review. Parkinsonism Relat Disord. 2011;17:413–7.

[14] Bugalho P, Correa B, Guimaraes J, et al. Set-shifting and behavioral dysfunction in primary focal dystonia. Mov Disord. 2008;23:200–6.

[15] Cakmakli GY, Oruckaptan H, Saka E, Elibol B. Reversible acute cognitive dysfunction induced by bilateral STN stimulation. J Neurol. 2009;256:1360–2.

[16] Camfield L, Ben-Shlomo Y, Warner T, the Epidemiological Study of Dystonia in Europe (ESDE) Collaborative Group. Impact of cervical dystonia on quality of life. Mov Disord. 2002;17:838–41.

[17] Caparros-Lefebvre D, Blond S, Pecheux N, et al. Evaluation neuropsychologique avant et apres stimulation thalamique chez 9 parkinsoniens. Rev Neurol (Paris). 1992;148:117–22.

[18] Castrioto A, Lhommee E, Moro E, Krack P. Mood and behavioural effects of subthalamic stimulation in Parkinson's disease. Lancet Neurol. 2014;13:287–305.

[19] Ceravolo R, Brusa L, Galati S, et al. Low frequency stimulation of the nucleus tegmenti pedunculopontini increases cortical metabolism in parkinsonian patients. Eur J Neurol. 2011;18:842–9.

[20] Combs HL, Folley BS, Berry DT, et al. Cognition and depression following deep brain stimulation of the subthalamic nucleus and globus pallidus pars internus in Parkinson's disease: a meta-analysis. Neuropsychol Rev. 2015;25:439–54.

[21] Contarino MF, Foncke EM, Cath DC, et al. Effect of pallidal deep brain stimulation on psychiatric symptoms in myoclonus-dystonia due to ε-sarcoglycan mutations. Arch Neurol. 2011;68:1087–8.

[22] Costa A, Carlesimo GA, Caltagirone C, et al. Effects of deep brain stimulation of the peduncolopontine area on working memory tasks in patients with Parkinson's disease. Parkinsonism Relat Disord. 2010;16:64–7.

[23] Czernecki V, Schupbach M, Yaici S, et al. Apathy following subthalamic stimulation in Parkinson disease: a dopamine responsive symptom. Mov Disord. 2008;23:964–9.

[24] Daniels C, Krack P, Volkmann J, et al. Risk factors for executive dysfunction after subthalamic nucleus stimulation in Parkinson's disease. Mov Disord. 2010;25:1583–9.

[25] Deuschl G, Schade-Brittinger C, Krack P, et al. A randomized trial of deep brain stimulation for Parkinson's disease. N Engl J Med. 2006;355:896–908.

[26] Dinkelbach L, Mueller J, Poewe W, et al. Cognitive outcome of pallidal deep brain stimulation for primary cervical dystonia: one year follow up results of a prospective multicenter trial. Parkinsonism Relat Disord. 2015;21:976–80.

[27] Dirnberger G, Jahanshahi M. Executive dysfunction in Parkinson's disease: a review. J Neuropsychol. 2013;7:193–224.

[28] Elgebaly A, Elfil M, Attia A, et al. Neuropsychologica performance changes following subthalamic versus pallidal deep brain stimulation in Parkinson's disease: a systematic review and meta-analysis. CNS Spectr. 2017;23:1–14.

[29] Emre M, Aarsland D, Brown R, et al. Clinical diagnostic criteria for dementia associated with Parkinson's disease. Mov Disord. 2007;22:1689–707.

[30] Fisher R, Salanova V, Witt T, et al. Electrical stimulation of the anterior nucleus of thalamus for treatment of refractory epilepsy. Epilepsia. 2010;51:899–908.

[31] Foley JA, Vinke RS, Limousin P, Cipolotti L. Relationship of cognitive function to motor symptoms and mood disorders in patients with isolated dystonia. Cogn Behav Neurol. 2017;30:16–22.

[32] Follett KA, Weaver FM, Stern M, et al. Pallidal versus subthalamic deep-brain stimulation for Parkinson's disease. N Engl J Med. 2010;362:2077–91.

[33] Foncke EM, Schuurman PR, Speelman JD. Suicide after deep brain stimulation of the internal globus pallidus for dystonia. Neurology. 2006;66:142–3.

[34] Francel P, Ryder K, Wetmore E, et al. Deep brain stimulation for Parkinson's disease: association between stimulation parameters and cognitive performance. Stereotact Funct Neurosurg. 2004;82:191–3.

[35] Frank MJ, Samanta J, Moustafa AA, Sherman SJ. Hold your horses: impulsivity, deep brain stimulation, and medication in parkinsonism. Science. 2007;318:1309–12.

[36] Georgiev D, Dirnberger G, Wilkinson L, et al. In Parkinson's disease on a probabilistic Go/NoGo task deep brain stimulation of the subthalamic nucleus only interferes with withholding of the most prepotent responses. Exp Brain Res. 2016;234:1133–43.

[37] Gisquet E. Cerebral implants and Parkinson's disease: a unique form of biographical disruption? Soc Sci Med. 2008;67:1847–51.

[38] Gratwicke J, Jahanshahi M, Foltynie T. Parkinson's disease dementia: a neural network perspective. Brain. 2015;138:1454–76.

[39] Haahr A, Kirkevold M, Hall EO, Østergaard K. From miracle to reconciliation: a hermeneutic phenomenological study exploring the experience of living with Parkinson's disease following deep brain stimulation. Int J Nurs Stud. 2010;47:1228–36.

[40] Haahr A, Kirkevold M, Hall EO, Østergaard K. Living with

advanced Parkinson's disease: a constant struggle with unpredictability. J Adv Nurs. 2011;67:408–17.

[41] Halbig TD, Gruber D, Kopp UA, et al. Pallidal stimulation in dystonia: effects on cognition, mood, and quality of life. J Neurol Neurosurg Psychiatry. 2005;76:1713–6.

[42] Halbig TD, Tse W, Frisina PG, et al. Subthalamic deep brain stimulation and impulse control in Parkinson's disease. Eur J Neurol. 2009;16:493–7.

[43] Hariz MI, Johansson F, Shamsgovara P, et al. Bilateral subthalamic nucleus stimulation in a parkinsonian patient with preoperative deficits in speech and cognition: persistent improvement in mobility but increased dependency: a case study. Mov Disord. 2000;15:136–9.

[44] Hariz GM, Limousin P, Tisch S, et al. Patients' perceptions of life shift after deep brain stimulation for primary dystonia—a qualitative study. Mov Disord. 2011;26:2101–6.

[45] Hely MA, Reid WGJ, Adena MA, et al. The Sydney multicenter study of Parkinson's disease: the inevitability of dementia at 20 years. Mov Disord. 2008;23:837–44.

[46] Houeto JL, Mesnage V, Mallet L, et al. Behavioural disorders, Parkinson's disease and subthalamic stimulation. J Neurol Neurosurg Psychiatry. 2002;72:701–7.

[47] Houeto JL, Mallet L, Mesnage V, et al. Subthalamic stimulation in Parkinson disease: behavior and social adaptation. Arch Neurol. 2006;63:1090–5.

[48] Jahanshahi M. Behavioural and psychiatric manifestations in Dystonia. In: Anderson K, Weiner W, Lang A, editors. Behavioural neurology of movement disorders. Advances in neurology, vol. 96. 2nd ed. Philadelphia: Lippincott Williams & Wilkins; 2005. p. 291–319.

[49] Jahanshahi M. Effects of deep brain stimulation of the subthalamic nucleus on inhibitory and executive control over prepotent responses in Parkinson's disease. Front Syst Neurosci. 2013;7:118.

[50] Jahanshahi M. Neuropsychological and neuropsychiatric features of idiopathic and DYT1 dystonia and the impact of medical and surgical treatment. Arch Clin Neuropsychol. 2017;32:888–905.

[51] Jahanshahi M, Marsden CD. Depression in torticollis: a controlled study. Psychol Med. 1988;18:925–33.

[52] Jahanshahi M, Marsden CD. Body concept, disability and depression in torticollis. Behav Neurol. 1990a;3:117–31.

[53] Jahanshahi M, Marsden CD. A longitudinal follow-up study of depression, disability and body concept in torticollis. Behav Neurol. 1990b;3:233–46.

[54] Jahanshahi M, Marsden CD. Living and coping with Parkinson's disease: a self-help guide for patients and their carers. London: Souvenir Press; 1998.

[55] Jahanshahi M, Torkamani M. The cognitive features of idiopathic and DYT1 dystonia. Mov Disord. 2017;32:1348–55.

[56] Jahanshahi M, Ardouin C, Brown RG, et al. The impact of deep brain stimulation on executive function in Parkinson's disease. Brain. 2000;123:1142–54.

[57] Jahanshahi M, Rowe J, Fuller R. Cognitive executive function in dystonia. Mov Disord. 2003;18:1470–81.

[58] Jahanshahi M, Czernecki V, Zurowski AM. Neuropsychological, neuropsychiatric, and quality of life issues in DBS for dystonia. Mov Disord. 2011;26:S63–78.

[59] Jahanshahi M, Torkamani M, Beigi M, et al. Pallidal stimulation for primary generalised dystonia: effect on cognition, mood and quality of life. J Neurol. 2014;261:164–73.

[60] Jahanshahi M, Obeso I, Baunez C, et al. Parkinson's disease, the subthalamic nucleus, inhibition, and impulsivity. Mov Disord. 2015a;30:128–40.

[61] Jahanshahi M, Obeso I, Rothwell JC, Obeso JA. A fronto-striato-subthalamic-pallidal network for goal-directed and habitual inhibition. Nat Rev Neurosci. 2015b;16:719–32.

[62] Kemmotsu N, Price CC, Oyama G, et al. Pre- and post-GPi DBS neuropsychological profiles in a case of X-linked dystonia-Parkinsonism. Clin Neuropsychol. 2011;25:141–59.

[63] Kiss ZH. Bilateral pallidal neurostimulation—long-term motor and cognitive effects in primary generalized dystonia. Nat Clin Pract Neurol. 2007;3:482–3.

[64] Kleiner-Fisman G, Liang GS, Moberg PJ, et al. Subthalamic nucleus deep brain stimulation for severe idiopathic dystonia: impact on severity, neuropsychological status, and quality of life. J Neurosurg. 2007;107:29–36.

[65] Kupsch A, Benecke R, Muller J, et al. Pallidal deep-brain stimulation in primary generalized or segmental dystonia. N Engl J Med. 2006;355:1978–90.

[66] L'hommee E, Klinger H, Thobois S, et al. Subthalamic stimulation in Parkinson's disease: restoring the balance of motivated behaviours. Brain. 2012;135:1463–77.

[67] Leimbach F, Gratwicke J, Foltynie T, Limousin P, Zrinzo L, Jahanshahi M. Impact of deep brain stimulation of the pedunculopontine nucleus on cognition in Parkinson's disease and progressive supranuclear palsy. Clin Parkinson Relat Disord. 2019;1:48–51.

[68] Lewis L, Butler A, Jahanshahi M. Depression in focal, segmental and generalized dystonia. J Neurol. 2008;255:1750–5.

[69] Lim SY, Evans AH, Miyasaki JM. Impulse control and related disorders in Parkinson's disease. Ann N Y Acad Sci. 2008;1142:85–107.

[70] Lim SY, O'Sullivan SS, Kotschet K, et al. Dopamine dysregulation syndrome, impulse control disorders and punding after deep brain stimulation surgery for Parkinson's disease. J Clin Neurosci. 2009;16:1148–52.

[71] Litvan I, Aarsland D, Adler CH, et al. MDS task force on mild cognitive impairment in Parkinson's disease: critical review of PD-MCI. Mov Disord. 2011;26:1814–24.

[72] Litvan I, Goldman JG, Troster AI, et al. Diagnostic criteria for mild cognitive impairment in Parkinson's disease: movement disorder society task force guidelines. Mov Disord. 2012;27:349–56.

[73] Loher TJ, Gutbrod K, Fravi NL, et al. Thalamic stimulation for tremor. Subtle changes in episodic memory are related to stimulation per se and not to a microthalamotomy effect. J Neurol. 2003;250:707–13.

[74] Maier F, Lewis CJ, Horstkoetter N, et al. Subjective perceived outcome of subthalamic deep brain stimulation in Parkinson's disease one year after surgery. Parkinsonism Relat Disord. 2016;24:41–7.

[75] Mallet L, Polosan M, Jaafari N, et al. Subthalamic nucleus stimulation in severe obsessive–compulsive disorder. N Engl J Med. 2008;359:2121–34.

[76] Martinez-Fernandez R, Pelissier P, Quesada J-L, et al. Postoperative apathy can neutralise benefits in quality of life after subthalamic stimulation for Parkinson's disease. J Neurol Neurosurg Psychiatry. 2016;87:311–8.

[77] Martinez-Martinez AM, Aguilar OM, Acevedo-Triana CA. Meta-analysis of the relationship between deep brain stimulation in patients with Parkinson's disease and performance in evaluation tests for executive brain functions. Parkinsons Dis. 2017;2017:9641392.

[78] McNeely HE, Mayberg HS, Lozano AM, Kennedy SH. Neuropsychological impact of Cg25 deep brain stimulation for treatment-resistant depression: preliminary results over 12 months. J Nerv Ment Dis. 2008;196:405–10.

[79] Muller J, Wissel J, Kemmler G, et al. Craniocervical dystonia questionnaire (CDQ-24): development and validation of a disease-specific quality of life instrument. J Neurol Neurosurg Psychiatry. 2004;75:749–53.

[80] Muslimovic D, Post B, Speelman JD, Schmand B. Cognitive profile of patients with newly diagnosed Parkinson disease. Neurology. 2005;65:1239–45.

[81] Obeso I, Wilkinson L, Rodríguez-Oroz MC, et al. Bilateral stimulation of the subthalamic nucleus has differential effects on reactive and proactive inhibition and conflict-induced slowing in Parkinson's disease. Exp Brain Res. 2013;226:451–62.

[82] Obeso I, Wilkinson L, Speekenbrink M, et al. The subthalamic nucleus alters the response threshold and controls speed-accuracy adjustments in situations of conflict: evidence from unilateral subthalamotomy in Parkinson's disease. Brain. 2014;137:1470–80.

[83] Odekerken VJJ, van Laar T, Staal MJ, et al. Subthalamic nucleus versus globus pallidus bilateral deep brain stimulation for advanced Parkinson's disease (NSTAPS study): a randomised controlled trial. Lancet Neurol. 2013;12:37–44.

[84] Owen T, Gimeno H, Selway R, Lin JP. Cognitive function in children with primary dystonia before and after deep brain

stimulation. Eur J Paediatr Neurol. 2015;19:48–55.

[85] Page D, Butler A, Jahanshahi M. Quality of life in focal, segmental, and generalized dystonia. Mov Disord. 2007;22:341–7.

[86] Pagonabarraga J, Kulisevsky J, Strafella AP, Krack P. Apathy in Parkinson's disease: clinical features, neural substrates, diagnosis, and treatment. Lancet Neurol. 2015;14:518–31.

[87] Papathanasiou I, MacDonald L, Whurr R, et al. Perceived stigma among patients with spasmodic dysphonia. J Med Speech-Lang Pathol. 1997;5:251–61.

[88] Papathanasiou I, MacDonald L, Whurr R, Jahanshahi M. Perceived stigma in spasmodic torticollis. Mov Disord. 2001;16:280–5.

[89] Parsons TD, Rogers SA, Braaten AJ, et al. Cognitive sequelae of subthalamic nucleus deep brain stimulation in Parkinson's disease: a meta-analysis. Lancet Neurol. 2006;5:578–88.

[90] Piacentini S, Romito L, Franzini A, et al. Mood disorder following DBS of the left amygdaloid region in a dystonia patient with a dislodged electrode. Mov Disord. 2008;23:147–50.

[91] Pillon B, Ardouin C, Dujardin K, et al. Preservation of cognitive function in dystonia treated by pallidal stimulation. Neurology. 2006;66:1556–8.

[92] Pinto S, Ferraye M, Espesser R, et al. Stimulation of the pedunculopontine nucleus area in Parkinson's disease: effects on speech and intelligibility. Brain. 2014;137:2759–72.

[93] Pote I, Torkamani M, Kefalopoulou ZM, et al. Subthalamic nucleus deep brain stimulation induces impulsive action when patients with Parkinson's disease act under speed pressure. Exp Brain Res. 2016;234:1837–48.

[94] Rahman S, Griffin HJ, Quinn NP, Jahanshahi M. Quality of life in Parkinson's disease: the relative importance of the symptoms. Mov Disord. 2008;23:1428–34.

[95] Ricciardi L, Piano C, Rita Bentivoglio A, Fasano A. Pedunculopontine nucleus stimulation in Parkinson's disease dementia. Biol Psychiatry. 2015;77:e35–40.

[96] Rieu I, Martinez-Martin P, Pereira B, De Chazeron I, Verhagen Metman L, Jahanshahi M, Ardouin C, Chéreau I, Brefel-Courbon C, Ory-Magne F, Klinger H, Peyrol F, Schupbach M, Dujardin K, Tison F, Houeto JL, Krack P, Durif F. International validation of a behavioral scale in Parkinson's disease without dementia. Mov Disord. 2015;30(5):705–13. https://doi.org/10.1002/mds.26223. Epub 2015 Mar 21.

[97] Romano R, Bertolino A, Gigante A, et al. Impaired cognitive functions in adult-onset primary cranial cervical dystonia. Parkinsonism Relat Disord. 2014;20:162–5.

[98] Saint-Cyr JA, Trépanier LL, Kumar R, et al. Neuropsychological consequences of chronic bilateral stimulation of the subthalamic nucleus in Parkinson's disease. Brain. 2000;123:2091–108.

[99] Schrag A, Jahanshahi M, Quinn N. What contributes to quality of life in patients with Parkinson's disease? J Neurol Neurosurg Psychiatry. 2000;69:308–12.

[100] Schuepbach WMM, Rau J, Knudsen K, et al. Neurostimulation for Parkinson's disease with early motor complications. N Engl J Med. 2013;368:610–22.

[101] Schupbach M, Gargiulo M, Welter ML, et al. Neurosurgery in Parkinson disease: a distressed mind in a repaired body? Neurology. 2006;66:1811–6.

[102] Scott R, Gregory R, Wilson J, et al. Executive cognitive deficits in primary dystonia. Mov Disord. 2003;18:539–50.

[103] Shahmoon S, Jahanshahi M. Optimizing psychosocial adjustment after deep brain stimulation of the subthalamic nucleus in Parkinson's disease. Mov Disord. 2017;32:1155–8.

[104] Smeding HMM, Goudriaan AE, Foncke EMJ, et al. Pathological gambling after bilateral subthalamic nucleus stimulation in Parkinson disease. J Neurol Neurosurg Psychiatry. 2007;78:517–9.

[105] Smeding HM, Speelman JD, Huizenga HM, et al. Predictors of cognitive and psychosocial outcome after STN DBS in Parkinson disease. J Neurol Neurosurg Psychiatry. 2011;82:754–60.

[106] Thevathasan W, Silburn PA, Brooker H, Coyne TJ, Khan S, Gill SS, et al. The impact of low-frequency stimulation of the pedunculopontine nucleus region on reaction time in parkinsonism. J Neurol Neurosurg Psychiatry. 2010;81(10):1099–104. https://doi.org/10.1136/jnnp.2009.189324.

[107] Thobois S, Ardouin C, L'homme E, et al. Non-motor dopamine withdrawal syndrome after surgery for Parkinson's disease: predictors and underlying mesolimbic denervation. Brain. 2010;133:1111–27.

[108] Torkamani M, Jahanshahi M. Neuropsychological and neuropsychiatric features of dystonia and the impact of medical and surgical treatment. In: Tröster AI, editor. Clinical neuropsychology and cognitive neurology of Parkinson's disease and other movement disorders. New York: Oxford University Press; 2014.p. 455–83.

[109] Tröster AI. Some clinically useful information that neuropsychology provides patients, care partners, neurolo-gists, and neurosurgeons about deep brain stimulation

[110] for Parkinson's disease. Arch Clin Neuropsychol. 2017;32:810–28.

[111] Tröster AI, Fields JA, Wilkinson SB, et al. Neuropsychological functioning before and after unilateral thalamic stimulating electrode implantation in Parkinson's disease. Neurosurg Focus. 1997;2:9.

[112] Tröster AI, Wilkinson SB, Fields JA, et al. Chronic electrical stimulation of the left ventrointermediate (Vim) thalamic nucleus for the treatment of pharmacotherapy-resistant Parkinson's disease: a differential impact on access to semantic and episodic memory? Brain Cogn. 1998;38:125–49.

[113] Tröster AI, Fields JA, Pahwa R, et al. Neuropsychological and quality of life outcome after thalamic stimulation for essential tremor. Neurology. 1999;53:1774–80.

[114] Tsai SZ, Lin SH, Lin SZ, et al. Neuropsychological effects after chronic subthalamic stimulation and the topography of the nucleus in Parkinson's disease. Neurosurgery. 2007;61:1024–30.

[115] Tyagi H, Apergis-Schoute AM, Akram H, et al. A randomized trial directly comparing ventral capsule and anteromedial subthalamic nucleus stimulation in obsessive compulsive disorder: clinical and imaging evidence for dissociable effects. Biol Psychiatry. 2019;85:726–34.

[116] Valldeoriola F, Regidor I, Minguez-Castellanos A, et al. Efficacy and safety of pallidal stimulation in primary dystonia: results of the Spanish multicentric study. J Neurol Neurosurg Psychiatry. 2010;81:65–9.

[117] Volkmann J, Daniels C, Witt K. Neuropsychiatric effects of subthalamic neurostimulation in Parkinson disease. Nat Rev Neurol. 2010;6:487–98.

[118] Voon V, Kubu C, Krack P, et al. Deep brain stimulation: neuropsychological and neuropsychiatric issues. Mov Disord. 2006;21(Suppl 14):S305–27.

[119] Voon V, Krack P, Lang AE, et al. A multicentre study on suicide outcomes following subthalamic stimulation for Parkinson's disease. Brain. 2008;131:2720–8.

[120] Wang JW, Zhang YQ, Zhang XH, et al. Cognitive and psychiatric effects of STN versus GPi deep brain stimulation in Parkinson's disease: a meta-analysis of randomized controlled trials. PLoS One. 2016;11:e0156721.

[121] Weaver FM, Follett KA, Stern M, et al. Randomized trial of deep brain stimulation for Parkinson disease: thirty-six-month outcomes. Neurology. 2012;79:55–65.

[122] Weintraub D. Dopamine and impulse control disorders in Parkinson's disease. Ann Neurol. 2008;64(Suppl 2):S93–100.

[123] Weintraub D, Duda JE, Carlson K, et al. Suicide ideation and behaviours after STN and GPi DBS surgery for Parkinson's disease: results from a randomised, controlled trial. J Neurol Neurosurg Psychiatry. 2013;84:1113–8.

[124] Williams A, Gill S, Varma T, et al. Deep brain stimulation plus best medical therapy versus best medical therapy alone for advanced Parkinson's disease (PD SURG trial): a randomised, open-label trial. Lancet Neurol. 2010;9:581–91.

[125] Witt K, Daniels C, Reiff J, et al. Neuropsychological and psychiatric changes after deep brain stimulation for Parkinson's disease: a randomised, multicentre study. Lancet Neurol. 2008;7:605–14.

[126] Witt K, Daniels C, Krack P, et al. Negative impact of borderline global cognitive scores on quality of life after subthalamic nucleus stimulation in Parkinson's disease. J Neurol Sci. 2011;310:261–6.

[127] Witt K, Granert O, Daniels C, et al. Relation of lead trajectory and electrode position to neuropsychological outcomes of subthalamic neurostimulation in Parkinson's disease: results from a randomized trial. Brain. 2013;136:2109–19.

[128] Woods SP, Fields JA, Lyons KE, et al. Neuropsychological and quality of life changes following unilateral thalamic deep brain stimulation in Parkinson's disease: a one-year follow-up. Acta Neurochir. 2001;143:1273–8.

[129] Xie Y, Meng X, Xiao J, et al. Cognitive changes following bilateral deep brain stimulation of subthalamic nucleus in Parkinson's disease: a meta-analysis. Biomed Res Int. 2016;2016:3596415.

[130] York MK, Wilde EA, Simpson R, Jankovic J. Relationship between neuropsychological outcome and DBS surgical trajectory and electrode location. J Neurol Sci. 2009;287:159–71.

[131] Zanini S, Moschella V, Stefani A, et al. Grammar improvement following deep brain stimulation of the subthalamic and the pedunculopontine nuclei in advanced Parkinson's disease: a pilot study. Parkinsonism Relat Disord. 2009;15:606–9.

第 10 章 伦理问题
Ethical Considerations

Dorothee Horstkötter　Guido de Wert　著
袁天硕　石　林　译　赵宝田　杨岸超　张建国　校

> **摘要**：自从 DBS 首次应用于人类以来，其已引发了许多关于伦理问题的顾虑，以及关于其重要性和可取性的广泛争论。伦理讨论的主要目标是指导和支持有关临床 DBS 治疗和相关医学研究中责任决策的制定，并提高人们对重要伦理问题的认识。
>
> 　　传统的医学伦理由尊重患者自主权、有利 / 不伤害和公正 3 个基本原则构成。而对 DBS 疗法而言，这些原则需要具体到关注"尊重自主权"到底意味着什么，什么是维护医疗有利性与不伤害原则，以及如何才能恪守公正。着重考量 DBS 疗法的风险和不良反应，以及与其潜在的替代疗法进行比较都是至关重要的。鉴于人们对 DBS 治疗精神类疾病的兴趣日益浓厚，对其伦理问题的研究已提上日程。大脑在人体中的特殊地位也引起了深刻的伦理学关注，特别是对于患者性格的潜在影响。DBS 研究中单独的伦理问题研究或整体的附加课题可促进产生新的系统性的伦理思想，从而可促进相关研究工作的推进和新颖应用的推出。

一、概述

脑深部电刺激（DBS）是治疗神经系统疾病和精神疾病的公认疗法，包括帕金森病、特发性震颤、肌张力障碍、癫痫及强迫症（OCD）。已有越来越多的研究将其作为治疗其他疾病的潜在疗法，包括抑郁症、神经性厌食症、Tourette 综合征（TS）和成瘾症（Holtzheimer 与 Mayberg，2011；Temel 等，2012）。

DBS 已经成为上述顽固性疾病患者的一种有效治疗方法，越来越多的运动障碍性疾病患者接受了手术治疗。但自从在人类中首次应用 DBS 以来，它还是引发了许多伦理方面的讨论和关注，并引发了关于脑深部电刺激的重要性和可行性的广泛争论。

有创性的大脑神经调控已经正式进入了医疗领域。如 Nuffield 生命伦理委员会（2013）所提出的，我们的大脑在人体中处于不同于其他器官的特殊地位。它的功能健全在我们的身体运作、自主活动、自我观念、人际交往，以及我们生活的方方面面，都发挥着核心作用。所以，神经调控引发并提出了其他生物医学技术所没有涉及的伦理学问题。尤其是针对 DBS 和其他神经调控技术可能影响个体性格、形象自我鉴定能力，以及自我身份认同等方面所提出的伦理问题（如 Baylis，2015；Bell 等，2009；Clausen，2010；Galert，2015；Glannon，2009；Nuffield Council on Bioethics，2013；Schechtman，2010；Schermer，2011；Synofzik，2015b；Witt 等，2013）。因此与大脑功能相关的疾病都面临着特殊的挑战。一方面，大脑的任何疾病或干扰都可能直接地、负面地影响着我们的个人性格和自我意识。这既强调了有效补救措施的必要性，也对相应治疗方法的探索施加了压力。但另一方面，格外的谨慎也是很有必要的。对于人脑的干预，通常对其作用和可能的不良反应尚不清楚，以及将如何影响目标条件、患者的其他特征，甚至是其身份或性格还有待讨论。

在这种背景下，DBS 自从诞生之日起就引发了许多伦理问题和疑虑，并引发了关于其重要性和可行性的广泛争论。伦理的主要目标是指导和支持临床治疗，以及医学研究中的责任决策的制定，并提高人们对重要伦理问题的认识。值得注意的是，伦理问题不仅包括潜在的问题和威胁，而且还包括可能的优势和受益。

传统的医学伦理由尊重患者自主权、有利/不伤害和公正3个基本原则构成。而对 DBS 疗法而言，这些原则需要具体关注"尊重自主权"到底意味着什么，什么是维护医疗有利性与不伤害原则，以及如何才能恪守公正（Beauchamp 与 Childress，2009；Bell 等，2009；Clausen，2010；Synofzik 与 Schlaepfer，2008）。考虑到 DBS 的风险和不良反应并将这种治疗与潜在的替代治疗（如心理治疗、药物治疗和其他类型的神经调节）进行比较都是至关重要的。鉴于人们对 DBS 治疗精神类疾病的兴趣日益浓厚，也已经做了大量的研究和试验性治疗，关于其伦理问题的研究也已提上日程（Fins 等，2011；Holtzheimer 和 Mayberg，2011；Synofzik，2015a）。

二、DBS 的医学伦理问题

根据 Beauchamp 和 Childress（2009）定义和描述的4项医学伦理原则可以很好地确定医疗伦理。这些内容涵盖了对自主权、有利性、不伤害和公正这4个方面。许多人认为最重要的原则是不伤害原则，"首先，不要造成伤害"。许多医疗行为不仅会产生积极的治疗效果，也可能伴随加重病情甚至伤害患者的不良反应。在实践当中，这意味着医生必须权衡可能的风险和收益，并只有在收益大于可预见的风险和负担的情况下，才有理由进行医学治疗。"尊重自主权"原则是指有自主能力的患者拥有并且应被给予自主决定的权利。即患者在被充分告知后，由患者来决定是否接受某种治疗，以及其他任何医疗程序。换言之，即便是违背医生的诚挚建议甚至是损害患者自身的医疗利益的，患者也可以选择拒绝（Emanuel 和 Emanuel，1992）。最后，"公正"指的是 DBS 的社会层面，要求即使在资源稀缺的情况下，也要公平的选择患者、平等的获得医疗设施、公平的分配财政及其他资源。以下内容将探讨在 DBS 的背景下这些道德要求意味着什么，如何实现这些需求，以及医生和护理人员可能面临的具体挑战。

（一）尊重自主权

每个人都享有身心健全的权利，这就要求他人不得在未经其知情和充分考虑后允许的情况下干预其身体或思想（Bell 等，2009；Clausen，2010）。对于有自主能力的患者来说，这种自主权意味着只有在医生已经告知他们的健康状况、治疗预后和所有治疗方案，并指出可能的益处和预期的效果，以及潜在的风险和不良反应之后，才可以开始治疗。由医生为患者指明治疗方法，并决定 DBS 是否适合患者当前状况（请参阅下面有关 DBS 的公正问题）。最后，还是由患者来决定是否接受这种（或任何一种）治疗。特别是如果能预见或担心出现严重的不良反应，患者则可能更愿意不采用 DBS 之类的治疗，即便疗效较差也宁愿选择其他治疗方式。这种自主权适用于手术开始，也适用于在整个手术过程中可能出现的各种问题或并发症，以及手术后期必须做出的任何进一步决定。当然，前提是医生提供的信息对于患者是可以理解的，这些信息包括医疗程序和要求，预期疗效及可能的不良反应。临床医生还应确保患者充分了解所提供的信息。而关于 DBS 则需要临床医生从各方面媒体报道中做出正确筛选（无论是正面的还是负面的），因为这些报道很容易左右患者的看法，使其产生不切实际的希望或毫无依据的恐惧（Gilbert 和 Ovadia，2011；Johansson 等，2013）。在某些情况下，尊重自主权还可能要求医生评估患者的决策能力（Glannon，2010）。就目前而言，患者的决策能力不是需要特别关注的问题，因为 DBS 目前最重要的适应证是运动障碍性疾病。但在不久的将来，如果 DBS 也可以用于治疗重度或难治性精神类疾病，那么患者的自主决策能力问题就会变得异常重要。

到目前为止，从伦理学的角度来看，DBS 对于现有疾病重度病例的治疗与其他重度疾病的治疗在伦理方面并无不同。但也必须认识到，一旦患者更加倾向于采用 DBS 治疗，与精神类药物治疗相比，在尊重自主权方面就存在了一些差异。当采用保守精神类药物治疗时，患者在治疗阶段保留自主权。即使患者已经初步认同了医生的治疗，他们也可以违背医生的建议，比如按照高于或低于建议频率来服药，甚至根本不服用药物（Leentjens 等，2016）。患者之所以这样做可能是因为他们想减轻可能出现的不良反应但又不敢告诉医生，甚至可能是为了体验多巴胺激动药导致的快感。但如果是通过电刺激治疗，这些情况则完全不同。患者刺激器参数的设置很大程度上由医生决定。他们没有或很少能自己调整设置参数。患者得到了症状上的缓解并为医生的专业性和责任心感到高兴。但这也限制了患者自己做出决定并直接、及时调整医疗方法可能性。虽然其中有医学原因导致这种情况，但临床医生应该认识到，这种设备依赖性会使患者对日常活动的自主权不断降低。从某种意义上讲，设备依赖性对医生和患者都提出了苛刻要求，所以 DBS 对良好的医患关系也提出了特殊要求。患者必须真实地告知他们遇到的各种问题和不良反应，医生有责任持续告知患者他们的健康状况，医疗机构也必须支持这种长期的医患关系。

（二）有利和不伤害

大多数治疗方法不仅具有针对性的治疗效果，还具有一些不良反应。有利和不伤害原则要求从一开始就必须确保预期的疗效超过任何可能出现的不良反应。这需要医生了解可能出现不良反应的种类和严重程度，以及可能出现不良反应的患者个人情况。结果就有学者认为，只有当那些低创伤疗法没有效果或效果不再明显的时候，才建议使用 DBS 这类创伤更大，患者负担更重的治疗方法（Kuhn 等，2009）。此外，必须充分告知患者预期疗效，并预期患者的生理、认知、情绪状态能够成功经受手术及配合术后护理（Bell 等，2009；Pollak，2013）。一些患者检查后发现其不能满足全部的手术标准，例如出现了早期认知功能障碍，这些患者应避免手术，但对一些很明确的例外情况，可在采取特殊手段或保障措施预防可能发生的不良事件的前提下安排手术（Kubu 和 Ford，2017）。所以，认真的选择患者对于手术和电刺激都是至关重要的，最好是由多学科团队来最终决定患者是否适合接受 DBS 手术（Kubu 和 Ford，2017）。

从有利和不伤害原则的角度来看，DBS 与其他有创和有潜在风险的疗法并无不同。尽管如此，DBS 疗法的许多作用和不良反应似乎也是独一无二的。一些运动障碍症状得到改善的患者却在社交和家庭生活中遭遇了严重的问题，并且出现了刺激依赖性的精神健康问题，甚至出现精神类疾病（Glannon，2009；Müller 和 Christen，2011；Schüpbach，2006；Volkmann 等，2010）。这就是所谓的"康复负担"现象（Gilbert，2012）。多年严重的运动障碍或强迫行为，使他们的家庭生活、社会交往，以及正常工作变得十分困难。经过 DBS 治疗后的立即好转，也使得患者和其家人必须去适应"正常"的生活。然而，这可能给一些人带来沉重的负担。因为一旦患者的运动障碍症状消失、刚能开始行走、对一些强迫性动作的需求减少，他们可能都不知道如何处理新的自由时间。因此有利和不伤害原则要求患者和家属既要事先做好准备并充分了解情况，又要提供充足的后期护理，这不仅要涵盖 DBS 的医学特征，而且还要考虑到更广泛的心理、家庭和社会层面。

除"康复负担"外，特别是DBS初期还观察到了刺激导致的和可调节的神经精神类症状，如（轻度）躁狂、冲动行为、性欲亢进和过度兴奋。如今随着人们对DBS靶点的解剖学研究不断深入，这些情况已很少发生。但正如Nuffield生物伦理委员会（2013年）所强调的那样，这些不良反应的产生也证明了大脑在人体的特殊地位，如何权衡风险和收益是相当复杂的。如果患者成功缓解了运动障碍疾病但却出现严重的神经精神类不良反应，那其将陷入进退两难的困境。这时可能无法"单纯"地权衡利弊。而是必须确定在当前情况下什么才是最需要解决的，因此什么才能被认为是"有利"，什么又被认为是"有害"。这时就需要患者当前在所给定的可能性和并发症下做出决定，对他们而言最有价值的是什么。反之，医生也应该尊重患者所认为的更有利或更安全。在这点上，有一个经常被人们引用和讨论的著名的荷兰案例（Leentjens等，2004）。这个案例以一种非常冷酷但清晰的方式阐明了上述伦理困境。该患者患有严重的帕金森病以至于卧床不起，但是在接受DBS治疗后，他恢复了良好的活动能力。但3年后，他被迫住进了精神病房。由于刺激导致的不良反应，患者出现了混乱、夸大和狂躁行为，引发了严重的家庭问题和财产纠纷，并丧失了自主决策能力。而且他的这些异常行为对于"经典"的精神类治疗没有反应，但调整刺激参数却有效。当患者适应了刺激参数后躁狂行为停止了，自主决策能力也恢复了，但原本的严重运动症状却开始复发并再次卧床不起。在这种时候，似乎无法在两种极端症状间达到一个令人满意的状态。结果就是，患者或是由于严重的PD而不得不进入疗养院，或是由于无法控制的躁狂而被迫送入精神病房，这使得患者极度痛苦，也使自己和他人陷入危险境地。从伦理学的角度，面对这种情形是很困难的，因为不清楚什么才是更有利或更安全。尽管处于进退两难的境地，但不做抉择也是不可能的和不负责的。在关机后患者和医生不应该仅是想趋利避

害，而是应该思考什么是好或更好，什么是差或更差。患者也要抉择未来几年要如何生活，要成为一个什么样的人（Bransen，2000；Taylor，1985）。最后患者选择了打开刺激器，选择了恢复运动功能而放弃了健全的心智，也被迫继续接受精神治疗。对于临床医生来说，这种"治疗"虽然解决了运动障碍，也同时剥夺了患者的自我决策能力。为了减轻这种精神症状带来的伤害，医生为患者安排了定期关机以恢复患者的自我决策能力，从而让患者能重新思考之前的选择。本案例中所讨论的身心健康之间的伦理困境也表明，为什么伦理不一定是最道德的选择，而是有条理的、理性的论证和思考。

（三）公正

医疗公正要求所有患者都按照同样的标准得到治疗，同时要考虑到经济限制和专业医疗中心实际提供所需护理及长期病后护理的能力（Bell等，2009）。这就意味着，在使用DBS治疗时必须优先考虑特定的患者群体。因此在面对实施手术的公平性时，仔细的选择患者在伦理上也是很重要的。所以，优先考虑那些症状最严重而且康复机会最大的患者似乎是最公平的。但显而易见，这两个要求很难同时满足。即使这样，也应该根据医学标准而不是年龄、财富、社会地位这些条件来选择接受DBS的患者。公正还要求一旦患者接受了DBS手术并植入了设备，必须保证患者的后续治疗和随访（Bell等，2009；Kubu和Ford，2017；Leentjens等，2016）。也有一些接受治疗的罕见病患者，能为他们提供帮助的医疗中心、从业医师都非常有限。这就需要那些提供DBS治疗罕见病或新适应证的中心来承担特殊的、长期的责任。

（四）DBS治疗精神类疾病

通过对运动障碍性疾病的治疗，我们发现了那些能影响患者情绪、思想和行为的不良反应。这些发现结合了最新的影像技术，促使了人们应用DBS治疗精神类疾病的探索（Clair等，

2018；Clausen，2010；Holtzheimer 和 Mayberg，2011）。如今 DBS 已被批准可用于 OCD 的治疗，并且针对抑郁症、成瘾、饮食失调、Tourette 综合征和攻击行为等多种精神疾病的研究也正在进行。考虑到 DBS 治疗精神类疾病（除 OCD 外）目前还处于研究阶段，所以这里的许多伦理学讨论都将集中在临床研究的伦理方面，特别是正在进行的试验的情况和对受试者的保护（见下一章节）。然而也有一些学者指出，一旦证明应用 DBS 治疗精神类疾病是安全有效的，并成为常规治疗方案的一种，那么则可能会出现一系列伦理问题（Glannon，2010；Kuhn 等，2009；Rabins 等，2009；Synofzik 和 Schlaepfer，2008）。在一定程度上，这些与上述运动障碍性疾病方面的医学伦理的要求相同。如果 DBS 想取得伦理上的合理性，其必须比以公认的心理疗法、药物疗法、消融手术疗法有着更大的好处或更少的风险。其治疗必须基于患者的知情同意，也要符合公正的标准规格。精神健康方面虽然在形式上有所相似，但也面临着特殊的挑战。

考虑到 DBS 有创性和高强度的特点，通常认为 DBS 是那些病情最重的、除此之外没有其他疗法的患者的最后治疗方案。尽管大多数患者在精神状态正常时都保持着决策能力，但如果患者的精神症状（如抑郁症等）加重或反复，患者的决策能力就会减低（Glannon，2008）。患有阿尔茨海默病的患者也会遇到类似的问题。到目前为止，应用 DBS 治疗阿尔茨海默病还处于研究阶段，其益处尚未可知。但如果病情进展到任何其他手段都不能延缓或减轻症状的时候，患者的认知能力也往往就无法帮他们决定是否参加 DBS 治疗了（Siegel 等，2017）。如果将 DBS 用于治疗成瘾症或药物滥用，在知情同意方面也会遇到一些问题。严重的成瘾患者往往在兴奋和戒断的状态中持续波动，这可能使他们失去了自我决策能力，从而无法判断 DBS 治疗的利弊（Carter 等，2011；Pisapia 等，2013）。而此时，自我决策能力却是决定是否开始 DBS 治疗的关键。而且有迹象表明，DBS 治疗精神类疾病往往需要花费数周或数月时间才会对刺激产生反应（如果有效的话），并达到最合理的刺激参数。因此患者不仅要具有能自主决定接受治疗的能力，而且还要有在后续一段时间内保持自主参与治疗的能力（Beeker 等，2017）。所以如果将 DBS 用于治疗精神类疾病，在尊重自主权方面将遇到特别的伦理学挑战。此外 DBS 的疗效不仅要与术前疾病所带来的负担进行比较，还应与替代方案对患者的影响进行比较，以确保 DBS 对患者是有益的，不会对患者造成过多伤害。Johansson 等（2013）在应用 DBS 治疗抑郁症的时候，发现了这种比较是多么的复杂。一方面，他们表明 DBS 相比损毁术破坏性更小；影响的脑组织更少，并且电刺激术后是可以调节的也是可逆的。在时空间方面 DBS 相比心理药理学更加特异，因为 DBS 仅作用于某一特定脑区而药物则是遍布全脑。另一方面，植入设备相当昂贵；并且手术依赖于很专业的医疗中心，对偏远地区的患者来说这也是一个问题；并且患者需要长期的甚至是终身的随访，这也会对患者带来沉重的负担。我们已经知道 DBS 在手术和刺激时也有很多的并发症和不良反应，也不得不承认 DBS 的治疗机制和长期风险仍有许多未知。所以，如何合理的衡量收益与风险，如何权衡各种影响，这些都是极其困难的。为此，最重要的是要考虑不同目标疾病的特殊性，以及患者的个体差异从而进行伦理审查。

例如，在患有神经性厌食症（AN）的患者中，需要特别注意这些患者不仅患有精神类疾病还存在严重的健康问题，瘦弱的身体可能会使他们接受 DBS 手术的风险高于其他患者（Müller 等，2015；Park 等，2017）。

在治疗精神类疾病方面，除了尊重自主权和风险利益权衡等医学伦理方面的问题外，还可能涉及更多问题。这些疾病影响着人们的思想、情绪和行为，也与一个人的性格或个人经历密切相关。在治疗运动障碍病的时候，DBS 对人情绪或感觉的影响属于无意的、意外的不良反应，也因此 DBS 在这方面受到诟病（Müller 和

Christen，2011；Schüpbach，2006）。但在治疗精神类疾病方面，个人性格或自我感受的改变并不一定是预期外的不良反应，而可能成为预期治疗目的的一部分。人们尝试通过改善情绪以治疗抑郁症，改变身材观念以治疗神经性厌食症，探索新的行为方式以治疗 OCD。DBS 确实可以促成这种改变，所以曾经的忧虑已不再存在，DBS 对于个人性格和自主权而言不是威胁而是帮助。但这也引起了进一步的担忧和关注。直接或通过刺激来改善情绪、思想、行为可能会导致新的问题，即当想要实现某种（期望的）改变时可直接绕过个人，不再需要心理发展或个人努力。传统的心理治疗法取决于患者的配合、积极努力，以及对自我形象的认知等。与之不同，刺激直接导致的自我和性格的改变存在着被动性。因此在治疗过程中，当患者的性格即将改变时，可能会使患者的自我形象丧失，并破坏他们的自主权。随之而来的问题就是，之后性格或行为是否比最初的性格更令人满意。此外，涉及被动性的问题不会依赖或支持自主权，而会直接削弱患者的自主权，所以这种被动性存在直接改变患者性格从而产生伦理质疑的风险（Focquaert 和 Schermer，2015）。到目前为止，这些问题都尚未得到充分的重视。但随着精神类疾病逐渐成为 DBS 治疗和研究的主流，这种疗法的道德显著性应受到伦理学监督。

三、DBS 的伦理研究

目前为止，唯一批准可用 DBS 治疗的精神类疾病就是 OCD。在美国，DBS 治疗 OCD 仅在"人道主义器材免除"条件下获得批准，在欧洲则获得了完整的 EC 批准。因此大部分 DBS 用于治疗精神类疾病的应用都是研究性的。这种情况下就伴随着很多伦理学问题，而且这方面的研究都要符合研究伦理的要求。一些国际性的人类医学研究指南确定了人体研究的规范框架，其中最著名的是世界医学协会（WMA）的《赫尔辛基宣言》（2013）和 ICH 临床实践指南（2016）。

医学研究的本质和核心是获取知识并为了未来患者的利益。所以医学研究可能会对当今的参与患者造成伤害。为了确保参与研究患者的利益，医学伦理学就有了扩展至人类医学研究方面的需要。为了符合伦理学要求，研究必须建立在参与者知情同意的基础上，必须有良好的风险-利益平衡，必须公平地选择受试者。日常实践中要求研究人员，要确保其研究具有科学或社会价值并具有科学依据，要适时关注任何敏感的受试者，尽可能地降低患者的研究风险和增加收益，要确保研究方案的独立审查，要充分告知参与者并让其做出自由选择（Emanuel 等，2000）。但对于 DBS，尤其是针对新适应证的研究，仍然面临着很多"经典"医学研究伦理所难以涵盖的问题（Nuffield Council on Bioethics，2013）。首先，研究往往不是按照科学的研究设计和方法进行的，而是在所谓试验性治疗的背景下进行的；其次，当 DBS 处于试验阶段时，情况往往是研究者对可能的结果难以确定、受试者丧失信心，相对风险和收益也难以衡量。

（一）试验性治疗的灰色地带

用于治疗精神类疾病的 DBS 通常作为对现有疗法无效或不再有效，并存在严重症状的某些患者最后的试验性治疗手段。虽然确实帮助某些患者减轻了他们的痛苦，并且从中也得到了重要的医学知识，但从科学兴趣和研究伦理的角度来看，试验性治疗却成了一个极具挑战性的灰色地带。它不同于常规的人体医学研究，因为它没有科学的研究设计，没有独立审查，也不一定会在科学期刊中报道；此外，试验性治疗没有任何依据，也没有遵循任何治疗方案，所以其也不同于常规治疗。因此，目前尚不清楚单个病例研究和报告、病例系列和小规模临床试验是否能可靠地提高我们的知识水平，也不清楚患者能否得到足够的保护。在此背景下，Nuffield 生物伦理委员会（2013）呼吁"应该明确具体的伦理准则，以指导临床医生和研究人员如何既能克服这些困难，又不会扼杀创造力"。国际神经外科协会鼓励研究者通过精心设计的随机对照试验以避免上述灰色地带（Nuttin 等，2014）。但是这可能并不总是可行的，因为即使在高度专业的 DBS 治疗中心，通常也只有很少的患者符合入组标准。因此，应用 DBS 治疗精神类疾病的这种试验性治疗很可能会持续下去。而当医疗伦理和研究伦理的要求都未能达到的时候，就需要对治疗方法负责。对于正规的试验，必须注册并公布研究结果。为了避免发表片面的阳性结果，所以对于试验性 DBS 也提出了类似的要求。为了避免这种发表偏倚，应该为新适应证的治疗建立中央病例登记系统，从而记录所有患者的任何一次试验性治疗结果（Synofzik，2015a）。此外，建立责任制出版惯例也至关重要（Schlaepfer 和 Fins，2010）。试验性治疗应始终作为个案或小病例系列而非作为一个成熟的研究项目进行报道。这样可以避免对研究结果的过度解读。此外避免"定向发表"也是很重要的，定向发表是指当得到积极结果并能表明治疗效果的时候才发表，而得到消极结果的时候则不发表。发表偏倚性结论不仅会导致对这种有潜力的治疗方法过度炒作（Gilbert 和 Ovadia，2011），失败经验的隐瞒也会使未来的患者或受试者承担不必要的风险。为了能够吸取经验教训，研究者必须负责任的对不理想的结果进行报道和批判性探讨（Smeets 等，2018），原则上杂志期刊也有责任接收这些结论并给予发表。

（二）DBS 研究中受试者保护方面的挑战

在当前 DBS 治疗精神类疾病的背景下，如果鼓励适当设立 RCT 研究可能会导致试验性治疗的减少。显然经典临床研究伦理的要求也适用于 DBS 研究（Clausen，2010；Emanuel 等，2000）。但由于各种原因，这些想法可能会受到挑战，尤其是关于 DBS 新适应证或应用于其他患者群体方面的研究。学者们对知情同意、有利的风险－利益平衡和公平的选择受试者这 3 点要求的可行性，以及不同伦理要求之间的固有困境表示担忧（Nuffield Council on Bioethics，2013）。DBS 研究是特别具有挑战性的，人们提出了专门的伦理标准来帮助研究者去克服这些挑战（Kuhn 等，2009；Lipsman 等，2010；Nuttin 等，2014；Rabins 等，2009）。

在知情同意方面，因为研究结果的不确定性通常很大，所以研究者可能无法将可能的风险、负担、不良反应全部合理的告知受试者。他们可能会告知患者医疗本身的不确定因素，但相较于其他绝大多数医学研究，这类研究存在更多的不确定性。另外一个可能损害参与者知情同意的方面是，那些被认为符合研究条件的受试者都是症状最严重并且始终无法治愈的患者。只要可能缓解痛苦，这些绝望的患者愿意接受任何方法，但这也使得他们失去了深思熟虑后做出决定的能力。此外，通常只有很少的医疗中心和专家能参与到 DBS 新适应证的试验性治疗。这也就使得受试者高度依赖于治疗他们的研究者，从而对受试者的自由、自主决策能力提出了挑战。严重的症状和极度的绝望也有让受试者产生治疗错觉的风险，这种错觉让患者以为向他们提供的所有东西都是能改善病情的，却没有理解这种创新性治疗方法或研究的试验特征（Appelbaum 等，1987）。知情同意方面的最后一个挑战来自成为当今 DBS 研究聚焦的疾病本身。严重的神经精神疾病会破坏受试者的自我决策能力。面对这些挑战，自主和知情要求的实现将会非常困难。

出于一些原因，权衡风险和收益也是一种很微妙的事情。尤其是在只能从有限的试点研究中获得初步数据的情况下，很难对预期收益做出明确的预测。而且有创手术总是伴随着风险，众所周知电刺激的不良反应可能影响认知、日常生活、整体生活质量。充分权衡可能的风险和收益的另一个复杂点在于，必须将 DBS 与其他的治疗方案（如心理疗法、心理药理学疗法或毁损术）进行比较。将这些替代治疗的效果和不良反应进行比较是很困难的，所以也不清楚什么才算做更大的风险和负担，哪些又是更安全和方便，是长期的 DBS 刺激还是只做一次的损毁术；是干预脑区更为特异的 DBS 还是影响范围更为广泛的心理药理学疗法；是通过 DBS 直接调节大脑和行为还是通过药物间接调控大脑？

公平的受试者选择近几年才受到重视，似乎存在着共识应该选择那些长期治疗效果不佳的成年患者（Rabins 等，2009）和有自我决策能力的患者（Nuttin 等，2014）。但因为 DBS 可能存在神经保护作用，一些学者则认为应该进行疾病早期治疗的研究，如帕金森病（Schermer，2011），或严重、长期的社会心理问题或教育问题，如青少年患者症状严重的抽动秽语综合征（TS）（Smeets 等，2018）。为了制定合理的伦理标准以解决这些研究伦理的复杂性，并为当今研究面临的各种状况提供可能的解决方案，有人提出将附加伦理或伦理子研究纳入研究 DBS 治疗各种精神类疾病效果和潜力的建议（Nuttin 等，2014），从而确定是否需要特殊的受试者保护措施，以及如何实施这些措施。如今这种伦理学研究已经在针对 DBS 治疗神经性厌食症的背景下进行，并且促使了"金标准框架"的制定，该框架明确了伦理学研究的具体要求并确定了纳入厌食症受试者的合理标准（Park 等，2017，2018）。此外，该框架还考虑到了疾病的致死性、患者群体较年轻、疾病的自我不和谐（ego-dystonic）特征，以及患者的不良体态。还针对不同疾病的 DBS 研究，制定了特别的伦理研究标准，比如成瘾（Carter 等，2011）、抑郁症（Christopher 和 Dunn，2015；Dunn 等，2011；Johansson 等，2013）、阿尔茨海默病（Siegel 等，2017）和青少年 TS 患者（Smeets 等，2018）。

四、DBS 与个人性格

综上所述，大脑是一种特殊的器官，是人类自我意识、自我形象、个人性格的生物学基础。在这种背景下，进行有关神经精神病学影响的病例研究（Leentjens 等，2004），以及对接受刺激的患者进行后续的报告和访谈研究（De Haan 等，2013；Gilbert，2018；Schüpbach，2006；Voigt，2018），这在直接和有创的干预大脑的可行性和合理性的伦理讨论中有着重要意义。如果 DBS 治疗不仅能改变患者的大脑功能和运动能力，也改变了患者的个人性格或原有性格，那么这种疗法可能就会产生伦理上的质疑（Baylis，2013；Gilbert 等，2017；Glannon，2009；Kraemer，2013；Witt 等，2013）。这种质疑不同于之前探讨的两难伦理窘境，即成功治疗疾病（如帕金森病）所带来的好处和新发生的精神类疾病（如躁狂或冲动）所带来的伤害和负担。而是患者将会觉得自己是陌生人或者对自己身体的某一部分感觉陌生。因此患者将失去真正的自我，不再表现出真实的行为，而是表现出受设备控制的行为。

在 DBS 疗法出现前人们就这类问题的一些方面就有过探讨。例如在起搏器和植入式心脏复律除颤仪（ICD）应用的早期阶段，就有过改变身体征象的报道；由于精神类药物治疗对人体的广泛影响，人们也对此进行了严格的讨论，如氟西汀（Prozac®）用于治疗抑郁症或哌甲酯（Ritalin®）用于治疗儿童 ADHD（Kramer，1993；Singh，2013）。这些讨论表明这些更深层次改变对于患者而言是真实、有影响的，但却是不全面的；他们仅是关注了患者的某一特定部位或一个方面，但没有在意是否形成新的性格或新的人格。

Schüpbach（2006）在一项关于 DBS 术后帕金森病患者的早期访谈研究中发现，在 29 名患者中有 19 名不认为自己还是同一个人，并且这些患者中有很大一部分都经历过这种困扰。最近，Gilbert 和同事证实了这一发现，并指出许多术后的 PD 患者有明显的自我疏离感，这是很麻烦的（Gilbert，2018；Gilbert 等，2017）。从伦理的角度来看，重要的是分析这些自我疏远和患者人格变化到底意味着什么。从定义上看，DBS 引起的自我认知或个人性格改变是否在伦理上存在问题，并且这些是否能构成对 DBS 产生质疑的理由（Gilbert 等，2018），或者无论这些改变何时出现，人们都要像面对其他改变人生的重大事件一样去学会适应？这时就需要注意，有些患者并没有这样的感受，有些患者觉得这些改变不会产生什么麻烦，有些患者甚至认为性格或身份的明显改变是积极的。例如，帕金森患者就属于后者，他们在恢复了运动能力后会倍感轻松，甚至感到高兴或幸福，并认为DBS使他们再次回到了得病前那种充满活力的状态。此外，强迫症患者有时也会说，是疾病抑制了他们的"真实自我"，而DBS使他们再次成为"真正的自己"（De Haan等，2013）。这种情况下，患者性格改变就不再是DBS应用的阻碍，一些患者也确实能从中受益，这是非常重要的（Müller等，2017）。

患者的直接观点和经验对于伦理反思至关重要（Snoek等，2019）。但在患者或研究参与者中进行"伦理民意调查"可能也不足以支持医生做出合理的伦理决策（Salloch等，2014）。为了进行规范的审议和充分的道德反思，清楚地理解这些探讨背后的概念也很重要。在这种意义上，Schechtman（2010）讨论了个人性格的不同含义，并将其用于DBS方面。她区分了所谓的数字身份和叙事身份。数字身份关系到一个人在生理和心理上随时间的连续性。数字身份的改变将发展出新的人格，心理上将与从前无关，从前的自传式记忆也将失去。至少有2个原因导致其成为严重的伦理问题。从前的人格在"伦理民意调查"中没有发言权，并被主动抹去，然后就会突然出现一个人，他没有记忆、经历、人际关系或任何有意义的社会因素。但即便是最严重的病例，最可疑和最复杂的患者也不会发展到这种地步。那些已知的改变和自我疏离感，其实指的是比较患者在手术和刺激前后自我和身体的体验，也指患者的社会关系和生活的其他方面。因此，发生改变的并不是患者的数字身份，而是会极大地影响患者的叙事身份，即他们对生活和经历的理解方式。从这方面讲，DBS和那些需要人们适应新的性格身份的重要事件很相似。每个人在生活中都会因为重大的"人生事件"，而一次甚至几次地调整自己的社会角色和个人身份。人们成了父母，患上了慢性疾病，事故中大难不死，在事业上起起落落或者至亲离世。尽管这些事件需要人们调整自己的叙事身份，但他们并不该因此受到谴责。所以由于DBS导致的个人叙述身份的改变也不应该成为伦理问题。重要的是要研究患者如何受到影响，如何经历其身份的变化，在日常生活中如何适应或应对这种变化。

关于个人性格的伦理讨论至少教会了我们3个重要的道理。第一，任何DBS治疗的成功不仅取决于大脑生理功能的改善和症状的缓解，还取决于对患者自我认知和社交生活的广泛影响。第二，手术意愿是很重要的，它关乎患者将如何经历性格的改变，能多好的去适应那些新的改变，以及他们将如何衡量"治愈的身体"与"治愈的思维"（如有）两者的价值（Gilbert等，2017）。第三，鉴于目前对这些问题的认识，临床医生有责任让患者和家属从一开始就做好面对这些困难的准备，所有的知情同意书里都应该对这些问题进行描述。并且医学中心应确保所提供的后续治疗不仅单纯在医疗方面，也要在患者心理健康和连贯性方面提供帮助和支持（Gilbert，2018）。

五、结论与展望

DBS治疗应该符合已有的医学伦理需求，既确保患者的自主权得到尊重，不伤害的前提下尽可能造福患者，从医疗角度考虑来选择患者并提供公正的治疗。除了用于治疗运动障碍疾病，DBS治疗精神类疾病的研究也在进行当中。这些研究面临很多根本性的挑战，需要从研究伦理的角度给予特别关注。DBS研究通常是试验性治疗而非严格设计的研究。这可能会阻碍学科的进展，导致发表偏倚，并危及患者的安全。所以建立多家专业治疗中心之间的国际合作将变得越来越重要，从而增加研究的可行性。通过中心试验登记注册能够可靠的涵盖该领域所有的试验和发现（无论结论是积极还是消极）。这方面，

DBS治疗Tourette患者的试验登记就是一个范例（Martinez-Ramirez等，2018）。独立的伦理子研究（Park等，2017）或整体附加项目（Nuttin等，2014）可以促进已有的研究工作或未来新适应证相关的系统的伦理学观念进步（Johansson等，2014）。此外，进行伦理反思对于所谓的新一代DBS的新式电刺激功能也是非常重要的（Goering等，2017）。

参考文献

[1] Appelbaum PS, Roth LH, Lidz CW, et al. False hopes and best data: consent to research and the therapeutic misconception. Hastings Cent Rep. 1987;17:20–4.

[2] Baylis F. 'I Am Who I Am'. On the perceived threats to personal identity from deep brain stimulation. Neuroethics. 2013;6:513–26.

[3] Baylis F. Neuroethics and identity. In: Clausen J, Levy N, editors. Handbook of neuroethics. Dordrecht: Springer Science; 2015. p. 367–72.

[4] Beauchamp TL, Childress JF. Principles of biomedical ethics. 6th ed. Oxford: Oxford University Press; 2009.

[5] Beeker T, Schlaepfer TE, Coenen VA. Autonomy in depressive patients undergoing DBS-treatment: informed consent, freedom of will and DBS' potential to restore it. Front Integr Neurosci. 2017;11:11.

[6] Bell E, Mathieu G, Racine E. Preparing the ethical future of deep brain stimulation. Surg Neurol. 2009;72:577–86.

[7] Bransen J. Alternatives of oneself: recasting some of our practical problems. Philos Phenomenol Res. 2000;60:381–400.

[8] Carter A, Bell E, Racine E, Hall W. Ethical issues raised by proposals to treat addiction using deep brain stimulation. Neuroethics. 2011;4:129–42.

[9] Christopher PP, Dunn LB. Risk and consent in neuropsychiatric deep brain stimulation: an exemplary analysis of treatment-resistant depression, obsessive-compulsive disorder, and dementia. In: Clausen J, Levy N, editors. Handbook of neuroethics. Dordrecht: Springer Science; 2015. p. 589–605.

[10] Clair A-H, Haynes W, Mallet L. Recent advances in deep brain stimulation in psychiatric disorders. F1000 Res. 2018;7:699.

[11] Clausen J. Ethical brain stimulation—neuroethics of deep brain stimulation in research and clinical practice. Eur J Neurosci. 2010;32:1152–62.

[12] De Haan S, Rietveld E, Stokhof M, Denys D. The phenomenology of deep brain stimulation-induced changes in OCD: an enactive affordance-based model. Front Hum Neurosci. 2013;7:653. https://doi.org/10.3389/fnhum.2013.00653.

[13] Dunn LB, Holtzheimer PE, Hoop JG, et al. Ethical issues in deep brain stimulation research for treatment-resistant depression: focus on risk and consent. AJOB Neurosci. 2011;2:29–36.

[14] Emanuel EJ, Emanuel LL. Four models of the physician-patient relationship. JAMA. 1992;267:2221–6.

[15] Emanuel EJ, Wendler D, Grady C. What makes clinical research ethical? JAMA. 2000;283:2701–11.

[16] Fins JJ, Mayberg HS, Nuttin B, et al. Misuse of the FDA's humanitarian device exemption In deep brain stimulation for obsessive-compulsive disorder. Health Aff. 2011;30:302–11.

[17] Focquaert F, Schermer M. Moral enhancement: do means matter morally? Neuroethics. 2015;8:139–51.

[18] Galert T. Impact of brain interventions on personal identity. In: Clausen J, Levy N, editors. Handbook of neuroethics. Dordrecht: Springer Science; 2015.p. 407–22.

[19] Gilbert F. The burden of normality: from 'chronically ill' to 'symptom free'. New ethical challenges for deep brain stimulation postoperative treatment. J Med Ethics. 2012;8:408–12.

[20] Gilbert F. Deep brain stimulation: inducing self-estrangement. Neuroethics. 2018;11:157–65.

[21] Gilbert F, Ovadia D. Deep brain stimulation in the media: over-optimistic portrayals call for a new strategy involving journalists and scientists in ethical debates. Front Integr Neurosci. 2011;5:16.

[22] Gilbert F, Goddard E, Viaña JNM, et al. I miss being me: phenomenological effects of deep brain stimulation. AJOB Neurosci. 2017;8:96–109.

[23] Gilbert F, Viaña JNM, Ineichen C. Deflating the 'DBS causes personality changes' bubble. Neuroethics. 2018:1–17. https://doi.org/10.1007/s12152-018-9373-8.

[24] Glannon W. Deep-brain stimulation for depression. HEC Forum. 2008;20:325–35. https://doi.org/10.1007/s10730-008-9084-3.

[25] Glannon W. Stimulating brains, altering minds. J Med Ethics. 2009;35:289–92.

[26] Glannon W. Consent to deep brain stimulation for neurological and psychiatric disorders. J Clin Ethics. 2010;21:104–11.

[27] Goering S, Klein E, Dougherty DD, Widge AS. Staying in the loop: relational agency and identity in next-generation DBS for psychiatry. AJOB Neurosci. 2017;8:59–70.

[28] Guideline for Good Clinical Practices of the ICH. ICH International Council for harmonisation of technical requirements for pharmaceuticals for human use. Integrated Addendum to ICH E6 (R1): Guideline for good clinical practice 2016. http://www.ich.org/fileadmin/Public_Web_Site/ICH_Products/Guidelines/Efficacy/E6/E6_R2__Step_4_2016_1109.pdf.Accessed 30 Sept 2018.

[29] Holtzheimer PE, Mayberg HS. Deep brain stimulation for psychiatric disorders. Annu Rev Neurosci. 2011;34:289–307.

[30] Johansson V, Garwicz M, Kanje M, et al. Beyond blind optimism and unfounded fears: deep brain stimulation for treatment resistant depression. Neuroethics. 2013;6:457–71.

[31] Johansson V, Garwicz M, Kanje M, et al. Thinking ahead on deep brain stimulation: an analysis of the ethical implications of a developing technology. AJOB Neurosci. 2014;5:24–33.

[32] Kraemer F. Authenticity or autonomy? When deep brain stimulation causes a dilemma. J Med Ethics. 2013;39:757–60.

[33] Kramer PD. Listening to Prozac. A psychiatrist explores antidepressant drugs and the remaking of the self. New York: Penguin Books; 1993.

[34] Kubu CS, Ford PJ. Clinical ethics in the context of deep brain stimulation for movement disorders. Arch Clin Neuropsychol. 2017;32:829–39.

[35] Kuhn J, Gaebel W, Klosterkoetter J, Woopen C. Deep brain stimulation as a new therapeutic approach in therapy-resistant mental disorders: ethical aspects of investigational treatment. Eur Arch Psychiatry Clin Neurosci. 2009;259:S135–41.

[36] Leentjens AF, Visser Vandewalle V, Temel Y, Verhey F. Manipuleerbare wilsbekwaamheid: een ethisch probleem bij elektrostimulatie van de nucleus subthalamicus voor ernstige ziekte van Parkinson. [Manipulation of mental competence: an ethical problem in case of electrical stimulation of the subthalamic nucleus for severe Parkinson's disease]. Ned Tijdschr Geneeskd. 2004;148:1394–8.

[37] Leentjens AF, Horstkötter D, De Wert G. Ethische overwegingen bij de behandeling met diepe hersenstimulaties [Ethical considerations in treatments with deep brain stimulation]. In: Temel Y, Leentjens AF, de Bie RM, editors. Handboek diepe hersenstimulatie bij neurologische en psychiatrische aandoeningen. Houten: Bohn Stafleu van Loghum; 2016. p. 67–75.

[38] Lipsman N, Bernstein M, Lozano AM. Criteria for the ethical conduct of psychiatric neurosurgery clinical trials. Neurosurg Focus. 2010;29:E9.

[39] Martinez-Ramirez D, Jimenez-Shahed J, Leckman JF, et al. Efficacy and safety of deep brain stimulation in Tourette syndrome: the International Tourette Syndrome Deep Brain Stimulation Public Database and Registry. JAMA Neurol. 2018;75:353–9.

[40] Müller S, Christen M. Deep brain stimulation in Parkinsonian patients—ethical evaluation of cognitive, affective, and behavioral sequelae. AJOB Neurosci. 2011;2:3–13.

[41] Müller S, Riedmüller R, Walter H, Christen M. An ethical

evaluation of stereotactic neurosurgery for anorexia nervosa. AJOB Neurosci. 2015;6:50–65.

[42] Müller S, Bittlinger M, Walter H. Threats to neurosurgical patients posed by the personal identity debate. Neuroethics. 2017;10:299–310.

[43] Nuffield Council on Bioethics. Novel neurotechnologies: intervening in the brain. London: Nuffield Council on Bioethics; 2013.

[44] Nuttin B, Wu H, Mayberg H, et al. Consensus on guidelines for stereotactic neurosurgery for psychiatric disorders. J Neurol Neurosurg Psychiatry. 2014;85:1003.

[45] Pacholczyk A. DBS makes you feel good!—why some of the ethical objections to the use of DBS for neuropsychiatric disorders and enhancement are not convincing. Front Integr Neurosci. 2011;5:14.

[46] Park RJ, Singh I, Pike AC, Tan JOA. Deep brain stimulation in anorexia nervosa: hope for the hopeless or exploitation of the vulnerable? The Oxford Neuroethics Gold Standard Framework. Front Psych. 2017;8:44.

[47] Park RJ, Scaife JC, Aziz TZ. Study protocol: using deep-brain stimulation, multimodal neuroimaging and neuroethics to understand and treat severe enduring anorexia nervosa. Front Psych. 2018;9:24.

[48] Pisapia JM, Halpern CH, Muller UJ, et al. Ethical considerations in deep brain stimulation for the treatment of addiction and overeating associated with obesity. AJOB Neurosci. 2013;4:35–46.

[49] Pollak P. Deep brain stimulation for Parkinson's disease—patient selection. Handb Clin Neurol. 2013;116:97–105.

[50] Rabins P, Appleby BS, Brandt J, et al. Scientific and ethical issues related to deep brain stimulation for disorders of mood, behavior and thought. Arch Gen Psychiatry. 2009;66:931–7.

[51] Salloch S, Vollmann J, Schildmann J. Ethics by opinion poll? The functions of attitudes research for normative deliberations in medical ethics. J Med Ethics. 2014;40:597–602.

[52] Schechtman MM. Philosophical reflections on narrative and deep brain stimulation. J Clin Ethics. 2010;21:133–9.

[53] Schermer M. Ethical issues in deep brain stimulation. Front Integr Neurosci. 2011;5:17.

[54] Schlaepfer TE, Fins JJ. Deep brain stimulation and the neuroethics of responsible publishing: when one is not enough. JAMA. 2010;303:775–6.

[55] Schüpbach MM. Neurosurgery in Parkinson disease: a distressed mind in a repaired body? Neurology. 2006;66:1811–6.

[56] Siegel AM, Barett MS, Bhati MT. Deep brain stimulation for Alzheimer's disease: ethical challenges for clinical research. J Alzheimers Dis. 2017;56:429–39.

[57] Singh I. Not robots: children's perspectives on authenticity, moral agency and stimulant drug treatments. J Med Ethics. 2013;39:359–66.

[58] Smeets AYJM, Duits AA, Horstkötter D, et al. Ethics of deep brain stimulation in adolescent patients with refractory Tourette syndrome: a systematic review and two case discussions. Neuroethics. 2018;11:143–55.

[59] Snoek A, de Haan S, Schermer M, Horstkötter D. On the Significance of the Identity Debate in DBS and the Need of an Inclusive Research Agenda. A Reply to Gilbert, Viaña and Ineichen. Neuroethics. 2019;1–10.https://doi.org/10.1007/s12152-019-09411-w.

[60] Synofzik M. Deep brain stimulation research ethics: the ethical need for standardized reporting, adequate trial design, and study registrations. In: Clausen J, Levy N, editors. Handbook of neuroethics. Dordrecht: Springer Science; 2015a. p. 621–33.

[61] Synofzik M. Ethical implications of brain stimulation. In: Clausen J, Levy N, editors. Handbook of neuroethics. Dordrecht: Springer Science; 2015b. p. 553–60.

[62] Synofzik M, Schlaepfer TE. Stimulating personality: ethical criteria for deep brain stimulation in psychiatric patients and for enhancement purposes. Biotechnol J. 2008;3:1511–20.

[63] Taylor C. The concept of a person. In: Taylor C, editor. Human agency and language. Philosophical papers 1. Cambridge: Cambridge University Press; 1985. p. 97–114.

[64] Temel Y, Hescham SA, Jahanshahi A, et al. Neuromodulation in psychiatric disorders. Int Rev Neurobiol. 2012;107:283–314.

[65] Voigt JS. Bodily felt freedom: an ethical perspective on positive aspects of deep brain stimulation. Neuroethics. 2018:1–13. https://doi.org/10.1007/s12152-018-9380-9.

[66] Volkmann J, Daniels C, Witt K. Neuropsychiatric effects of subthalamic neurostimulation in Parkinson disease. Nat Rev Neurol. 2010;6:487.

[67] Witt K, Kuhn J, Timmermann L, et al. Deep brain stimulation and the search for identity. Neuroethics. 2013;6:499–511.

[68] World Medical Association. Declaration of Helsinki. Ethical principles for medical research involving human subjects. 2013. https://www.wma.net/policiespost/wma-declaration-of-helsinki-ethical-principlesfor-medical-research-involving-human-subjects/. Accessed 30 Sept 2018.

第 11 章　脑深部电刺激患者围术期管理
Organization of Care for Patients Treated by Deep Brain Stimulation

Rianne A. J. Esselink　Mark L. Kuijf　著
陈颖川　张　华　译　杨岸超　张建国　校

> **摘要**：脑深部电刺激（DBS）是治疗运动障碍疾病和精神障碍疾病的一种选择，其过程复杂，需要多学科协作。成功的 DBS 手术及其预后取决于诸多因素，其中，以患者为中心的围术期管理非常重要。团队成员应该赋予明确的任务和职责，应该经历良好的工作培训。在患者及其照看者需要对各方面问题咨询时，特别是对于手术的客观预期，团队的沟通应该是快速便捷的。因此，需要针对患者咨询、评估、手术及术后护理整个流程制定一套全面的多学科方案，所有参与治疗的人员的任务和责任都应在方案中明确说明。
>
> 最后，DBS 中心应具有创新精神，并愿意对团队培训和物资器材持续投入。

一、概述

当考虑使用 DBS 治疗神经系统疾病或精神障碍疾病时，该疾病通常已处于较为复杂的阶段，因此往往会转诊至 DBS 专业中心。对于 DBS 专业中心，一支训练有素、经验丰富的跨学科团队是必不可少的。虽然，DBS 不再被认为是最后的干预手段，尤其对于运动障碍疾病来说，但是，DBS 团队依旧应该非常熟悉疾病的其他可选方案，也必须充分告知 DBS 手术的所有的风险和并发症，手术风险和并发症可能影响个别患者的手术结果。理想情况下，DBS 多学科团队应该包括功能神经外科医生、神经内科医生、神经放射科医生、麻醉科医生、精神科医生、神经心理科医生、手术室成员和专科护士。必要时，神经生理学家和全科医生也应该参与围术期管理。

在 DBS 中心，通过全面的术前评估来筛选适合 DBS 手术的患者。随后，需要多学科团队制定决策方案。手术本身是一个按部就班的过程，不同中心的手术方法也有所不同。术后，当患者出院时，将对 DBS 系统进行程控，与生活方式、活动变化和心理影响的相关问题需要医护人员系统的专业性的解释。手术前后，神经外科医生是主要负责医生，神经内科医生或精神科医生充当顾问。之后的随访与治疗，神经内科医生或精神科医生应该起到主要作用。在本章中，参与 DBS 围术期管理的神经内科医生或精神科医生被称为 DBS 专家。

二、DBS 患者的选择和咨询

患者的选择是手术良好预后的关键因素。在运动障碍疾病中，超过 30% 的效果不佳的 DBS 手术是由于患者选择不当（Okun 等，2005）。患者选择是基于个体化风险 – 获益评估。

患者应该符合手术适应证，不存在手术禁忌证。DBS 的一般性的纳入标准和排除标准见表 11-1。对于不同疾病特殊的纳入标准和排除标准将在相应章节中讨论。

如果患者符合 DBS 手术条件，应该向患者提供有关 DBS 治疗的风险、获益和流程的相关信息，其他可供选择的治疗方案也应该一并告知。可以在治疗方案选择过程中使用患者决策辅助工具，可以提高患者的满意度及其预后（Elwyn 等，2012）。DBS 专家和专科护士经常在治疗方案选择阶段提供的信息内容总结在表 11-2。

关于手术疗效、潜在的相关不良事件、手术流程、术后影响，患者及照顾者应该具有合理的预期。DBS 团队应该反复交代相关事项，确保患者及照顾者已充分理解。对于 DBS 手术全部流程，从术前筛选到最终程控参数设定，需要整个团队充分的耐心、努力及合作。合理的预期与患者及照顾者的满意度密切相关。如果 DBS 专家评估后认为患者可以进行手术，就可以开始进行术前筛选。

三、术前筛选

详细的术前筛选通常需要在日间病房或者住院进行。术前筛选的主要目的是明确手术指征和

表 11-1　DBS 的常规纳入和排除标准

DBS 的纳入标准
- 诊断明确
- 符合特定疾病的纳入标准
- 最佳治疗方案和其他非手术治疗方案疗效不理想或不满意
- 最佳治疗方案和其他非手术治疗方案存在禁忌证或严重不良反应

DBS 的排除标准
- 符合特定疾病的排除标准
- 痴呆或严重认知障碍（除非痴呆本身是手术的指征）
- 现在或既往严重精神障碍（除非精神障碍本身是手术的指征）
- 总体健康状况差，明显增加手术风险
- 年龄在 70—75 岁以上是相对禁忌证
- MRI 显著异常，明显增加手术风险
- 患者缺乏充分的术后照顾，应对能力不足，如智力残疾、精神障碍或其他个人情况

手术风险。在入院之后，应该反复向患者和照顾者告知 DBS 手术流程、疗效和潜在的不良事件。表 11-3 是需要反复告知的项目列表。同样，也应该与患者及照顾者充分沟通对手术的预期。建议以下专业人员参与术前筛选，包括 DBS 专家（取决于诊断）、神经外科医生、专科护士、（神经）心理科医生、麻醉科医师，以及全科医生和其他医学专家。

疾病的严重程度应该进行量化测评。对于帕金森病（Parkinson disease，PD），可以用运动障碍学会帕金森病综合评量表（movement

表 11-2　术前与患者沟通的相关事项

- DBS 无法治愈疾病本身，只是改善疾病的特定症状，也意味着在随访期间可能会出现新的症状
- 手术适应证和禁忌证
- 短期和长期的获益
- DBS 术后症状改善不明显
- 最常见的不良事件和严重不良事件
- 治疗方案（筛选、手术、术后随访）
- 运作良好的社会支持系统的重要性
- 手术流程
- 术后随访：通常 3~6 个月，如果需要 DBS 参数和药物调整，可以适度延长
- DBS 术后功能改善或减退的影响，患者及照顾者需要时间重建身体、心理和社会交往的平衡
- DBS 术后身体状况对日常生活、社会交往及工作的影响
- DBS 术后认知、情绪和行为的变化对患者自身、照顾者及其社交环境的影响（有关更多详细信息，请参见第 9 章）
- 禁止驾驶的问题
- 生活方式的问题
- 更换电池的问题
- 重视与患者及照顾者沟通手术疗效的预期
- 重视与患者及照顾者沟通治疗过程的预期

表 11-3　术前筛查需检查项目

- 疾病严重程度（用药期间和非用药期间）
- 脑部 MRI
- 常规术前检查，如血液检查（包括凝血状态）、心电图
- 神经心理评估
- 精神科医生或神经心理医生评估情绪、行为、人格和应对方式等方面，由照顾者提供的病史也应作为筛选的一部分
- 麻醉评估

disorder society unified Parkinson disease rating scale，MDS-UPDRS）进行测评。对于其他 DBS 适应证，需要运用相关疾病的评分量表。虽然症状的严重程度测评相对主观，但是，如果测评结果证明药物治疗可以改善症状，DBS 手术通常对症状的影响也是正向的。当依据疾病严重程度分级作为手术治疗的依据时，以 PD 为例，可将药物"关期"MDS-UPDRS-Ⅲ（motor）评分 25 作为术前筛选的下限。在决定手术之前，应该对 MRI 进行充分评估，明确是否存在穿刺路径和靶点本身的结构异常，明确是否会阻碍电极植入。应该由麻醉科医师评估患者是否适合手术，包括凝血状态的评估和完善心电图明确心脏功能。因为高血压会增加手术颅内出血的风险（Gorgulho 等，2005），在筛选过程中，应特别关注血压。

一套完整的神经心理评估可以明确患者是否具有足够的认知储备，也可以明确患者是否已处于痴呆前期。这一点非常重要，因为手术具有加重认知障碍的风险。应该关注情绪、应对方式和行为方式异常的筛选。对于精神疾病的患者（如强迫症），术前筛选最好在临床中进行，因为对患者强迫行为的观察所获取的信息，可能对术后出现的问题有所提示。例如，患者反复清洗的行为可能会导致伤口感染。通过这种方式，我们可以预见这些将影响手术预后的行为。

四、多学科团队评估

术前测评的结果和指标应该在多学科会议上讨论。在大多数中心，会议参与者至少包括 1 名 DBS 专家、1 名神经外科医生、1 名神经心理科医生、1 名专科护士和 1 名精神科医生。由于手术和电刺激可能产生的不良事件，该会议讨论重点在于权衡手术获益和潜在风险。此外，会议需要讨论患者和照顾者对手术预期是否合理，如果手术预期过高，建议进一步沟通。如果多学科团队术前评估会议对于手术决策达成共识后，随后选择最合适的靶点，以及正式预约手术。评估结果应该与患者及照顾者充分交代。手术医生参与并充分告知手术获益、手术风险及并发症，完成手术知情同意。

五、手术流程

DBS 手术技术将在第 4 章中讨论。功能神经外科从 20 世纪开始，在清醒状态下进行立体定向毁损手术中，使用电极尖端进行电刺激。这种方法可以准确定位和最终确定需要毁损的靶点位置。目前，可以粗略分为清醒手术和全麻手术两种方式。在局麻下进行的清醒手术，允许术中进行试验性刺激评估手术疗效及不良反应。为了术中测试宏刺激对疾病症状的疗效，需要在手术前一天停用治疗疾病的相关药物。长效药物应在手术前几周逐渐减少。这样的停药流程通常用于 PD。对于全麻下进行 DBS 手术，没有停药的必要。在上述两种手术方式中，都可以使用微电极记录（MER）。这两种方法的选择取决于手术适应证和 DBS 中心的偏好。全身麻醉下的手术大多应用于肌张力障碍和精神障碍疾病。在清醒手术期间，往往需要专科护士在手术过程中持续监测患者状况。

无论是清醒手术还是全麻手术，感染预防措施、停止或交替抗凝治疗、影像扫描、手术器械

和设备等，这些术前准备的诸多事项应该在团队中分工明确（见第 7 章）。

六、术后阶段

术后 24h 内，应密切监测生命体征和神经系统功能。监测重点是手术相关并发症，如生命体征、颅内出血、谵妄、跌倒和相关疾病症状。术后根据指导严格执行用药方案。患者通常可以在手术后 1 周内出院，如果住院期间程控 DBS 系统，可以适当延长住院时间。

在患者出院时，患者和照顾者应当得到口头或是书面的出院告知信息（表 11-4）。这些信息可以由专科护理提供。也有必要充分解释术后患者面对的诸多限制。

表 11-4　术后出院告知患者和照顾者的信息

- DBS 中心的联系方式（电话号码和电子邮件地址）
- 如有特殊问题和疑问，请联系 DBS 中心（书面的；如适用，数字的）
- DBS 识别卡（包括患者数据、DBS 系统数据和 DBS 中心联系信息）
- 患者信息，包括患者程控器或"遥控器"的说明（书面的；如适用，数字的）
- 禁驾期（如适用）
- 生活方式问题

七、DBS 程控和手术后管理

（一）DBS 程控

DBS 程控的具体方法将在第 8 章中讨论。刺激器的程控通常在手术后 2~4 周进行，因为此时微毁损效应已逐渐消退。在首次程控过程中，所有电极的触点都要进行临床疗效评价和不良反应阈值测定，即所谓的"电极定位"。每个触点将设置固定的脉冲宽度和频率进行测试，随着逐渐增加电压，顺序记录临床疗效和不良反应，以便在日后的调控中使用。对于肌张力障碍、癫痫和精神疾病的患者，DBS 程控采用不同的方法。因为临床疗效一般延迟产生，需要术后较长时间的随访观察，首次调控主要测定不良

反应阈值。程控过程通常在神经内科医生或精神科医生指导下，由专科护士或病例随访人员完成。当开启刺激器之后，需要向患者和照顾者解释如何使用患者程控仪和远程调控，并提供使用手册。通过患者程控仪，患者可以在预先设定的刺激参数范围内进行自行调整。术后 3~6 个月需要在 DBS 中心进行多次复诊，逐步调整刺激参数以达到最佳刺激参数设置和药物治疗方案。在复诊中，要特别关注疗效、不良反应、不良事件及其处理。每次复诊都应该测定 DBS 系统阻抗和电量。

（二）手术后管理

一旦最佳的程控参数设定之后，可以由推荐来诊的神经内科医生或精神科医生进行复诊随访。依然建议在 DBS 中心进行不太频繁的随访，主要检查 DBS 设备的剩余电量和阻抗。如果电池耗尽，应该安排更换。普通刺激器需要每 3~5 年更换，可充电刺激器则需要 15~20 年更换。刺激器更换手术应在 DBS 中心进行。

在长期随访期间，DBS 中心有必要提供便捷的随访预约，以解决 DBS 相关专业问题、生活方式问题、相关诊治建议、刺激参数调整或任何可能出现的硬件相关问题。

（三）长期随访

DBS 的并发症和不良反应并不少见，包括手术相关并发症（出血、感染、移位等）、硬件相关并发症（电极断裂、刺激器故障等）和靶点刺激相关的不良反应（Bhatia 等，2001）。一旦这些手术的和刺激的相关并发症和不良反应出现，随即采取相应措施处理。DBS 团队应该提前做好准备，有不同的医疗专业人员可以提供紧急的医疗咨询来解决相关问题（Farris 和 Giroux，2013）。

八、社会支持

除了关注 DBS 术后的疗效和可能的不良反

应外，还应特别关注病情变化对患者及其社交的总体影响。术后需要时间来调整身体和精神状态的变化，无论这些变化是积极的还是消极的，这些对于患者自己、他们的伴侣、其他家庭成员及亲朋好友来说，都是比较复杂的。患者需要在日常生活、社交、休闲活动及工作中，不断地尝试什么事能做，什么事不能做。如果患者、家属或其亲戚朋友在应对患者术后各种情况时遇到困难，应考虑向心理科医生、社工、公司医生、康复科医生咨询。

九、生活方式问题

在手术前后和出院前，应该向患者和照顾者强调术后具体的限制和规定。虽然DBS是一种术后限制相对较少的外科治疗，但是患者、照顾者和全科医生需要充分了解植入DBS系统后的相关风险。此前已经报道过，一些操作或行为可能损害DBS设备，有时甚至导致脑组织损伤（Henderson等，2005）。建议（书面和口头）告知患者以下事项。

- 建议患者佩戴DBS识别卡，识别卡上有DBS医学中心和DBS设备公司的联系方式。
- 患者和照顾者应向医生、物理治疗师、口腔科医生和其他医疗专业人员说明已植入DBS设备。
- 植入DBS设备后，无法进行MRI检查，或者仅在DBS中心的特定条件下才能进行MRI。如果需要进行MRI扫描，应将患者转至DBS中心。每一种植入设备都有它自己的MRI限制。DBS中心需要时常更新MRI兼容性指南。植入DBS设备后进行MRI检查的风险包括设备部件发热，主要源于电极和电路开放，发热可以造成的组织损伤。这可能会导致严重的永久性的损伤，包括昏迷、瘫痪和死亡。发热也可能导致电极破损、硬件重置、断开连接和重新编程。根据植入的DBS设备，并且只有在专门的DBS中心使用特定的指南情况下，才能进行MRI检查（Rezai等，2005）。在MRI检查前后，需要进行刺激参数记录、阻抗测试，以及在双极配置中关闭DBS至0 V。如果发现阻抗增加，不应该进行MRI检查，应明确阻抗增加的原因（如电极断裂、失去连接；见前述）。MRI是否可以进行取决于DBS系统、DBS制造商、MRI特征和特殊线圈的可用性。较低的磁场强度并不会降低发热的风险，甚至可能增加发热的风险（Baker等，2005）。

- 应避免物理治疗师经常使用的热敷疗法。短波脉冲治疗，如用于治疗肾结石的体外冲击波碎石术，会对DBS装置周围的组织造成损害，应该尽量避免。
- 在手术过程中，应关闭DBS设备。需要电热凝设备的手术过程应仅使用双极。因为，在单极使用中，潜在的电路可能导致组织损伤或DBS设备损坏。
- 为避免心电图检查时出现伪影，DBS系统可暂时关闭（可由患者或照顾者操作）。
- 最好避免使用机场检测系统。患者可以出示DBS患者识别卡或从DBS中心带来明确避免使用检测系统的声明。
- 在非常罕见的情况下，强磁场，如发电厂或无线电发射设备，理论上可能会关闭或中断DBS设备。
- 如武术、蹦极、跳伞、射击等极限活动及运动会破坏DBS设备，游泳也尽量避免。

十、多学科DBS团队和设备的管理

DBS治疗是一种复杂的、终身的、多学科的治疗，对整个流程进行充分的管理是非常重要的。DBS中心需要综合性的多学科协作方案，涵盖从患者被建议手术治疗到手术后管理全过程。在该方案中需要记录所有参与治疗的人员的任务和责任。一个多学科团队通常包括功能神经外科医生、神经内科医生、神经放射科医生、麻醉科医生、精神科医生、神经心理科医生、专科护士和手术室团队成员。必要时，神经生理学家和全科医生也应该参与围术期管理中。所有的团队成员都应该接受良好的培训。团队成员、患者及照看者能够清楚地知道每个多学科团队成员的任务和责任。建议 DBS 团队中的每个学科至少有 2 名专业人员。在 DBS 中心，对于病例选择、手术本身、随访，以及诸如更换电池、感染或刺激的急性不良反应等紧急问题，应该有一个良好的综合性管理设计。临床专科之间不应有沟通壁垒。轻松的跨学科交流对良好的围术期管理至关重要。

应该对所有团队成员进行定期教育和培训，既要有本专业的单学科培训，更要有涉及多学科的培训。

为了患者的安全，手术设备应定期进行安全检查，并保证定期数据备份。严格管理植入设备的物流。书面或数字的患者信息应该及时和便于获得。当开始 DBS 手术或调整 DBS 流程时，应该进行前瞻性风险分析和建模分析以达到最佳实施效果。

十一、结果评价

建议定期评价 DBS 不同流程的结果。应重视临床预后数据测评、不同流程适应证和患者满意度。结果评价应采用症状、功能和生活质量评定量表，并应记录术后至少 1 年内的不良反应和并发症。这些评价结果应在定期的团队会议上与多学科团队成员共享。应该鼓励团队成员和患者提出可能的改进意见。应根据这些评价对流程进行适当的更改。

十二、结论

DBS 是一个复杂的治疗过程，应该在专门的医学中心由专业的多学科团队进行。围术期管理方案需要清晰界定全部流程（从病例入选到终身随访），并且必须明确每个团队成员的任务和职责。多学科团队成员应该接受良好的培训，既要有本专业的单学科培训，更要有涉及多学科的培训。务必保证定期的团队会议、持续的培训教育、结果的评估及改进，以及开放的团队氛围。此外，清晰的管理、透明的流程、团队成员之间的信任也是必不可少的。

在 DBS 手术前，多学科团队参与术前评估和决策，并通过提供最新的疗效信息调整患者和照看者对手术的预期。在 DBS 手术过程中，保证手术中影像资料清晰、器械完备、设备运行良好。在 DBS 手术后，参与患者术后的医疗和社会支持，并能够处理可能出现的并发症和不良反应。DBS 中心和专家之间的协作可以提高流程效率和改善患者体验。

参考文献

[1] Baker KB, Nyenhuis JA, Hrdlicka G, et al. Neurostimulation systems: assessment of magnetic field interactions associated with 1.5- and 3-Tesla MR systems. Magn Reson Imaging. 2005;21:72–7.

[2] Bhatia R, Dalton A, Richards M, et al. The incidence of deep brain stimulator hardware infection: the effect of change in antibiotic prophylaxis regimen and review of the literature. Br J Neurosurg. 2001;25:625–31.

[3] Elwyn G, Frosch D, Thomson R, et al. Shared decision making: a model for clinical practice. J Gen Intern Med. 2012;27:1361–7.

[4] Farris S, Giroux M. Retrospective review of factors leading to dissatisfaction with subthalamic nucleus deep brain stimulation during long-term management. Surg Neurol Int. 2013;4:69.

[5] Gorgulho A, De Salles AA, Frighetto L, Behnke E. Incidence of hemorrhage associated with electrophysiological studies performed using macroelectrodes and microelectrodes in functional neurosurgery. J Neurosurg. 2005;102:888–96.

[6] Henderson JM, Tkach J, Phillips M, et al. Permanent neurological deficit related to magnetic resonance imaging in a patient with implanted deep brain stimulation electrodes for Parkinson's disease: case report. Neurosurgery. 2005;57:E1063.

[7] Okun MS, Tagliati M, Pourfar M, et al. Management of referred deep brain stimulation failures: a retrospective analysis from 2 movement disorders centers. Arch Neurol. 2005;62:1250–5.

[8] Rezai AR, Baker KB, Tkach JA, et al. Is magnetic resonance imaging safe for patients with neurostimulation systems used for deep brain stimulation? Neurosurgery. 2005;57:1056–62.

第二篇

神经病学
Neurology

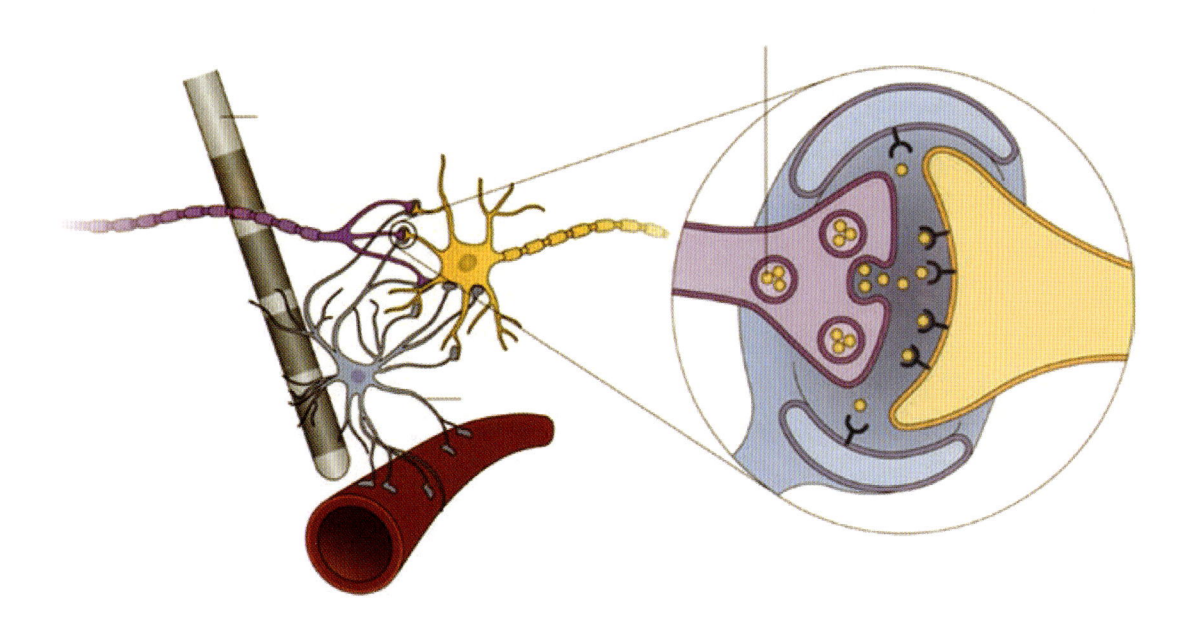

第 12 章 脑深部电刺激治疗帕金森病
Deep Brain Stimulation for Parkinson's Disease

Timo R.ten Brinke　Martijn Beudel　Rob M.A.de Bie　**著**
陈颖川　张　华　**译**　杨岸超　张建国　**校**

> **摘要**：脑深部电刺激（deep brain stimulation, DBS）是治疗晚期帕金森病（Parkinson disease, PD）公认的有效方法。治疗 PD 最常用的 2 个靶点是底丘脑核（subthalamic nucleus，STN）和苍白球内侧部（internal globus pallidus, GPi）。DBS 对于治疗顽固性震颤、药物反应性运动症状波动和异动特别有效。通常，DBS 对运动症状的最佳疗效与多巴胺能药物一样好，但更稳定。成功进行 DBS 治疗的 3 个基本要素包括最佳的患者选择、准确的 DBS 电极位置，以及包括程控和药物调整在内的术后管理。

一、概述

帕金森病（PD）是第二常见的神经退行性疾病。其核心特征是运动迟缓、伴随静止性震颤、僵直或两者兼有（Kalia 和 Lang，2015）。大多数患者还具有非运动症状，如睡眠功能障碍、自主神经功能障碍（如便秘、尿急和直立性低血压）、嗅觉减退、认知功能减退和精神障碍（如抑郁症、焦虑症和精神错乱）（Schapira 等，2017）。尽管运动症状是诊断 PD 的先决条件，但非运动症状也可能占主导地位。该疾病大多老年起病，平均发病年龄为 60 岁。在 65—75 岁的人群中，PD 的患病率为 425/10 万，并且随着年龄的增长而增加（Pringsheim 等，2014）。

（一）病理生理

PD 的病因尚未十分清楚。PD 的神经病理学特征是神经元丢失、黑质色素脱失和路易体形成（Fahn，2018）。尽管尚不清楚 α 突触核蛋白的功能，但它在 PD 的病理生理学中的关键作用似乎无可辩驳，因为路易体中有丰富的 α 突触核蛋白的聚集体，PD 的遗传特征与 α 突触核蛋白形成或降解相关因素有关（Spillantini 等，1997；Singleton，2003；Fahn，2018）。PD 的典型症状是由于多巴胺能神经元变性导致黑质 – 纹状体系统中多巴胺能神经环路功能障碍引起的。黑质、纹状体（尾状核、壳状核和伏隔核）、屏状核、苍白球和底丘脑核一起形成基底节。它们通常被认为是与运动、动眼、认知，以及边缘系统相关环路的组成部分（Afifi，1994）。很明显，基底节系统是一个复杂且分布广泛的神经元网络，通过轴突的分支联络形成网络，以多种路径影响基底节的输出核团（Graybiel，2008；Redgrave 等，2010；Nelson 和 Kreitzer，2014）（另见第 2 章，解剖学）。除了基底节功能受损外，PD 病理改变会逐渐扩散到整个大脑，从脑干到颞叶皮质，从旧皮质到新皮质，从运动前区域到感觉相关区域逐渐扩散。这个过程在诸如自主神经功能障碍、精神症状和认知功能减退等"非多巴胺能"症状中起重要作用（Braak 等，2003；Alves 等，2005；Hawkes 等，2009；Lieberman 和 Krishnamurthi，2013；Rietdijk 等，2017）。

（二）保守治疗

PD 仍然无法治愈。对症治疗主要包括用左旋多巴加外周脱羧酶抑制药或连同多巴胺激动药补充多巴胺缺乏。这些药物可以显著改善运动迟缓和僵硬，但震颤的改善往往差强人意。

在疾病发展了 4~6 年后，患者可能会出现症状波动（Calabresi 等，2010；Aquino 和 Fox，2015）。最初，这些波动与左旋多巴摄入量呈现明显的时间相关性，并且可以通过调整药物来减少症状波动。然而，随着疾病的进展，可能会出现其他不良反应，例如与药物相关的不自主运动（如异动）或精神症状（如幻觉和偏执妄想）。服用左旋多巴后交替出现显著的症状改善（可能伴有不自主运动）和症状显著的现象称为反应性波动。将药物疗效显著的时间（即患者可以自由活动）称为"开期"，并将症状显著（即药物疗效较少或没有）的时间称为"关期"。从"开期"到"关期"的过渡可能要花费一些时间（如 15min 或更长时间），被称为"疗效衰减期"。随着疾病的进展，运动状态下的反应性波动可能会突然激增，如果使用更复杂的用药计划，药物疗效与左旋多巴的时间相关性可能会消失。

有几种药理学方法可以解决运动症状的波动。基本思想是稳定连续的多巴胺能刺激。这些策略大部分并没有进行随机对照研究相互比较，因此，并没有足够的循证数据来支持某一种治疗方案（Fox 等，2018）。下文提及的策略并未刻意排序，也不完整。一种策略是调整左旋多巴在每日中的服用次数，例如，从每日 3 次至每日 5 次。另一种策略是使用左旋多巴长效制药或增加多巴胺受体激动药（如罗匹尼罗、普拉克索或罗替高汀），可以按照左旋多巴等效剂量添加或换算多巴胺受体激动药（Fox 等，2018）。多巴胺受体激动药更易引起不良反应，例如恶心、幻觉、精神症状、冲动控制障碍和嗜睡（Stowe 等，2008）。其他策略包括添加一种酶抑制药（该酶催化将多巴胺分解为无活性的代谢物），从而增加左旋多巴作用的持续时间。可以使用儿茶酚 -O- 甲基转移酶（catechol-O-methyltransferase inhibitors, COMT）抑制药，如恩他卡朋或奥匹卡朋（Müller，2015）和单胺氧化酶 -B（monoamine-oxidase-B inhibitors，MAO-B）抑制药，如司来吉兰或雷沙吉兰（Schapira，2011）。如果添加 COMT 或 MAO-B 抑制药后异动增加，则可能需要降低左旋多巴的剂量。对于难以控制的异动，可以尝试使用金刚烷胺（Pereira da Silva-Júnior 等，2005）。

除了运动症状会随着疾病进展而越来越复杂，还会逐渐出现非运动症状，将会导致生活不能自理和幸福感严重降低（Bhidayasiri 和 Wolters，2008）。非运动症状出现时间和范围各不相同，差异很大。

（三）进阶治疗

自 20 世纪 90 年代以来，DBS 已被证明是治疗晚期 PD 的有效方法（Limousin 等，1995）。几项随机对照试验（RCT）已经证实，对于减轻症状和提高生活质量，DBS 比最佳药物治疗更有效（Spottke 等，2002；Deuschl 等，2006；Schuepbach 等，2013；Becerra 等，2016）。对于 DBS 治疗 PD 运动症状，主要靶点是底丘脑核（subthalamic nucleus, STN）和苍白球内侧核（globus pallidus internus, GPi）。在 PD 患者中，出现帕金森症状时，STN 电生理活动的特征性变化，包括放电频率增加和爆发性电活动增强（Albin 等，1989；Hassani 等，1996）。在 STN 中，可以观察到与临床震颤同步的相关神经元电信号，这些细胞被称为震颤细胞（Levy 等，2000，2002）。患者主动运动及 STN 的高频刺激不仅能够缓解震颤，还可以减少与震颤相关的神经元电活动。大约 50% 的 STN 神经元的放电模式伴随主动或被动运动而变化，并且这些与运动有关的神经元大多数位于 STN 的背外侧和背侧，这里是 STN-DBS 的最佳靶点区域（Williams 等，2005；Coenen 等，2008）。同样，当患者出现帕金森症状时，GPi 后部和腹侧电活动也会增强（Williams 等，2005）。

出现药物相关的运动症状波动的患者可以进行持续空肠内左旋多巴输注（continuous intrajejunal levodopa infusion，CLI）和持续皮下阿扑吗啡输注（continuous subcutaneous apomorphine infusion，CAI）的治疗，具有一定疗效（Espay，2010；Worth，2013；Antonini 等，2018）。尚未对这 3 种治疗方法（DBS、CLI 和 CAI）通过随机对照研究进行比较。目前已完成的研究使用了不同的结果指标、实验设计和随访时间，难以进行相互比较。关于治疗相关不良反应的比较同样知之甚少。当前，根据下列具体情况进行治疗方法的选择，包括设备特点（如脑外科手术与佩戴泵）、特定症状的疗效差异、不良反应、治疗的可获得性、患者的偏好，以及医生的经验（表 12-1）（Antonini 等，2018）。对于治疗方法的选择，国家之间和国家内部也存在很大的差异（Antonini 等，2018）。

部分 PD 患者症状表现以震颤为主，意味着静止性和（或）姿势性震颤是疾病起始最主要的症状，仅伴有轻度的运动迟缓和僵直（Rajput 等，2009；Thenganatt 和 Jankovic，2014）。对于这组患者，疾病进展和日常生活受限的进展并不迅速，这主要是因为运动迟缓、步态和姿势不稳对日常生活的影响更大，而震颤为主的 PD 患者上述症状并不突出（Thenganatt 和 Jankovic，2014）。尽管使用较高剂量的多巴胺替代疗法，并且有相当多的患者确实会产生效果，但震颤改善并不明显（Sethi，2008）。在这些情况下，可以尝试使用其他药物治疗，如抗胆碱能药（最好 ≤ 60 岁）和普萘洛尔（Marjama-Lyons 和 Koller，2000）。如果治疗仍不能改善震颤，除了 GPi 和 STN DBS 以外，还可以选择对丘脑腹侧中间核（ventral intermediate nucleus，VIM）进行手术（Marjama-Lyons 和 Koller，2000；Reinacher

表 12-1 帕金森病药物相关的运动症状波动 3 种疗法的治疗特点

	脑深部电刺激（DBS）	CAI	CLI
	将电脉冲施加于大脑的靶点区域	通过皮下放置的针头给药	通过 PEG 管向十二指肠给药
单一或联合治疗	• DBS 联合口服药物	• CAI 联合口服药物	• CLI 可以用作单一疗法
可能的不良反应和风险	• 脑出血 • 术后感染 • 谵妄 • 认知障碍 • 行为改变 • 言语障碍 • 技术问题或电池耗尽导致重新操作 • 平衡和步态问题	• 注射部位皮下痛性结节 • 恶心 • 出汗 • 低血压 • 心力衰竭 • 多巴胺失调综合征和冲动控制障碍	• PEG 管阻塞 • 恶心 • PEG 管进入部位周围发炎 • 腹壁开口周围泄漏 • PEG 管的位移 • 便秘 • 直立性低血压
可能的缺点	• 神经外科手术固有的风险 • 无法进行测试治疗 • 一些系统与 MRI 不兼容 • 在通过金属探测器时可能会出现问题 • 每 5~9 年需要更换一次电池	• 患者必须在白天携带泵 • 每天放置皮下针头并连接泵，清洁泵，插入部位皮肤护理 • 注射部位皮下痛性结节 • 泵可能存在的问题/故障 • 数年后通常需要另一种治疗	• 患者必须在白天携带泵 • 每天需要连接和断开泵的连接，清洁管道，插入部位皮肤护理 • 放置 PEG 管需要进行手术 • 泵可能存在的问题/故障
可能的优势	• 与持续皮下注射阿扑吗啡和 CLI 相比，没有日常限制，无须携带外部泵	• 无须手术 • 许多患者都可以选择 • 可以测试治疗	• 许多患者都可以选择 • 可以测试治疗

DBS. 脑深部电刺激；CAI. 持续皮下阿扑吗啡输注；CLI. 持续空肠内左旋多巴/卡比多巴输注；PEG. 经皮内镜下胃造口术；MRI. 磁共振成像

等，2018）。考虑到大多数以震颤为主的PD患者最终也会出现运动迟缓，因此多数DBS团队更倾向于进行STN DBS，但前提是不存在禁忌证（如认知障碍）。

二、手术选择

当考虑进行DBS治疗PD时，多学科团队参与的病例筛选非常重要。该团队将进行术前评估，如症状严重程度、症状波动、异动的存在，以及可能的药物不良反应（Rodriguez等，2007）。除了确定患者是否适合使用DBS外，团队还必须调整患者及照顾者可能提出的不切实际的高期望。

（一）DBS术前筛选

评估DBS的适应证，需要评估"开"期和"关"期的症状严重程度、药物不良反应，以及认知和精神状况。大多数DBS团队使用MDS-统一帕金森病评价量表（movement disorders society unified PD rating scale，MDS-UPDRS）和异动评分量表（Goetz等，2008）来评估。通常，在多巴胺能药物停药后的隔夜清晨评估"关"期症状的严重性，早晨服用第一种药物后1h评估药物"开"期症状程度。为了使患者快速达到"开"期状态，患者可以在早晨禁食后服用短效左旋多巴，如左旋多巴/苯并呋喃糖苷分散片100/25 mg，剂量比平时晨起首次剂量高一点（例如，左旋多巴等效剂量为平时首次剂量的120%～150%）。药物"关"期、"开"期评估是筛选PD DBS适应证的基础，因为对左旋多巴反应良好的症状很可能对DBS反应良好（Rodriguez等，2007）。关于临界值，存在很大差异。通常在30%～50%（Welter等，2002；Morishita等，2011；Schuepbach等，2013）。

为了评估DBS手术的安全性和可行性，可以进行脑MRI（评估血管系统、脑萎缩和意外的结构异常，如脑膜瘤）、实验室检查、心电图和麻醉评估。此外，在许多DBS中心，在手术前进行神经心理筛查，因为认知障碍可能在DBS手术后加重（Rodriguez等，2007；Foley等，2018）。合并精神疾病，如抑郁症或精神错乱，以及认知障碍会使手术和程控变得更加复杂。此外，存在这些共病的情况下，很难确定哪一种症状对患者的日常生活影响最大。一些精神障碍可能会给清醒手术带来问题，如活动性精神病和创伤后应激障碍。在特定的情况下，建议在进行DBS之前由精神科医生进行评估。

在决定进行手术之前，需要特别关注患者和家属对DBS的疗效和可能的不良反应的预期，这一点非常重要，因为超过30%的手术失败是由于患者选择不当（Okun等，2005）。预期有时是不切实际的，例如，患者要求行DBS手术，但尚未接受患病的事实，期待着DBS术后一切恢复正常。

同样重要的是，需要事先告知患者和家属手术流程、DBS的预期疗效，以及症状不能改善的可能性、潜在的不良反应、电极路径（包括微损毁效应）、单极测试（mapping session）和随着时间延长程控参数逐渐增加，还有必要的调整服药时间表（参见第8章：程控）。当刺激参数达到最佳设置时，不需要定期调整，这可能会使患者感到困惑，因为这与术前药物方案经常调整的情况相反。

运动障碍DBS团队通常由1名运动障碍疾病专业的神经内科医生、1名进行DBS手术的神经外科医生、1名精神科医生、1名神经心理科医生和1名专门从事PD和DBS术后护理的专科护士组成。我们将在下面讨论DBS在PD中的适应证和禁忌证。

（二）药物相关的运动症状波动

DBS治疗PD最重要的适应证是由药物相关的运动症状波动引起的功能障碍，如肌张力障碍和疼痛，以及药物难治性震颤（Duker和Espay，2013）。DBS的适应证和禁忌证见表12-2。由于DBS潜在的最大效应或多或少等于多巴胺能药物治疗的最大效应，因此手术后的功能障碍一般

表 12-2 DBS 治疗帕金森病的适应证和禁忌证

适应证
- 药物相关的运动症状波动和由运动迟缓、疼痛、肌张力障碍和（或）异动引起的功能障碍
- 药物难治性震颤

禁忌证
- 药物作用期严重功能障碍（如姿势不稳）
- 严重的认知障碍（如 Mattis dementia rating scale 得分＜120）（Matteau 等，2011）
- 精神病或抑郁症
- 神经外科手术的禁忌证，如不能停用抗凝血药、严重高血压和吞咽困难

不太可能优于术前最佳药物治疗阶段的功能障碍（Williams 等，2010）。但是功能性神经外科手术（如 DBS 和损毁）对于药物难治性震颤非常有效，可以超过多巴胺能药物治疗的最大效应。震颤将在下一段中讨论。与口服多巴胺能药物（尤其是左旋多巴）治疗不同，DBS 的作用是稳定的、昼夜连续的，能够有效减少症状波动。在临床实践中，这意味着在"关期"帕金森症状得到有效改善，而"开期"症状可能变化很少或是没有变化，但是，DBS 术后"开期"异动可能减少（Williams 等，2010）。

（三）震颤

震颤是 DBS 的一个适应证。对于那些使用了最大剂量的药物，仍然存在致残性震颤的患者来说也是如此，因为与服用多巴胺能药物相比，DBS 可能会改善症状（Morishita 等，2011）。这是因为 DBS 对震颤的影响与多巴胺能（和其他）药物对震颤的影响并不相关（Zaidel 等，2010）。

（四）异动

DBS 可以直接减少异动（Krack 等，1998；Wu 等，2001）。这对于剂峰异动和双相异动均有效。

（五）行为障碍

多年以来，与 PD 相关的行为障碍，如焦虑、冲动控制障碍和多巴胺能药物成瘾，被许多人认为是 DBS 治疗的禁忌证。但是，精神症状也可能与运动症状类似。一些文献报道了 DBS 术后出现行为障碍或是原有症状恶化（Lim 等，2009），其发生机制可能是直接刺激效应（Sensi 等，2004；Smeding 等，2006）或 DBS 术后药物调整（Smeding 等，2006）。据文献报道，高多巴胺能现象，如冲动控制障碍和多巴胺能药物成瘾，在开始或维持 DBS 治疗后得到改善，精神症状本身并不应该被视为禁忌证（Lhommee 等，2018）。

（六）DBS 不能或只能轻微改善症状

患者对 DBS 反应较差的症状，包括步态障碍、自主神经功能障碍或构音障碍，部分患者以上述症状为主要表现。选择 DBS 与否不应该单独考虑这些症状，因为预期的功能改善并不明显。

（七）适合做 DBS 的年龄

DBS 手术没有绝对的年龄限制，但年龄越大，伴随的并发症和认知功能障碍越多，DBS 的风险也越大。年龄较大的 PD 患者左旋多巴反应降低（服用药物前后的运动功能差异），因此 DBS 治疗获益较少（Weaver 等，2009）。然而，对于年龄＞70 岁，左旋多巴反应明显，且有 DBS 治疗适应证，其他身体状态健康的患者，可以考虑手术治疗。

（八）合适的 DBS 时机

在早期运用阶段，患者选择 DBS 手术的时间较晚，通常在所有其他治疗方案都失败之后。渐渐地，患者接受手术的时间逐渐提前。对于这种变化，EARLYSTIM 试验起到了关键作用。在这项临床试验中，入选标准为起病至少 4 年和具

有运动症状波动的患者，使用的药物可能只有1~2个。试验的平均病程为7.5年。经过2年的随访，STN DBS 患者采用 PD 问卷（PDQ-39）对生活质量的健康相关指标进行评估，表明有显著提高（Jenkinson 等，1995），而单独采用最佳药物治疗方案的患者（Deuschl 等，2013）则无显著提高（$P < 0.05$）。目前，DBS 不再被认为是最后的治疗手段，可以更早地运用于运动症状波动的治疗。

三、靶点选择

多种因素影响 PD 患者 DBS 的靶点选择。在不同的临床试验中发现 GPi 和 STN DBS 在效果上的差异将在本章后面讨论，但是在 PD 患者中选择 DBS 靶点的一些注意事项讨论如下。

（一）底丘脑核

STN DBS 或多或少模仿了多巴胺能药物的作用，对运动迟缓、震颤、僵直和疼痛有改善的作用（Limousin 等，1998）。如果这些症状中至少有一种导致残疾，可以考虑 STN DBS。STN 也是治疗 PD 药物难治性震颤的合适靶点。随着疾病的进展，其他症状，如运动迟缓，可能成为功能障碍的主要因素（Pfeiffer，2016）。

STN DBS 可能增加异动，甚至可能在"非运动期"诱发异动（Zheng 等，2010）。一般来说，这被认为是一种积极的现象，因为它证实了 DBS 触点位于 STN 里面。因为 STN DBS 术后每日服用的多巴胺能药物可减少 30%~50%（Deuschl 等，2006；Weaver 等，2012；Odekerken 等，2013），与药物相关的不自主运动可能逐渐减少或消失。STN DBS 术后减少多巴胺能药物治疗可能出现低多巴胺能症状，如冷漠、抑郁和焦虑。在多巴胺激动药戒断综合征（Dopamine agonist withdrawal syndrome，DAWS）被广泛认知之前（Patel 等，2017），一些团队在手术后短时间内大量减少并停用了多巴胺激动药，这可能诱发了多巴胺激动药戒断综合征。然而，重要的是，最近的一项 RCT 结果表明，因为运动症状而接受 DBS 手术的患者常选用 STN 靶点，更易于出现药物诱发致残性高多巴胺能状态和神经精神症状波动（Lhommee 等，2018）。在 STN 和 GPi DBS 两组之间出现术后行为障碍的概率差别不大（Weaver 等，2012；Odekerken 等，2013）。

（二）苍白球内侧部

与 STN 一样，GPi 也是 PD 药物难治性震颤的合适靶点，而且，随着疾病的进展，其他症状可能会成为未来致残的主要因素（Pfeiffer，2016）。当刺激 GPi 时，与 STN DBS 相比，需要更高的电流幅度，这可能加快电池消耗，而且，与 STN DBS 相比，GPi DBS 术后多巴胺能药物减量较少（Odekerken 等，2013）。GPi DBS 可以直接减轻对侧异动（Krack 等，1998；Wu 等，2001）。

（三）丘脑腹侧中间核

对于以震颤为主的 PD，如果不能选择 STN DBS 和 GPi DBS，例如患者是老年人并且有认知障碍，则可以考虑选择 VIM 作为手术靶点。通过射频消融或 MRI 引导的聚焦超声手术进行的 VIM 丘脑毁损术，只能进行单侧手术，因为双侧手术具有明显不良反应（Alomar 等，2017）。然而，VIM DBS 可以进行双侧或毁损对侧手术（Lozano，2000；Schuurman 等，2000）。

四、手术方式

PD 患者的 DBS 靶点主要涉及 STN 和 GPi，在某些情况下涉及 VIM。脚桥核（pedunculo-pontine，PPN）仅是正在研究的靶点。选择特定靶点的参数已在上一节中给出。鉴于精确放置 DBS 电极是取得良好手术效果的最重要的预测指标之一，因此将 DBS 电极放置在正确的位置至关重要（Welter 等，2014）。DBS 电极的植入属于立体定向手术，后续通过皮下"隧道"置入延长导线，以及锁骨下置入脉冲发生器。第4章（技术方面）详细描述了植入过程和植入后的验证过程。在以下部分中，将讨论靶点的详细解剖结构、术中发现与临床结果之间的关系及主要争议。

（一）底丘脑核

底丘脑核是皮质下结构，其解剖学尺寸为9mm（长）×10mm（宽）×3mm（高）（Patil等，2012）。STN在冠状面、矢状面和轴面都是斜向的，这使得对其尺寸的估计依赖于视角。此外，1.5T-MRI发现的STN与尸体解剖后的STN尺寸不同（Mavridis等，2013）。在电场强度为3.0T时，关于STN的功能和解剖描述的差异，文献提供了不同的报告。一些研究显示了显著的一致性（Mavridis等，2013），而另一些研究则差异性很大（Verhagen等，2016）。考虑到这些差异，神经生理微电极记录（MER）对于正确描绘STN是具有特殊价值，特别是当只有场强度较低的MRI图像或CT图像可用时。考虑到存在与进行多通道MER记录有关的医源性风险，尤其是颅内出血的风险，需要特别重视与谨慎（Binder等，2005）。

目前STN最常使用可视化（"直接"）定位，在立体定向空间中，相对于连合中点的典型坐标为：x = 12 mm，y = 2 mm（后方）和z = 4 mm（Andrade-Souza等，2005；Rabie等，2016）。考虑到患者间的异质性，基于MRI图像的直接定位靶点方法更为准确。然而，尽管MRI序列的不断发展和MRI场强的持续增强，STN本身仍然很难在MRI上直接可视。可以使用MR上可视的红核（red nucleus，RN）作为直接定位的替代。RN在T_2加权像上明显低信号的结构，位于STN的后内方。可以使用RN间接定位STN，已有报告比较了直接和间接定位STN的结果（Andrade-Souza等，2005）。

在定位STN靶点之后是STN核团内亚区的定位。虽然STN核团内没有严格的功能划分，但传入和传出纤维存在功能上的差别，分别是位于STN背外侧、中央和腹内侧的运动、联络和边缘亚区（Haynes和Haber，2013）。以STN背外侧运动亚区作为靶点可以获得最佳的运动症状改善，而位于其他区域的电极，尤其是STN边缘亚区的电极会导致不良反应的产生（Welter等，2014）。除了基于MRI直接定位STN的背外侧区域外，MER记录可以作为指导（Gross等，2006）。使用MER，可以检测到STN和周围组织的单神经元放电。常规在预定靶点上方约6mm处开始MER，然后将MER微电极以0.5~1mm的步距移动到靶点或更深处。这条路径最常以记录到丘脑电活动开始，在这里几乎检测不到神经元放电，然后到达未定带，出现单峰值。随后，检测到代表STN背侧边界的神经元放电明显增加。这种放电活动在整个STN中持续存在，当到达STN的下界时逐渐消失（Gross等，2006）。STN下方是黑质网状部（SN），神经元放电相似，然而，在STN和SN之间，神经元放电的显著下降是最常见的。

STN背（前）外侧是内囊、丘脑及其上界的未定带，内侧是第三对脑神经纤维。由于毗邻这些结构，使得微小的电极偏移将导致疗效不佳和不良反应增加。避免这种情况的一种方法是术中使用宏刺激测试疗效阈值和不良反应阈值。可能出现的典型不良反应是眼动障碍、构音障碍和因为定位太靠内或太靠外而引起的肌肉强直性收缩。因此，术中测试不同电压下DBS电极路径上不同深度的疗效和不良反应是非常有用的。常规的术中测试在药物"关"期状态进行，主要包括对侧肢体运动症状及体征、动眼神经功能、语言功能和不自主运动的评估。然而，围术期临床试验指出，通过术中试验性刺激只能预测小部分患者的最终疗效和不良反应（Blume等，2017）。因此，术中测试应该使用非常低的不良反应阈值和只能作为粗略的疗效评价。一般情况下，术中测试的时间窗较短，主要原因是患者疲劳而不能配合，无法评估过多的电极位置。此外，要认识到在围术期刺激中洗脱效应的重要性，这是患者所特有的，而且随着病程的延长而减少的

（Cooper 等，2013）。

（二）苍白球内侧部靶点

苍白球内侧部（globus pallidus, GPi）是豆状核的一部分，豆状核还包括苍白球外侧部（globus pallidus, GPe）和壳核。值得注意的是，豆状核与其说是一个功能结构，不如说是一个解剖学术语。GPi 位于 GPe 的内侧位置。和 STN 一样，可以采用直接和间接的方法来定位 GPi。以联合中点为原点，GPi 的坐标为 x：侧方 20～22 mm, y：后方 2 mm, z：下方 1～2 mm（Schaltenbrand 和 Wahren，1977）。早期的实验室工作发现，只有调节 GPi 的感觉运动（后腹侧和外侧）区域才能缓解对侧肢体运动症状（Taha 等，1996）。

与 STN 相比，GPi 在 MRI 上更明显，通常应用 T_1WI 而不是 T_2WI（Nowacki 等，2015）。但是，与 STN 一样，MER 记录结果可能与影像定位有出入（Baker 等，2010）。GPi 路径中的 MER 典型信号，表现为壳核没有神经元放电，在壳核和 GPe 的边界有零星的尖峰活动，在 GPe 中爆发性电活动，在 GPi 中存在连续的尖峰活动，随后，GPi 以下出现散在尖峰活动（Vitek 等，2009）。根据 MER 结果并结合术前影像，确定在 GPi 进行宏刺激测试的位置。

GPi 的内侧和腹侧被内囊和视束包绕。鉴于这种解剖学架构，在术中测试时可以考虑以下方面，包括音量和发音、面部或对侧肢体的强直性收缩及视觉相关表现。

（三）VIM 靶点

与 GPi 或 STN 不同，VIM 通常是不可视的。这与它在 MRI 上的低可视性有关，尽管一些更新的 MRI 序列可以解决这个问题（Vassal 等，2012）。VIM 的间接定位是通过可视化的相邻结构来实现的，如内囊或第三脑室，并使用相对于丘脑高度和连合中点的距离。与 VIM 不可视化所致的定位困难相比，震颤是在所有对 DBS 有反应的运动症状中最容易进行术中评估的。因此，术中测试对 VIM DBS 治疗非常重要。除此之外，MER 记录也很有帮助。对于 VIM 的 MER 是基于（被动）运动进行的。VIM 是通过 MER 中与手部相对应的运动区域来定义的，位于丘脑腹侧核边界前 2～4mm 处（Gross 等，2006），后者是由对触觉刺激有反应的神经生理学定义的相关区域。

最近的一项双盲研究结果表明，在（特发性）震颤患者中，与 VIM DBS 相比，底丘脑后区（posterior subthalamic, PSA），包括未定带（zona incerta, ZI）DBS 同样有效，且能耗更低（Barbe 等，2018）。同样的道理也适用于 PD 患者，刺激 ZI 可显著减少震颤，可与 VIM 刺激相媲美（Blomstedt 等，2018）。考虑到一个 DBS 电极可以同时刺激 VIM 和 PSA，术中发现可以务实地确定个体患者震颤抑制的最佳靶点。

（四）DBS 步骤的争议

尽管 DBS 现在已经在临床上应用了数十年，但是关于最佳手术方案仍存在争议。在前面的部分中，已经涉及了其中一些问题。一个重要的问题是，在全身麻醉下进行 DBS 手术是否和在局部麻醉清醒状态下进行的结果近似，因为清醒状态下可以进行术中测试。由于 MRI 技术的发展，手术步骤已大大改善，许多 DBS 手术团队已更改其手术流程，开始在全身麻醉下进行 DBS 手术。尽管单独的队列研究报告了在全身麻醉和局部麻醉下进行的手术结果类似，但目前正在进行的随机对照的"head-to-head"临床研究结果尚未发表（Holewijn 等，2017）。同样，与没有 MER 的手术相比，使用多通道 MER 的手术更容易引起出血（Zrinzo 等，2012）。然而，对是否使用 MER 的手术团队进行比较，均能有效的缓解 PD 症状（Foltynie 等，2011）。迄今为止，尚未进行有或没有 MER 的 DBS 手术之间的直接比较。因为 MER 所致出血的发生率相对较低，所以进行两者比较的临床研究将需要大量样本。手术方法的其他最新进展包括运用 DWI 纤维素成像技术进行 DBS 电极植入手术（Akram 等，

2017）和无框架机器人辅助 DBS 电极植入手术（Ho 等，2019）。

五、DBS 的结果

自 20 世纪 90 年代以来，DBS 已被证明是晚期 PD 的有效治疗方法（Limousin 等，1995）。

（一）STN DBS

如果左旋多巴治疗能够缓解运动迟缓、僵直、疼痛和震颤，STN DBS 也可以减轻上述症状，也可能对语言和步态产生积极的影响（表 12-3）（Bronstein 等，2011）。最初，STN DBS 可诱发异动。在清醒状态下的手术过程中，通过术中测试刺激，可以观察到异动，这就证实了测试电极的接触点在 STN 的运动亚区（Houeto 等，2003）。STN DBS 术后，随着时间的推移，往往通过减少多巴胺能药物，异动可以得到改善。随着多巴胺能药物治疗的减少，尤其是左旋多巴高剂量"脉冲式"给药的减少，产生异动的阈值药物剂量和 DBS 产生异动的阈值也将会升高（Espay 和 Lang，2017）。

几项随机对照试验证实，对于治疗药物相关的运动症状波动的 PD 患者，DBS 比最佳药物治疗更能有效地减轻症状（Fahn 等，1987）和提高疾病相关生活质量（Spottke 等，2002；Schuepbach 等，2013；Becerra 等，2016）。在一个德国大型临床试验中，以及在一个法德联合大型临床试验（"早期刺激"试验）中，STN DBS 与术后 2 年的最佳治疗进行了比较（Deuschl 等，2006；Schuepbach 等，2013）。在 EARLYSTIM 试验中，招募了早期运动并发症的患者（Schuepbach 等，2013）。这个试验入选标准主要包括：病程≥ 4 年；使用 UPDRS 运动部分评估，多巴胺能药物使运动体征改善 50% 以上；≤ 3 年的运动症状波动或异动；UPDRS 日常生活活动部分（第二部分）得分＞ 6 分；轻度至中度的社会和职业功能障碍（Schuepbach 等，2013）。因此，该研究表明，DBS 可以有效地提高疾病早期的生活质量（Schuepbach 等，2013）。值得注意的是，虽然所有的临床试验都表明 DBS 对临床症状由显著疗效，但这些临床试验都没有对主要结果进行双盲评估（Deuschl 等，2006；Schuepbach 等，2013）。

（二）GPi DBS

GPi DBS 同样能够改善运动迟缓、僵直、疼痛和震颤（表 12-3）。GPi DBS 可直接阻断异动。在 GPi 的特定区域，DBS 可能会加重 PD 症状（Bonifati 等，2016）。支持 GPi 作为 DBS 靶点的原因可能是其强大的异动抑制和相对容易程控（Williams 等，2014）。

（三）GPi DBS vs. STN DBS

由于 20 世纪 80—90 年代苍白球毁损术在治疗 PD 方面的成功，GPi 最初被广泛认为是 DBS 最合适的治疗靶点。随后，STN 作为治疗 PD 的靶点开始流行，引发了关于治疗 PD 的最佳靶点的讨论（Williams 等，2014）。这引发了一些由不同手术团队进行的 head-to-head 的比较。在一项临床试验中，与 STN DBS 相比，GPi DBS 减轻了非药物期的帕金森症状（Odekerken 等，2013）。在更大型的临床试验中，GPi DBS 和 STN DBS 在减轻药物"关"期帕金森症状严重程度方面同样有效（Weaver 等，2012）。在这两项试验中，STN DBS 手术后每日多巴胺能药物总量减少，GPi DBS 手术后用药量没有变化（Weaver 等，2012；Odekerken 等，2013）。

2005 年发表的一项小型盲法随机对照试验的结果也表明，STN 和 GPi DBS 对运动症状和异动同样有效（Anderson 等，2005）。然而，STN DBS 似乎与认知、情绪和行为问题更加相关（Anderson 等，2005）。在一项大型临床试验［veterans affairs cooperative studies program（CSP）-468 VA］研究中，255 名患者被随机分组到接受药物治疗或接受 DBS 两组，而接受 DBS 治疗的患者被随机分组到 GPi DBS 和 STN DBS 两组，进行为期 6 个月的比较（Follett 等，

表 12-3 脑深部电刺激治疗帕金森病的随机对照试验结果

实验	靶点	患者数量	随访时间（个月）	手术年龄（岁）	术前药物治疗时间	UPDRS Ⅱ 减少（%）	UPDRS Ⅲ 减少（%）	LED 减少（%）	异动减少（%）	生活质量提高（%）
Anderson 等（2005）	STN	12	12	61	15.6	25.9	48	38	43.5	N/A
	GPi	11	12	54	10.3	18	39	3	89	N/A
Deuschl 等（2006）	STN	156	6	60.5	13	39	40	50	40	22.7
Esselink 等（2004）	STN	20	6	61	12	46.3	48.5	33	56.3	23.2[a]
Follett 等（2010）	STN	147	24	61.9	11.1	15.5	33	31.5	44	8.7
	GPi	152	24	61.8	11.5	17.3	39.3	17.9	72.7	11.6
Okun 等（2012）	STN	136	12	60.6	12.1	N/A	37.5	34.3	50	17.0
Odekerken 等（2016）	STN	63	12	60.9	9.5	32.9	45.7	43.5	20.8	19.4
	GPi	65	12	59.1	18	21.8	26	15.6	16.7	12.3
Schuepbach 等（2013）	STN	124	24	52.9	7.3	41.3	49.3	65.1	71.4	26.4
Weaver 等（2012）	STN	70	36	60.7	11.3	6.2	30.5	35.6	55.4	8.0
	GPi	89	36	60.4	11.4	8.6	34.1	17.8	73	5.6
Williams 等（2010）	STN	174	12	59	11.5	26	35.7	N/A	50	13.3

PD. 帕金森病；STN. 底丘脑核；Gpi. 苍白球内侧部；UPDRS. 统一 PD 评估量表；LED. 等效左旋多巴剂量
a. 使用 PDQL

2010）。在最初随机分组接受药物治疗的 134 名患者中，有 117 名随后进入 DBS 手术，并随机分配给 GPi 或 STN DBS。由于一项中期分析表明，255 名患者的样本量足以进行药物治疗和 DBS 的比较，因此其余 61 名患者被随机分配为直接接受 GPi 或 STN DBS 治疗（共 299 名患者）（Follett 等，2010）。术后 24 个月，在对 DBS 指标进行盲法设计的情况下，患者 GPi DBS 和 STN DBS 术后运动症状改善相近。在规模较小的另一项临床试验（Netherlands subThalamic 和 pallidal stimulation，STAPS）研究中，65 例患者被随机分配到 GPi DBS 组，63 例分配到 STN DBS 组（Odekerken 等，2013）。1 年后的主要结果无统计学显著性差异，主要结果为残疾（按非药物期和药物期加权），以及认知、情绪和行为不良反应。然而，次级结果测量显示，与 GPi 组相比，STN 组在标准化非药物期的 UPDRS Ⅲ 评分和功能障碍有更大的改善。在这两项研究中，GPi DBS 组和 STN DBS 组在不良事件数量上没有差异（Follett 等，2010；Odekerken 等，2013）。STN DBS 组的多巴胺能药物使用比 GPi DBS 组下降更多，STN DBS 组的刺激强度明显低于 GPi DBS 组。在 VA 试验和 NSTAPS 试验中，随访至术后 3 年，总体来说，两项研究对于 2 个靶点的长期结果与之前试验结果相似（Follett 等，2010；Odekerken 等，2013）。

六、不良反应

构音障碍、强直性肌肉收缩、步态不稳、共轭眼球偏转和感觉异常等不良反应可能会影响 DBS 的有效性（Pollo 等，2014）。这些不良反应可能是由于刺激电流累及 STN、GPi 和 VIM 周围相邻结构造成的（Cubo 等，2014；Pollo 等，2014）。可能的不良反应及其相应核团的"解剖"关系见图 12-1。构音障碍和姿势反射障碍可能是疾病进展的结果，但也可能是由于 DBS 所致。需要认识到构音障碍和平衡问题如果是由于逐渐增加 DBS 参数所引起的，就不能单纯地认为疾病发展是罪魁祸首。STN 和 GPi DBS 也可能导致认知、情绪和行为问题（Anderson 等，2005；Okun 等，2009；Castrioto 等，2014）。认知、情绪和行为执行问题可能直接由 DBS 引起，与相邻的边缘和额叶回路的刺激有关。STN DBS 手术后多巴胺能药物的减少较为常见，可能会激发冷漠和抑郁情绪（Lhommee 等，2018）。多巴胺激动药使用的突然减少可能会引发多巴胺撤药综合征（Dopamine agonist withdrawal syndrome，DAWS），如果没有及时发现 DAWS，可能需要 2 年才能解决（Patel 等，2017）。虽然 DBS 可能伴有行为障碍不良反应，但行为障碍也可以作为 DBS 手术改善运动症状之外的另一个适应证（Lhommée 等，2018）。毕竟，与持续的最佳医疗护理相比，STN DBS 患者的情绪和行为障碍在整体水平上改善更多。在更大的随机对照研究中，STN DBS 和 GPi DBS 在术后认知、情绪和行为障碍方面没有差异（Weaver 等，2012；Odekerken 等，2013）。

七、微损毁效应

在 DBS 手术操作中测试电极和最终植入电极可能会导致脑组织的微小损伤，并在这些区域引起短暂的水肿。患者可能由于这些（微）损伤而出现暂时性的不良反应，如面部无力、构音障碍和行为改变（如轻躁狂），但也可能出现 PD 症状减轻或异动加重（Maltête 等，2008；Gago 等，2009；Groiss 等，2009）。水肿相关的症状由特定的 DBS 靶点和周围结构决定。微毁损效应临床症状缓解需要 1~2 天的时间达到峰值，然后逐渐消退，并可能持续 4 周（Maltete 等，2008）。STN 和 GPi DBS 电极放置后短暂性 PD 症状减轻程度是 DBS 疗效的预测因子（Maltete 等，2008）。必须事先告知患者，当微损伤效应逐渐消失时，这并不意味着"DBS 不再有效"。"水肿可能影响较大范围，导致更严重的局灶性神经症状，但会自行消散（Maltete 等，2008）。"

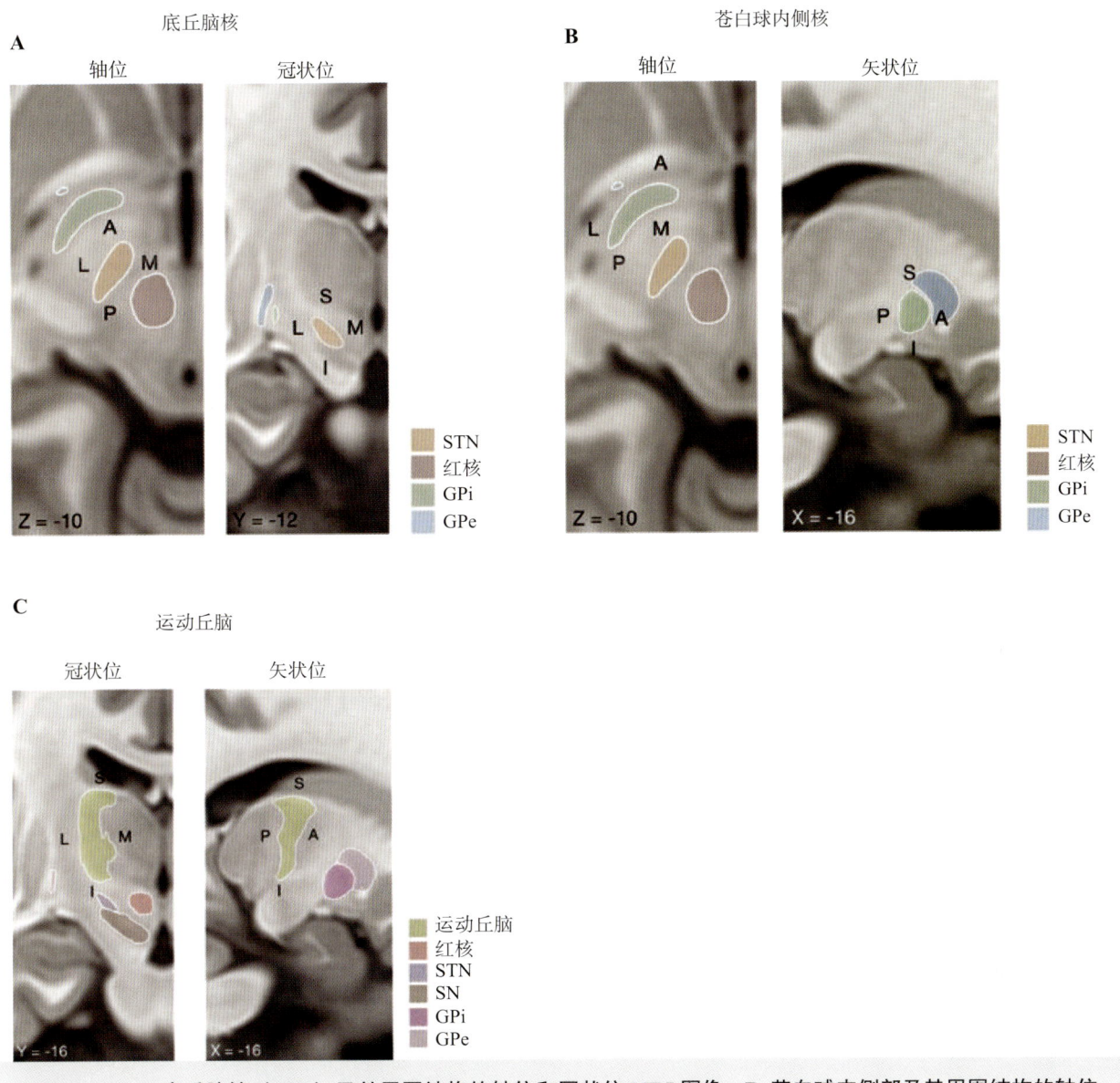

▲ 图 12-1　**A.** 底丘脑核（STN）及其周围结构的轴位和冠状位 **MRI** 图像；**B.** 苍白球内侧部及其周围结构的轴位和矢状位 **MRI** 图像；**C.** 运动丘脑（包括丘脑腹中核）及其周围结构的冠状面和矢状面 **MRI** 图像

STN. 底丘脑核；GPi. 苍白球内侧部；GPe. 苍白球外侧部；SN. 黑质；RN. 红核；A: 前；P: 后；L: 外；M: 内；S: 上；I: 下；图像生成使用 Lead DBS（Horn 和 Kühn，2015），附加 3D 丘脑重建（Ilinsky 等，2018）

八、程控

程控的详细描述在第 8 章中提供。

（一）单极刺激测试

DBS 术中和术后影像学检查可指导在慢性刺激过程中使用的电极触点的选择。尽管如此，对于最终的触点选择，单极刺激测试也是必要的（另见第 8 章）。首先，对每个触点的阻抗进行测量，以测试 DBS 硬件的完整性。在单极测试期间，每个触点的症状（运动迟缓、僵硬和震颤）减轻的阈值和不良反应的阈值均予以测定。实际上，患者需要处于非药物状态才能评估 PD 症状。对每一个触点给予标准参数（例如，60μs 和 130Hz），刺激强度小幅度增加（0.5V 和 0.5mA），进而评估 PD 症状和不良反应（如构音障碍、感觉异常和紧张性收缩）。然后可以选择在PD症状减轻的低阈值与不良反应的高阈值（即具有最大治疗窗口的阈值）之间选择最佳平衡的触点，开始慢性刺激。全面的单极刺激测试非常耗时，可能需要1.5h。由于微损毁效应可能会改善药物"关"期帕金森症状的严重程度，从而掩盖了真正的DBS效应，因此，如果在手术后数周进行单极刺激测试，结果更为准确。

在单极刺激测试中，需要意识到，DBS对症状的缓解所需的时间因患者而异，并且每种症状可能有所不同。例如，刚接通刺激后数秒内强直可能消失，而震颤可能需要数分钟至数小时，运动迟缓需要数分钟至数天（Temperli等，2003；Cooper等，2011，2013）。打开DBS后，异动充分显现可能需要几分钟到几天的时间。类似地，DBS关闭后症状重新出现也可能需要几分钟到几天，对于各种症状也各有不同（Temperli等，2003；Cooper等，2011，2013）。在进行单极刺激测试时必须考虑这些现象。

（二）程控

如果确定了最佳的刺激触点，慢性刺激可以从低到中电压或电流开始，例如1.0或1.5V或mA。然后，每4～6周安排一次定期随访，进行程控和调整PD药物。在少数情况下，以一个触点为负极、以脉冲发生器外壳为正极的方式无法达到令人满意的效果时，必须探索更复杂的程控方式，例如双极刺激或双单极刺激。在第8章中，将更详细地讨论程控。大多数患者在4～6个月后达到稳定（Wagle Shukla等，2017）。PD的典型设置见表12-4。对于STN DBS患者，可能需要将多巴胺能药物减少30%～50%（Weaver等，2012；Odekerken等，2013）。一般来说，GPi DBS对多巴胺能药物每日剂量影响很小。在大多数患者中，程控参数不需要在6个月期间内定期调整。在每次程控随访时记录刺激参数和阻抗。较新的DBS系统有多种选择，可以对不同的刺激参数设置进行编码（如方案A、方案B、方案C），患者可以选择和尝试不同的方案，以评估每个方案的疗效和不良反应。还有一种选择是，根据所使用的系统，为患者设定一个范围，在这个范围内，患者可以降低或增加刺激强度（电压或电流）。

由于疾病异质性，DBS程控有时会非常复杂，并且随着时间的推移会出现多种症状（包括震颤、运动迟缓、异动、情绪、焦虑）、疾病进展、复杂的用药时间表，以及左右电极可能会有不同的DBS效果，并且左右电极的作用可能会相互影响（如左电极或右电极分别打开时没有构音障碍，但如果两个电极都打开，则存在构音障碍）。对患者和医生来说，只见树木不见森林会使程控过程更加困难。在这些情况下，停用PD药物一晚后，使用MDS-UPDRS Ⅲ评估下述4种情况下的症状可能是有帮助的，药物"关"期和DBS"关"期（off-drug with DBS off），药物"关"期和DBS"开"期（off-drug with DBS on），药物"开"期和DBS"关"期（on-drug with DBS off），药物"开"期和DBS"开"期（on-drug with DBS on）。

（三）长期随访

STN和GPi DBS对运动迟缓、强直和震颤的疗效是长期的（Limousin和Foltynie，2019）。但是，非多巴胺能症状不但对DBS治疗反应差，而且会逐渐进展。几年后，患者可能会出现认知障碍、幻觉、构音障碍、姿势反射障碍、冻结和自主神经功能障碍，这些症状目前很难治疗。在此阶段，患者可能看起来不像典型的PD患者，一方面缺乏多巴胺反应性运动症状波动，而另一方面又具有构音障碍和平衡、步态问题（Fasano等，2010；Yamamoto等，2017）。在长期的DBS治疗中，多达15%的患者在随访10年后可能出现硬件相关问题。这些问题是多种多样的，包括硬件感染、导线周围组织破溃、延长导线断裂、twiddler综合征（由于脉冲发生器的扭曲导致引线收紧）、感染，以及在更换电池的手术中意外切断延长导线（Blomstedt和Hariz，2005）。

表 12-4 典型的脑深部电刺激参数

	幅度	频率	脉冲宽度
STN
Deuschl 等（2006）	2.9±0.6V	139±18Hz	63±7.7μs
Esselink 等（2004）	中位数 2.3V（1.4～3.5）	中位数 145Hz（100～130）	中位数 60μs（60～90）
Follett 等（2010）	3.16V	165Hz	75.9μs
Okun 等（2012）	2.3mA	151.1Hz	74μs
Odekerken 等（2016）	2.6±0.6V	135.0±20.8Hz	63.9±9.6μs
Schuepbach 等（2013）	2.8±0.7V	142±27Hz	66±13μs
GPI
Follett 等（2010）	3.95V	168Hz	95.7μs
Odekerken 等（2016）	2.9±0.5V	137.5±20.0Hz	73.0±23.8μs
VIM
Parihar 等（2015）（18 例药物难治性震颤 PD 患者的回顾性分析）	3.3±0.9V	164±27.2Hz	98±41.7μs
Pahwa 等（2006）（8 例双侧 DBSPD 患者的 5 年随访研究中，仅有 20% 的患者接受单极刺激）	4.4V	166Hz	138μs

九、结论

脑深部电刺激是治疗 PD 的有效方法。它可以显著改善顽固性震颤、运动症状波动和异动。成功进行 DBS 治疗的 3 个基本要素包括最佳的患者选择、准确的 DBS 电极植入，以及包括程控和药物调整在内的术后管理。当满足上述条件，运动症状的改善能够与术前最佳多巴胺能药物治疗相媲美，而且疗效更加稳定。

参考文献

[1] Afifi AK. Topical review: basal ganglia: functional anatomy and physiology. Part 2. J Child Neurol. 1994;9(4):352–61.

[2] Akram H, et al. Subthalamic deep brain stimulation sweet spots and hyperdirect cortical connectivity in PD. Neuroimage. 2017;158:332–45.

[3] Albin RL, Young AB, Penney JB. The functional anatomy of basal ganglia disorders. Trends Neurosci. 1989;12(10):366–75.

[4] Alomar S, et al. Speech and language adverse effects after thalamotomy and deep brain stimulation in patients with movement disorders: a meta-analysis. Mov Disord. 2017;32(1):53–63.

[5] Alves G, et al. Progression of motor impairment and disability in Parkinson disease: a population-based study. Neurology. 2005;65(9):1436–41.

[6] Anderson VC, et al. Pallidal vs subthalamic nucleus deep brain stimulation in parkinson disease. Arch Neurol. 2005;62(4):554.

[7] Andrade-Souza YM, et al. Comparison of three methods of targeting the subthalamic nucleus for chronic stimulation in PD. Neurosurgery. 2005;56(2 Suppl):360–8;discussion 360-8.

[8] Antonini A, et al. Developing consensus among movement disorder specialists on clinical indicators for identification and management of advanced PD: a multi-country Delphi-panel approach. Curr Med Res Opin. 2018;34(12):2063–73.

[9] Aquino CC, Fox SH. Clinical spectrum of levodopa-induced complications. Mov Disord. 2015;30(1): 80–9.

[10] Baker KB, et al. Somatotopic organization in the internal segment of the globus pallidus in PD. Exp Neurol. 2010;222(2):219–25.

[11] Barbe MT, et al. DBS of the PSA and the VIM in essential tremor: a randomized, double-blind, crossover trial. Neurology. 2018;91(6):e543–50.

[12] Becerra JE, et al. Economic analysis of deep brain stimulation in Parkinson disease: systematic review of the literature. World Neurosurg. 2016;93:44–9.

[13] Bhidayasiri R, Wolters E. Management of non-motor symptoms in advanced Parkinson disease. J Neurol Sci. 2008;266(1–2):216–28.

[14] Binder DK, Rau GM, Starr PA. Risk factors for hemorrhage during microelectrode-guided deep brain stimulator implantation for movement disorders. Neurosurgery. 2005;56(4):722–32; discussion 722-32.

[15] Blomstedt P, Hariz MI. Hardware-related complications of deep brain stimulation: a ten year experience. Acta Neurochir. 2005;147(10):1061–4.

[16] Blomstedt P, et al. Deep brain stimulation in the caudal zona incerta versus best medical treatment in patients with PD: a randomised blinded evaluation. J Neurol Neurosurg Psychiatry. 2018;89(7):710–6.

[17] Blume J, et al. Intraoperative clinical testing overestimates the therapeutic window of the permanent DBS electrode in the subthalamic nucleus. Acta Neurochir. 2017;159(9):1721–6.
[18] Bonifati V, et al. Movement disorders induced by deep brain stimulation. Parkinsonism Relat Disord. 2016;25:1–9.
[19] Braak H, et al. Staging of brain pathology related to sporadic PD. Neurobiol Aging. 2003;24(2):197–211.
[20] Bronstein JM, et al. Deep brain stimulation for Parkinson disease: an expert consensus and review of key issues. Arch Neurol. 2011;68(2):165.
[21] Calabresi P, et al. Levodopa-induced dyskinesias in patients with PD: filling the bench-to-bedside gap. Lancet Neurol. 2010;9(11):1106–17.
[22] Castrioto A, et al. Mood and behavioural effects of subthalamic stimulation in PD. Lancet Neurol. 2014;13(3):287–305.
[23] Coenen VA, et al. What is dorso-lateral in the subthalamic Nucleus (STN)?—a topographic and anatomical consideration on the ambiguous description of today's primary target for deep brain stimulation (DBS) surgery. Acta Neurochir. 2008;150(11):1163–5.
[24] Cooper SE, et al. Return of bradykinesia after subthalamic stimulation ceases: relationship to electrode location. Exp Neurol. 2011;231(2):207–13.
[25] Cooper SE, et al. Association of deep brain stimulation washout effects with Parkinson disease duration. JAMA Neurol. 2013;70(1):95.
[26] Cubo R, Åström M, Medvedev A. Target coverage and selectivity in field steering brain stimulation. In: 36th Annual International Conference of the IEEE Engineering in Medicine and Biology Society, EMBC 2014, vol. 1; 2014. pp. 522–5.
[27] Deuschl G, et al. A randomized trial of deep-brain stimulation for PD. N Engl J Med. 2006;355(9):896–908.
[28] Deuschl G, et al. Neurostimulation for PD with early motor complications. N Engl J Med. 2013;368(21):2037–8.
[29] Duker AP, Espay AJ. Surgical treatment of Parkinson disease: past, present, and future. Neurol Clin. 2013;31(3):799–808.
[30] Espay AJ. Management of motor complications in Parkinson disease: current and emerging therapies. Neurol Clin. 2010;28(4):913–25.
[31] Espay AJ, Lang AE. Common myths in the use of levodopa in parkinson disease. JAMA Neurol. 2017;74(6):633.
[32] Esselink RAJ, et al. Unilateral pallidotomy versus bilateral subthalamic nucleus stimulation in PD: a randomized trial. Neurology. 2004;62(2):201–7.
[33] Fahn S. The 200-year journey of Parkinson disease: Reflecting on the past and looking towards the future. Parkinsonism Relat Disord. 2018;46:S1–5.
[34] Fahn S, Elton R, program members UPDRS. Unified Parkinsons disease rating scale. In: Recent developments in Parkinsons disease, vol. 2. Florham Park, NJ: Macmillan Healthcare Information; 1987. p. 153–63.
[35] Fasano A, et al. Motor and cognitive outcome in patients with PD 8 years after subthalamic implants. Brain. 2010;133(9):2664–76.
[36] Foley JA, et al. Standardised neuropsychological assessment for the selection of patients undergoing DBS for PD. Parkinsons Dis. 2018;2018:4328371.
[37] Follett KA, et al. Pallidal versus subthalamic deep-brain stimulation for PD. N Engl J Med. 2010;362(22):2077–91.
[38] Foltynie T, et al. MRI-guided STN DBS in PD without microelectrode recording: efficacy and safety. J Neurol Neurosurg Psychiatry. 2011;82(4):358–63.
[39] Fox SH, et al. International Parkinson and movement disorder society evidence-based medicine review: update on treatments for the motor symptoms of PD. Mov Disord. 2018;33(8):1248–66.
[40] Gago MF, et al. Transient disabling dyskinesias: a predictor of good outcome in subthalamic nucleus deep brain stimulation in PD. Eur Neurol. 2009;61(2):94–9.
[41] Goetz CG, et al. Movement Disorder Society—sponsored revision of the Unified PD Rating Scale (MDS-UPDRS): scale presentation and clinimetric testing results. Mov Disord. 2008;23(15):2129–70.
[42] Graybiel AM. Habits, rituals, and the evaluative brain. Annu Rev Neurosci. 2008;31(1):359–87.
[43] Groiss SJ, et al. Deep brain stimulation in PD. Ther Adv Neurol Disord. 2009;2(6):20–8.
[44] Gross RE, et al. Electrophysiological mapping for the implantation of deep brain stimulators for PD and tremor. Mov Disord. 2006;21(S14):S259–83.
[45] Hassani OK, Mouroux M, Féger J. Increased subthalamic neuronal activity after nigral dopaminergic lesion independent of disinhibition via the globus pallidus. Neuroscience. 1996;72(1):105–15.
[46] Hawkes CH, Del Tredici K, Braak H. PD. Ann N Y Acad Sci. 2009;1170(1):615–22.
[47] Haynes WIA, Haber SN. The organization of prefrontal-subthalamic inputs in primates provides an anatomical substrate for both functional specificity and integration: implications for Basal Ganglia models and deep brain stimulation. J Neurosci. 2013;33(11): 4804–14.
[48] Ho AL, et al. Frameless robot-assisted deep brain stimulation surgery: an initial experience. Oper Neurosurg. 2019;17(4):424–31.
[49] Holewijn RA, et al. General anesthesia versus local anesthesia in StereotaXY (GALAXY) for PD: study protocol for a randomized controlled trial. Trials. 2017;18(1):417.
[50] Horn A, Kühn AA. Lead-DBS: a toolbox for deep brain stimulation electrode localizations and visualizations. Neuroimage. 2015;107:127–35.
[51] Houeto J-L, et al. Subthalamic stimulation in Parkinson disease. Arch Neurol. 2003;60(5):690.
[52] Ilinsky I, et al. Human motor thalamus reconstructed in 3D from continuous sagittal sections with identified subcortical afferent territories. eNeuro. 2018;5(3):ENE URO.0060-18.2018.
[53] Jenkinson C, et al. Self-reported functioning and well-being in patients with PD: comparison of the Short-form Health Survey (SF-36) and the PD Questionnaire (PDQ-39). Age Ageing. 1995;24(6):505–9.
[54] Kalia LV, Lang AE. Parkinson Dis. Lancet. 2015;386(9996):896–912.
[55] Krack P, et al. Opposite motor effects of pallidal stimulation in PD. Ann Neurol. 1998;43(2):180–92.
[56] Levy R, et al. High-frequency synchronization of neuronal activity in the subthalamic nucleus of parkinsonian patients with limb tremor. J Neurosci. 2000;20(20):7766–75.
[57] Levy R, et al. Dependence of subthalamic nucleus oscillations on movement and dopamine in PD. Brain. 2002;125(Pt 6):1196–209.
[58] Lhommée E, et al. Behavioural outcomes of subthalamic stimulation and medical therapy versus medical therapy alone for PD with early motor complications (EARLYSTIM trial): secondary analysis of an open-label randomised trial. Lancet Neurol. 2018;17(3):223–31.
[59] Lieberman A, Krishnamurthi N. Is there room for non-dopaminergic treatment in Parkinson disease? J Neural Transm. 2013;120(2):347–8.
[60] Lim S-Y, et al. Dopamine dysregulation syndrome, impulse control disorders and punding after deep brain stimulation surgery for PD. J Clin Neurosci. 2009;16(9):1148–52.
[61] Limousin P, Foltynie T. Long-term outcomes of deep brain stimulation in Parkinson disease. Nat Rev Neurol. 2019;15(4):234–42.
[62] Limousin P, et al. Bilateral subthalamic nucleus stimulation for severe PD. Mov Disord. 1995;10(5):672–4.
[63] Limousin P, et al. Electrical stimulation of the subthalamic nucleus in advanced PD. N Engl J Med. 1998;339(16):1105–11.
[64] Lozano AM. Vim thalamic stimulation for tremor. Arch Med Res. 2000;31(3):266–9.
[65] Maltête D, et al. Microsubthalamotomy: an immediate predictor of long-term subthalamic stimulation efficacy in Parkinson disease. Mov Disord. 2008;23(7):1047–50.
[66] Marjama-Lyons J, Koller W. Tremor-predominant Parkinson's disease. Drugs Aging. 2000;16(4):273–8.
[67] Matteau E, Dupré N, Langlois M, et al. Mattis Dementia Rating Scale 2. Am J Alzheimer's Dis Other Dementiasr. 2011;26(5):389–98.
[68] Mavridis I, Boviatsis E, Anagnostopoulou S. Anatomy of the human subthalamic nucleus: a combined morphometric study. Anat Res Int. 2013;2013:319710.
[69] Morishita T, et al. DBS candidates that fall short on a levodopa challenge test: alternative and important indications. Neurologist. 2011;17(5):263–8.

[70] Müller T. Catechol-O-Methyltransferase inhibitors in PD. Drugs. 2015;75(2):157–74.
[71] Nelson AB, Kreitzer AC. Reassessing models of basal ganglia function and dysfunction. Annu Rev Neurosci. 2014;37:117–35.
[72] Nowacki A, et al. Using MDEFT MRI sequences to target the GPi in DBS surgery. PLoS One. 2015;10(9):e0137868.
[73] Odekerken VJJ, et al. Subthalamic nucleus versus globus pallidus bilateral deep brain stimulation for advanced PD (NSTAPS study): a randomised controlled trial. Lancet Neurol. 2013;12(1):37–44.
[74] Odekerken VJJ, et al. GPi vs STN deep brain stimulation for Parkinson disease: three-year follow-up. Neurology. 2016;86(8):755–61.
[75] Okun MS, et al. Management of referred deep brain stimulation failures: a retrospective analysis from 2 movement disorders centers. Arch Neurol. 2005;62(8):1250–5.
[76] Okun MS, et al. Cognition and mood in PD in subthalamic nucleus versus globus pallidus interna deep brain stimulation: the COMPARE trial. Ann Neurol. 2009;65(5):586–95.
[77] Okun MS, et al. Subthalamic deep brain stimulation with a constant-current device in PD: an openlabel randomised controlled trial. Lancet Neurol. 2012;11(2):140–9.
[78] Pahwa R, et al. Long-term evaluation of deep brain stimulation of the thalamus. J Neurosurg. 2006;104(4):506–12.
[79] Parihar R, et al. Comparison of VIM and STN DBS for Parkinsonian resting and postural/action tremor. In: Tremor and other hyperkinetic movements, vol. 5. New York: Center for Digital Research and Scholarship; 2015. p. 321.
[80] Patel S, et al. Dopamine agonist withdrawal syndrome (DAWS) in a tertiary Parkinson disease treatment center. J Neurol Sci. 2017;379:308–11.
[81] Patil PG, et al. The anatomical and electrophysiological subthalamic nucleus visualized by 3-T magnetic resonance imaging. Neurosurgery. 2012;71(6):1089–95.
[82] Pereira da Silva-Júnior F, et al. Amantadine reduces the duration of levodopa-induced dyskinesia: a randomized, double-blind, placebo-controlled study. Parkinsonism Relat Disord. 2005;11(7):449–52.
[83] Pfeiffer RF. Non-motor symptoms in PD. Parkinsonism Relat Disord. 2016;22:S119–22.
[84] Pollo C, et al. Directional deep brain stimulation: an intraoperative double-blind pilot study. Brain. 2014;137(Pt 7):2015–26.
[85] Pringsheim T, et al. The prevalence of PD: a systematic review and meta-analysis. Mov Disord. 2014;29(13):1583–90.
[86] Rabie A, Verhagen Metman L, Slavin K. Using "Functional" target coordinates of the subthalamic nucleus to assess the indirect and direct methods of the preoperative planning: do the anatomical and functional targets coincide? Brain Sci. 2016;6(4):65.
[87] Rajput AH, et al. Course in Parkinson disease subtypes: a 39-year clinicopathologic study. Neurology. 2009;73(3):206–12.
[88] Redgrave P, et al. Goal-directed and habitual control in the basal ganglia: implications for PD. Nat Rev Neurosci. 2010;11(11):760–72.
[89] Reinacher PC, et al. One pass thalamic and subthalamic stimulation for patients with Tremor-Dominant Idiopathic Parkinson Syndrome (OPINION): protocol for a randomized, active-controlled, double-blinded pilot trial. JMIR Res Protocols. 2018;7(1):e36.
[90] Rietdijk CD, et al. Exploring Braak's hypothesis of PD. Front Neurol. 2017;8:37.
[91] Rodriguez RL, et al. Pearls in patient selection for deep brain stimulation. Neurologist. 2007;13(5):253–60.
[92] Schaltenbrand G, Wahren W. Atlas for stereotaxy of the human brain. Thieme; 1977.
[93] Schapira AHV. Monoamine oxidase B inhibitors for the treatment of Parkinson's disease. CNS Drugs. 2011;25(12):1061–71.
[94] Schapira AH, Ray Chaudhuri K, Jenner P. Non-motor features of Parkinson disease. Nature Publishing Group; 2017, p. 18.
[95] Schuepbach WMM, et al. Neurostimulation for PD with early motor complications. N Engl J Med. 2013;368(7):610–22.
[96] Schuurman PR, et al. A comparison of continuous thalamic stimulation and thalamotomy for suppression of severe tremor. N Engl J Med. 2000;342(7):461–8.
[97] Sensi M, et al. Explosive-aggressive behavior related to bilateral subthalamic stimulation. Parkinsonism Relat Disord. 2004;10(4):247–51.
[98] Sethi K. Levodopa unresponsive symptoms in Parkinson disease. Mov Disord. 2008;23(S3):S521–33.
[99] Singleton AB. Synuclein Locus triplication causes PD. Science. 2003;302(5646):841.
[100] Smeding HMM, et al. Neuropsychological effects of bilateral STN stimulation in Parkinson disease: a controlled study. Neurology. 2006;66(12):1830–6.
[101] Spillantini MG, et al. α-synuclein in Lewy bodies. Nature. 1997;388(6645):839–40.
[102] Spottke EA, et al. Evaluation of healthcare utilization and health status of patients with PD treated with deep brain stimulation of the subthalamic nucleus. J Neurol. 2002;249(6):759–66.
[103] Stowe R, et al. Dopamine agonist therapy in early PD. Cochrane Database Syst Rev. 2008;(2):CD006564.
[104] Taha JM, et al. Characteristics and somatotopic organization of kinesthetic cells in the globus pallidus of patients with PD. J Neurosurg. 1996;85(6):1005–12.
[105] Temperli P, et al. How do parkinsonian signs return after discontinuation of subthalamic DBS? Neurology. 2003;60(1):78–81.
[106] Thenganatt MA, Jankovic J. Parkinson disease subtypes. JAMA Neurol. 2014;71(4):499.
[107] Vassal F, et al. Direct stereotactic targeting of the ventrointermediate nucleus of the thalamus based on anatomic 1.5-T MRI mapping with a white matter attenuated inversion recovery (WAIR) sequence. Brain Stimul. 2012;5(4):625–33.
[108] Verhagen R, Schuurman PR, van den Munckhof P, Contarino MF, de Bie RMA, Bour LJ. Comparative study of microelectrode recording-based STN location and MRI-based STN location in low to ultra-high field (7.0 T) T2-weighted MRI images. J Neural Eng. 2016;13(6):066009.
[109] Vitek JL, et al. Microelectrode-guided pallidotomy: technical approach and its application in medically intractable PD. J Neurosurg. 2009;88(6):1027–43.
[110] Wagle Shukla A, et al. DBS programming: an evolving approach for patients with PD. Parkinsons Dis. 2017;2017:1–11.
[111] Weaver FM, et al. Bilateral deep brain stimulation vs best medical therapy for patients with advanced Parkinson disease: a randomized controlled trial. JAMA. 2009;301(1):63–73.
[112] Weaver FM, et al. Randomized trial of deep brain stimulation for Parkinson disease: thirty-six-month outcomes. Neurology. 2012;79(1):55–65.
[113] Welter ML, et al. Clinical predictive factors of subthalamic stimulation in PD. Brain. 2002;125(3):575–83.
[114] Welter M-L, et al. Optimal target localization for subthalamic stimulation in patients with Parkinson disease. Neurology. 2014;82(15):1352–61.
[115] Williams ZM, et al. Timing and direction selectivity of subthalamic and pallidal neurons in patients with Parkinson disease. Exp Brain Res. 2005;162(4):407–16.
[116] Williams A, et al. Deep brain stimulation plus best medical therapy versus best medical therapy alone for advanced PD (PD SURG trial): a randomised, open-label trial. Lancet Neurol. 2010;9(6):581–91.
[117] Williams NR, Foote KD, Okun MS. STN vs. GPi deep brain stimulation: translating the rematch into clinical practice. Move Dis Clin Pract. 2014;1(1):24–35.
[118] Worth PF. When the going gets tough: how to select patients with PD for advanced therapies. Pract Neurol. 2013;13(3):140–52.
[119] Wu YR, et al. Does stimulation of the GPi control dyskinesia by activating inhibitory axons? Mov Disord. 2001;16(2):208–16.
[120] Yamamoto T, et al. Long term follow-up on quality of life and its relationship to motor and cognitive functions in PD after deep brain stimulation. J Neurol Sci. 2017;379:18–21.
[121] Zaidel A, et al. Levodopa and subthalamic deep brain stimulation responses are not congruent. Mov Disord. 2010;25(14):2379–86.
[122] Zheng Z, et al. Stimulation-induced dyskinesia in the early stage after subthalamic deep brain stimulation. Stereotact Funct Neurosurg. 2010;88(1):29–34.
[123] Zrinzo L, et al. Reducing hemorrhagic complications in functional neurosurgery: a large case series and systematic literature review. J Neurosurg. 2012;116(1):84–94.

第 13 章 震颤
Tremor

Alfonso Fasano　Volker Arnd Coenen　著
王　垚　张　弨　译　朱冠宇　杨岸超　张建国　校

> **摘要**：震颤是一种最常见的运动障碍疾病。尽管药物治疗通常有效或容易控制，但对于药物治疗不敏感的患者，却严重影响其生活质量，甚至使其致残。在这种情况下，可以考虑手术治疗，因为手术治疗震颤通常是非常有效的。目前，有 4 种外科治疗方法可供选择，包括脑深部电刺激、丘脑射频毁损术、放射外科和共聚焦超声。震颤的外科治疗需要考虑专科医师擅长手术方式的选择、患者的选择、术后的处理，以及处理不可预见的不良反应。就目前而言，因为具有良好的疗效和安全性，DBS 仍然是最有效的治疗方案。

一、概述

震颤是一种最常见的运动障碍疾病，它属于一种运动亢奋症状，被定义为"身体某部位的不自主、有节奏、振荡似的运动"（Deuschl 等，1998；Bhatia 等，2018）。国际帕金森与运动障碍病学会震颤小组最近回顾了震颤的分类方法，并借鉴肌张力障碍的分类方法，将震颤用两维度法进行分类，维度 1 指的是一种特定的临床表现（表 13-1），并且可以分为孤立性震颤（震颤是唯一的异常症状）和合并性震颤（存在其他异常的神经或系统症状）。将维度 1 扩展开来，维度 2 进一步定义了维度 1 所描述的病因学条件，获得性、遗传性或特发性（家族性或散发）（Bhatia 等，2018）。大多数震颤仅根据维度 1 的内容就足以确定是否可以行手术治疗；表 13-2 列出了诊断震颤的主要临床表现。

排在"增强性生理性震颤"之后，原发性震颤（ET）是第二常见的震颤综合征（维度 1）（Espay 等，2017；Fasano 等，2018b）。历史上，它被认为是成人中最常见的运动障碍病，患病率为 0.5%～5%（Louis 和 Ferreira，2010），尽管现在人们知道 ET 是一种极其具有异质性的疾病，其可能是由多种不明因素引起的综合征（Fasano 等，2018b）。尽管 ET 十分复杂，但其对药物和外科治疗的反应是可预测的。很多治疗手段在远期观察来看，存在较大的变异性，这可能是由上述提到疾病的异质性引起的。

二、脑深部电刺激治疗原发性震颤的预后

自 1991 年首次报道 6 例 ET 患者病情得到持续改善以来，DBS 已成为治疗严重的、药物难治性 ET 最常见的手术方式（Benabid 等，1991）。DBS 治疗 ET 在 1993 由 EC 批准，在 1997 年由美国食品药品管理局（FDA）批准（见第 1 章）。

表 13-1　可用于震颤分类的病史、临床表现和实验室检查结果（Bhatia 等，2018）

病史特点	起病年龄 • 婴儿：出生至 2 岁 • 儿童：3—12 岁 • 青少年：13—20 岁 • 青年：21—45 岁 • 中年：46—60 岁 • 老年：>60 岁 短暂的发作和演变 既往病史 家族史 • 有 / 没有 / 不详 酒精或药物过敏史 • 有 / 没有 / 不详
震颤的临床表现	肢体累及分布 • 局灶性（只有 1 个部位受累） • 节段性（上半身或下半身的 2 个或多个相邻身体部位受累） • 偏侧震颤（半侧躯体受累） • 全身性（上半身和下半身均受累） • 直立性震颤（站立时下肢或躯干受累） 发作的激活条件 • 休息时 • 活动时 　– 动力性（简单活动、意向运动、特定任务） 　– 姿势性（位置依赖、位置独立） 　– 等长收缩性震颤 震颤频率 • ＜4Hz • 4～8Hz • 8～12Hz • ＞12Hz
并发症	• 全身性疾病表现 • 神经系统疾病表现 • 轻度症状（例如，双足步态受损，轻度 / 可疑的张力障碍）
实验室检查	• 电生理检查（针刺或表面肌电图、手负重和不负重时的肌电图记录和肌肉加速度的傅里叶分析、多个肢体肌电图的傅里叶和相干分析） • 结构像检查（MRI 或者 CT） • 受体显像（多巴胺和 5- 羟色胺转运体显像紊乱或缺乏综合征） • 血清和组织生物标志物

EMG. 肌电图检查；MRI. 磁共振成像；CT. 计算机断层扫描术

（一）丘脑腹侧中间核

丘脑腹侧中间核［ventral intermediate（Vim）nucleus］是 DBS 治疗 ET 的经典靶点（图 13-1）。一些研究表明，单侧 Vim-DBS 可在短期内显著减少震颤。在单侧 Vim-DBS 下，整体震颤减少率在 53.4%～62.8%（图 13-2）。单侧 DBS 可显著改善上肢和任务时的动作性震颤，震颤评分

表 13-2　主要震颤综合征的诊断标准

原发性震颤	• 以双侧上肢活动性震颤为表现的孤立性震颤综合征至少 3 年，其他部位（如头部、发声或下肢）有或无震颤，无其他神经症状，如肌张力障碍、共济失调或帕金森病
原发性震颤加	• 具有 ET 特征的震颤同时合并其他不确定的神经症状，如串联步态受损、可疑的张力障碍性姿势、记忆障碍或其他轻微的神经症状；合并静止性震颤的 ET 也属于此类
孤立节段性姿势或运动性震颤综合征	• 孤立性局灶性震颤（发声、头部），增强性生理震颤
孤立静息性震颤综合征	• 震颤通常发生在上肢、下肢或偏侧肢体，也可能发生在其他地方（如嘴唇、下巴或舌头）
孤立局灶性震颤	• 孤立性发声震颤是指发声器官的可见和（或）可听见的震颤。孤立性头部震颤是指头部在点头、摇头或其他可变方向上的摇晃。腭震颤的特征是软腭以 0.5～5Hz 有节奏的运动。孤立的任务和特定位置的震颤发生在做特定的任务或姿势的时候（如果与其他神经症状相关，它可能是原发性或症状性的）。其他包括遗传性颏震颤、孤立性下颌震颤、孤立性舌震颤、兔唇综合征和微笑时震颤
直立性震颤	• 原发性直立性震颤是一种发生在站立时的全身性高频（13～18Hz）孤立性震颤综合征。通常使用肌电图和加速计来确认震颤频率。假性直立性震颤的特征是站立时震颤的频率 < 13Hz（也被称为缓慢直立性震颤、直立时震颤、站立时震颤等）
肌张力障碍性震颤综合征	• 此震颤综合征以震颤和肌张力障碍同时存在为主要的神经症状。受肌张力障碍影响的身体部位出现的震颤被称为肌张力障碍性震颤。如果肌张力障碍和震颤出现在不同的身体部位，这称为与肌张力障碍相关的震颤
震颤合并帕金森病	• 典型的帕金森病震颤是一种 4～7Hz 的手、下肢、下颌、舌头或脚的静止性震颤，患者同时患有帕金森病（运动迟缓和强直）。其他类型的震颤可能在帕金森病患者中共存，如姿势性或运动性震颤，其频率与静息性震颤相同或更高
意向性震颤	• 运动性震颤，频率 < 5Hz，有或无其他局灶性症状，通常由小脑丘脑通路的病变引起
Holmes 震颤	• 通常由近端和远端的肌肉低频（< 5Hz）有节律的收缩引起的一种静息、姿势和意向性震颤的综合征
肌节律	• 一种罕见的 1～4Hz 频率的震颤，通常累及头部及四肢的肌肉，在静息和活动时均可见。其通常与局灶性的脑干症状有关
功能性震颤（又名心因性震颤）	• 震颤不是由器质性神经系统疾病引起的，其特征是易分心、频率捕捉现象或对抗性肌肉协同活动 • 原发性腭震颤在大多数情况下是功能性的
不确定震颤综合征	• 不符合上述所定义的任何一类综合征，需要进一步观察的一类综合征

EMG. 肌电图检查

修改自 Bhatia 等，2018

的下降幅度为 38.2%～78.9%（Graff-Radford 等，2010；Huss 等，2015）。在长达 5 年的长期随访中，数据显示单侧 Vim-DBS 患者上肢活动性震颤缓解良好（评分降幅为 60.3%～75%）（Pahwa 等，2006；Blomstedt 等，2007）。Vim-DBS 还能改善 ET 患者的日常生活。单侧 DBS 患者中，第 1 年 ADL 改善率为 57.9%～82%，5 年后改善率为 32.3%～51%（Lyons 等，1998；Obwegeser 等，2000；Pahwa 等，2006；Blomstedt 等，2007；Nazzaro 等，2012）。

现有的关于 DBS 长期疗效的研究较少，总体上都证实大多数受试者的震颤可以得到持续改善，失去最初疗效的患者比例较小（所谓的"脱落者"，见后述）（Rehncrona 等，2002；

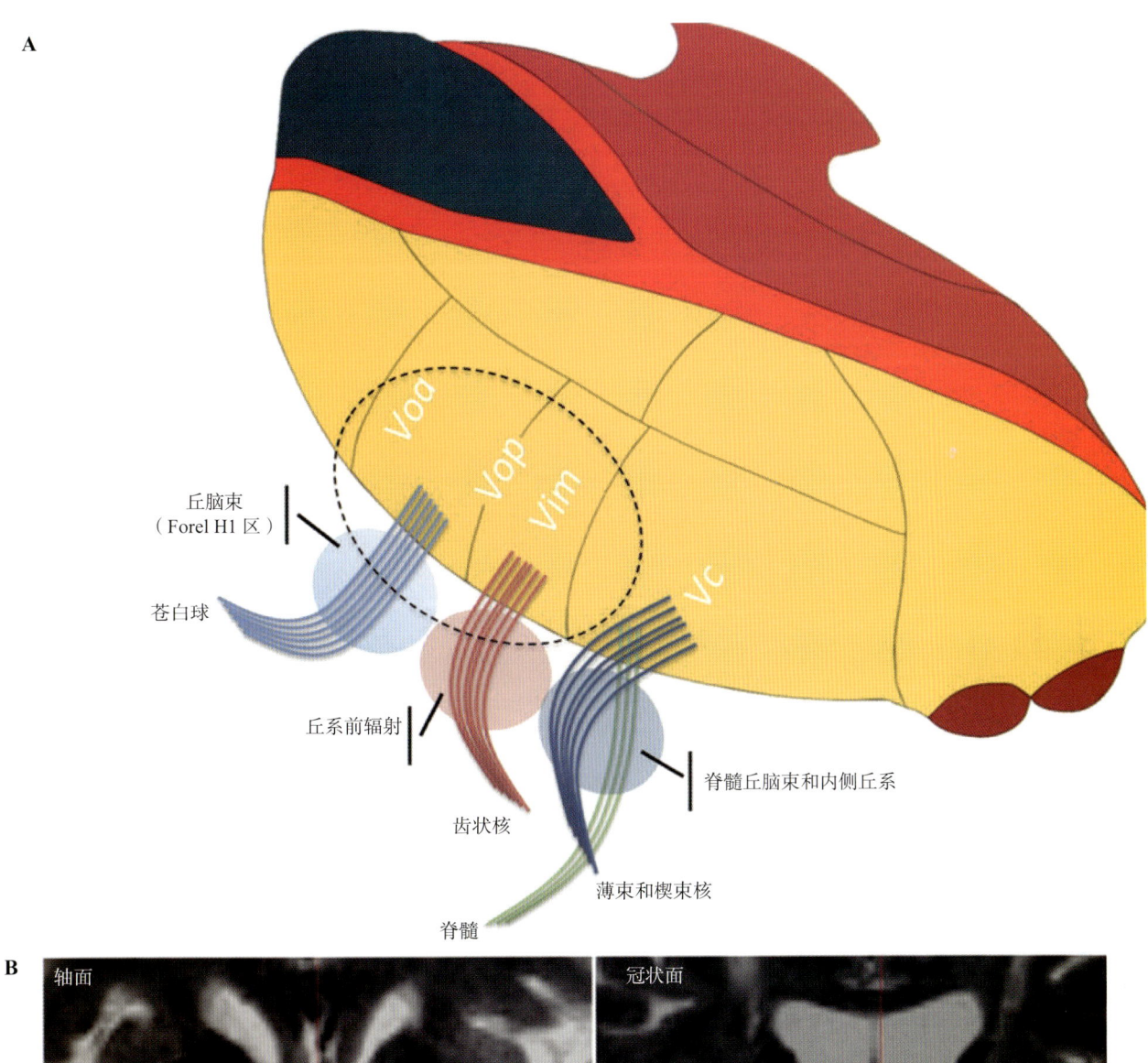

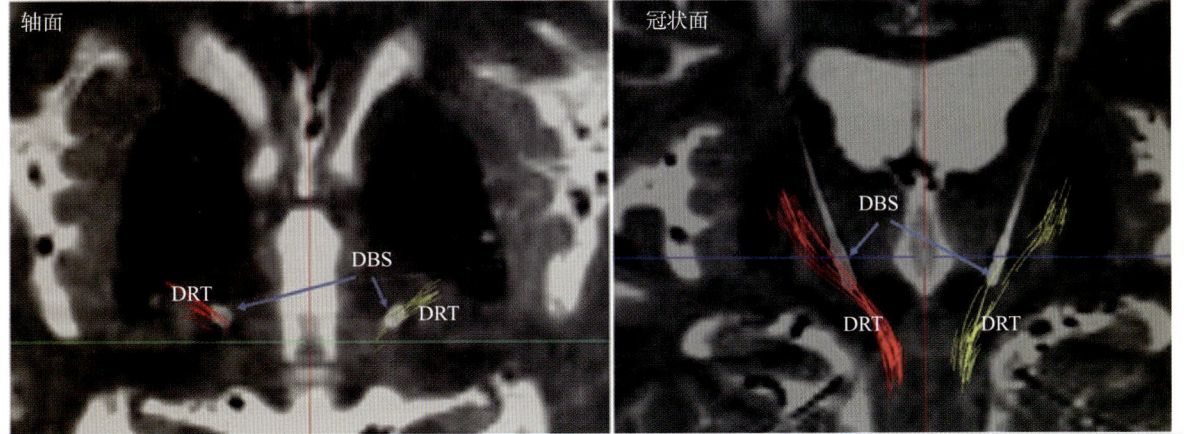

▲ 图 13-1　**A**. 震颤手术的外科解剖。运动丘脑接受来自小脑和苍白球的传入纤维。虚线椭圆显示震颤综合征的主要靶点。丘脑腹侧中间核（Vim）作为可选择的靶点是因为它通过齿状红核丘脑束（**DRT**，又称小脑丘脑束）从小脑齿状核接收无意识本体感觉信息。近年来，由于丘脑下的白质是许多轴突汇入丘脑核团之前汇聚的解剖瓶颈，使得人们对它产生了极大的兴趣。这些区域包括丘脑束和丘系前辐射（Raprl），这些都属于未定带的一部分，这一区域被定义为丘脑后区（**PSA**），在解剖学上与 **DRT** 的远端投射汇合；**B**. 原发性震颤的纤维束定位图。左图为轴面图，显示与术后 **MRI-CT** 融合的解剖结构（白色圆点为 **DBS** 电极伪影）。小脑丘脑束（又称齿状红核丘脑束）的投射图，分别用红色和黄色纤维束表示。右图为冠状面，显示在一个复杂的近端和躯干震颤的病例中，**DBS** 电极进入丘脑底区域的深度

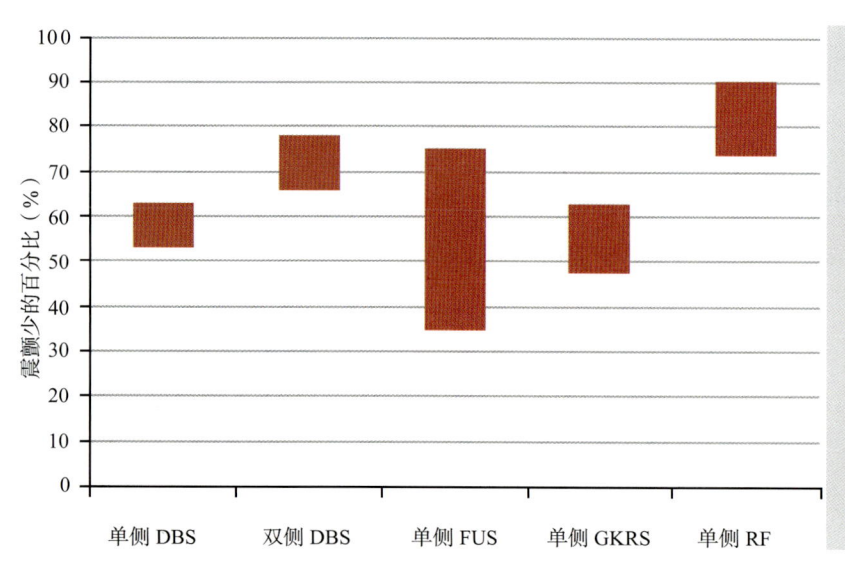

图 13-2 不同神经外科手术方式对原发性震颤的疗效

DBS 数据来源于 53 个病例研究（40 个 Vim-DBS 的病例研究，13 个 PSA/cZI-DBS 的研究），其中包括 1093 例患者（913 例 Vim-DBS，180 例 PSA/cZI-DBS）。大多数手术是单侧进行的（637 例 Vim，121 例 PSA/cZI），双侧 DBS 包括 276 例 Vim，59 例 PSA/cZI）。双侧手术大多是在一次手术中完成。其他的手术方式由于是有创的，故只行单侧手术（经许可转载，引自 Dallapiazza 等，2018）
DBS. 脑深部电刺激；FUS. 共聚焦超声丘脑切除术；GKRS. 伽马刀放射丘脑切除术；RF. 射频丘脑切除术

Baizabal-Carvallo 等，2013）。在术后 6 年，尽管仍然有显著的改善，但是改善率下降到平均 50%，（表 13-3）。一项最新的研究报告了 ET 患者术后长达 18 年的有效随访结果，平均改善率从术后 1 年时的 66% 下降到最晚随访时的 48%，尽管在亚组分析中，这种改善率的下降并不显著（Cury 等，2017）。

DBS 是唯一可以安全地进行双侧操作的手术。它实际上最开始是用来治疗做过丘脑切除术的震颤患者（Benabid 等 1987）。双侧 Vim-DBS 是安全的，并且由于两侧都接受了治疗，因此可以使得整体震颤减轻达到最大化，这对患有头部震颤的患者来说是特别有意义的。双侧 Vim-DBS 使整体震颤减少 66%~78%（图 13-2）（Pahwa 等，2006；Pilitsis 等，2008；GraffRadford 等，2010；Nazzaro 等，2012；Huss 等，2015；Cury 等，2017）。此外，双侧 Vim-DBS 对轴性震颤、头颈部震颤和发声震颤有较好的改善作用（Obwegeser 等，2000；Sydow，2003；Mandat 等，2011）。据报道，DBS 植入 5 年后，头部震颤改善率高达 75%，发声震颤改善率达 60%（Sydow，2003）。有趣的是，尽管双侧丘脑 DBS 可以使震颤总体减轻，但一些研究表明，与单侧治疗相比，在致残或生活质量方面几乎没有差别（Huss 等，2015）。

有趣的是，Vim-DBS 似乎也影响潜在的小脑功能障碍（表 13-4）。虽然过度刺激诱发共济失调，但低振幅电刺激也能改善震颤和小脑受累引起的轻度亚临床症状（Herzog 等，2007；Fasano 等，2010，2012b）。

（二）其他靶点

小脑丘脑束（CTT）- 在文献中常被称为齿状红核丘脑束（DRT），在震颤回路中被认为是重要的结构（Coenen 等，2011，2014），所以丘脑后区（PSA）/ 不定带尾侧（cZI）成了 ET 患者电刺激的靶点（图 13-1）。虽然关于 PSA/cZI 电刺激的病例报道的数量较少，但它仍被认为是一个有效并且高效率的靶点，因为它对 DBS 系统的能耗需求较低（Barbe 等，2011）。也有人认为其对 ET 患者的轻度共济失调（Herzog 等，2007）及近端肢体的症状（Murata 等，2003）有更好的疗效。

系列病例报道显示，在第 1 年内，单侧 PSA/cZI-DBS 使震颤整体减少了 62%~95%（Blomstedt 等，2010，2011）。而双侧电刺激可以使震颤减轻了 75.9%~80.1%（Plaha 等，2004；Plaha 等，2008）。在植入后的 5 年内，单侧 DBS 的改善率（52.4%~81%）和双侧 DBS 的改善率（73.8%）相差无几（Plaha 等，2011）。术后 1 年左右，单侧和双侧 PSA/cZI-DBS 对于上肢震颤

第13章 震颤 Tremor

表13-3 DBS治疗ET的临床疗效及安全性

文 献	例数[a]	随访时间（年）	疗效（改善的百分比%）	脱落者（例数）	不良反应
Koller 等（2001）	25	3.3	50.0% vs. 基线 45.5% vs. "关"	最初队列中49例患者中有5例：3个月后（2例者）、6个月后（1名患者）、12个月后（2例患者）和24个月后（1例患者在DBS术后3个月已重新植入）	1例患者效果不理想，另1例患者电极移位（导致无效）
Rehncrona 等（2002）	13（1）	6.5±0.3	47.1% vs. 基线[b] 47.1% vs. "关"[b]	0	无
Sydow（2003）[d]	19（7）	6.5±0.6	56.6% vs. 基线[e] 45.9% vs. "关"[e]	0（使震颤加重）	38例患者中有40个不良反应报告。构音障碍在双侧电刺激中更常见
Putzke 等（2004）	13（NA）	3	88.4% vs. 基线 86.2% vs. "关"	75个触点（原始队列中的52名患者）中，8个触点因"无效"而需要重新定位	双侧丘脑刺激更易出现构音障碍、平衡困难、吞咽困难和流涎
Pahwa 等（2006）	26（8）	5	49.6% vs. 基线[f] 50.7% vs. "关"[f]	2	6例导线断裂
Blomstedt 等（2007）	19（0）	7.2±0.75	44.1% vs. 基线[b] 44.4% vs. "关"[b]	2例因更改诊断（肌张力障碍和小脑震颤）而被排除在初始队列之外	ET患者随机分为DBS组和ET随机分为丘脑切除组者：1/6有轻度步态共济失调；ET患者随机分为丘脑切除组者：1/4有认知障碍，1/4存在构音障碍
Schuurman 等（2008）	6	5	6个月时震颤得到抑制，3例患者出现轻、中度震颤复发	0/6 ET患者，0/19 PD患者和3/5 MS患者纳入同一系列	总人数的23.5%出现了硬件问题
Zhang 等（2010）	12（不详）	7.6	67.7%[c]	在最初的队列中，有2例患者由于不良反应而停止使用DBS	
Fytagoridis 等（2012）	18（2）	4.0±0.8	52.4% vs. 基线 51.4% vs. "关"	0（靶点为cZi）	
Nazzaro 等（2012）	22	7~12	31.2% vs. 基线	2/42例患者（DBS后2~7年）和3/22例患者（DBS后7~12年）因DBS无效而调整电极位置	不详
Shih 等（2013）	45（21）	4.7±2.9	不详	33例（3例因诊断改正为小脑共济失调而被排除在初始队列之外）	
Baizabal-Carvallo 等（2013）	13（7）	11.0±1.3	44.1% vs. "关"（开放阶段）[b] 44.4% vs. "关"（双盲阶段）[b]	1	23%出现硬件相关并发症。双侧刺激更易出现构音障碍和共济失调

(续表)

文 献	例数[a]	随访时间（年）	疗效（改善的百分比 %）	脱落者（例数）	不良反应
Borretzen 等（2014）[g]	36	6.0	VAS: 8.5%（DBS 后），7.4%（最近一次随访）	不详	构音障碍（65%）、共济失调（35%）、头痛（35%）、感觉异常（23%）、味觉异常（31%）
Rodriguez Cruz 等（2016）	14（11）	7.7±3.8	50.1% vs. 基线	2 例因电极位置错误而导致早期无效，从而被排除在初始队列之外	
Cury 等（2017）	12	13.2±2.8	33.5% vs. 基线 48% vs. "关"	0	感觉异常（17%）[h]、构音障碍（17%）、步态不稳和共济失调（10%）、丘脑出血（3.9%）
Eisinger 等（2018）	47（6）	4	Vim: 68%～92% vs. 基线[b] cZi: 33%～76% vs. 基线[b]	0	
Sandoe 等（2018）	31（3）	3.3±2.7	44.2% vs. 基线[b]	10 例（2 例早期脱落）	9.6% 有一个或多个手术相关并发症
Paschen 等（2019）	20（20）	5.9±0.6	22.0% vs.DBS 术后 1 年[f] 42.6% vs. "关"[f]	0	

cZi. 不定带尾侧；DBS. 脑深部电刺激；ET. 原发性震颤；MS. 多发性硬化；VAS. 视觉模拟量表

a. 括号内为双侧电刺激例数；b. 该部分研究在刺激对侧对震颤评分中的 A 和分项 B 进行了测试；c. 该部分研究对侧震颤评分中的 A 部分和 B 部分进行了选择，而后进行了测试；d.（Limousin 等 1999）的随访；e. 该部分研究仅进行了震颤评分 A 部分的测试；f. 该部分研究进行了全部震颤评分的测试；g. 基于 26 名患者的问卷式的不良反应调查（也包括患有其他震颤疾病的患者）；h. 包括整个队列（也包括患有其他震颤疾病的患者）的随访时间

表 13-4 丘脑 DBS 对 ET 患者小脑受累亚临床征象的影响

功 能	小脑通路	效 果	参考文献
眨眼条件反射	内侧	+	Kronenbuerger 等（2008）
嗅觉	?	-	Kronenbuerger 等（2010）
适应性运动控制（抓取）	外侧	-	Chen 等（2005）
上肢共济失调（激动-拮抗偶联）	外侧	=	Zackowski 等（2002）
上肢共济失调（辨距障碍）	外侧	+	Herzog 等（2007）
下肢共济失调	外侧	+	Fasano 等（2010，2012b）
步态	内+外侧	+	Fasano 等（2010，2012b）
平衡	内侧	-/+	Ondo 等（2006）

-.变差；+.改善；-/+.可变的；=.无变化；?.未知；DBS.脑深部电刺激；ET.原发性震颤

（单侧：87%~89% 改善，双侧：68% 改善）和 ADL（单侧：66.1%~66% 改善，双侧：68% 改善）的改善效果类似（Plaha 等，2004；Blomstedt 等，2010，2011）。

其他有报道的靶点包括丘脑腹侧核的前部、后部（Voa、Vop）和底丘脑核（STN）（Kobayashi 等，2003；Meng 等，2013）。这些核团治疗震颤的总体疗效和安全性都很好。但是由于发表文章的数量较少，可能会带来一定的偏倚。这些核团对于治疗例如小脑震颤等疾病可能存在一些困难（见后述）。

（三）DBS 的个体化成像：弥散张量成像（DTI）纤维束成像辅助靶点定位

个体解剖变异的存在使得行 DBS 或者毁损术时，术前定位从单纯地依靠连合中间点（MCP）转变为利用磁共振成像（MRI）直接定位靶点。STN 的靶点定位通常依靠 T_2 加权像。最新的进展是引入了 DTI 纤维追踪辅助 DBS 定位（Coenen 等，2011，2012）。震颤症状的术中快速变化可以很容易地用于评估进一步的手术计划，以确定"使震颤减少的最佳解剖位置"。可能许多震颤症状的基础是 CTT，因为它连接了 3 个经典的震颤靶点（Vim、PSA 和 cZi）（Coenen 等，2014）。现在有许多研究使用这项技术来识别和定位个体震颤解剖，以及改善手术效果（Sammartino 等，2016；Fenoy 和 Schiess，2017）。目前正在研究全身麻醉下使用单独一个靶点治疗震颤（Sajonz 等，2016）和利用纤维追踪技术联合刺激 DRT 和 STN 治疗帕金森病震颤的方法（Coenen 等，2017；Reinacher 等，2018）。

（四）自适应 DBS

目前，DBS 的治疗是一个开环控制系统，在这个系统中，持续的刺激作用于大脑的某一个靶区（见第 5 章）。自适应 DBS（aDBS）是一个由相关生物标记物（如脑内局部场电位活动或惯性震颤数据）反馈的闭环系统。这种方法目前已进入临床阶段，特别是对帕金森病患者（Fasano 等，2017b）。2010 年，当震颤部位的肌电活动被发现能有效地成为闭合刺激回路的反馈指标时，aDBS 对 ET 的作用就被认为是有效的（Graupe 等，2010）。这一方法在帕金森合并震颤患者中验证有效（Malekmohammadi 等，2016）。理论上，aDBS 有许多优点，特别是较低的电池消耗，更好的安全性（Reich 等，2016）并且可能对震颤有更高的疗效等。据推测，只有当刺激发生在震颤的某一特定阶段（Cagnan 等，2017）时，才能更好地抑制震颤。

(五)并发症

丘脑 DBS 并非没有潜在的并发症(表13-5)。电极置入可导致严重的脑出血,发生率占 0.5%~1.5%。此外,还存在伤口感染(1.7%~5.4%)和硬件相关并发症的风险,如电极断裂或移位(1.4%~3.8%)(Fenoy 和 Simpson,2014)。DBS 手术的其他不良反应可能与手术时的置入效应有关,也可能与设备打开后的刺激有关。通常情况下,置入的不良反应在手术后几周内消退;然而,当设备打开时,与刺激相关的不良反应可以持续存在。当电刺激引起神经系统不良反应时,可以对参数进行调整,保持对震颤效果的同时尽量减少对神经系统的影响。

丘脑 DBS 最常见的神经不良反应是刺激性构音障碍和共济失调。多项研究表明,与单侧 DBS 相比,这些不良反应更常见于双侧 DBS。据报道,11%~38.5% 的单侧 DBS 患者存在构音障碍(Barbe 等,2014;Alomar 等,2017),而双侧 DBS 患者的发生率为 22%~75%(Pahwa 等,2006;Baizabal-Carvallo 等,2013;Matsumoto 等,2016)。发声过弱也常见于 DBS 的患者中,其中双侧 DBS 出现的概率更大(单侧 5%,双侧 18.8%)(Alomar 等,2017)。双侧丘脑 DBS 的共济失调发生率(56%~85.7%)也高于单侧(9.1%~16.7%)(Peng-Chen 等,2013;Alomar 等,2017)。其他不常见的潜在不良反应包括短暂性偏瘫(单侧:4.5%,双侧:6.7%)和感觉异常(单侧:4.5%~45%,双侧:5.9%)(Zhang 等,2010;PengChen 等,2013)。也有报告称患者语言流利性下降,但工作记忆和认知抑制却没有下降(Pedrosa 等,2014)。PSA/cZI-DBS 的潜在不良反应与 Vim-DBS 相似,尽管一些研究者认为 PSA/cZI-DBS 可能比 Vim-DBS 更安全(Plaha 等,2004)。PSA/cZI 的安全性可能依赖于能量传递较少,因为该区域的轴突对刺激非常敏感,因此在底丘脑靶区需要较少的电流刺激即可达到目的。

三、"脱落者":耐受还是进展

有证据表明,随着时间的推移,震颤的抑制效果会逐渐减弱。虽然 Vim-DBS 在短期内可以很好地缓解震颤和改善生活质量,但随着时间的推移,其效益逐渐下降(表 13-3)。在这种情况下,DBS 装置可以重新程控以进一步控制震颤,尽管结果并不总是令人满意,特别是当刺激引起的不良反应限制了增加刺激强度的可能性时(Picillo 等,2016;Sandoe 等,2018)。尽管震颤可能逐渐进展,Vim-DBS 在长期看仍有利于大多数患者,这一点可以通过比较 DBS 开和关的效果来得到证明(Favilla 等,2012)。

然而,在 0%~73% 的患者中(Shih 等,2013),人们不再感觉 DBS 可以发挥任何作用,这就提出了一个问题,即这些"脱落者"出现的原因是否是由于疾病进展而不是刺激丧失了作用(即耐受性)。

Benabid 等首先提出了耐受的概念,因为他们观察到随着时间的推移,丘脑电刺激在 ET 中不如 PD 引起的震颤有效(Benabid 等,1994)。

表 13-5 ET 患者不同丘脑手术常见的暂时性和永久性并发症出现概率

	单侧 DBS	双侧 DBS	MRI 引导的超声共聚焦	伽马刀放射手术	射频手术
构音障碍	11%~39%	22%~75%	0%	1%~3%	4.6%~29%
共济失调	9%~17%	56%~85%	23%	0%~17%	5%~27%
感觉异常	5%~45%	5.9%	14%~25%	1%~9%	6%~42%
偏瘫	4.5%	6.7%	2%~7%	0%~8%	0%~34%

DBS. 脑深部电刺激;MRI. 磁共振成像
经许可转载,引自 Dallapiazza 等,2018

虽然长期 Vim 刺激无效的原因尚不清楚，但 DBS 对 ET 患者逐渐丧失作用现在已被经常报道。它可能因为疾病的自然进展及其他外科因素（如电极位置和距 CTT 的距离）（Pilitsis 等，2008；Louis 等，2011；Favilla 等，2012；Sandoe 等，2018）。至于疾病进展，ET 是一种异质性疾病，通常提示着一种进行性小脑疾病（Fasano 等，2018b）；有时 DBS 疗效不佳或无效迫使临床医生进一步研究震颤病因（Fasano 等，2017a）。帕金森病震颤的良好长期预后也很好地说明了 ET 的疾病是进展的（Benabid 等，1994；Hariz 等，2008），因为帕金森病震颤是一种随着疾病进展而稳定或改善的症状。不幸的是，没有一项比较 ET 患者 DBS 术后和非 DBS 的随机长期研究可提供这方面的解释。

最后，关于耐受性的假设，是早期关于 ET 药物治疗的文献中提出的，目前尚未在 DBS 患者中证实（Calzetti 等，1990；Hariz 等，1999）。一些作者提出了在夜间关机以避免耐受性出现的方法，同样的，这种方法也从未被证明是有效的。

最近，长期电刺激可能导致可逆性共济失调的假设产生了一个观点，即震颤会随着时间推移而加重意味着其是可逆性小脑震颤（Reich 等，2016）。虽然这一假设很有趣，但它的可能性较小，因为即使在 DBS 诱发的共济失调消退后，刺激关闭后几天，仍观察到震颤复发。此外，一些研究发现射频丘脑切除术后震颤也会复发。例如，Akbostanci 等报告了 5 例因震颤复发而再次手术治疗，得到了满意的效果（Akbostanci 等，1999）。MRI 引导下的超声共聚焦术后的复发病例提示，早期的复发可能是由于毁损灶过小（Fasano 等，2018a），而晚期的复发，可能是由于疾病进展所致。

四、其他非 ET 的震颤的综合征

（一）帕金森病

自 1987 年首次报道单侧丘脑切除术治疗帕金森病（PD）相关震颤以来，帕金森病（PD）相关震颤成了 DBS 手术的第一个适应证（Benabid 等，1987；Benabid 等，1991）。许多随访时间较短和少量样本的长期随访的（长达 5～6 年）研究评估了 Vim-DBS 在治疗 PD 震颤的效果，相关研究都是小样本的研究（8～38 人），报道的 PD 平均改善率为 54%～85%（Rehncrona 等，2002；Hariz 等，2008）。最近，这一结果在一个随访了 10 年以上的队列研究中被证实（Cury 等，2017）。总的来说，帕金森病相关震颤的长期治疗效果要比 ET 好，这可能是由于帕金森病进展会使震颤自然改善所致（Sandoe 等，2018）。

STN 和苍白球内侧部（GPi）也是可以改善 PD 的其他基本症状的有效靶点，因此在有致残性震颤的 PD 患者中应作为首选，而 Vim-DBS（和丘脑切除术）仍然可作为无法行 STN 或 GPi-DBS 的 PD 患者的有效选择，例如老年患者（70—75 岁以上）或有明显认知障碍或精神共病的患者（尤其不适合选择 STN）（图 13-3）（Fasano 等，2012a）。

（二）肌张力障碍性震颤

对于肌张力障碍患者，没有已发表的前瞻性试验将震颤作为主要观察指标。数据量较少，Fasano 等在 2014 年将其做了归纳。总的来说，GPi-DBS 在改善张力障碍姿势和相关震颤方面是有效的，而丘脑 DBS 只能改善震颤。丘脑（也可单侧）可作为非肌张力障碍患者（如斜颈）和（或）肌张力障碍背景下严重运动性震颤患者的选择靶点（图 13-4）。据报道，有少数患者在丘脑手术（丘脑切除术或 DBS）后出现肌张力障碍症状加重，可能类似于丘脑梗死后出现的肌张力障碍性手部疼痛（所谓的"丘脑手"）的临床情况（个人观察）。

（三）其他罕见的震颤

表 13-6 列出了 DBS 术的所有适应证和靶点。除了少数报道外（Oliveria 等，2017），这些研究绝大多数都是回顾性研究，并且每个研究报道的

```
                    ┌──────────────┐
                    │  PD 合并震颤  │
                    └──────┬───────┘
                           ↓
                    ┌──────────────────┐
                    │ 治疗僵直/运动迟缓 │
                    │（多巴胺激动药或左旋多巴）│
                    └──────────────────┘
```

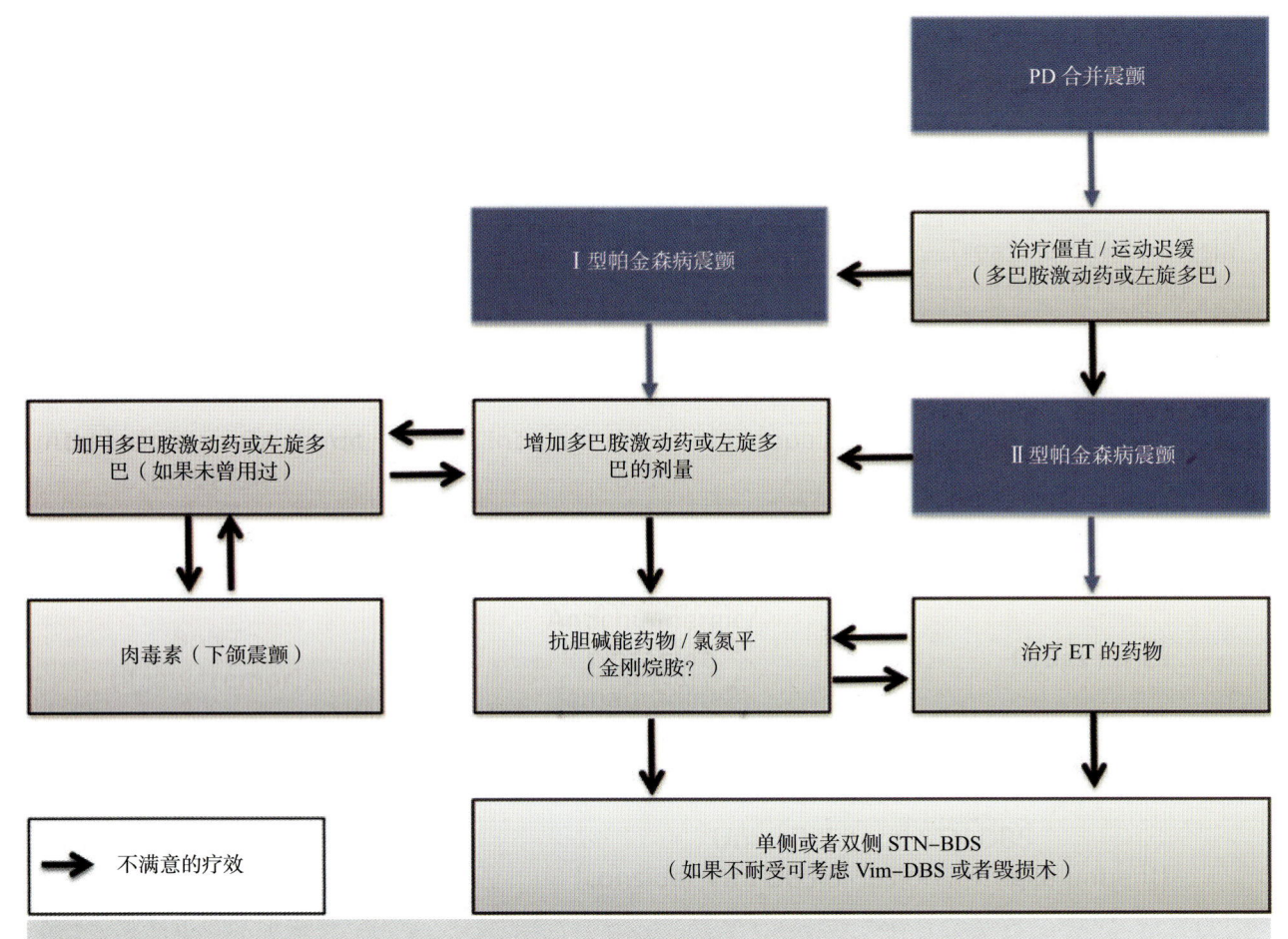

▲ 图 13-3　帕金森病震颤的治疗流程

患者的运动迟缓和僵直应接受初步治疗。运动性震颤可能对多巴胺能药物没有反应，必要时可以尝试使用治疗震颤的药物进行额外辅助治疗。在疾病进展缓慢，且已震颤为主的 PD 老年患者中，若其他症状不是其不能自理的原因，可以考虑 Vim-DBS 进行治疗。STN 是年轻患者的可选靶点，因为它的刺激可以改善疾病的所有基本症状；当震颤不是唯一的残疾来源时，GPi 可以是耐受力较差的患者的有效选择（Martino 等，2016）

DBS. 脑深部电刺激；Gpi. 苍白球内侧部；PD. 帕金森病；STN. 底丘脑核；Vim. 丘脑腹侧中间核

病例数较少。最常见的震颤综合征是脆性 X 相关震颤/共济失调综合征、Holmes 震颤和多发性硬化相关震颤。根据经验，这些综合征会表现出不同临床症状的共济失调，由于 DBS 对共济失调的效果不佳，所以这些综合征的手术预后都不太令人满意。因此，即使有报告称震颤得到改善时，这也不一定是功能性改善。由于这些症状对于多数传统靶点都比较耐受，人们探索了多种代替 Vim 的靶点（表 13-6）。

五、患者的选择

关于震颤患者是否适合行 DBS 手术的决定是复杂并且需要多方面考虑的。在选择患者时，必须考虑 2 个主要因素，包括患者和震颤（表 13-7）（Fasano 等，2009）。

（一）患者相关因素

1. 年龄

Vim-DBS 的病例报道中通常包括高达 80 岁或以上的受试者。然而，尽管从公布的数据中没有足够的证据表明丘脑 DBS 的结果受年龄的影响，但是我们认为 DBS 的理想候选者年龄是 75 岁以下。采取这种观点的主要原因是老年人的手术风险较高。

2. 致残和功能改善

从实用的角度出发，如果震颤严重干扰进

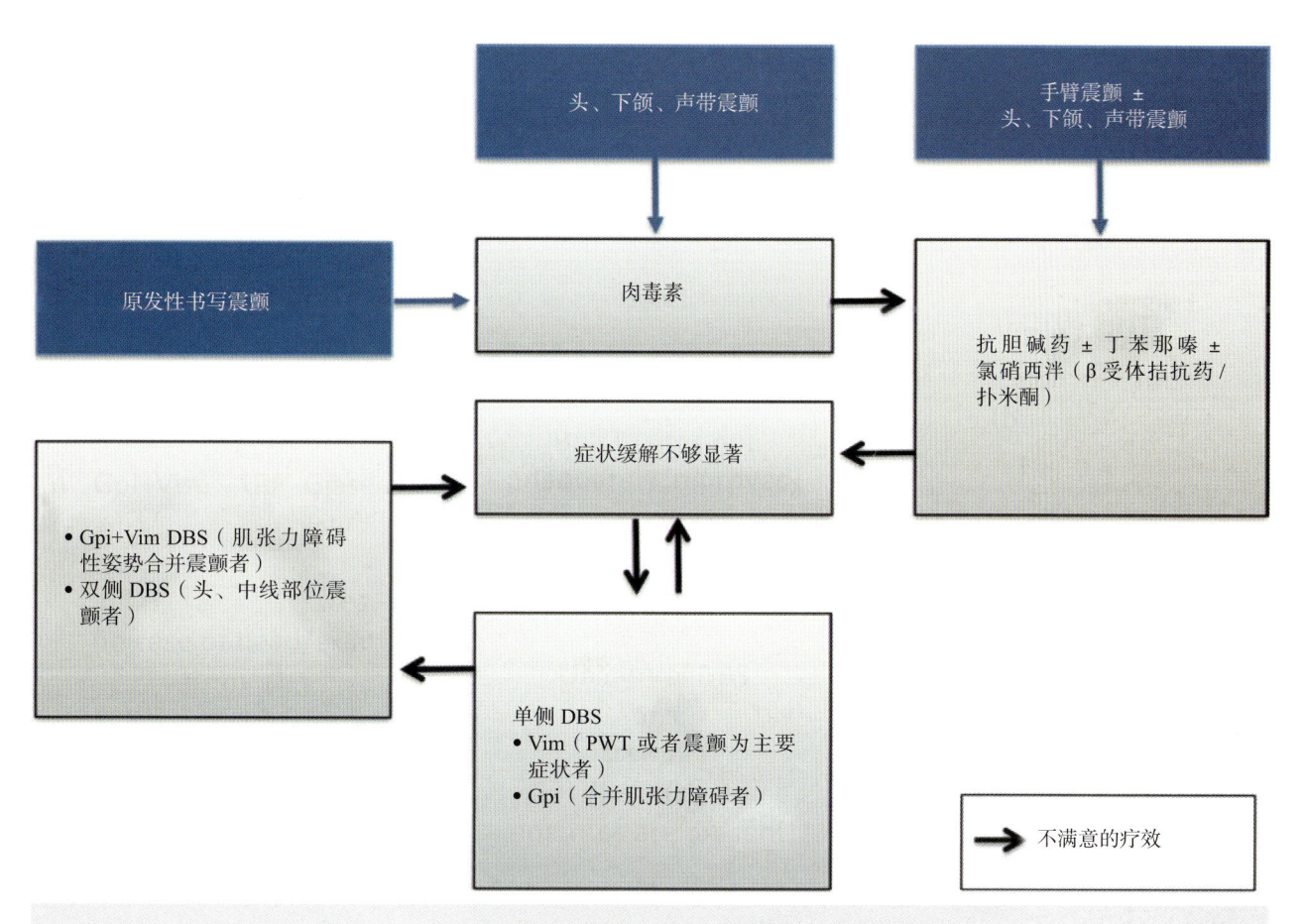

▲ 图 13-4 肌张力障碍性震颤和原发性书写震颤（PWT）的治疗流程

肉毒素是治疗轴性（头部或声带）震颤最有效的方法。然而，除了 PWT 外，四肢震颤首选药物治疗，肉毒素可作为添加治疗（在药物治疗存在不能改善的一些症状时，可用肉毒素治疗）。当震颤引起的残疾的风险大于手术的风险时应考虑手术治疗。四肢震颤可采用单侧手术，而头部震颤应为双侧。至于 DBS 的靶点选择，Vim 和 Gpi 是最常用的靶点，如何选择靶点基于患者的症状以震颤（Vim）还是肌张力障碍姿势（Gpi）为主。其他目标（Vop、STN 和周围区域）可能在非常特定的情况下被考虑（Martino 等，2016）

DBS. 脑深部电刺激；Gpi. 苍白球内侧部；PWT. 原发性书写震颤；STN. 底丘脑核；Vim. 丘脑腹侧中间核；Vop. 丘脑腹外侧核

食、饮水和书写，或者在发声或头部震颤的患者中，震颤会影响日常交流，那么残疾是不可接受的。另一方面，残疾有时完全源于震颤对社交的影响，例如当它是社交耻辱。患者的选择是个体化的，这取决于患者的状况、就业能力、人际关系和对功能改善的期望。减少震颤幅度本身不应是 DBS 手术的最终目标。对患者来说，最重要的结果是功能的改善。减少震颤但不能改善肢体功能的手术（如残存共济失调或改善效果微弱）对患者的益处是值得怀疑的。

3. 全身性共病

虽然缺乏正式的研究，但严重的系统性共病应被视为 DBS 的禁忌证。这些疾病包括所有明显降低预期寿命或严重损害 DBS 的效果或增加手术风险的疾病。

4. 神经系统共病

痴呆、严重精神病、严重人格障碍和酗酒通常被认为是 DBS 的禁忌证。在进行手术前，应先有效的治疗严重的抑郁和焦虑。在非痴呆患者中，丘脑 DBS 被认为是一种相对安全的治疗方法，因为只会导致轻微的语言记忆和语言流畅性下降，而没有证据表明会导致其他负面的神经心理后果。由于构音障碍和吞咽困难是丘脑 DBS 的常见不良反应，在考虑到患者术前就出现这些症状时应谨慎选择。

表 13-6　DBS 手术治疗罕见震颤综合征的靶点及疗效

疾病名称	靶点（例数）	预　后	参考文献
共济失调动眼神经性失用症 2	• 双侧 Gpi（1）	+（肌张力障碍性震颤）	Oyama 等（2014）
小脑震颤（酒精）	• 双侧 RN（1）	-	Lefranc 等（2014）
小脑震颤（卒中）	• 单侧 DN（1）	+（推测对共济失调也有效）	Teixeira 等（2015）
Holmes 震颤（卒中、创伤）	• 单侧 Vim（12） • Vim 和 STN（9） • Vop/Zi（8） • 单侧 Gpi（7） • 双侧 Vim（5） • 单侧 Vim 和 Gpi（5） • 单侧 Vim/Vop 和 Voa/Vop（3） • 单侧 Vim 和 Gpi 苍白球切开术（1） • 双侧 Zi（1） • 单侧 LF（1） • 单侧 Voa/Zi（1） • Voa/Vop 和 STN（1）	效果好（轻微意向性震颤）可能 Gpi 产生的效果更好	Sitsapesan 等（2014）和 Artusi 等（2018）
Klinefelter 综合征	• Vim（3）	+	Koegl-Wallner 等（2014）
MS 综合征	• 单侧 Vim（96） • 双侧 Vim（28） • 双侧 Vop/Zi（22） • 单侧 Vop/Zi（12） • 单侧 Vim/Vop 和 Voa/Vop（12） • 单侧 Vim 和 STN（5） • 双侧 Zi（4） • 双侧 Vim 和 STN（2） • Vim 和 PSA（1） • Voa 和 Vim（1）	+（尤其是在多靶点刺激和刺激 Zi/PSA 时）	Artusi 等（2018）的综述
神经性震颤	• 双侧 Vim（9） • 单侧 Vim（4） • 单侧 PSA（1）	+（一个亚组中出现了耐受）	Artusi 等（2018）的综述
眼腭震颤	• 双侧 RN（1）	-	Wang 等（2009）
直立性震颤	• 双侧 Vim（16） • 单侧 Vim（1）	+（双侧）	Merola 等（2017）
SCA2	• Vim（1）	+	Oyama 等（2014）
SCA6	• 单侧 Vim（1） • 双侧 Vim（1）	+（对共济失调没有作用，需要较高刺激参数）	Hashimoto 等（2018）
SCA17	• 双侧 Gpi（1）	+（肌张力障碍性震颤）	Oyama 等（2014）
SCA31	• 双侧 Vim（1）	+（共济失调无效，需要刺激参数较高）	Hashimoto 等（2018）
SCA35	• 单侧 Vim（1）	-	Fasano 等（2017a）
XFATS	• 双侧 Vim（4） • 单侧 Vim（2） • 双侧 PSA/Vim（1） • 双侧 Vim 和双侧 STN（1） • 单侧 PSA（1） • Vop/Zi（1）	+（共济失调也有效，单侧刺激更安全）	Artusi 等（2018）的综述

-. 无效；/. 同一电极刺激多个靶点，或者 2 个电极刺激多个靶点；+. 有改善；DN. 齿状核；FXTAS. 脆性 X 染色体相关震颤 / 共济失调综合征；Gpi. 苍白球内侧部；LF. 豆状束；MS. 多发性硬化；PSA. 后丘脑区域；Raprl. 丘系前放射；RN. 红核；SCA. 脊髓小脑共济失调；STN. 底丘脑核；Vim. 丘脑腹侧中间核；Voa. 丘脑腹前核；Vop. 丘脑腹外侧核；Zi. 未定带

表 13-7　选择考虑使用 DBS 的震颤患者的主要纳入和排除标准

纳入标准	• 生理年龄＜ 75 岁 • 震颤严重影响生活（如干扰进食，饮水和书写） • 药物难治性震颤［单用或联合使用普萘洛尔，托吡酯和（或）扑米酮达最高耐受剂量；在 PD 震颤情况下左旋多巴达到最高耐受剂量］ • 震颤姿势（图 13-5）
排除标准	• 降低预期寿命的系统性并发症 • 侵入性神经外科手术的禁忌证（如不受控制的糖尿病、凝血病、免疫缺陷） • 神经系统并发症（痴呆、重度共济失调、重度构音障碍和吞咽困难） • 精神类并发症（严重的精神疾病、严重的人格障碍、酗酒、无法控制的严重抑郁症和焦虑症）

DBS. 脑深部电刺激；PD. 帕金森病

5. 既往震颤手术史

在先前接受过震颤手术的患者中，关于 DBS 的报道很少。然而，在既往单侧苍白球切除术或丘脑切除术的患者中，已有行单侧和双侧 DBS（Fasano 等，2018a）后疗效较好的报道，尽管当对侧存在既往手术损伤时，经常会出现不良反应。

6. 术前应考虑的事项

一般认为，DBS 应考虑用于严重受药物难治性震颤影响的患者。一种可行的方法是在考虑 DBS 之前，用严格的循证方法，对每个患者的特定震颤进行双盲研究，测试所有已证明有效的药物。然而，这类研究对于许多类型的震颤并不适用。β 受体阻滞药、托吡酯和普利米酮单独或以最高耐受剂量联合使用是大多数震颤的一线药物治疗手段，但帕金森病相关震颤除外，多巴胺能药物是其主要的治疗药物（表 13-3）。然而，单靠药物往往不足以控制严重的症状，并可能产生不良的不良反应（Zesiewicz 等，2005）。此外，即使在低剂量或标准剂量下，患者也常常对抗震颤药物不耐受。因此，每位患者都必须在潜在获益和 DBS 潜在风险之间取得平衡。

（二）震颤相关因素

在考虑 DBS 时，必须考虑几个与震颤相关的因素：①患者是什么样的震颤？②对一个特定的患者来说，手术有效的机会有多大？③在特定情况下手术的结果如何？这些方面已在上文和表 13-6 中讨论过。对于一个特定的患者来说，最难回答的问题是他的症状是震颤还是共济失调，因为震颤多被认为是可以通过 DBS 而改善，而共济失调则不能。图 13-5 总结了影响手术结果的主要震颤的症状学特征。

六、替代 DBS 的神经外科治疗方法

初级运动皮质的神经调控治疗目前已有一些初步的结果（Moro 等，2011；Picillo 等，2015）。然而，从 20 世纪 50 年代，消融即被认为是有效的，可以用来替代 DBS。射频（RF）丘脑切除术是历史最长的一种外科治疗方法（Cooper 1959；Sweet 等，1960）。最近，为了在不穿透颅骨的情况下进行丘脑切除术，发展了"微创"技术，单侧伽马刀放射外科（GKRS）（Young 等，2001；Lim 等，2010；Witjas 等，2015；Niranjan 等，2017）和 MRI 介导的超声共聚焦技术（MRgFUS）（Lipsman 等，2013；Elias 等，2013；Chang 等，2014；Elias 等，2016；Gallay 等，2016；Zaaroor 等，2018；Kim 等，2017）。这些技术被认为可以显著降低震颤的严重程度，尽管每个患者的预后都有很大的差异。表 13-8 列出了用 RF、GKRS 或 MRgFUS 进行丘脑切除术的特点；图 13-2 和表 13-9 分别列出了它们的短期和长期临床结果。

丘脑手术的并发症包括短暂或永久性感觉障碍、偏瘫、构音障碍、共济失调、步态障碍、意识障碍和认知能力下降等（表 13-5）。有趣的是，

▲ 图 13-5 手术后震颤反应的预测因素

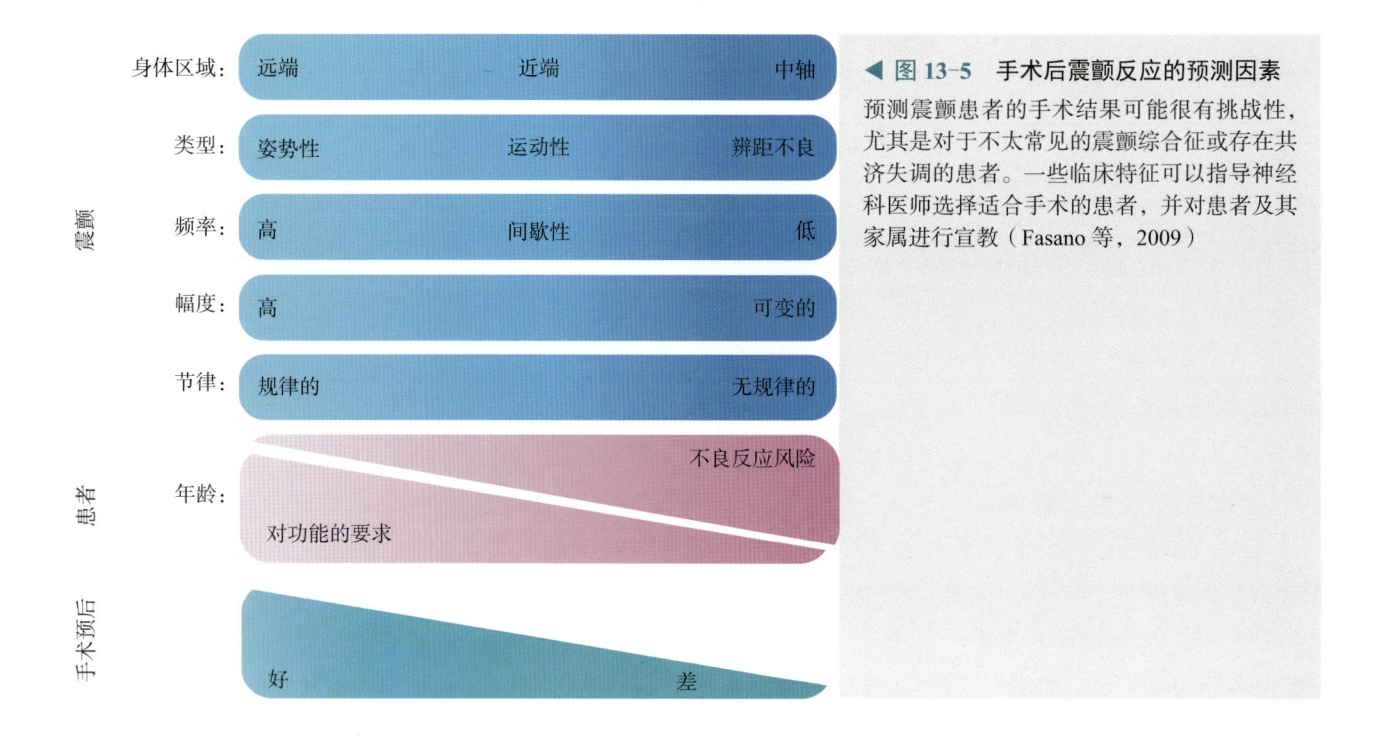

预测震颤患者的手术结果可能很有挑战性，尤其是对于不太常见的震颤综合征或存在共济失调的患者。一些临床特征可以指导神经科医师选择适合手术的患者，并对患者及其家属进行宣教（Fasano 等，2009）

一些 GKRS 患者术后数年观察到延迟的不良反应，包括在接受心房颤动抗凝治疗区域发生出血性卒中（Lim 等，2010；Rothstein，2010），以及由于术腔的逐渐扩大而引起的复杂的不自主运动（Siderowf 等，2001）。

有几位作者认为，虽然文献的报道仅限于少数 ET 患者，但目前的技术可以安全地进行分期双侧丘脑切除术（Dallapiazza 等，2018）。

七、如何选择手术方式

目前，4 种手术方式可供震颤患者选择，外科医生通常会建议和使用逻辑上可行或最熟悉的治疗方法；然而，每种治疗方法都有其优点和局限性（表 13-8）。

在比较 RF 丘脑切除术和 DBS 治疗震颤的研究中，RF 的患者早期手术并发症和永久性神经不良反应的发生率更高（Pahwa 等，2001；Schuurman 等，2000，2008）。作比较通常是困难的，特别是参考回顾性研究，因为非 DBS 患者经常有需要抗凝的严重医学共病（可在 GK 期间继续抗凝治疗），拒绝接受 DBS 手术，或之前接受了不成功的 DBS 或 RF 手术（Lim 等，2010；Young 等，2010；Ohye 等，2012；Kooshkabadi 等，2013；Witjas 等，2015；Kim 等，2017；Niranjan 等，2017；Tuleasca 等，2017）。最后，从世界范围内多年的经验来看，手术方式的选择依据有很大的不同，特别是从治疗的长期结果来看。例如，近年来 MRgFUS 治疗的患者数量在稳步增加，而在以后 MRgFUS 的长期疗效和不良反应将会变得更加清楚。

图 13-6 显示了震颤患者接受治疗的一般流程。

八、结论

总之，DBS 可作为严重的药物难治性震颤患者的治疗选择，其具有良好的手术风险收益比，并且对改善功能有较高的期望。几乎所有类型的震颤都可以接受手术治疗。ET 和 PD 引起的震颤术后改善的可能性很大，而脊髓小脑退行性变、肌张力障碍、多发性硬化、创伤、多发性神经病或脑卒中引起的震颤的治疗效果较为不确定（有时效果较差）。

表 13-8 神经外科技术治疗震颤的主要特点

	DBS	RF[a]	MRIg-FUS[a]	GKRS[a]
框架的应用	有[b]	有	有	有
理发	部分	部分	全部	不需要
颅骨钻孔	需要	需要	不需要	不需要
全麻	需要	不需要	不需要	不需要
靶点确认	MER、电刺激、术中临床评价	MER、电刺激、检查病灶、术中临床评价	检查病灶、磁共振热图、术中临床评价	间接解剖定位
治疗起效时间	立即/延迟（程控时间）	立即	立即	延迟（平均4个月后）
可调节	是	否	否	否
可逆	是[c]	否	否	否
双侧治疗	可以	不可以	不可以	可以
置入物	有	无	无	无
世界范围的经验	>30年	>50年	5年	>15年
长期治疗数据	有	有	无	有（少量报道）
证据级别（OCEM）	2	2~4	1	4
其他注意事项	需要设备维护（如更换电池）和程控；手术后不能进行磁共振检查[d]	颅骨的穿透；丰富的经验	颅骨密度过高、不能做磁共振检查，以及既往颅脑手术病史者不适合	放射所致的不良反应可能逐渐加重
颅内出血风险	有	有	无？	无
感染风险	有	有	无	无
硬件故障风险	有	无	无	无
短暂不良反应出现的风险[e]	有	有	有	有
永久不良反应出现的风险[e]	无	有	有	有（延迟出现）
理想的手术候选人	需要长期调整的年轻患者，只有需要双侧或中线震颤控制的患者才有可能选择	不能定期就诊的患者（如精神病患者）、身体条件差的患者（不能全身麻醉的老年患者）	感染风险高或不能定期就诊的患者（如精神病患者）。以前做过脑部手术的患者不适合接受该治疗	有出血风险（如抗凝治疗）、感染风险高或不能定期就诊（如精神病）的患者

DBS. 脑深部电刺激；GKRS. 伽马刀放射手术；MER. 电生理监测；MRI. 磁共振成像；MRIg-FUS.MRI引导下共聚焦超声；OCEM. 牛津循证医学中心；RF. 射频

a. 单侧丘脑切除术；b. 可以用小框架（神经导航）进行；c. 手术的并发症（如脑卒中）不可逆；d. 与设备的生产厂家有关；e. 非术中并发症（如脑卒中）引起的感觉异常、感觉丧失、虚弱、共济失调、视野缺陷、言语和吞咽困难

表 13-9 在现有的长期研究（3 年以上）中，丘脑切除术治疗非帕金森病性震颤的临床疗效和安全性统计表

参考文献	手术方式	治疗疾病	N[a]	最长随访时间（年）	脱落者
Nagaseki 等（1986）	RF	ET	21（5）	4.7±3.0	0
Shahzadi 等（1995）	RF	ET/MS/CT	21（3）/33/21	• ET：5 例患者随访了 1～7 年，5 例患者随访超过 7 年 • MS：4 例患者随访了 2～4 年 • CT：11 例患者随访了 1～5 年	9 例 ET 患者（42.8%）、15 例 MS 患者（45.4%）、10 例 CT 患者（47.6%）丧失部分疗效
Kondziolka 等（2008）	GKRS	ET	31	3（中位数）	0
Schuurman 等（2008）	RF	ET/MS	4/4	5	0
Niranjan 等（2017）	GKRS	ET	28	4.5（中位数）	3 例震颤复发
Park 等（2019）	MRgFUS	ET	12	4	0

CT. 非 MS 的小脑震颤；ET. 原发性震颤；GKRS. 伽马刀放射手术；MRgFUS.MRI 引导下共聚焦超声；MS. 多发性硬化；RF. 射频
a. 括号内为行双侧手术的病例数

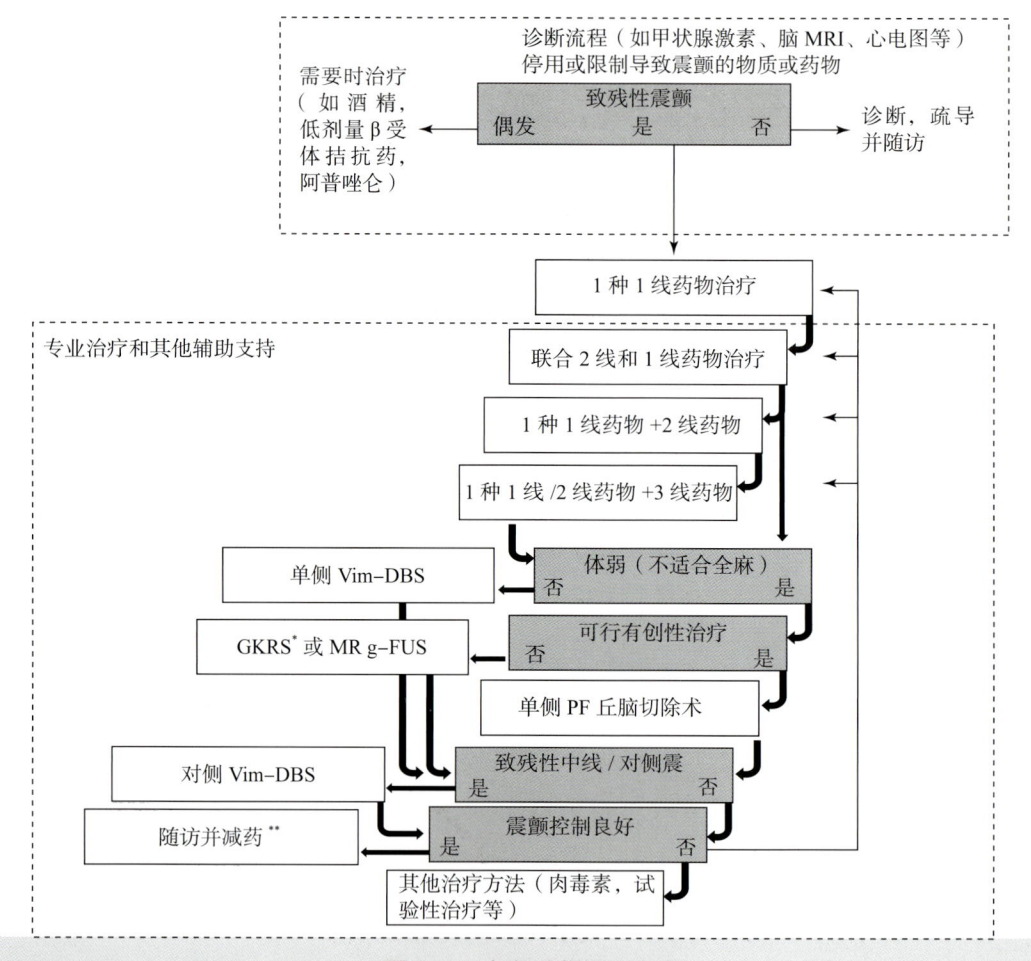

▲ 图 13-6　如何选择手术方式

对于肢体震颤患者，单侧手术（DBS 或消融）有时可能足以避免致残。如果双侧肢体、头部、声音或躯干震颤，必须进行双侧手术。其他研究较少的靶点包括 Zi，特别是其尾侧部分（Raprl），丘脑的 Vop 和 Voa 核（Rohani 和 Fasano，2017）
DBS. 脑深部电刺激；GKRS. 伽马刀放射手术；MRgFUS.MR 引导下共聚焦超声；Raprl. 丘系前放射；RF. 射频；Vim. 丘脑腹侧中间核；Voa. 丘脑腹前核；Vop. 丘脑腹外侧核
*. 有严重出血风险的患者可考虑（如持续抗凝）；**. 减药可导致中线 / 对侧震颤恶化

在几乎所有类型的震颤中，手术的主要靶点是外侧丘脑的 Vim 核，肌张力障碍性震颤和帕金森病震颤除外，其首选靶点分别是 GPi 和 STN。双侧手术通常效果更好，尤其以头部、声音或躯干震颤为主要症状时。但是，在某些情况下可以考虑单侧手术。静息性震颤和上肢姿势性震颤极有可能随着 Vim 的刺激而得到改善。如果以意向性震颤或近端肢体震颤为主，手术成功率会略有下降，因此最近提出了更多新的靶点。

参考文献

[1] Akbostanci MC, Slavin KV, Burchiel KJ. Stereotactic ventral intermedial thalamotomy for the treatment of essential tremor: results of a series of 37 patients. Stereotact Funct Neurosurg. 1999;72:174–7.

[2] Alomar S, King NKK, Tam J, Bari AA, Hamani C, Lozano AM. Speech and language adverse effects after thalamotomy and deep brain stimulation in patients with movement disorders: a meta-analysis. Mov Disord. 2017;32:53–63.

[3] Artusi CA, Farooqi A, Romagnolo A, et al. Deep brain stimulation in uncommon tremor disorders: indications, targets, and programming. J Neurol. 2018;265:2473–93.

[4] Baizabal-Carvallo JF, Kagnoff MN, Jimenez-Shahed J, Fekete R, Jankovic J. The safety and efficacy of thalamic deep brain stimulation in essential tremor: 10 years and beyond. J Neurol Neurosurg Psychiatry. 2013;85:567–72.

[5] Barbe MT, Liebhart L, Runge M, et al. Deep brain stimulation of the ventral intermediate nucleus in patients with essential tremor: Stimulation below intercommissural line is more efficient but equally effective as stimulation above. Exp Neurol. 2011;230:131–7.

[6] Barbe MT, Dembek TA, Becker J, et al. Individualized current-shaping reduces DBS-induced dysarthria in patients with essential tremor. Neurology. 2014;82:614–9.

[7] Benabid AL, Pollak P, Louveau A, Henry S, de Rougemont J. Combined (thalamotomy and stimulation) stereotactic surgery of the VIM thalamic nucleus for bilateral Parkinson disease. Appl Neurophysiol. 1987;50:344–6.

[8] Benabid AL, Pollak P, Gervason C, et al. Long-term suppression of tremor by chronic stimulation of the ventral intermediate thalamic nucleus. Lancet. 1991;337:403–6.

[9] Benabid AL, Pollak P, Hoffman D. Chronic high frequency stimulation in Parkinson's disease. In: Koller WC, Paulson GW, editors. Therapy of Parkinson's disease. 2nd ed. New York: Marcel Dekker; 1994. p. 381–482.

[10] Bhatia KP, Bain P, Bajaj N, et al. Consensus Statement on the classification of tremors. from the task force on tremor of the International Parkinson and Movement Disorder Society. Mov Disord. 2018;33:75–87.

[11] Blomstedt P, Hariz GM, Hariz MI, Koskinen LOD. Thalamic deep brain stimulation in the treatment of essential tremor: a long-term follow-up. Br J Neurosurg. 2007;21:504–9.

[12] Blomstedt P, Sandvik U, Tisch S. Deep brain stimulation in the posterior subthalamic area in the treatment of essential tremor. Mov Disord. 2010;25:1350–6.

[13] Blomstedt P, Sandvik U, Hariz MI, et al. Influence of age, gender and severity of tremor on outcome after thalamic and subthalamic DBS for essential tremor. Parkinsonism Relat Disord. 2011;17:617–20.

[14] Borretzen MN, Bjerknes S, Saehle T, et al. Long-term follow-up of thalamic deep brain stimulation for essential tremor—patient satisfaction and mortality. BMC Neurol. 2014;14:120.

[15] Cagnan H, Pedrosa D, Little S, et al. Stimulating at the right time: phase-specific deep brain stimulation. Brain. 2017;140:132–45.

[16] Calzetti S, Sasso E, Baratti M, Fava R. Clinical and computer-based assessment of long-term therapeutic efficacy of propranolol in essential tremor. Acta Neurol Scand. 1990;81:392–6.

[17] Chang WS, Jung HH, Kweon EJ, Zadicario E, Rachmilevitch I, Chang JW. Unilateral magnetic resonance guided focused ultrasound thalamotomy for essential tremor: practices and clinicoradiological outcomes. J Neurol Neurosurg Psychiatry. 2014;86:257–64.

[18] Chen H, Smith M, Shadmehr R. Effects of deep brain stimulation on adaptive control of reaching. Conf Proc IEEE Eng Med Biol Soc. 2005;5:5445–8.

[19] Coenen VA, Madler B, Schiffbauer H, Urbach H, Allert N. Individual fiber anatomy of the subthalamic region revealed with diffusion tensor imaging: a concept to identify the deep brain stimulation target for tremor suppression. Neurosurgery. 2011;68:1069–75; discussion 1075-1066.

[20] Coenen VA, Schlaepfer TE, Allert N, Mdler B. Diffusion tensor imaging and neuromodulation: DTI as key technology for deep brain stimulation. In: Emerging horizons in neuromodulation: new frontiers in brain and spine stimulation. 1st ed. Amsterdam: Elsevier; 2012. p. 28.

[21] Coenen VA, Allert N, Paus S, Kronenburger M, Urbach H, Madler B. Modulation of the cerebellothalamo-cortical network in thalamic deep brain stimulation for tremor: a diffusion tensor imaging study. Neurosurgery. 2014;75:657–69; discussion 669-670.

[22] Coenen VA, Varkuti B, Parpaley Y, et al. Postoperative neuroimaging analysis of DRT deep brain stimulation revision surgery for complicated essential tremor. Acta Neurochir. 2017;159:779–87.

[23] Cooper IS. Dystonia musculorum deformans alleviated by chemopallidectomy and chemopallidothalamectomy. Arch Neurol Psychiatry. 1959;81:5.

[24] Cury RG, Fraix V, Castrioto A, et al. Thalamic deep brain stimulation for tremor in Parkinson disease, essential tremor, and dystonia. Neurology. 2017;89:1416–23.

[25] Dallapiazza RF, Lee DJ, De Vloo P, et al. Outcomes from stereotactic surgery for essential tremor. J Neurol Neurosurg Psychiatry. 2018;90:474–82.

[26] Deuschl G, Bain P, Brin M. Consensus statement of the Movement Disorder Society on Tremor. Ad Hoc Scientific Committee. Mov Disord. 1998;13(Suppl 3):2–23.

[27] Eisinger RS, Wong J, Almeida L, et al. Ventral intermediate nucleus versus Zona incerta region deep brain stimulation in essential tremor. Mov Disord Clin Pract. 2018;5:75–82.

[28] Elias WJ, Huss D, Voss T, et al. A pilot study of focused ultrasound thalamotomy for essential tremor. N Engl J Med. 2013;369:640–8.

[29] Elias WJ, Lipsman N, Ondo WG, et al. A randomized trial of focused ultrasound thalamotomy for essential tremor. N Engl J Med. 2016;375:730–9.

[30] Espay AJ, Lang AE, Erro R, et al. Essential pitfalls in "essential" tremor. Mov Disord. 2017;32:325–31.

[31] Fasano A, Herzog J, Deuschl G. Selecting appropriate tremor patients for DBS. In: Bain P, Aziz T, Liu X, Nandi D, editors. Deep brain stimulation. Oxford: Oxford University Press; 2009.

[32] Fasano A, Herzog J, Raethjen J, et al. Gait ataxia in essential tremor is differentially modulated by thalamic stimulation. Brain. 2010;133:3635–48.

[33] Fasano A, Daniele A, Albanese A. Treatment of motor and non-motor features of Parkinson's disease with deep brain stimulation. Lancet Neurol. 2012a;11:429–42.

[34] Fasano A, Herzog J, Raethjen J, et al. Lower limb joints kinematics in essential tremor and the effect of thalamic stimulation. Gait Posture. 2012b;36:187–93.

[35] Fasano A, Bove F, Lang AE. The treatment of dystonic tremor: a systematic review. J Neurol Neurosurg Psychiatry. 2014;85:759–69.

[36] Fasano A, Hodaie M, Munhoz RP, Rohani M. SCA 35 presenting as isolated treatment-resistant dystonic hand tremor. Parkinsonism

Relat Disord. 2017a;37:118–9.

[37] Fasano A, Lozano AM, Cubo E. New neurosurgical approaches for tremor and Parkinson's disease. Curr Opin Neurol. 2017b;30:435–46.

[38] Fasano A, De Vloo P, Llinas M, et al. Magnetic resonance imaging-guided focused ultrasound thalamotomy in Parkinson tremor: reoperation after benefit decay. Mov Disord. 2018a;33:848–9.

[39] Fasano A, Lang AE, Espay AJ. What is "essential" about essential tremor? A diagnostic placeholder. Mov Disord. 2018b;33:58–61.

[40] Favilla CG, Ullman D, Wagle Shukla A, Foote KD, Jacobson CE, Okun MS. Worsening essential tremor following deep brain stimulation: disease progression versus tolerance. Brain. 2012;135:1455–62.

[41] Fenoy AJ, Simpson RK. Risks of common complications in deep brain stimulation surgery: management and avoidance. J Neurosurg. 2014;120:132–9.

[42] Fenoy AJ, Schiess MC. Deep brain stimulation of the Dentato-Rubro-thalamic tract: outcomes of direct targeting for tremor. Neuromodulation. 2017;20:429–36.

[43] Fytagoridis A, Sandvik U, Åström M, Bergenheim T, Blomstedt P. Long term follow-up of deep brain stimulation of the caudal zona incerta for essential tremor. J Neurol Neurosurg Psychiatry. 2011;83:258–62.

[44] Fytagoridis A, Sandvik U, Astrom M, Bergenheim T, Blomstedt P. Long term follow-up of deep brain stimulation of the caudal zona incerta for essential tremor. J Neurol Neurosurg Psychiatry. 2012;83:258–62.

[45] Gallay MN, Moser D, Rossi F, et al. Incisionless transcranial MR-guided focused ultrasound in essential tremor: cerebellothalamic tractotomy. J Therapeut Ultrasound. 2016:4.

[46] Graff-Radford J, Foote KD, Mikos AE, et al. Mood and motor effects of thalamic deep brain stimulation surgery for essential tremor. Eur J Neurol. 2010;17:1040–6.

[47] Graupe D, Basu I, Tuninetti D, Vannemreddy P, Slavin KV. Adaptively controlling deep brain stimulation in essential tremor patient via surface electromyography. Neurol Res. 2010;32:899–904.

[48] Hariz MI, Shamsgovara P, Johansson F, Hariz G, Fodstad H. Tolerance and tremor rebound following long-term chronic thalamic stimulation for Parkinsonian and essential tremor. Stereotact Funct Neurosurg. 1999;72:208–18.

[49] Hariz MI, Krack P, Alesch F, et al. Multicentre European study of thalamic stimulation for parkinsonian tremor: a 6 year follow-up. J Neurol Neurosurg Psychiatry. 2008;79:694–9.

[50] Hashimoto T, Muralidharan A, Yoshida K, et al. Neuronal activity and outcomes from thalamic surgery for spinocerebellar ataxia. Ann Clin Transl Neurol. 2018;5:52–63.

[51] Herzog J, Hamel W, Wenzelburger R, et al. Kinematic analysis of thalamic versus subthalamic neurostimulation in postural and intention tremor. Brain. 2007;130:1608–25.

[52] Huss DS, Dallapiazza RF, Shah BB, Harrison MB, Diamond J, Elias WJ. Functional assessment and quality of life in essential tremor with bilateral or unilat- eral DBS and focused ultrasound thalamotomy. Mov Disord. 2015;30:1937–43.

[53] Kim M, Jung NY, Park CK, Chang WS, Jung HH, Chang JW. Comparative evaluation of magnetic resonance-guided focused ultrasound surgery for essential tremor. Stereotact Funct Neurosurg. 2017;95:279–86.

[54] Kobayashi K, Katayama Y, Kasai M, Oshima H, Fukaya C, Yamamoto T. Localization of thalamic cells with tremor-frequency activity in Parkinson's disease and essential tremor. Acta Neurochir Suppl. 2003;87:137–9.

[55] Koegl-Wallner M, Katschnig-Winter P, Pendl T, et al. Tremor associated with Klinefelter syndrome--a case series and review of the literature. Parkinsonism Relat Disord. 2014;20:323–7.

[56] Koller WC, Lyons KE, Wilkinson SB, Troster AI, Pahwa R. Long-term safety and efficacy of unilateral deep brain stimulation of the thalamus in essential tremor. Mov Disord. 2001;16:464–8.

[57] Kondziolka D, Ong JG, Lee JYK, Moore RY, Flickinger JC, Lunsford LD. Gamma Knife thalamotomy for essential tremor. J Neurosurg. 2008;108:111–7.

[58] Kooshkabadi A, Lunsford LD, Tonetti D, Flickinger JC, Kondziolka D. Gamma Knife thalamotomy for tremor in the magnetic resonance imaging era. J Neurosurg. 2013;118:713–8.

[59] Kronenbuerger M, Tronnier VM, Gerwig M, et al. Thalamic deep brain stimulation improves eyeblink conditioning deficits in essential tremor. Exp Neurol. 2008;211:387–96.

[60] Kronenbuerger M, Zobel S, Ilgner J, et al. Effects of deep brain stimulation of the cerebellothalamic pathways on the sense of smell. Exp Neurol. 2010;222:144–52.

[61] Lefranc M, Manto M, Merle P, et al. Targeting the red nucleus for cerebellar tremor. Cerebellum. 2014;13:372–7.

[62] Lim S-Y, Hodaie M, Fallis M, Poon Y-Y, Mazzella F, Moro E. Gamma knife thalamotomy for disabling tremor. Arch Neurol. 2010;67:584–8.

[63] Limousin P, Speelman JD, Gielen F, Janssens M. Multicentre European study of thalamic stimulation in parkinsonian and essential tremor. J Neurol Neurosurg Psychiatry. 1999;66:289–96.

[64] Lipsman N, Schwartz ML, Huang Y, et al. MR-guided focused ultrasound thalamotomy for essential tremor: a proof-of-concept study. Lancet Neurol. 2013;12:462–8.

[65] Louis ED, Ferreira JJ. How common is the most common adult movement disorder? Update on the worldwide prevalence of essential tremor. Mov Disord. 2010;25:534–41.

[66] Louis ED, Agnew A, Gillman A, Gerbin M, Viner AS. Estimating annual rate of decline: prospective, longitudinal data on arm tremor severity in two groups of essential tremor cases. J Neurol Neurosurg Psychiatry. 2011;82:761–5.

[67] Lyons KE, Pahwa R, Busenbark KL, Tröster AI, Wilkinson S, Koller WC. Improvements in daily functioning after deep brain stimulation of the thalamus for intractable tremor. Mov Disord. 1998;13:690–2.

[68] Malekmohammadi M, Herron J, Velisar A, et al. Kinematic adaptive deep brain stimulation for resting tremor in Parkinson's disease. Mov Disord. 2016;31:426–8.

[69] Mandat T, Koziara H, Rola R, Bonicki W, Nauman P. Thalamic deep brain stimulation in the treatment of essential tremor. Neurol Neurochir Pol. 2011;45:37–41.

[70] Martino D, Espay AJ, Fasano A, Morgante F. Rhythmical involuntary movements (tremor and tremor-like conditions). In: Disorders of movement: a guide to diagnosis and treatment. Berlin: Springer-Verlag; 2016. p. 207–63.

[71] Matsumoto JY, Fossett T, Kim M, et al. Precise stimulation location optimizes speech outcomes in essential tremor. Parkinsonism Relat Disord. 2016;32:60–5.

[72] Meng FG, Kao CC, Chen N, et al. Deep brain stimulation of the subthalamic nucleus for essential tremor. Chin Med J (Engl). 2013;126:395–6.

[73] Merola A, Fasano A, Hassan A, et al. Thalamic deep brain stimulation for orthostatic tremor: a multicenter international registry. Mov Disord. 2017;32:1240–4.

[74] Moro E, Schwalb JM, Piboolnurak P, et al. Unilateral subdural motor cortex stimulation improves essential tremor but not Parkinson's disease. Brain. 2011;134:2096–105.

[75] Murata JI, Kitagawa M, Uesugi H, et al. Electrical stimulation of the posterior subthalamic area for the treatment of intractable proximal tremor. J Neurosurg. 2003;99:708–15.

[76] Nagaseki Y, Shibazaki T, Hirai T, et al. Long-term follow-up results of selective VIM-thalamotomy. J Neurosurg. 1986;65:296–302.

[77] Nazzaro JM, Pahwa R, Lyons KE. Long-term benefits in quality of life after unilateral thalamic deep brain stimulation for essential tremor. J Neurosurg. 2012;117:156–61.

[78] Niranjan A, Raju SS, Kooshkabadi A, Monaco E, Flickinger JC, Lunsford LD. Stereotactic radiosurgery for essential tremor: Retrospective analysis of a 19-year experience. Mov Disord. 2017;32:769–77.

[79] Obwegeser AA, Uitti RJ, Turk MF, Strongosky AJ, Wharen RE. Thalamic stimulation for the treatment of midline tremors in essential tremor patients. Neurology. 2000;54:2342–4.

[80] Ohye C, Higuchi Y, Shibazaki T, et al. Gamma knife thalamotomy for Parkinson disease and essential tremor. Neurosurgery. 2012;70:526–36.

[81] Oliveria SF, Rodriguez RL, Bowers D, et al. Safety and efficacy of dual-lead thalamic deep brain stimulation for patients with treatment-refractory multiple sclerosis tremor: a single-centre,

randomised, single-blind, pilot trial. Lancet Neurol. 2017;16:691–700.
[82] Ondo WG, Almaguer M, Cohen H. Computerized posturography balance assessment of patients with bilateral ventralis intermedius nuclei deep brain stimulation. Mov Disord. 2006;21:2243–7.
[83] Oyama G, Thompson A, Foote KD, et al. Deep brain stimulation for tremor associated with underlying ataxia syndromes: a case series and discussion of issues. Tremor Other Hyperkinet Mov (N Y). 2014;4:228.
[84] Pahwa R, Lyons KE, Wilkinson SB, et al. Comparison of thalamotomy to deep brain stimulation of the thalamus in essential tremor. Mov Disord. 2001;16:140–3.
[85] Pahwa R, Lyons KE, Wilkinson SB, et al. Long-term evaluation of deep brain stimulation of the thalamus. J Neurosurg. 2006;104:506–12.
[86] Park YS, Jung NY, Na YC, Chang JW. Four-year follow-up results of magnetic resonance-guided focused ultrasound thalamotomy for essential tremor. Mov Disord. 2019;34:727–34.
[87] Paschen S, Forstenpointner J, Becktepe J, et al. Long-term efficacy of deep brain stimulation for essential tremor: an observer-blinded study. Neurology. 2019;92(12):e1378–86.
[88] Pedrosa DJ, Auth M, Pauls KAM, et al. Verbal fluency in essential tremor patients: the effects of deep brain stimulation. Brain Stimulation. 2014;7:359–64.
[89] Peng-Chen Z, Morishita T, Vaillancourt D, et al. Unilateral thalamic deep brain stimulation in essential tremor demonstrates long-term ipsilateral effects. Parkinsonism Relat Disord. 2013;19:1113–7.
[90] Picillo M, Moro E, Edwards M, Di Lazzaro V, Lozano AM, Fasano A. Subdural continuous theta burst stimulation of the motor cortex in essential tremor. Brain Stimul. 2015;8:840–2.
[91] Picillo M, Lozano AM, Kou N, Munhoz RP, Fasano A. Programming deep brain stimulation for tremor and dystonia: the Toronto Western Hospital algorithms.Brain Stimul. 2016;9:438–52.
[92] Pilitsis JG, Metman LV, Toleikis JR, Hughes LE, Sani SB, Bakay RAE. Factors involved in long-term efficacy of deep brain stimulation of the thalamus for essential tremor. J Neurosurg. 2008;109:640–6.
[93] Plaha P, Patel NK, Gill SS. Stimulation of the subthalamic region for essential tremor. J Neurosurg. 2004;101:48–54.
[94] Plaha P, Khan S, Gill SS. Bilateral stimulation of the caudal zona incerta nucleus for tremor control. J Neurol Neurosurg Psychiatry. 2008;79:504–13.
[95] Plaha P, Javed S, Agombar D, et al. Bilateral caudal zona incerta nucleus stimulation for essential tremor: outcome and quality of life. Journal of Neurology. Neurosurg Psychiatry. 2011;82:899–904.
[96] Putzke JD, Wharen RE Jr, Obwegeser AA, et al. Thalamic deep brain stimulation for essential tremor: recommendations for long-term outcome analysis. Can J Neurol Sci. 2004;31:333–42.
[97] Rehncrona S, Johnels B, Widner H, Törnqvist A-L, Hariz M, Sydow O. Long-term efficacy of thalamic deep brain stimulation for tremor: double-blind assessments. Mov Disord. 2002;18:163–70.
[98] Reich MM, Brumberg J, Pozzi NG, et al. Progressive gait ataxia following deep brain stimulation for essential tremor: adverse effect or lack of efficacy? Brain. 2016;139:2948–56.
[99] Reinacher PC, Amtage F, Rijntjes M, et al. One pass thalamic and subthalamic stimulation for patients with tremor-dominant idiopathic Parkinson syndrome (OPINION): protocol for a randomized, active-controlled, double-blinded pilot trial. JMIR Res Protoc. 2018;7:e36.
[100] Rodriguez Cruz PM, Vargas A, Fernandez-Carballal C, Garbizu J, De La Casa-Fages B, Grandas F. Long-term thalamic deep brain stimulation for essential tremor: clinical outcome and stimulation parameters. Mov Disord Clin Pract. 2016;3:567–72.
[101] Rohani M, Fasano A. Focused ultrasound for essential tremor: review of the evidence and discussion of current hurdles. Tremor Other Hyperkinet Mov (N Y). 2017;7:462.
[102] Rothstein TL. A late complication of gamma knife radiosurgery. Rev Neurol Dis. 2010;7:150–1; discussion 157-159.
[103] Sajonz BE, Amtage F, Reinacher PC, et al. Deep brain stimulation for tremor tractographic versus traditional (DISTINCT): study protocol of a randomized controlled feasibility trial. JMIR Res Protoc. 2016;e244:5.
[104] Sammartino F, Krishna V, King NKK, et al. Tractography-based ventral intermediate nucleus targeting: novel methodology and intraoperative validation. Mov Disord. 2016;31:1217–25.
[105] Sandoe C, Krishna V, Basha D, et al. Predictors of deep brain stimulation outcome in tremor patients. Brain Stimul. 2018;11:592–9.
[106] Schuurman PR, Bosch DA, Bossuyt PMM, et al. A comparison of continuous thalamic stimulation and thalamotomy for suppression of severe tremor. N Engl J Med. 2000;342:461–8.
[107] Schuurman PR, Bosch DA, Merkus MP, Speelman JD. Long-term follow-up of thalamic stimulation versus thalamotomy for tremor suppression. Mov Disord. 2008;23:1146–53.
[108] Shahzadi S, Tasker RR, Lozano A. Thalamotomy for essential and cerebellar tremor. Stereotact Funct Neurosurg. 1995;65:11–7.
[109] Shih LC, LaFaver K, Lim C, Papavassiliou E, Tarsy D. Loss of benefit in VIM thalamic deep brain stimulation (DBS) for essential tremor (ET): How prevalent is it? Parkinsonism Relat Disord. 2013;19:676–9.
[110] Siderowf A, Gollump SM, Stern MB, Baltuch GH, Riina HA. Emergence of complex, involuntary movements after gamma knife radiosurgery for essential tremor. Mov Disord. 2001;16:965–7.
[111] Sitsapesan HA, Holland P, Oliphant Z, et al. Deep brain stimulation for tremor resulting from acquired brain injury. J Neurol Neurosurg Psychiatry. 2014;85:811–5.
[112] Sweet WH, Mark VH, Hamlin H. Radiofrequency lesions in the central nervous system of man and cat. J Neurosurg. 1960;17:213–25.
[113] Sydow O. Multicentre European Study of thalamic stimulation in essential tremor: a six year follow up. J Neurol Neurosurg Psychiatry. 2003;74:1387–91.
[114] Teixeira MJ, Cury RG, Galhardoni R, et al. Deep brain stimulation of the dentate nucleus improves cerebellar ataxia after cerebellar stroke. Neurology. 2015;85:2075–6.
[115] Tuleasca C, Witjas T, Najdenovska E, et al. Assessing the clinical outcome of Vim radiosurgery with voxel-based morphometry: visual areas are linked with tremor arrest! Acta Neurochir. 2017;159:2139–44.
[116] Wang D, Sanchez J, Foote KD, et al. Failed DBS for palliation of visual problems in a case of oculopalatal tremor. Parkinsonism Relat Disord. 2009;15:71–3.
[117] Witjas T, Carron R, Krack P, et al. A prospective single-blind study of Gamma Knife thalamotomy for tremor. Neurology. 2015;85:1562–8.
[118] Young RF, Jacques DB, Mark R, Copcutt B. 794 Gamma Knife medial thalamotomy for treatment of chronic pain: long-term results. Neurosurgery. 2001;49:534.
[119] Young RF, Li F, Vermeulen S, Meier R. Gamma Knife thalamotomy for treatment of essential tremor: long-term results. J Neurosurg. 2010;112:1311–7.
[120] Zaaroor M, Sinai A, Goldsher D, Eran A, Nassar M, Schlesinger I. Magnetic resonance–guided focused ultrasound thalamotomy for tremor: a report of 30 Parkinson's disease and essential tremor cases. J Neurosurg. 2018;128:202–10.
[121] Zackowski KM, Bastian AJ, Hakimian S, et al. Thalamic stimulation reduces essential tremor but not the delayed antagonist muscle timing. Neurology. 2002;58:402–10.
[122] Zesiewicz TA, Elble R, Louis ED, et al. Practice parameter: therapies for essential tremor: report of the quality standards Subcommittee of the American Academy of Neurology. Neurology. 2005;64:2008–20.
[123] Zhang K, Bhatia S, Oh MY, Cohen D, Angle C, Whiting D. Long-term results of thalamic deep brain stimulation for essential tremor. J Neurosurg. 2010;112:1271–6.

第 14 章 肌张力障碍
Dystonia

Maria Fiorella Contarino　Joachim K.Krauss　著
赵宝田　张　凯　译　王　垚　杨岸超　张建国　校

> **摘要**：肌张力障碍是一种复杂的、具有多种临床特征的综合征。描述肌张力障碍的临床特点和准确的诊断都具有一定挑战性，需要较深的专业知识，而这对于选择适当的药物和手术治疗至关重要。
>
> 全身型肌张力障碍的首选治疗方案是口服药物治疗，尤其是抗胆碱能类药物。然而，药物治疗的效果往往会因其不良反应而受到影响。尽管肉毒杆菌神经毒素对治疗局灶型或节段型肌张力障碍的疗效是确切且安全的，仍有部分患者对这类药物完全无反应，或药效随时间推移而逐渐消失。
>
> 在对药物和肉毒素耐受患者的治疗上，脑深部电刺激已成为一种重要的治疗方案，靶点位于苍白球内侧部（GPi）的腹后外侧部。
>
> 与帕金森病或特发性震颤不同，肌张力障碍的脑深部电刺激（DBS）的程控面临着一些特殊的问题，因为它对症状的改善存在明显的延迟。此外，目前对慢性刺激的程序设定尚未达成共识，脉冲宽度和刺激频率在不同中心间差异较大。由于所需的刺激强度较高，可考虑使用可充电的植入性脉冲发生器。
>
> 有可靠的证据显示，DBS 对单纯特发性和遗传性肌张力障碍的疗效往往优于复合性继发性获得性肌张力障碍，虽然在后者当中仍有少数的病例疗效很好，但有少数患者的 DBS 疗效远比预期差。除此之外，即使接受 DBS 手术后患者的长期生活质量得以提升，且运动症状显著改善，但仍有一些患者对疗效不够满意。因此，对于术前评估和术后管理提出了更高的要求，包括心理和社会层面。
>
> 考虑到这种疾病较为罕见且临床症状复杂，只有经验丰富的团队才能够开展 DBS 治疗。

一、背景

（一）定义和分类

肌张力障碍是在多种疾病中表现出的一类综合征。"肌张力障碍"这一术语是由德国的神经病学家 Hermann Oppenheim 在 1911 年率先提出的。得益于影像技术的日益进步和基因方面的学术发现（Van Egmond 等，2017），该运动障碍性疾病逐渐被人们所熟知。肌张力障碍可能发生在儿童或成人中，涉及身体多个部位，而临床表现与这些受累部位间的关系错综复杂。因此，在临床上诊断肌张力障碍和准确对其定义都比较困难

（Van Egmond 等，2019）。

对肌张力障碍的最新定义为："是一种持续性或间断性肌肉收缩引起的异常运动（多为重复性）或姿势障碍的运动障碍性疾病"（Albaneses 等，2013）。在描述肌张力障碍综合征的临床特征时，需要结合患者的发病年龄、受累部位，以及起病的顺序，也要判断属于单纯性的肌张力障碍，还是与其他神经系统或系统性疾病的临床表现有关（即复合性肌张力障碍）（Albanese 等，2013）。过去很长一段时间，多将肌张力障碍划分为特发性和获得性，但最新的概念中引入了遗传性肌张力障碍（Lohmann 和 Klein，2017），这类疾病的症状多与基因相关。

肌张力障碍的表现多种多样，可分为：①局灶型，即局限于单一部位（如斜颈）；②节段型；③可引起严重功能障碍的全身型。肌张力障碍也可由某些心因性的病因引起（即功能性肌张力障碍）。依据病因，可将肌张力障碍分为3类，包括特发性、遗传性和获得性。

（二）患病率和发病率

由于临床表现复杂，发病严重程度各不相同，仍有许多患者没有被确诊，故很难得到准确的患病率和发病率。有调查数据显示，特发性肌张力障碍的患病率为16/10万，年发病率为1.07/10万（Steeves 等，2012）。

（三）单纯性肌张力障碍

这类患者只表现出肌张力障碍的症状，其中肌张力障碍性震颤也被视为肌张力障碍的特征之一。

1. 特发性

特发性单纯性肌张力障碍又可分为，局灶型（包括活动诱发的类型）、节段型和全身型。该类型通常在影像学上无明显异常，病因也不明确。

2. 遗传性

研究发现了越来越多的遗传性肌张力障碍（Lohmann 和 Klein，2017）。最常见的遗传性肌张力障碍有 DYT1 相关肌张力障碍（TOR1A 基因）和 DYT7 相关肌张力障碍（THAP1 基因），这两种均属于不完全外显的常染色体显性遗传。无论何种类型，通常会在儿童期起病，从四肢开始，进展为全身受累，往往造成患者无法自理。DYT6 相关肌张力障碍通常引起颈部和喉部肌肉受累，造成语言功能受损，上述临床特征在其他类型的肌张力障碍中并不常见。

3. 获得性

只有少部分获得性肌张力障碍表现为单纯性肌张力障碍。其中包括药物引起的迟发性肌张力障碍，是由长期使用经典的安定类抗精神病药物、抗焦虑/抑郁类药物，以及抗癫痫药（Zádori 等，2015）引起的。迟发性肌张力障碍患者可表现出多种不同的临床症状，通常会累及中轴部位的肌肉。这类疾病常表现为固定的肌张力障碍姿势，也可伴有较多的时相性"异动症样"活动。迟发性肌张力障碍的典型表现是面部运动障碍，有时可扩展至颈部甚至身体躯干。

（四）复合性肌张力障碍

复合性肌张力障碍，通常伴有其他的神经系统疾病或其中某些疾病的特征。这些神经性的症状或综合征常伴随其他运动障碍性疾病，如帕金森病和肌阵挛，或多发性神经病、痉挛等综合征。

1. 特发性与遗传性的复合性肌张力障碍

复合性肌张力障碍中包括伴肌阵挛肌张力障碍。对于这种疾病，肌张力障碍与肌阵挛可出现在相同部位，也可在不同部位出现（Roze 等，2018）。肌阵挛肌张力障碍可能属于特发性，也可由 SGCE 基因（DYT11）的突变引起。另一种复合性肌张力障碍为脑组织铁沉积性神经变性（NBIA），是以铁蓄积于基底节为主要特征的一组异质性疾病。在该类型中，肌张力障碍通常伴有痉挛、神经精神症状或视网膜变性。这些疾病中最常见的是由 PANK2 基因突变所引起的泛酸激酶相关神经变性（PKAN）。PKAN2 的典型特征为儿童期起病，呈进行性病程，以苍白球铁沉积为特征，可出现典型的"虎眼"征。

在其他复合性肌张力障碍中，有时主要的临床表现为帕金森综合征。如 X 连锁肌张力障碍 - 帕金森综合征，被命名为 DYT3（DYT/PARK-TAF1 或 Lubag），以及由于 ATP1A3 基因突变引起的起病迅速的肌张力障碍 - 帕金森综合征（RODP），被命名为 DYT12。在肝豆状核变性等综合征中，由于 ATP7B 基因突变，铜的全身性蓄积不仅引起肌张力障碍，还引起精神症状和肝损害。

2. 获得性复合性肌张力障碍

获得性复合性肌张力障碍包括出生时或出生后脑损伤引起的各种综合征。在这些类型中，肌张力障碍通常伴随其他运动障碍性疾病，有时伴痉挛或小脑症状，具体表现取决于致病性病变的大小和位置。壳核或基底节区的创伤性或脑血管病变可导致累及一侧半身的肌张力障碍综合征（偏身型肌张力障碍）。脑性瘫痪（CP），往往因围产期缺氧，引起症状复杂的肌张力障碍综合征，常伴有不同程度的痉挛和小脑症状。肌张力障碍本身的症状和其他系统受累引起的症状之间，有时是难以区分的（Eggink 等，2017）。

二、肌张力障碍的病理生理学

肌张力障碍的病理生理学基础在很大程度上尚不清楚。由于在人类和动物模型中基底节区域的病变可能导致肌张力障碍，推测基底神经节可能发挥了一定作用（Jinnah 等，2005；Guehl 等，2009）。此外，临床观察发现，刺激感觉系统可暂时改善肌张力障碍症状，神经生理学和功能影像数据也提示，其内在机制与感觉区及联合区域相关（感觉运动皮质、运动前区、顶叶皮质）（Zoons 等，2011）。据推测，感觉运动整合受损可能是异常运动或姿势产生和维持的原因（Konczak 和 Abbruzzese，2013）。近年来功能性研究指出，机制可能涉及皮质通路、脑干和小脑，进而造成整个脑网络模式的紊乱（Lehéricy 等，2013；Egger 等，2007；Neychev 等，2011）。

三、治疗方法的选择与 DBS 靶点位置

制定肌张力障碍的治疗方案时，需要综合考虑诊断、临床表现和年龄等因素（Jankovic 等，2013）。肌张力障碍比较罕见且临床表现和分类复杂多样，因此针对各类肌张力障碍治疗方法的随机对照试验数目不多。

（一）药物治疗

对于一些罕见形式的肌张力障碍，存在特异性治疗方法，如左旋多巴治疗多巴反应性肌张力障碍，或锌和铜螯合剂治疗 Wilson 病出现的肌张力障碍（Roubertie 等，2012）。先天性代谢紊乱的患者有时可表现出罕见形式的肌张力障碍。我们应该利用生化或基因技术做出诊断，并采取适当的特异性治疗方案。

全身型肌张力障碍首选口服药物治疗。抗胆碱能药（如苯海索）对 40%～50% 的患者有效。儿童可使用相对高剂量的药物，效果良好，而由于成人用药的不良反应较多，药物剂量不宜太高。巴氯芬可口服或通过植入式可再填充设备鞘内给药，尤其适用于伴有痉挛和下肢受累的类型（Woon 等，2007；Roubertie 等，2012）。苯二氮䓬类药物（如氯硝西泮）常可改善肌阵挛或肌张力障碍性震颤，而丁苯那嗪和氯氮平适用于药物诱发的肌张力障碍。有时会使用抗惊厥药（如加巴喷丁）或联合使用上述这些药物。这些药物对症状的改善是暂时性的，疗效有限。

（二）肉毒杆菌毒素

已有高级别证据说明，肉毒杆菌神经毒素（BoNT）A 和 B 对于局灶型或节段型肌张力障碍有效，且不良反应发生率较低（Contarino 等，2017）。BoNT 的疗效是通过局部化学传导阻滞形成的。通常情况下，疗效在 3～5 天出现，2～4 周后达到峰值，持续 3～6 个月。有时由于 BoNT 治疗仅产生局部效应，一些肌张力障碍患者首次治疗无效（首次无应答者），或初期

有效而后期疗效不佳（再次无应答者）。耐药性产生的原因包括治疗方法不当，肌张力障碍的内在机制复杂或产生了中和抗体（Contarino 等，2016）。

（三）支持性治疗

物理治疗对于改善肌肉控制能力和减少持续性收缩非常重要，可延长 BoNT 疗效的持续时间，提高治疗效果（Delnooz 等，2009）。目前存在几种不同的物理疗法，但没有证据指示何种方案效果最好（Van Den Dool 等，2019）。肌张力障碍患者可能存在精神疾病，如反应性或原发性抑郁和焦虑（Fabbrini 等，2010）。支持性的心理治疗有助于改善生活质量，也能够让患者意识到治疗的效果。特定的一些行为治疗可能适用于功能性肌张力障碍。

（四）脑深部电刺激

上述治疗方案无效或疗效较差的患者，可考虑接受脑深部电刺激（DBS）。

四、手术选择

（一）总体原则

由于肌张力障碍诊断和治疗复杂，应该由经验丰富的团队决定患者是否适合接受 DBS 手术。适应证的选择对手术结果至关重要。分类方面，应清楚地辨别单纯性和混合性，以及其中的特发性、遗传性和获得性肌张力障碍，以得到准确的诊断。尤其应注意鉴别病因，排除可通过药物等方法治疗的肌张力障碍，以及很可能效果不佳的复杂的进展性综合征，还要有丰富的临床经验，以识别罕见的功能性肌张力障碍。术前需进行完整的检查，包括脑影像及其他检查。影像可用于辅助诊断，有些受损伤的脑区虽与肌张力障碍的症状无直接关联，也可通过影像被发现。利用脑磁共振成像（MRI）也可以发现脑萎缩，进而评估手术风险。

对临床表现的评估，目的是筛选出伴有残疾的肌张力障碍患者。尤其对于复合性肌张力障碍，接受 DBS 后其相关症状（如痉挛或共济失调）很可能不会改善，该情况在有功能性障碍的患者中经常出现。

医护人员应该与患者共同讨论后确定合适的手术时机。一方面，只有当患者的症状非常严重时，才值得承担手术可能存在的风险；但另一方面，若早在发生持续性的肌肉挛缩和骨骼畸形及社交能力下降之前进行手术，手术的预后更好（Isaias 等，2008）。

DBS 术后的肌张力障碍患者的抑郁和焦虑症的患病率较高（Hälbig 等，2005），曾有极少数的自杀病例的报道。因此，在术前评估中排除活动性抑郁症或其他禁忌的精神疾病非常重要。这类疾病可能常见于某些特定类型的肌张力障碍（Van Tricht 等，2012；Contarino 等，2011）。

最后，患者和护理人员应致力于提供准确的信息，以期在临床实践中获得满意的疗效。

（二）DBS 手术适应证的选择

20 世纪 90 年代末，出现了以苍白球为靶点的 DBS 手术（Krauss 等，1999；Kumar 等，1999；Coubes 等，2000），该手术对于单纯性肌张力障碍（原命名为"原发性肌张力障碍"）的患者效果最好（Albanese 等，2019）。"原发性肌张力障碍"又包括了特发性和遗传性肌张力障碍，因此过去的报道通常还包含复合性肌张力障碍（Sasikumar 等，2019）。而早在 1999 年就已有苍白球 DBS 治疗颈部肌张力障碍的报道（Krauss 等，1999），随后 DBS 治疗全身型肌张力障碍得到关注，会议中展示的视频可看出其对症状显著的改善。最初误认为与躯干受累的肌张力障碍相比，伴肢体症状的肌张力障碍 DBS 的效果更明显，但后续研究未能证明这一观点（表 14-1）。之后有报道提出，虽然慢性刺激后肌张力障碍中的强直成分可能需要数月的时间才得到改善，但在刺激起始期便可改善某些时相性成分（Krause 等，2004）。

表 14-1 DBS 治疗肌张力障碍的常见适应证

单纯性	特发性和遗传性	单基因（如 DYT1、DYT6）
	获得性	药物诱发（迟发型）
复合性	特发性和遗传性	• 伴肌阵挛的肌张力障碍（如 SGCE 所致） • NBIA（如 PKAN） • X 连锁肌张力障碍 – 帕金森综合征 • 迅速进展型肌张力障碍 – 帕金森综合征 • Wilson 病
	获得性	• 脑性瘫痪 • 创伤性 • 出血性 / 缺氧性

PKAN. 泛酸激酶相关神经退行性病变；SGCE. ε– 肌聚糖；NBIA. 神经变性伴脑铁蓄积

一般而言，虽然部分患者可从手术中获益，大多数获得性（"继发性"）肌张力障碍患者的 DBS 疗效逊于特发性和遗传性肌张力障碍。虽然有报道称 MRI 阴性患者的手术效果不如 MRI 阳性。之后类似的研究较少，手术的疗效可能与病损的部位、大小有关。

通常获得性肌张力障碍患者 DBS 的疗效并不好，但其中的单纯性迟发性肌张力患者接受 DBS 后效果很好。在这种肌张力障碍的患者中，并未观察到脑部病变。

除此之外，当神经退行性疾病的患者出现肌张力障碍时，疾病通常呈进展性。在这种情况下，疗效可能会随时间推移逐渐减弱。另一个问题是获得性肌张力障碍的临床表现背后存在多种原因，但由于其罕见性，相关结果仅见于病例报告这一类论文中，也许是因为阴性结果不容易发表所造成的偏移。

与其他类型的肌张力障碍相同，应由患者和护理人员告诉我们哪些是术后决定生活质量的因素，并将手术指征建立在改善这些指标的基础上。

五、手术方式

在过去 20 年中，脑深部电刺激已成为肌张力障碍的一种重要的、得到认可的治疗方式。它出现于 20 世纪 90 年代，此后全球约 15 000 名患者接受了该手术。在此我们将对其发展历程及适应证作一概述。若想了解更深入的信息，可参考以下资料（Moro 等，2011；Dressler 等，2018），其中也包含其他手术方式。

在 20 世纪 60—70 年代，射频毁损术治疗肌张力障碍尝试了将多个丘脑核团作为靶点（Loher 等，2004），目前 DBS 的主要靶点是 GPi 腹后外侧核。刺激 GPi 可显著改善肌张力障碍的主要临床表现，且不良反应相对较少。近期报道称，DBS 对治疗轻微运动迟缓和步态问题，尤其是成年的节段型肌张力障碍患者效果较好，但其机制尚不清晰（Blahak 等，2011a；b；Schrader 等，2011），这一现象促使人们开始寻找新的靶点。在过去几年中，有研究将底丘脑核（Ostrem 等，2011，2017；Deng 等，2017；Zhan 等，2018）和丘脑核团（Pauls 等，2014；Wolf 等，2019）作为潜在的靶点，但尚未得到更广泛的关注。未来研究的难点在于明确腹外侧核中哪个区域是最理想的靶点——前部［即根据 Hassler 分区中的腹 – 嘴前核（Voa）］或后部［腹中间核（Vim）］，抑或是中间区域［过去称为腹 – 嘴后核（Vop）的区域］。

以 GPi 为靶点的立体定向脑深部电极植入术

可在清醒或全身麻醉下进行。伴有严重全身性肌张力障碍或肌张力障碍风暴的患者及儿童患者只能选择全麻手术（Ben-Haim 等，2016）。可通过立体定向核磁共振成像直接定位靶点，也可通过使用基于前-后连合的立体定向坐标系间接定位靶点。预定的腹侧后外侧 GPi 的坐标为：x = 20，y = + 3，z = -4。微电极记录是识别 GPi 感觉运动功能（sensorimotor GPi）的重要手段，对于确定靶点下界有重要意义（Alam 等，2015）。

对于所有接受 DBS 手术的患者，术后必须进行影像学检查，目的是排除颅内出血和记录电极位置以便于后续的 DBS 程控。已有研究证实了立体定向 CT 和非立体定向 MR 的价值。

手术不良反应与其他植入电极的运动障碍性疾病相似（Jitkritsadakul 等，2017）。最严重的并发症是有临床症状的出血，发生率约为 1%。早期，人们认为相比于其他运动障碍性疾病，肌张力障碍患者可能更容易发生电极或延伸导线断裂（Parkin 等，2001；Krause 等，2004），随后便意识到这是因为连接器放在颈部，放在其他部位即可解决（Jitkritsadakul 等，2017）。

对于颈部肌张力障碍、全身型肌张力障碍或偏身型肌张力障碍患者，均可以将 GPi 中的相同区域作为 DBS 长期刺激的靶点。直到近期才发现"最佳靶点"的位置位于 GPi 内。该靶点位于腹侧 GPi 的一个区域内，刺激这一区域会同时影响苍白球传出通路中的豆状襻和豆状束（Reich 等，2019）。有证据显示，诱发运动迟缓出现的"热点"区域与所谓的"最佳靶点"之间有较多重叠。

（一）肌张力障碍的 DBS 程控

与帕金森病或特发性震颤相比，肌张力障碍中的 DBS 程控情况特殊，其对肌张力障碍症状的影响有延迟性。因此，必须全程记录基线水平和症状严重时的情况（通过录像记录），在植入神经刺激系统后数天或数周内对 IPG 进行程序设计。时相性肌张力障碍患者有时会出现轻度的"顿抑效应"现象。

该如何设计肌张力障碍的慢性刺激程序，尚未达成共识，建议在术后早期和晚期分别进行设置（Kupsch 等，2011；Tagliati 等，2011；Picillo 等，2016）。通常我们用单极模式对 4 触点电极的触点进行阻抗检查，治疗阈值和可诱发不良反应的阈值也达成了共识。由于肌张力障碍症状改善通常会延迟，限制了对治疗效果的检测。各个中心所采用的刺激模式包括单极和双极。一般而言，选择 130Hz 或更高的频率作为早期刺激，脉冲宽度通常设定为 60～420μs，但脉冲宽度设置在各中心差异较大，初始电压或电流通常高于帕金森病的苍白球 DBS 的设置。

在术后早期随访时，可每隔 3 个月进行 1 次程控。在慢性刺激的最初几个月内逐渐增加刺激量对部分患者有效。在少数患者中，使用了更复杂的刺激程序，例如交错刺激或循环模式刺激。较低频率的刺激可以改善 DBS 的运动迟缓的不良反应，但从长期来看，许多患者需要恢复到 130Hz 的刺激以维持疗效。

（二）DBS 治疗肌张力障碍的机制

DBS 治疗肌张力障碍的机制是复杂的，并且改善还存在延迟，可能涉及基底节环路中可塑性适应不良、抑制性改变和病理性振荡活动（Ruge 等，2011a,b；Barow 等，2014）。

六、DBS 的疗效

（一）单纯性肌张力障碍

1. 特发性

许多前期研究集中于儿童和成人的全身型肌张力障碍（Bereznai 等，2002；Krauss 等，2003；Coubes 等，2004；Krauss 等，2004）。

根据 Burke Fahn 和 Marsden（BFM）运动量表评估，大多数研究显示有效率为 60%～90%。在大规模的研究中，研究对象通常包括全身型和节段型肌张力障碍患者（Isaias 等，2011）。第一项对结局设盲的多中心研究是 2005 年发表的法国 SPIDY 研究（Vidailhet 等，2005）。在纳入 22 名全身型肌张力障碍患者的前瞻性试验中，对患者进行了 3 年随访，结果 BFM 运动评分显著改善（降低 25.3 分），同时 BFM 残疾评分也显著改善（降低 5.1 分）（Vidailhet 等，2007）。

Kupsch 等在 2006 年发表的研究，为双侧苍白球 DBS 治疗全身型和节段型肌张力障碍的有效性提供了 I 级证据（Kupsch 等，2006）。该研究纳入了 40 名患者，前瞻性、随机地分配至刺激组和假性刺激组并观察 3 个月。对刺激组患者的苍白球给予低于无法引起其注意的刺激，其 BFM 运动评分降低 15.8 分，而假性刺激组降低 1.4 分。随访结果显示，疗效长期维持，且 BFM 运动评分和 BFM 残疾评分的平均改善率均为 60%（Volkmann 等，2012）。

多年来，已经有几项关于苍白球 DBS 治疗全身型和节段型肌张力障碍疗效的 Meta 分析（Andrews 等，2010；Moro 等，2017）。Moro 等的分析纳入了 24 项研究中的 523 名患者，结果显示 BFM 运动评分和 BFM 残疾评分的平均改善率分别为 65% 和 59%。

几项前期性研究证实了苍白球 DBS 治疗颈部肌张力障碍的安全性和有效性（Krauss 等，1999；Parkin 等，2001）。在西方国家，过去几年 DBS 几乎取代了其他的手术治疗方案，如选择性外周神经阻滞和肌肉切开术。早期研究显示，根据多伦多西部痉挛性斜颈评定量表（TWSTRS）的评分，苍白球 DBS 对其的改善率，如肌张力障碍严重程度 38%、疼痛 50%、功能性残疾 54%。随后，几项前瞻性临床试验验证了这些结果（Kiss 等，2007；Skogseid 等，2012）。一项包括 62 名患者的多中心、前瞻性、随机假刺激对照试验也提供了 I 级证据，经过 3 个月的治疗，刺激组中肌张力障碍的 TWSTRS 严重度评分降低 26%，而假刺激对照组仅降低了 6%（Volkmann 等，2014）。在研究的开放期，经过 6 个月的慢性刺激，TWSTRS 严重程度改善了 28%，疼痛改善了 51%，功能障碍评分改善了 51%。其他研究中，5 年随访时盲态视频评估显示改善程度与前述结果类似，其中 TWSRTS 运动评分降低 48%（Walsh 等，2013）。由于前期试验结果较理想，在德国开展了一项早期刺激研究，目前已开始招募患者，该研究旨在比较苍白球 DBS 与肉毒杆菌毒素注射的疗效。

根据几项小规模研究，双侧苍白球 DBS 对于 Meige 综合征效果良好（Capelle 等，2003；Ostrem 等，2007；Blomstedt 等，2008；Ghang 等，2010）。一项多中心回顾性研究证实，早期随访时 BFM 运动评分改善 45%，38.8 个月后平均改善 53%（Reese 等，2011），言语、吞咽，以及眼睑痉挛显著改善。这样的疗效在其他类型的节段型或局灶型肌张力障碍较为少见。在苍白球 DBS 治疗肌张力障碍性躯干前曲症（Capelle 等，2011；Reese 等，2014）和苍白球及丘脑 DBS 治疗书写痉挛和职业性肌张力障碍的研究中，改善率与前述相当（Cho 等，2009）。

2. 遗传性

单纯性全身型和节段型肌张力障碍 DBS 疗效的差异可能与潜在的不同遗传因素有关（Jinnah 等，2017）。有证据表明，苍白球 DBS 治疗伴随 TOR1A 突变（DYT1）的肌张力障碍比其他基因突变类型疗效更好。

在 TOR1A 突变患者的研究中，观察到了一致性良好的积极的结果（Cif 等，2010；Panov 等，2013）。一般而言，此类患者比单纯性特发性肌张力障碍患者的疗效出现得更早、更明显。对携带 TOR1A 突变的重度全身型肌张力障碍儿童，苍白球 DBS 可作为一线治疗方案。

苍白球 DBS 对携带 THAP1 突变（DYT6）的患者的疗效往往较差（Panov 等，2012；Brüggemann 等，2015；Groen 等，2010）。在 DYT1 和非 DYT 肌张力障碍的正面比较中，DYT6 肌张力障碍患者的 BFM 运动量表改善较少，早期随访时改善 32%，长期随访时改善达到 42%。然而在该研究中，与非 DYT 患者相比，该增益仍然明显较少（42% vs. 61%）。

3. 获得性

对苍白球 DBS 治疗肌张力障碍的研究显示，

迟发性肌张力障碍与"原发性肌张力障碍"的疗效相当（Trottenberg 等，2001），该结果得到了随后几个研究的证实（Capelle 等，2010；Chang 等，2010）。根据一篇纳入 95 名患者的文献综述，其中包括一些病例报告和病例数较少的研究，慢性刺激后 BFM 运动评分平均改善约为 70%（Gruber 和 Kupsch，2018）。来自法国的一项多中心对照研究报告了约 50% 的持续改善率，无情绪恶化或精神性疾病（Pouclet-Courtemanche 等，2016）。最近的一项假性刺激随机对照试验显示，在 3 个月随访时，相比于假性刺激组 12% 的改善率，实验组 BFM 运动评分改善了 23%，但差异无显著性（Gruber 等，2018）。在研究的开放阶段的第 6 个月，平均改善达到 42%。

（二）复合性肌张力障碍

1. 特发性和遗传性

各种定义明确的遗传性肌张力障碍，常伴随其他运动障碍性疾病（例如肌阵挛肌张力障碍或 NBIA，可能是特发性或继发于基因异常），DBS 治疗对于它们的效果不同。疗效不仅取决于肌张力障碍的改善，还取决于 DBS 对其他运动障碍性疾病、神经或精神症状所致残疾的影响。

DBS 在肌阵挛性肌张力障碍中的疗效得到了各项研究的一致认可，依据传统，该类肌张力障碍被命名为 DYT11 单基因肌张力障碍。GPi 和丘脑均被作为慢性刺激的靶点，有时两者同时作为靶点。苍白球 DBS 可显著改善肌阵挛和肌张力障碍，但与丘脑 DBS 相比，对肌张力障碍的作用更明显（Rughani 和 Lozano，2013）。在一项对多电极植入患者的研究中，丘脑和苍白球组合 DBS 在 8 名患者中有 6 名取得了更好的疗效（Gruber 等，2010）。关于 DBS 对肌阵挛性肌张力障碍相关精神症状的影响，根据现有数据得到的结论并不一致（Contarino 等，2011）。

X 连锁肌张力障碍 - 帕金森综合征（DYT3）患者接受苍白球 DBS 后，肌张力障碍和帕金森综合征均得到改善（Patel 等，2014）。一项观察性、前瞻性队列研究对 16 名患者进行了设盲视频评分，在 6 个月随访时，BFM 运动评分改善 59%，统一帕金森病评定量表（UPDRS）Ⅲ 评分平均改善 27%，长期随访中疗效保持良好（Brüggemann 等，2018）。

由于肌张力障碍可能是 NBIA 的突出症状，尤其是在最常见的 PKAN 亚型中，苍白球 DBS 已成为一种治疗方案（Castelnau 等，2005；Timmermann 等，2010）。近期一项使用独立数据的 Meta 分析，共纳入了 99 名 DBS 患者的信息。总体而言，1 年随访时 BFM 运动评分平均改善 26%（De Vloo 等，2019）。值得注意的是，年长的非典型 PKAN 患者（平均年龄 31 岁）的表现优于典型 PKAN 患者（平均年龄 11 岁），BFM 运动评分改善分别为 45% 和 16%。肌张力障碍越严重的患者改善越明显。

关于苍白球 DBS 对起病迅速的肌张力障碍 - 帕金森综合征（DYT12）的疗效的研究较少。大多数病例报告表明，苍白球 DBS 对这种罕见疾病的疗效有限（Deutschländer 等，2005）。

2. 获得性

DBS 治疗在获得性肌张力障碍中的应用，多见于肌张力障碍/运动障碍或"舞蹈手足徐动症"脑瘫（"choreoathetotic" cerebral palsy），这些疾病通常也与痉挛和其他神经症状有关（Elia 等，2018）。早期研究发现苍白球 DBS 的疗效存在很大差异（Krauss 等，2003；Koy 等，2013）。随后研究发现，运动评分的改善与主观改善程度并不一致。对于低龄儿童或成年患者，应该如何选择 DBS 的手术时机仍不清楚。法国的一项多中心、前瞻性、开放试验中，系统地研究了 13 名肌张力障碍/异动症样 - 舞蹈手足徐动症脑瘫（dystonic/dyskinetic or choreoathetotic cerebral palsy）成人患者的疗效（Vidailh 等，2009）。在 12 个月随访时，BFM 运动评分平均改善 24%，但存在很大的个体差异。虽然 4 名患者的改善范围为 39%~55%，但另外 4 名患者改善 < 20%，视为治疗无效。在对 20 项 DBS 治疗脑瘫研究的系统性综述中，手术年龄与临床疗效之间没有

相关性（Koy 等，2013）。术前肌张力障碍越严重，慢性 DBS 的术后改善程度越小。一些团队在肌张力障碍脑瘫的低龄患者中推广了苍白球 DBS 的使用，而一些其他团队并不认同这一观点（Gimeno 等，2014；Koy 等，2017；Elkaim 等，2019）。

对继发于创伤或脑血管病变的基底神经节病变导致的偏身型肌张力障碍，运用苍白球和丘脑 DBS 治疗的案例较少。意外的是，某些报道中出现了显著而持续的改善，但另一些报道中结果不同（Loher 等，2000；Slow 等，2015）。

对 DBS 治疗获得性肌张力障碍的疗效进行评价时，除了症状严重程度的相关量表，还应参考其他因素。除了残疾和生活质量的变化，还需要考虑患者的个体特点，可能需要重新定义这些重度残疾患者治疗的"成功"或"失败"（Gimeno 和 Lin，2017）。由于某些类型的肌张力障碍罕见，可能要通过不同民族之间的合作来实现这一目标。

（三）长期随访和生活质量

与帕金森病或特发性震颤不同，接受 DBS 手术之后，大多数患者的病程不再继续进展，或进展非常迟缓。虽然几个月后刺激疗效才完全展现出来，但之后几年，大多数患者出现了进行性改善（Loher 等，2008；Cif 等，2013；Volkmann 等，2012；Meoni 等，2017）。对于慢性苍白球 DBS 治疗期间，肌张力障碍复发或进展的少数患者，可以考虑植入额外的苍白球电极（Cif 等，2012），慢性苍白球 DBS 的长期疗效通常比术后 1-2 年更明显。令人费解的是，在术后早期停止刺激后，数分钟至数小时内肌张力障碍可能会复发（Grips 等，2007），但术后多年再停止刺激时，症状并不会马上出现（Cif 等，2013）。考虑到慢性刺激对神经可塑性的影响，DBS 可作为一种疾病修饰疗法，在疾病早期选择接受 DBS 也是合理的，而不只是保守治疗无效或效果不佳时。

在特发性和遗传性肌张力障碍患者中，通过标准评定量表（如 BFM 或 TWSTRS）评估得到的肌张力障碍严重程度和相关残疾改善情况，通常与生活质量的改善相当（Blahak 等，2008；Mueller 等，2008；Isaias 等，2009）。最近的数据表明，通过非疾病特异性量表（如 SF 36）评估的生活质量改善，在慢性刺激开始后维持了 10 年以上（Hogg 等，2018）。值得注意的是，不同遗传背景患者之间的运动改善差异，并不一定导致长期随访时生活质量的显著差异（Isaias 等，2011；Hogg 等，2018）。

如上所述，评价 DBS 的实际疗效及其对获得性肌张力障碍患者生活质量的改善具有一定难度。而在少数研究中，应用 SF 36 证实了一些分项评分的改善（Vidailhet 等，2009），其他评分表包括加拿大职业性量表或患者自我评定量表（Krauss 等，2003；Gimeno 和 Lin 2017）。

（四）非应答患者和疗效预测

在 DBS 治疗肌张力障碍的大量研究中，有小部分患者经过长期的 DBS 治疗后无效，包括原发性和继发性的治疗无效，前者定义为在标准肌张力障碍运动评定量表的改善率 < 25%，后者定义为治疗初期有效而后期疗效减退。此外，尽管有时根据评定量表得出了"客观"有效的结论，但有可能患者对疗效并不满意。

一项纳入 11 个中心的 22 名单纯性特发性或遗传性肌张力障碍患者的研究显示，治疗无效患者中半数存在电极放置位置有误及其他问题（Pauls 等，2017），除此之外，有 5 名患者存在固定性的畸形，2 名患者存在精神性疾病。

经证实，最重要的预后因素包括手术年龄和患病时间（Andrews 等，2010；Isaias 等，2011）。由于遗传因素发挥着主要作用，至少在慢性刺激的前几年，建议对接受 DBS 肌张力障碍患者进行基因检测（Jinnah 等，2017）。

七、DBS 治疗肌张力障碍的不良反应

导线断裂、皮肤糜烂和感染等硬件相关

并发症的发生率与其他运动障碍性疾病相似（itkritsadakul 等，2017）。当电极过于靠近内囊时，可能会出现内囊刺激反应（肌肉抽搐、构音障碍、眼球运动异常），导致无法达到最佳电流。总体而言，苍白球刺激对于情绪和认知功能是安全的（Pillon 等，2006；Meoni 等，2015）。

由于刺激强度较高，植入的脉冲发生器需要尽早更换电池，有时在两年后即需要更换（Blahak 等，2011a；b）。对于这些患者，电池寿命长达 15 年的可充电植入式脉冲发生器（IPG）是更好的选择（Perez 等，2017）。在苍白球 DBS 术后的前几年由于 IPG 的电量突然耗尽，可导致肌张力障碍的复发，因此常需要预先更换 IPG（Grips 等，2007）。在少数情况下，可能进展成危及生命的肌张力障碍风暴（Ben-Haim 等，2016）。

慢性 DBS 治疗肌张力障碍的罕见的不良反应是出现轻度帕金森症状，如小写症、运动迟缓和步态变化（Tisch 等，2007；Berman 等，2009；Blahak 等，2011a；b；Schrader 等，2011）。肌张力障碍的显著改善可能掩盖这些不良反应，只有通过仔细的针对性检查才能观察到。少数情况会表现为帕金森综合征（Schrader 等，2011）。这些不良反应在节段型比全身型肌张力障碍更常见，之前未受累的肢体可能会出现运动迟缓。研究发现，DBS 对手指敲击速度存在频率特异性调节，在高频刺激下恶化，在较低频率下得到改善（Huebl 等，2015）。在一项对 71 名肌张力障碍患者进行的队列研究中，6 名患者由起步困难发展为步长缩短，直至出现冻结态和慌张步态而跌倒（Schrader 等，2011）。这些不良反应的潜在机制尚未完全阐明，可能与皮质发育、神经信号改变之间存在复杂的相互作用（Huebl 等，2015；Mahlknecht 等，2018）。

不良反应中运动障碍发生的频率尚不明确，而这很大程度上取决于刺激强度。值得注意的是，虽未得到大规模的多中心、前瞻性试验证实，但有时可通过详细的检查而发现。在一项对 10 名节段型肌张力障碍患者进行的研究中，原本没有注意到患者步态的任何变化，但是采用慢性苍白球 DBS 时平均步长减少了约 10%，且步态的变异率（variability）明显降低（Wolf 等，2016）。在对 37 名接受慢性苍白球 DBS 治疗并随访至少 5 年的患者进行的问卷调查中，患者的运动障碍并发症包括声音低沉（30%）、表情缺乏（8%）或冻结步态（8%）（Hogg 等，2018）。在最近的一项研究中，与未接受刺激的肌张力障碍患者相比，接受慢性苍白球刺激的肌张力障碍患者的运动迟缓更显著，UPDRS 的轴性运动分项评分较高，而 2 组之间的震颤和强直分项评分没有差异（Mahlknecht 等，2018）。

出乎意料的是，慢性苍白球 DBS 患者中，也观察到了过度运动的现象（Wloch 等，2017），而这有可能与电极位置更靠近苍白球外侧有关。

八、结论

DBS 治疗肌张力障碍具有挑战性。由于各种肌张力障碍综合征的个体差异大、症状复杂且相对罕见，开展临床工作需要在该领域具备较深的专业知识。因此，建议由多学科团队共同做出决策，如决定哪些患者适合接受 DBS、何时进行手术，以及选择哪里作为靶点。

医疗团队应该综合考虑患者和医护人员的预期、治疗的优势与不足，以帮助患者实现预期的治疗目标。

最后，术前评估和术后管理不应只关注于运动症状，还应重点考察影响着生活质量的社会和心理因素，这一点至关重要。

参考文献

[1] Alam M, Schwabe K, Lütjens G, Capelle HH, Manu M, von Wrangel C, Müller-Vahl K, Schrader C, Scheinichen D, Blahak C, Heissler HE, Krauss JK. Comparative characterization of single cell activity in the globus pallidus internus of patients with dystonia or Tourette syndrome. J Neural Transm. 2015;122(5):687–99.

[2] Albanese A, Bhatia K, Bressman SB, DeLong MR, Fahn S, Fung VSC, et al. Phenomenology and classification of dystonia: a consensus update. Mov Disord. 2013;28:863–73.

[3] Albanese A, Di Giovanni M, Lalli S. Dystonia: diagnosis and

[4] Andrews C, Aviles-Olmos I, Hariz M, Foltynie T. Which patients with dystonia benefit from deep brain stimulation? A metaregression of individual patient outcomes. J Neurol Neurosurg Psychiatry. 2010;81(12):1383–9.

[5] Barow E, Neumann WJ, Brücke C, Huebl J, Horn A, Brown P, Krauss JK, Schneider GH, Kühn AA. Deep brain stimulation suppresses pallidal low frequency activity in patients with phasic dystonic movements. Brain. 2014;137(Pt 11):3012–24.

[6] Ben-Haim S, Flatow V, Cheung T, Cho C, Tagliati M, Alterman RL. Deep brain stimulation for status dystonicus: a case series and review of the literature. Stereotact Funct Neurosurg. 2016;94(4):207–15.

[7] Bereznai B, Steude U, Seelos K, Botzel K. Chronic high-frequency globus pallidus internus stimulation in different types of dystonia: a clinical, video, and MRI report of six patients presenting with segmental, cervical, and generalized dystonia. Mov Disord. 2002;17:138–44.

[8] Berman BD, Starr PA, Marks WJ Jr, Ostrem JL. Induction of bradykinesia with pallidal deep brain stimulation in patients with cranial-cervical dystonia. Stereotact Funct Neurosurg. 2009;87:37–44.

[9] Blahak C, Wöhrle JC, Capelle HH, Baezner H, Grips E, Weigel R, Kekelia K, Krauss JK. Health-related quality of life in segmental dystonia is improved by bilateral pallidal stimulation. J Neurol. 2008;255: 178–82.

[10] Blahak C, Capelle HH, Baezner H, Kinfe TM, Hennerici MG, Krauss JK. Micrographia induced by pallidal DBS for segmental dystonia: a subtle sign of hypokinesia? J Neural Transm. 2011a;118:549–53.

[11] Blahak C, Capelle HH, Baezner H, Kinfe TM, Hennerici MG, Krauss JK. Battery lifetime in pallidal deep brain stimulation for dystonia. Eur J Neurol. 2011b;18(6):872–5.

[12] Blomstedt P, Tisch S, Hariz MI. Pallidal deep brain stimulation in the treatment of Meige syndrome. Acta Neurol Scand. 2008;118:198–202.

[13] Brüggemann N, Kühn A, Schneider SA, Kamm C, Wolters A, Krause P, Moro E, Steigerwald F, Wittstock M, Tronnier V, Lozano AM, Hamani C, Poon YY, Zittel S, Wächter T, Deuschl G, Krüger R, Kupsch A, Münchau A, Lohmann K, Volkmann J, Klein C. Shortand long-term outcome of chronic pallidal neurostimulation in monogenic isolated dystonia. Neurology. 2015;84(9):895–903.

[14] Brüggemann N, Domingo A, Rasche D, Moll CKE, Rosales RL, Jamora RDG, Hanssen H, Münchau A, Graf J, Weissbach A, Tadic V, Diesta CC, Volkmann J, Kühn A, Münte TF, Tronnier V, Klein C. Association of pallidal neurostimulation and outcome predictors with X-linked dystonia parkinsonism. JAMA Neurol. 2018;76(2):211–6.

[15] Capelle HH, Weigel R, Krauss JK. Bilateral stimulation of the globus pallidus for treatment of blepharospasm-oromandibular dystonia (Meige syndrome). Neurology. 2003;60:2017–8.

[16] Capelle HH, Blahak C, Schrader C, Baezner H, Kinfe TM, Herzog J, Dengler R, Krauss JK. Chronic deep brain stimulation in patients with tardive dystonia without a history of major psychosis. Mov Disord. 2010;25:1477–81.

[17] Capelle HH, Schrader C, Blahak C, Fogel W, Kinfe TM, Bäzner H, Krauss JK. Deep brain stimulation for camptocormia in dystonia and Parkinson's disease. J Neurol. 2011;258:96–103.

[18] Castelnau P, Cif L, Valente EM, Vayssiere N, Hemm S, Gannau A, Digiorgio A, Coubes P. Pallidal stimulation improves pantothenate kinase-associated neurodegeneration. Ann Neurol. 2005;57(5):738–41.

[19] Chang EF, Schrock LE, Starr PA, Ostrem JL. Long-term benefit sustained after bilateral pallidal deep brain stimulation in patients with refractory tardive dystonia. Stereotact Funct Neurosurg. 2010;88(5):304–10.

[20] Cho CB, Park HK, Lee KJ, Rha HK. Thalamic deep brain stimulation for writer's cramp. J Korean Neurosurg Soc. 2009;46(1):52–5.

[21] Cif L, Vasques X, Gonzalez V, Ravel P, Biolsi B, Collod-Beroud G, Tuffery-Giraud S, Elfertit H, Claustres M, Coubes P. Long-term follow-up of DYT1 dystonia patients treated by deep brain stimulation: an open-label study. Mov Disord. 2010;25(3):289–99.

[22] Cif L, Gonzalez-Martinez V, Vasques X, Corlobé A, Moura AM, Bonafé A, Coubes P. Staged implantation of multiple electrodes in the internal globus pallidus in the treatment of primary generalized dystonia. J Neurosurg. 2012;116(5):1144–52.

[23] Cif L, Ruge D, Gonzalez V, Limousin P, Vasques X, Hariz MI, Rothwell J, Coubes P. The influence of deep brain stimulation intensity and duration on symptoms evolution in an OFF stimulation dystonia study. Brain Stimul. 2013;6(4):500–5.

[24] Contarino MF, Foncke EM, Cath DC, Schuurman PR, Speelman JD, Tijssen MA. Effect of pallidal deep brain stimulation on psychiatric symptoms in myoclonus-dystonia due to epsilon-sarcoglycan mutations. Arch Neurol. 2011;68:1087–8.

[25] Contarino MF, Smit M, van den Dool J, Volkmann J, Tijssen MA. Unmet needs in the management of cervical dystonia. Front Neurol. 2016;7:165. eCollection 2016. Erratum in: Front Neurol. 2016 Dec 19;7:232.

[26] Contarino MF, Van Den Dool J, Balash Y, Bhatia K, Giladi N, Koelman JH, Lokkegaard A, Marti MJ, Postma M, Relja M, Skorvanek M, Speelman JD, Zoons E, Ferreira JJ, Vidailhet M, Albanese A, Tijssen MA. Clinical practice: evidence-based recommendations for the treatment of cervical dystonia with Botulinum toxin. Front Neurol. 2017;8:35.

[27] Coubes P, Roubertie A, Vayssiere N, Hemm S, Echenne B. Treatment of DYT1-generalized dystonia by stimulation of the internal globus pallidus. Lancet. 2000;355:2220–1.

[28] Coubes P, Cif L, El Fertit H, Hemm S, Vayssiere N, Serrat S, Picot MC, Tuffery S, Claustres M, Echenne B, Frerebeau P. Electrical stimulation of the globus pallidus internus in patients with primary generalized dystonia: long-term results. J Neurosurg. 2004;101(2):189–94.

[29] De Vloo P, Lee DJ, Dallapiazza RF, Rohani M, Fasano A, Munhoz RP, Ibrahim GM, Hodaie M, Lozano AM, Kalia SK. Deep brain stimulation for pantothenate kinase-associated neurodegeneration: a meta-analysis. Mov Disord. 2019;34(2):264–73.

[30] Delnooz CC, Horstink MW, Tijssen MA, van de Warrenburg BP. Paramedical treatment in primary dystonia: a systematic review. Mov Disord. 2009;18:231–40.

[31] Deng ZD, Li DY, Zhang CC, Pan YX, Zhang J, Jin H, Zeljec K, Zhan SK, Sun BM. Long-term follow-up of bilateral subthalamic deep brain stimulation for refractory tardive dystonia. Parkinsonism Relat Disord. 2017;41:58–65.

[32] Deutschländer A, Asmus F, Gasser T, Steude U, Bötzel K. Sporadic rapid-onset dystonia-parkinsonism syndrome: failure of bilateral pallidal stimulation. Mov Disord. 2005;20(2):254–7.

[33] Dressler D, Altenmüller E, Krauss JK, editors. Treatment of dystonia. Cambridge: Cambridge University Press; 2018.

[34] Egger K, Mueller J, Schocke M, Brenneis C, Rinnerthaler M, Seppi K, et al. Voxel bases morphometry reveals specific gray matter changes in primary dystonia. Mov Disord. 2007;22:1538–42.

[35] Eggink H, Kremer D, Brouwer OF, Contarino MF, van Egmond ME, Elema A, Folmer K, van Hoorn JF, van de Pol LA, Roelfsema V, Tijssen MAJ. Spasticity, dyskinesia and ataxia in cerebral palsy: are we sure we can differentiate them? Eur J Paediatr Neurol. 2017;21(5):703–6.

[36] Elia AE, Bagella CF, Ferré F, Zorzi G, Calandrella D, Romito LM. Deep brain stimulation for dystonia due to cerebral palsy: a review. Eur J Paediatr Neurol. 2018;22(2):308–15.

[37] Elkaim LM, Alotaibi NM, Sigal A, Alotaibi HM, Lipsman N, Kalia SK, Fehlings DL, Lozano AM, Ibrahim GM, North American Pediatric DBS Collaboration. Deep brain stimulation for pediatric dystonia: a meta-analysis with individual participant data. Dev Med Child Neurol. 2019;61(1):49–56.

[38] Eltahawy HA, Saint-Cyr J, Giladi N, Lang AE, Lozano AM. Primary dystonia is more responsive than secondary dystonia to pallidal interventions: outcome after pallidotomy or pallidal deep brain stimulation. Neurosurgery. 2004;54(3):613–9.

[39] Fabbrini G, Berardelli I, Moretti G, Pasquini M, Bloise M, Colosimo C, et al. Psychiatric disorders in adultonset focal dystonia: a case-control study. Mov Disord. 2010;25:459–65.

[40] Ghang JY, Lee MK, Jun SM, Ghang CG. Outcome of pallidal deep brain stimulation in Meige syndrome. J Korean Neurosurg Soc. 2010;48: 134–8.

[41] Gimeno H, Lin JP. The international classification of functioning (ICF) to evaluate deep brain stimulation neuromodulation in childhood dystonia-hyperkinesia informs future clinical & research priorities in a multidisciplinary model of care. Eur J Paediatr Neurol. 2017;21(1):147–67.

[42] Gimeno H, Tustin K, Lumsden D, Ashkan K, Selway R, Lin JP. Evaluation of functional goal outcomes using the Canadian Occupational Performance Measure (COPM) following Deep Brain Stimulation (DBS) in childhood dystonia. Eur J Paediatr Neurol. 2014;18(3):308–16.

[43] Grips E, Blahak C, Capelle HH, Bazner H, Weigel R, Sedlaczek O, Krauss JK, Wohrle JC. Patterns of reoccurrence of segmental dystonia after discontinuation of deep brain stimulation. J Neurol Neurosurg Psychiatry. 2007;78(3):318–20.

[44] Groen JL, Ritz K, Contarino MF, van de Warrenburg BF, Aramideh M, Foncke EM, van Hilten JJ, Schuurman PR, Speelman JD, Koelman JH, de Bie RM, Baas F, Tijssen MA. DYT6 dystonia: mutation screening, phenotype, and response to deep brain stimulation. Mov Disord. 2010;25(14):2420–7.

[45] Gruber D, Kupsch A. Deep brain stimulation for tardive dystonia. In: Dressler D, Altenmüller E, Krauss JK, editors. Treatment of dystonia. Cambridge: Cambridge University Press; 2018. p. 372–7.

[46] Gruber D, Kühn AA, Schoenecker T, Kivi A, Trottenberg T, Hoffmann KT, Gharabaghi A, Kopp UA, Schneider GH, Klein C, Asmus F, Kupsch A. Pallidal and thalamic deep brain stimulation in myoclonus-dystonia. Mov Disord. 2010;25(11):1733–43.

[47] Gruber D, Südmeyer M, Deuschl G, Falk D, Krauss JK, Mueller J, Müller JU, Poewe W, Schneider GH, Schrader C, Vesper J, Volkmann J, Winter C, Kupsch A, Schnitzler A, DBS Study Group for Dystonia. Neurostimulation in tardive dystonia/dyskinesia: a delayed start, sham stimulation-controlled randomized trial. Brain Stimul. 2018;11:1368–77.

[48] Guehl D, Cuny E, Ghorayeb I, Michelet T, Bioulac B, Burbaud P. Primate models of dystonia. Prog Neurobiol. 2009;87:118–31.

[49] Hälbig TD, Gruber D, Kopp UA, Schneider GH, Trottenberg T, Kupsch A. Pallidal stimulation in dystonia: effects on cognition, mood and quality of life. J Neurol Neurosurg Psychiatry. 2005;76:1713–6.

[50] Hogg E, During E, Tan E, Athreya K, Eskenazi J, Wertheimer J, Mamelak AN, Alterman RL, Tagliati M. Sustained quality-of-life improvements over 10 years after deep brain stimulation for dystonia. Mov Disord. 2018;33(7):1160–7.

[51] Huebl J, Brücke C, Schneider GH, Blahak C, Krauss JK, Kühn AA. Bradykinesia induced by frequency-specific pallidal stimulation in patients with cervical and segmental dystonia. Parkinsonism Relat Disord. 2015;21(7):800–3.

[52] Isaias IU, Alterman RL, Tagliati M. Outcome predictors of pallidal stimulation in patients with primary with primary dystonia: the disease duration. Brain. 2008;131:1895–902.

[53] Isaias IU, Alterman RL, Tagliati M. Deep brain stimulation for primary generalized dystonia: long-term outcomes. Arch Neurol. 2009;66:465–70.

[54] Isaias IU, Alterman RL, Tagliati M. Factors predicting protracted improvement after pallidal DBS for primary dystonia: the role of age and disease duration. J Neurol. 2011;258:1469–76.

[55] Jankovic J. Medical treatment of dystonia. Mov Disord. 2013;28(7):1001–12.

[56] Jinnah HA, Hess EJ, Ledoux MS, Sarma N, Baxter MG, Delong MR. Rodent models for dystonia research: characteristics, evaluation, and utility. Mov Disord. 2005;20:283–92.

[57] Jinnah HA, Alterman R, Klein C, Krauss JK, Moro E, Vidailhet M, Raike R. Deep brain stimulation for dystonia: A novel perspective on the value of genetic testing. J Neural Transm. 2017;124:417–30.

[58] Jitkritsadakul O, Bhidayasiri R, Kalia SK, Hodaie M, Lozano AM, Fasano A. Systematic review of hardware-related complications of deep brain stimulation: do new indications pose an increased risk? Brain Stimul. 2017;10(5):967–76.

[59] Kiss ZH, Doig-Beyaert K, Eliasziw M, Tsui J, Haffenden A, Suchowersky O, Functional and Stereotactic Section of the Canadian Neurosurgical Society; Canadian Movement Disorders Group. The Canadian multicentre study of deep brain stimulation for cervical dystonia. Brain. 2007;130(Pt 11):2879–86.

[60] Konczak J, Abbruzzese G. Focal dystonia in musicians: linking motor symptoms to somatosensory dysfunction. Hum Neurosci. 2013;7:297.

[61] Koy A, Hellmich M, Pauls KA, Marks W, Lin JP, Fricke O, Timmermann L. Effects of deep brain stimulation in dyskinetic cerebral palsy: a meta-analysis. Mov Disord. 2013;28(5):647–54.

[62] Koy A, Weinsheimer M, Pauls KAM, Kühn AA, Krause P, Huebl J, Schneider GH, Deuschl G, Erasmi R, Falk D, Krauss JK, Lütjens G, Schnitzler A, Wojtecki L, Vesper J, Korinthenberg J, Coenen VA, Visser-Vandewalle V, Hellmich M, Timmermann L, GEPESTIM consortium. German registry of paediatric deep brain stimulation in patients with childhood-onset dystonia (GEPESTIM). Eur J Ped Neurol. 2017;21: 136–46.

[63] Krause M, Fogel W, Kloss M, Rasche D, Volkmann J, Tronnier V. Pallidal stimulation for dystonia. Neurosurgery. 2004;55(6):1361–8.

[64] Krauss JK, Pohle T, Weber S, Ozdoba C, Burgunder JM. Bilateral stimulation of globus pallidus internus for treatment of cervical dystonia. Lancet. 1999;354(9181):837–8.

[65] Krauss JK, Loher TJ, Weigel R, Capelle HH, Weber S, Burgunder JM. Chronic stimulation of the globus pallidus internus for treatment of non-dYT1 generalized dystonia and choreoathetosis: 2-year follow up. J Neurosurg. 2003;98:785–92.

[66] Krauss JK, Yianni J, Loher TJ, Aziz TZ. Deep brain stimulation for dystonia. J Clin Neurophysiol. 2004;21:18–30.

[67] Kumar R, Dagher A, Hutchison WD, Lang AE, Lozano AM. Globus pallidus deep brain stimulation for generalized dystonia: clinical and PET investigation. Neurology. 1999;53(4):871–4.

[68] Kupsch A, Benecke R, Muller J, Trottenberg T, Schneider GH, Poewe W, Eisner W, Wolters A, Muller JU, Deuschl G, Pinsker MO, Skogseid IM, Roeste GK, Vollmer-Haase J, Brentrup A, Krause M, Tronnier V, Schnitzler A, Voges J, Nikkhah G, Vesper J, Naumann M, Volkmann J, Deep-Brain Stimulation for Dystonia Study Group. Pallidal deep-brain stimulation in primary generalized or segmental dystonia. N Engl J Med. 2006;355(19):1978–90.

[69] Kupsch A, Tagliati M, Vidailhet M, Aziz T, Krack P, Moro E, Krauss JK. Early postoperative management of DBS in dystonia: programming, response to stimulation, adverse events, medication changes, evaluations, and troubleshooting. Mov Disord. 2011;26(S1):S37–53.

[70] Lehéricy S, Tijssen MA, Vidailhet M, Kaji R, Meunier S. The anatomical basis of dystonia: current view using neuroimaging. Mov Disord. 2013;28(7):944–57.

[71] Loher TJ, Hasdemir MG, Burgunder JM, Krauss JK. Long-term follow-up study of chronic globus pallidus internus stimulation for posttraumatic hemidystonia. J Neurosurg. 2000;92:457–60.

[72] Loher T, Pohle T, Krauss JK. Functional stereotactic surgery for treatment of cervical dystonia. Review of the experience from the lesional era. Stereotact Funct Neurosurg. 2004;82(1):1–13.

[73] Loher TJ, Capelle H-H, Kaeling-Lang A, et al. Deep brain stimulation for dystonia: outcome at long-term follow-up. J Neurol. 2008;255:881–4.

[74] Lohmann K, Klein C. Update on the genetics of dystonia. Curr Neurol Neurosci Rep. 2017;17(3):26.

[75] Mahlknecht P, Georgiev D, Akram H, Brugger F, Vinke S, Zrinzo L, Hariz M, Bhatia KP, Hariz GM, Willeit P, Rothwell JC, Foltynie T, Limousin P. Parkinsonian signs in patients with cervical dystonia treated with pallidal deep brain stimulation. Brain. 2018;14:3023–34.

[76] Meoni S, Zurowski M, Lozano AM, Hodaie M, Poon YY, Fallis M, Voon V, Moro E. Long-term neuropsychiatric outcomes after pallidal stimulation in primary and secondary dystonia. Neurology. 2015;85(5):433–40.

[77] Meoni S, Fraix V, Castrioto A, Benabid AL, Seigneuret E, Vercueil L, Pollak P, Krack P, Chevrier E, Chabardes S, Moro E. Pallidal deep brain stimulation for dystonia: a long term study. J Neurol Neurosurg Psychiatry. 2017;88(11):960–7.

[78] Moro E, Albanese A, Krauss JK, Metman LV, Vidailhet M, Hariz MI. Deep brain stimulation for dystonia: the state of the art. Mov Disord. 2011;26(S1):S1–S78.

[79] Moro E, LeReun C, Krauss JK, Albanese A, Lin JP, Walleser Autiero S, Brionne TC, Vidailhet M. Efficacy of pallidal

stimulation in isolated dystonia: a systematic review and meta-analysis. Eur J Neurol. 2017;24:552–60.

[80] Mueller J, Skogseid IM, Benecke R, Kupsch A, Trottenberg T, Poewe W, Schneider GH, Eisner W, Wolters A, Müller JU, Deuschl G, Pinsker MO, Roeste GK, Vollmer-Haase J, Brentrup A, Krause M, Tronnier V, Schnitzler A, Voges J, Nikkhah G, Vesper J, Naumann M, Volkmann J. Deep-Brain Stimulation for Dystonia Study Group: pallidal deep brain stimulation improves quality of life in segmental and generalized dystonia: results from a prospective, randomized sham-controlled trial. Mov Disord. 2008;23:131–4.

[81] Neychev VK, Gross RE, Lehéricy S, Hess EJ, Jinnah HA. The functional neuroanatomy of dystonia. Neurobiol Dis. 2011;42:185–201.

[82] Oppenheim H. About a rare spasm disease of childhood and young age (Dysbasia lordotica progressiva, dystonia musculorum deformans). Neurologische Centralblatt. 1911;30:1090–107.

[83] Ostrem JL, Marks WJ, Volz MM, Heath SL, Starr PA. Pallidal deep brain stimulation in patients with cranial-cervical dystonia (Meige syndrome). Mov Disord. 2007;22:2885–1891.

[84] Ostrem JL, Racine CA, Glass GA, Grace JK, Volz MM, Heath SL, Starr PA. Subthalamic nucleus deep brain stimulation in primary cervical dystonia. Neurology. 2011;76(10):870–8.

[85] Ostrem JL, San Luciano M, Dodenhoff KA, Ziman N, Markun LC, Racine CA, de Hemptinne C, Volz MM, Heath SL, Starr PA. Subthalamic nucleus deep brain stimulation in isolated dystonia: a 3-year follow-up study. Neurology. 2017;88(1):25–35.

[86] Panov F, Tagliati M, Ozelius LJ, Fuchs T, Gologorsky Y, Cheung T, Avshalumov M, Bressman SB, Saunders-Pullman R, Weisz D, Alterman RL. Pallidal deep brain stimulation for DYT6 dystonia. J Neurol Neurosurg Psychiatry. 2012;83(2):182–7.

[87] Panov F, Gologorsky Y, Connors G, Tagliati M, Miravite J, Alterman RL. Deep brain stimulation in DYT1 dystonia: a 10-year experience. Neurosurgery. 2013;73(1):86–93; discussion 93.

[88] Parkin S, Aziz T, Gregory R, Bain P. Bilateral internal globus pallidus stimulation for the treatment of spasmodic torticollis. Mov Disord. 2001;16(3):489–93.

[89] Patel AJ, Sarwar AI, Jankovic J, Viswanathan A. Bilateral pallidal deep brain stimulation for X-linked dystonia-parkinsonism. World Neurosurg. 2014;82(1-2):241.e1–4.

[90] Pauls KA, Hammesfahr S, Moro E, Moore AP, Binder E, El Majdoub F, Fink GR, Sturm V, Krauss JK, Maarouf M, Timmermann L. Deep brain stimulation in the ventrolateral thalamus/subthalamic area in dystonia with head tremor. Mov Disord. 2014;29(7):953–9.

[91] Pauls KAM, Krauss JK, Kämpfer CE, Kühn AA, Schrader C, Südmeyer M, Allert N, Benecke R, Blahak C, Boller JK, Fink GR, Fogel W, Liebig T, El Majdoub F, Mahlknecht P, Kessler J, Mueller J, Voges J, Wittstock M, Wolters A, Maarouf M, Moro E, Volkmann J, Bhatia KP, Timmermann L. Causes of failure of pallidal deep brain stimulation in cases with pre-operative diagnosis of isolated dystonia. Parkinsonism Relat Disord. 2017;43:38–48.

[92] Perez J, Gonzalez V, Cif L, Cyprien F, Chan-Seng E, Coubes P. Rechargeable or nonrechargeable deep brain stimulation in dystonia: a cost analysis. Neuromodulation. 2017;20(3):243–7.

[93] Picillo M, Lozano AM, Kou N, Munhoz RP, Fasano A. Programming deep brain stimulation for tremor and dystonia: the Toronto Western Hospital Algorithms. Brain Stimul. 2016;9(3):438–52.

[94] Pillon B, Ardouin C, Dujardin K, Vittini P, Pelissolo A, Cottencin O, Vercueil L, Houeto JL, Krystkowiak P, Agid Y, Destée A, Pollak P, Vidailhet M, French SPIDY Study Group. Preservation of cognitive function in dystonia treated by pallidal stimulation. Neurology. 2006;66(10):1556–8.

[95] Pouclet-Courtemanche H, Rouaud T, Thobois S, Nguyen JM, Brefel-Courbon C, Chereau I, Cuny E, Derost P, Eusebio A, Guehl D, Laurencin C, Mertens P, Ory-Magne F, Raoul S, Regis J, Ulla M, Witjas T, Burbaud P, Rascol O, Damier P. Long-term efficacy and tolerability of bilateral pallidal stimulation to treat tardive dyskinesia. Neurology. 2016;86(7):651–9.

[96] Reese R, Gruber D, Schoenecker T, Baezner HJ, Blahak C, Capelle HH, Falk D, Herzog J, Pinsker MO, Schneider GH, Schrader C, Deuschl G, Mehdorn HM, Kupsch A, Volkmann J, Krauss JK. Long-term clinical outcome in Meige syndrome treated with internal pallidum deep brain stimulation. Mov Disord. 2011;26:691–8.

[97] Reese R, Knudsen K, Falk D, Mehdorn HM, Deuschl G, Volkmann J. Motor outcome of dystonic camptocormia treated with pallidal neurostimulation. Parkinsonism Relat Disord. 2014;20(2):176–9.

[98] Reich MM, Horn A, Lange F, Roothans J, Paschen S, Runge J, Wodarg F, Pozzi NG, Witt K, Nickl RC, Soussand L, Ewert S, Maltese V, Wittstock M, Schneider GH, Coenen V, Mahlknecht P, Poewe W, Eisner W, Helmers AK, Matthies C, Sturm V, Isaias IU, Krauss JK, Kühn AA, Deuschl G, Volkmann J. Probabilistic mapping of the antidystonic effect of pallidal neurostimulation: a multicentre imaging study. Brain. 2019;142(5):1386–98.

[99] Roubertie A, Mariani LL, Fernandez-Alvarez E, Doummar D, Roze E. Treatment for dystonia in childhood. Eur J Neurol. 2012;19(10):1292–9.

[100] Roze E, Lang AE, Vidailhet M. Myoclonus-dystonia: classification, phenomenology, pathogenesis, and treatment. Curr Opin Neurol. 2018;31(4):484–90.

[101] Ruge D, Cif L, Limousin P, Gonzalez V, Vasques X, Hariz MI, Coubes P, Rothwell JC. Shaping reversibility? long-term deep brain stimulation in dystonia: the relationship between effects on electrophysiology and clinical symptoms. Brain. 2011a;134:2106–15.

[102] Ruge D, Tisch S, Hariz MI, Zrinzo L, Bhatia KP, Quinn NP, Jahanshahi M, Limousin P, Rothwell JC. Deep brain stimulation effects in dystonia: time course of electrophysiological changes in early treatment. Mov Disord. 2011b;26(10):1913–21.

[103] Rughani AI, Lozano AM. Surgical treatment of myoclonus dystonia syndrome. Mov Disord. 2013;28(3):282–7.

[104] Sasikumar S, Albanese A, Krauss JK, Fasano A. Implementation of the current dystonia classification from 2013 to 2018. Mov Disord Clin Pract. 2019;6(3):250–3.

[105] Schrader C, Capelle HH, Kinfe TM, Blahak C, Bazner H, Lutjens G, Dressler D, Krauss JK. GPi-DBS may induce a hypokinetic gait disorder with freez-ing of gait in patients with dystonia. Neurology. 2011;77(5):483–8.

[106] Skogseid IM, Ramm-Pettersen J, Volkmann J, Kerty E, Dietrichs E, Røste GK. Good long-term efficacy of pallidal stimulation in cervical dystonia: a prospective, observer-blinded study. Eur J Neurol. 2012;19(4):610–5.

[107] Slow EJ, Hamani C, Lozano AM, Poon YY, Moro E. Deep brain stimulation for treatment of dystonia secondary to stroke or trauma. J Neurol Neurosurg Psychiatry. 2015;86(9):1046–8.

[108] Steeves TD, Day L, Dykeman J, Jette N, Pringsheim T. The prevalence of primary dystonia: a systematic review and meta-analysis. Mov Disord. 2012;27:1789–96.

[109] Tagliati M, Krack P, Volkmann J, Aziz T, Krauss JK, Kupsch A, Vidailhet AM. Long-term management of DBS in dystonia: response to stimulation, adverse events, battery changes, and special considerations. Mov Disord. 2011;26(S1):S54–62.

[110] Timmermann L, Pauls KA, Wieland K, Jech R, Kurlemann G, Sharma N, Gill SS, Haenggeli CA, Hayflick SJ, Hogarth P, Leenders KL, Limousin P, Malanga CJ, Moro E, Ostrem JL, Revilla FJ, Santens P, Schnitzler A, Tisch S, Valldeoriola F, Vesper J, Volkmann J, Woitalla D, Peker S. Dystonia in neurodegeneration with brain iron accumulation: outcome of bilateral pallidal stimulation. Brain. 2010;133(Pt 3):701–12.

[111] Tisch S, Rothwell JC, Bhatia KP, Quinn N, Zrinzo L, Jahanshahi M, Ashkan K, Hariz M, Limousin P. Pallidal stimulation modifies after-effects of paired associative stimulation on motor cortex excitability in primary generalised dystonia. Exp Neurol. 2007;206(1):80–5.

[112] Trottenberg T, Paul G, Meissner W, Maier-Hauff K, Taschner C, Kupsch A. Pallidal and thalamic neurostimulation in severe tardive dystonia. J Neurol Neurosurg Psychiatry. 2001;70(4):557–9.

[113] van den Dool J, Visser B, Koelman JHTM, Engelbert RHH, Tijssen MAJ. Long-term specialized physical therapy in cervical dystonia: outcomes of a randomized controlled trial. Arch Phys Med Rehabil. 2019;100:1417–25.

[114] van Egmond ME, Lugtenberg CHA, Brouwer OF, Contarino MF, Fung VSC, Heiner-Fokkema MR, van Hilten JJ, van der Hout AH, Peall KJ, Sinke RJ, Roze E, Verschuuren-Bemelmans CC,

Willemsen MA, Wolf NI, Tijssen MA, de Koning TJ. A post hoc study on gene panel analysis for the diagnosis of dystonia. Mov Disord. 2017;32(4):569–75.

[115] van Egmond ME, Contarino MF, Lugtenberg CHA, Peall KJ, Brouwer OF, Fung VSC, Roze E, Stewart RE, Willemsen MA, Wolf NI, de Koning TJ, Tijssen MA. Variable interpretation of the dystonia consensus classification items compromises 1st solidity. Mov Disord. 2019;34(3):317.

[116] Van Tricht MJ, Dreissen YE, Cath D, Dijk JM, Contarino MF, van der Salm SM, et al. Cognition and psychopathology in myoclonus-dystonia. J Neurol Neurosurg Psychiatry. 2012;83(8):814–20.

[117] Vidailhet M, Vercueil L, Houeto JL, Krystkowiak P, Benabid AL, Cornu P, Lagrange C, Tézenas du Montcel S, Dormont D, Grand S, Blond S, Detante O, Pillon B, Ardouin C, Agid Y, Destée A, Pollak P, French Stimulation du Pallidum Interne dans la Dystonie (SPIDY) Study Group. Bilateral deep-brain stimulation of the globus pallidus in primary generalized dystonia. N Engl J Med. 2005;352(5):459–67.

[118] Vidailhet M, Vercueil L, Houeto JL, Krystkowiak P, Lagrange C, Yelnik J, Bardinet E, Benabid AL, Navarro S, Dormont D, Grand S, Blond S, Ardouin C, Pillon B, Dujardin K, Hahn-Barma V, Agid Y, Destée A, Pollak P. French SPIDY Study Group. Bilateral pallidal deep-brain stimulation in primary generalised dystonia: a prospective 3 year follow-up study. Lancet Neurol. 2007;6(3):223–9.

[119] Vidailhet M, Yelnik J, Lagrange C, Fraix V, Grabli D, Thobois S, Burbaud P, Welter ML, Xie-Brustolin J, Braga MC, Ardouin C, Czernecki V, Klinger H, Chabardes S, Seigneuret E, Mertens P, Cuny E, Navarro S, Cornu P, Benabid AL, Le Bas JF, Dormont D, Hermier M, Dujardin K, Blond S, Krystkowiak P, Destee A, Bardinet E, Agid Y, Krack P, Broussolle E, Pollak P, French SPIDY-2 Study Group. Bilateral pallidal deep brain stimulation for the treatment of patients with dystonia-choreoathetosis cerebral palsy: a prospective pilot study. Lancet Neurol. 2009;8(8):709–17.

[120] Volkmann J, Wolters A, Kupsch A, Müller J, Kühn AA, Schneider GH, Poewe W, Hering S, Eisner W, Müller JU, Deuschl G, Pinsker MO, Skogseid IM, Roeste GK, Krause M, Tronnier V, Schnitzler A, Voges J, Nikkhah G, Vesper J, Classen J, Naumann M, Benecke R, DBS Study Group for Dystonia. Pallidal deep brain stimulation in patients with primary generalised or segmental dystonia: 5-year follow-up of a randomised trial. Lancet Neurol. 2012;11(12):1029–38.

[121] Volkmann J, Mueller J, Deuschl G, Kuhn AA, Krauss JK, Poewe W, Timmermann L, Falk D, Kupsch A, Kivi A, Schneider GH, Schnitzler A, Sudmeyer M, Voges J, Wolters A, Wittstock M, Muller JU, Hering S, Eisner W, Vesper J, Prokop T, Pinsker M, Schrader C, Kloss M, Kiening K, Boetzel K, Mehrkens J, Skogseid IM, Ramm-Pettersen J, Kemmler G, Bhatia KP, Vitek JL, Benecke R, DBS Study Group for Dystonia. Pallidal neurostimulation in patients with medication-refractory cervical dystonia: a randomised, sham-controlled trial. Lancet Neurol. 2014;13(9):875–84.

[122] Walsh RA, Sidiropoulos C, Lozano AM, Hodaie M, Poon YY, Fallis M, Moro E. Bilateral pallidal stimulation in cervical dystonia: blinded evidence of benefit beyond 5 years. Brain. 2013;136(Pt 3):761–9.

[123] Wloch A, Blahak C, Abdallat M, Heissler HE, Wolf ME, Krauss JK. Development of hyperkinesias after long-term pallidal stimulation for idiopathic segmental dystonia. Tremor Other Hyperkinet Mov (N Y). 2017;19(7):480.

[124] Wolf ME, Capelle HH, Bäzner H, Hennerici MG, Krauss JK, Blahak C. Hypokinetic gait changes induced by bilateral pallidal deep brain stimulation for segmental dystonia. Gait Posture. 2016;49:358–63.

[125] Wolf ME, Blahak C, Saryyeva A, Schrader C, Krauss JK. Deep brain stimulation for dystonia-choreoathetosis in cerebral palsy: Pallidal versus thalamic stimulation. Parkinsonism Relat Disord. 2019;63:209–12.

[126] Woon K, Tsegaye M, Vloeberghs MH. The role of intrathecal baclofen in the management of primary and secondary dystonia in children. Br J Neurosurg. 2007;21:355–8.

[127] Zádori D, Veres G, Szalárdy L, Klivényi P, Vécsei L. Drug-induced movement disorders. Expert Opin Drug Saf. 2015;14(6):877–90.

[128] Zhan S, Sun F, Pan Y, Liu W, Huang P, Cao C, Zhang J, Li D, Sun B. Bilateral deep brain stimulation of the subthalamic nucleus in primary Meige syndrome. J Neurosurg. 2018;128(3):897–902.

[129] Zoons E, Booij J, Nederveen AJ, Dijk JM, Tijssen MA. Structural, functional and molecular imaging of the brain in primary focal dystonia—a review. Neuroimage. 2011;56:1011–20.

第15章 癫痫
Epilepsy

Kai Lehtimäki　Jukka Peltola　著
赵宝田　张　凯　译　王　垚　杨岸超　张建国　校

> **摘要**：丘脑前核（ANT）脑深部电刺激（DBS）是一种新兴的难治性局灶性癫痫治疗选择，已被美国食品药品管理局（Food and Drug Administration，FDA）和欧洲当局批准。这种疗法基于以下假设，癫痫发作通过直接或间接涉及丘脑前核的神经通路传播，并最终导致意识中断。高频电刺激该网络有望抑制或阻止癫痫传播。这一假设得到了实验数据和初步研究的支持。SANTE试验显示ANT-DBS具有抗癫痫作用，与假刺激组相比，刺激组3个月后癫痫发作减少。长期非盲刺激显示出明显的治疗效果，2年和5年时中位癫痫发作减少分别为56%和69%。报告的有效率，定义为癫痫发作减少50%以上的患者百分比，ANT-DBS似乎比迷走神经电刺激（vagus nerve stimulation，VNS）效果更好，但并无直接比较这两种疗法的试验证实。在已发表的试验中，治疗效果明显的主要患者群体包括额叶和颞叶癫痫，其中以发作期伴有意识障碍的局灶性癫痫为主。精准定位丘脑前核似乎是获得良好预后的关键，而精神方面的不良反应与刺激深部结构有关。从外科角度来看，丘脑前核定位具有一定的挑战性，因为它相对于常见的立体定向标志的位置是可变的，并且邻近脑脊液腔。因此，推荐使用MRI直接定位丘脑前核。

一、概述

药物难治性癫痫的治疗仍然是一个重大的挑战。根据世界卫生组织的报告，癫痫占全球疾病负担的1%。众所周知，1/3的癫痫患者不能通过抗癫痫药物（antiepileptic drug，AED）控制癫痫发作。这些难治性癫痫患者不太可能从额外的抗癫痫药物试验中获益。通常认为这些患者具有切除手术或神经调控的指征。根据国际指南，癫痫手术的术前评估应在两种AED治疗无效后进行，以确定是否存在切除性手术可能。手术切除病变可使1/2的患者癫痫发作得到控制，其中颞叶切除术后效果较非颞叶切除效果更好。尽管在某些病例中，癫痫灶切除是一种选择，但不适合手术切除的患者群体庞大且差异性很大。直到最近，迷走神经电刺激一直是唯一的替代手术疗法，它可以降低近一半患者癫痫发作频率或严重程度。然而，难治性癫痫患者中不适合手术切除且对VNS反应不佳的比例很高，因此需要额外的治疗方案。

由于DBS在运动障碍疾病治疗中的成功，它被认为是难治性癫痫的一种治疗选择。理论上，DBS能够调节大脑中几乎任何深部的神经元结构。丘脑前核是局灶性癫痫患者的脑深部电刺激大型随机对照试验（SANTE 试验）的唯一深部靶点。ANT-DBS 在 2018 年被 FDA 批准为局灶性难治性癫痫的辅助治疗。

丘脑前核是边缘系统的一部分，在结构上与其他丘脑核团通过一层薄而不完整的白质层分隔开。ANT 包括 4 个亚核（前内侧核、前腹核、前背核和背外侧核）。ANT 与额叶皮质、扣带回、下托和内侧颞叶皮质（如内嗅皮质和嗅周皮质）相互联系，这些皮质进一步投射到海马。因此，ANT 在 Papez 环路中是一个中继站，Papez 环路是神经元的功能性多突触环路，首先从海马经穹窿和丘脑乳头束到达 ANT，再到扣带、下托和海马。此外，ANT 还与次级运动皮质和视觉皮质有联系。

从功能上讲，ANT 的前内侧亚核（AM）可以将海马和间脑的信号传递到前额叶皮质。因此，AM 涉及高级认知功能，如执行功能。前腹核系统（AV）维持海马的 θ 活动，参与学习和记忆。最后，前背核系统（AD）是一个涉及空间和注意定位的头部方向系统。

到额叶前部的投射是丘脑前辐射（anterior thalamic radiation，ATR）的一部分，可以通过弥散张量成像（diffusion tensor imaging，DTI）和纤维追踪显示。组织学上已证实了到扣带回的纤维束，它们在尾状核的外侧和上部与扣带束相连。

由于 ANT 与一些经常参与癫痫发作产生或传播的大脑结构联系密切，它被视为 DBS 的潜在靶点。简单来说，其作用机制与在运动障碍疾病中的作用机制类似，高频刺激的目的是使异常的神经元放电正常化，从而减轻神经元网络的异常振荡。这一过程抑制了癫痫活动的传播和产生，但确切的机制仍不明确。

除了丘脑前核外，目前研究常用的靶点还有丘脑中央中核（centromedian nucleus of the thalamus，CM）和海马（hippocampus，HIP）。CM-DBS 用于治疗全面性癫痫，HIP-DBS 用于治疗颞叶癫痫。然而，由于缺乏随机对照试验的疗效证据，CM-DBS 和 HIP-DBS 目前仍处于试验治疗阶段。

二、手术选择

目前，没有明确的证据表明特定类型的局灶性癫痫对 ANT-DBS 的反应比其他类型的局灶性癫痫更佳。SANTE 试验纳入了额叶癫痫和颞叶癫痫，它们对 ANT-DBS 的反应均较好。Lee 和 Lehtimäki 等的研究纳入的患者主要是多灶性癫痫或额颞叶癫痫。这两项研究的结果都与 SANTE 试验相当，本章稍后将对此进行更详细的讨论。相反，在 Krishna 等的研究中，也包括了全面性癫痫患者。该研究报告了一个不太成功的长期结果。在另一项研究中，人们发现，DBS 植入前难治性癫痫患者的神经心理学特征可能预测预后，执行功能和注意力受损预示预后不良。有趣的是，在最近的一份报告中，我们发现了 VNS 和 DBS 的一些相似之处。早期中止 VNS 治疗的患者对 ANT-DBS 的反应与对 VNS 的反应相似。在临床实践中，伴有频繁（至少每月 1 次）的致残性发作的成人局灶性难治性癫痫患者通常是 ANT-DBS 治疗的最佳候选者。虽然没有明确的年龄上限，但大多数手术患者的年龄在 18—60 岁。伴有活动性精神病通常是该手术禁忌证。进一步的随访研究是必需的，以便为目前 ANT-DBS 的患者选择提供明确的建议，以及直接比较 DBS 和 VNS 的效果。

三、手术方法

（一）立体定向解剖学

ANT 是一个具有挑战性的立体定向靶点。这是因为它在侧脑室底壁的独特位置，它的前、上、内侧被脑脊液包围。ANT 的前部和上部偶尔出现相对较大的静脉，即丘脑纹状体静脉与脉络膜上静脉连接形成的大脑内静脉。根据 Schaltenbrand 图谱矢状面定位，ANT 的立体定向坐标为前后连合间径中点前 0～2mm，外 5～6mm，上 12mm。应当注意的是，这些坐标并不代表同一图谱其他方向上同一的解剖点。

ANT位置相对于传统的立体定向标志（及2个半球之间）变异度高。Mottonen等使用3T MRI的研究发现，与Schaltenbrand图谱相比，ANT的可识别边界确实有很大的不同，许多患者ANT的位置更靠前、靠上、靠外。将ANT的横截面投影相对于前后连合间径中点分析时发现，个体患者之间的重叠出乎意料地小（图15-1）。用一系列坐标可以更好地描述ANT的立体定向坐标（前后连合间径中点外4～7mm，前0～5mm，上10～15mm）。显然，巨大的解剖变异限制了传统的间接基于图谱的间接定位。

（二）ANT影像

ANT由不完整的薄白质层环绕，即内髓板和外髓板。乳头丘脑束是连接海马、乳头体和ANT的白质纤维束。T_1加权MPRAGE序列或STIR序列中可以观察到乳头丘脑束。典型的ANT影像如图15-2所示。重要的是，在1.5T MRI和3T MRI中均可充分地辨别这些结构。利用这些解剖标志，我们可以克服ANT靶点的解剖变异。带立体定向框架扫描T_1影像可以定位ANT，但是无立体定向框架3T磁共振也可以更好地可视化ANT。

（三）直接定位

如何根据可视的解剖标志来确定神经刺激的最佳靶点是ANT靶点定位的关键问题。在SANTE试验中，采用术后核磁检查确认靶点位置，确保电极刺激双侧ANT。最近的两项单中心研究均解决了这个问题。在我们的研究所，我们发现当电极触点位于ANT的前、外、上方，略高于乳头丘脑束终点时，治疗效果较好。当电极触点位于ANT的后、下方，或在ANT外时，治疗效果差（图15-3）。Krishna等计算了一组治疗有效患者的激活组织体积（volume of activated tissue，VAT），发现VAT与略高于乳头丘脑束终点的ANT区域重合。综上所述，ANT的刺激部位似乎对治疗结果至关重要。这一发现确实表明，刺激ANT和（或）与ANT相连的神经元结构产生的抗癫痫作用是特异性的。

（四）手术技术

在初步研究和随后的SANTE试验中，额叶经侧脑室路径均取得成效。然而，许多神经外科医生认为，这项技术容易产生位置偏移（由于穿透了侧脑室），并有发生脑室内出血的风险（脑室内偶尔出现大血管）。建议使用更偏外的侧脑室外路径替代。然而，使用侧脑室外路径将电极触点置于ANT具有一定的挑战。最近的多中心注册数据表明，一些欧洲神经外科中心更常选择侧脑室外路径。进一步详细分析发现，侧脑室外路径与ANT内植入触点数量显著减少相关（图15-4）。ANT和丘脑纹状体静脉之间的解剖关系似乎是侧脑室外入路成功的主要决定因素。由于ANT通常在轴面向侧脑室内突出，当入点在冠状缝水平时，丘脑纹状体静脉通常位于ANT中心的直线上。因此，可以相对一致地定位ANT的下方和后方，而无法定位ANT的中部。到目前为止，尚无不同的手术路径和在ANT内电极植入成功率与治疗结果相关的数据。此外，一些患者使用了侧脑室外后入路。这一路径入点在顶叶交界区的非语言皮质，并且避免了穿透侧脑室。通过这种入路，电极触点在ANT内沿前后轴线排列（与之相对的是，经侧脑室入路电极触点沿上下轴线排列）。目前，只有额叶经侧脑室入路有大规模长期疗效随访数据（图15-5）。经侧脑室入路的手术方法不同于传统的运动障碍疾病，其主要原因是该手术有意地穿透了侧脑室。因此，为了防止电极移位，必须使用套管针。

（五）微电极记录

微电极记录（microelectrode registration，MER）是一种术中技术，用于术中确认所需靶点位置，尤其是在运动障碍疾病中。在目标结构神经元放电模式典型的情况下，例如底丘脑核（STN），MER可以确认电极进入目标核团。同样地，有人提出了可以确认电极进入ANT的方法。从侧

第 15 章 癫痫
Epilepsy

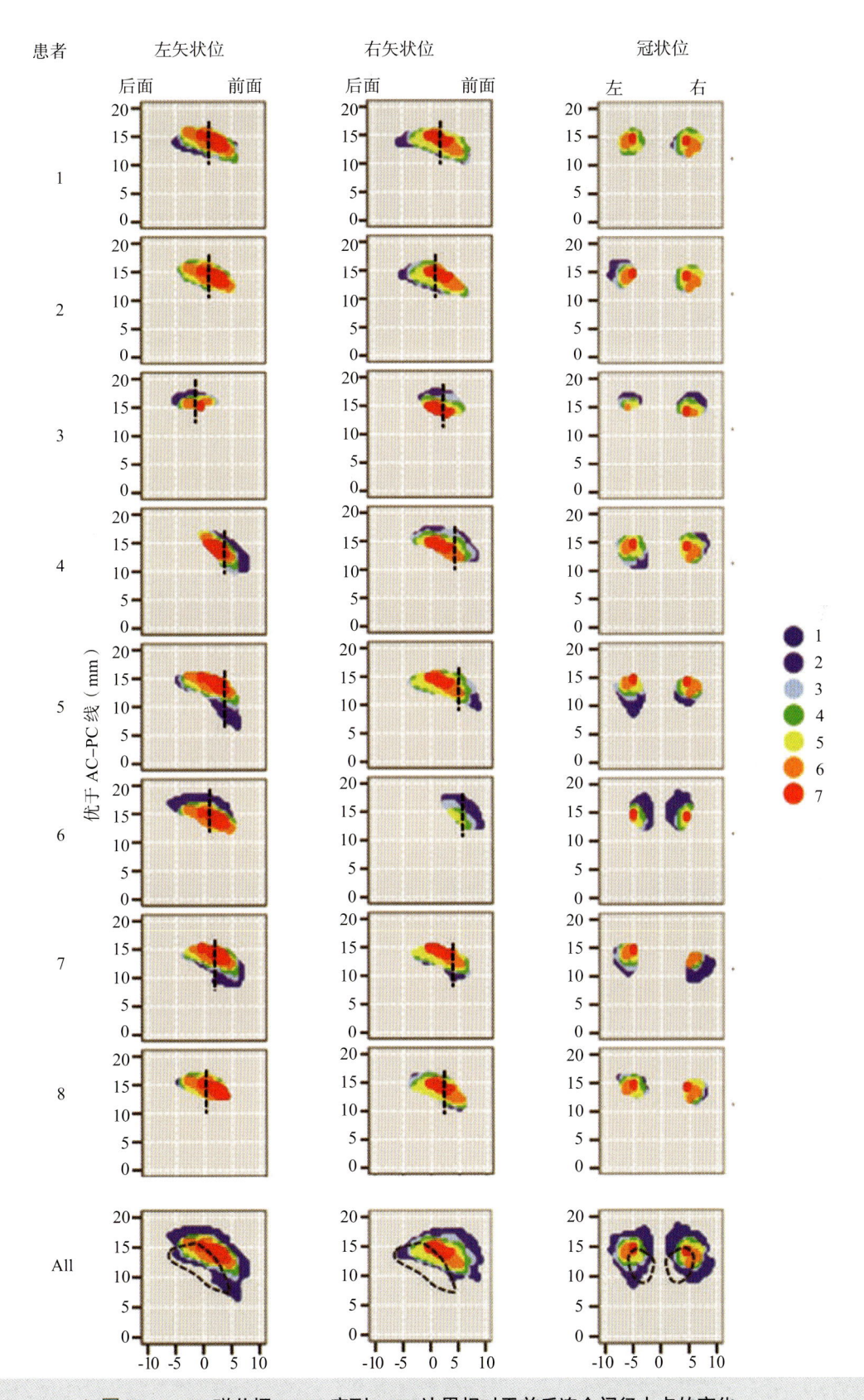

▲ 图 15-1 3T 磁共振 STIR 序列 ANT 边界相对于前后连合间径中点的变化
颜色编码表示个体之间的重叠程度。虚线描绘了乳头丘脑束水平的冠状面（患者 1~8）。最下方图像中的虚线表示基于 Schaltenbrand 图谱的 ANT 边界

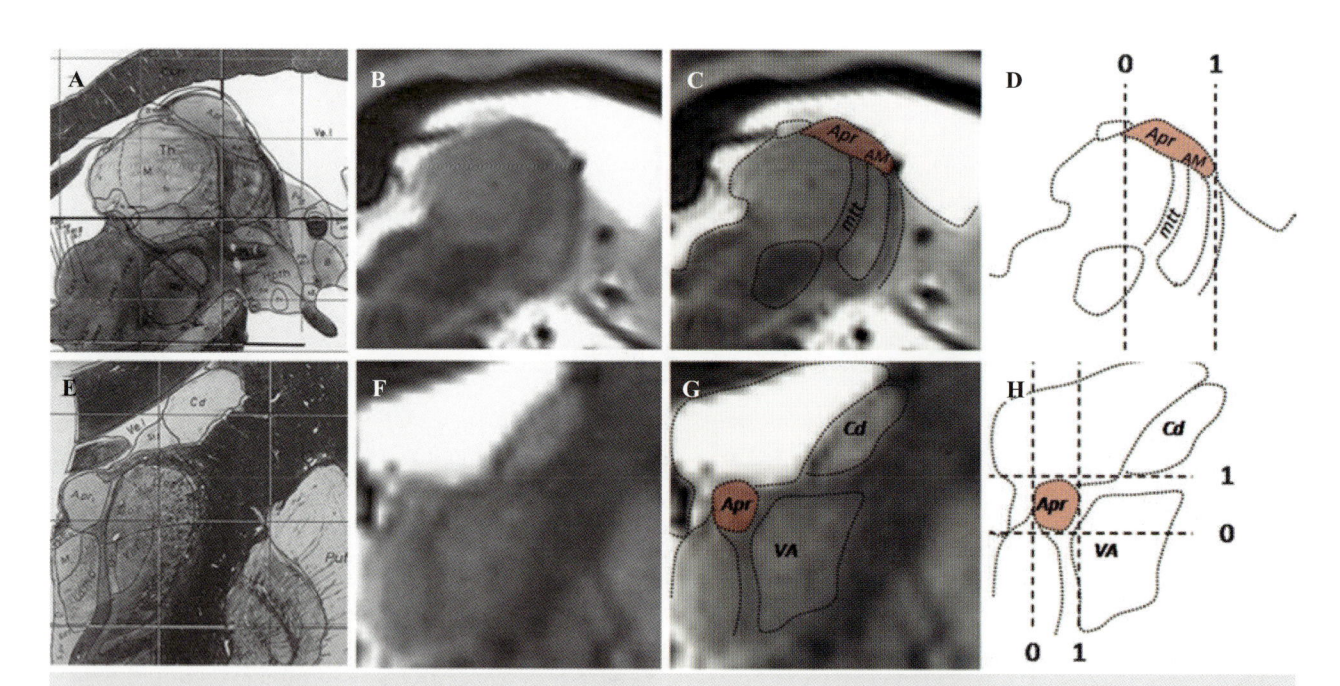

▲ 图 15-2 ANT 在 3T 磁共振中所示，在一定程度上与 Schaltenbrand 图谱矢状位和冠状位的位置相关联。图中展示了基于可视化 ANT 边界的坐标系原理

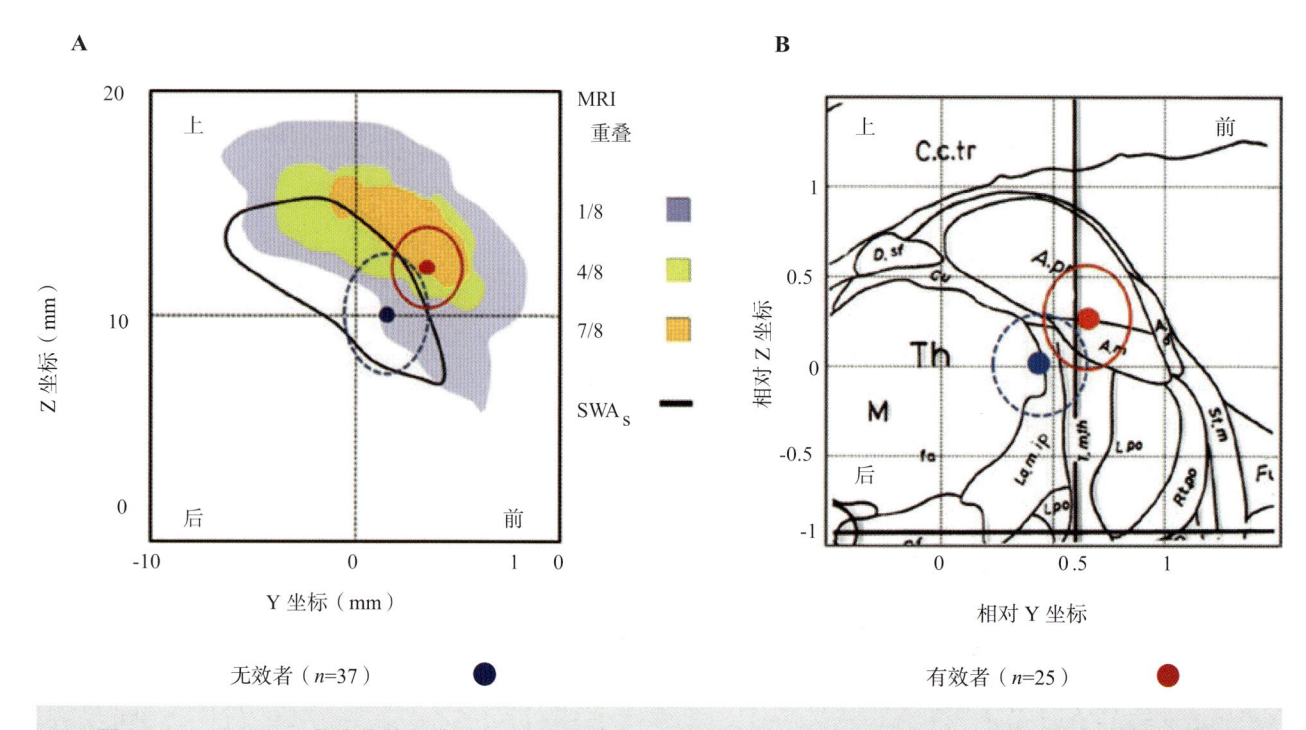

▲ 图 15-3 ANT-DBS 临床疗效与基于 3T 磁共振确定的电极触点在 ANT 的位置相关，间接坐标确定的刺激区域通常位于 ANT 的后下方，无法获得较好临床疗效

第 15 章 癫痫
Epilepsy

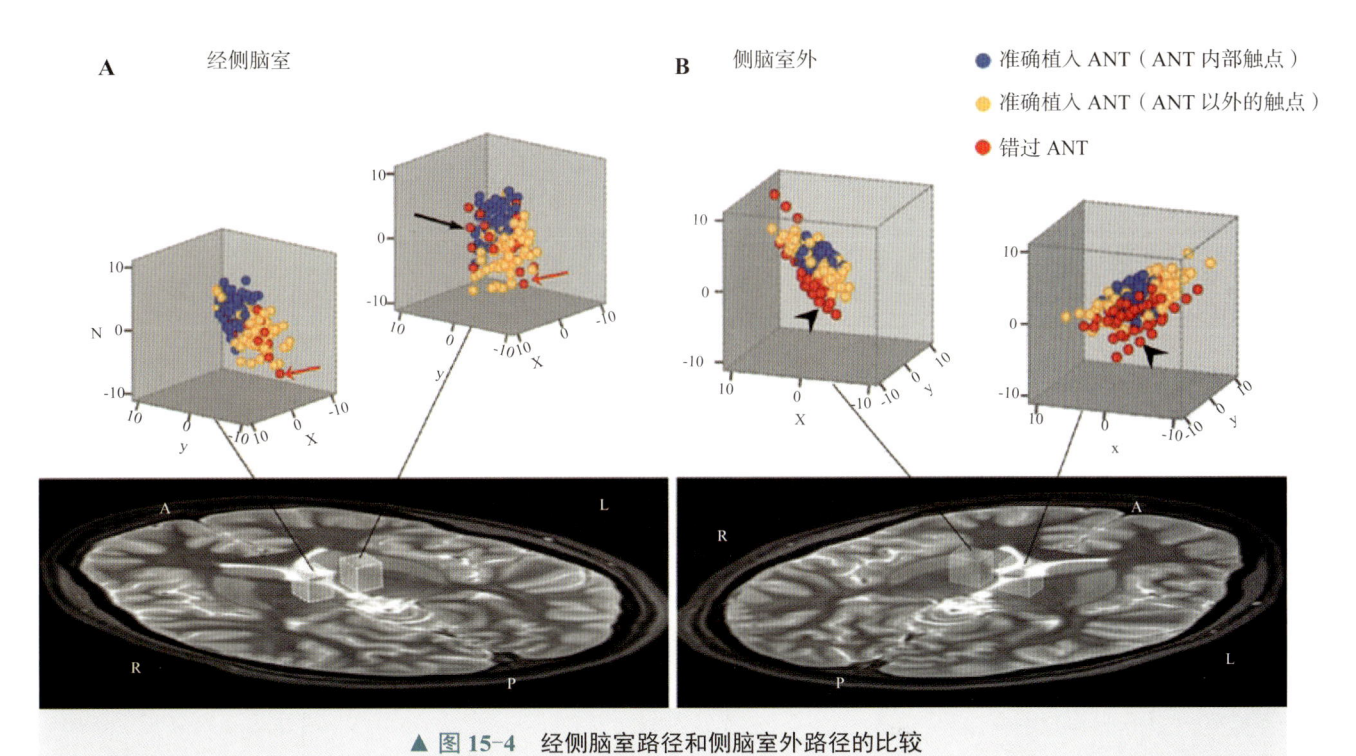

▲ 图 15-4 经侧脑室路径和侧脑室外路径的比较

A. 经侧脑室路径植入的典型异位是放置位置过深或偏向脑脊液腔内侧；B. 侧脑室外路径植入比较常见的异位是偏 ANT 后方和下方

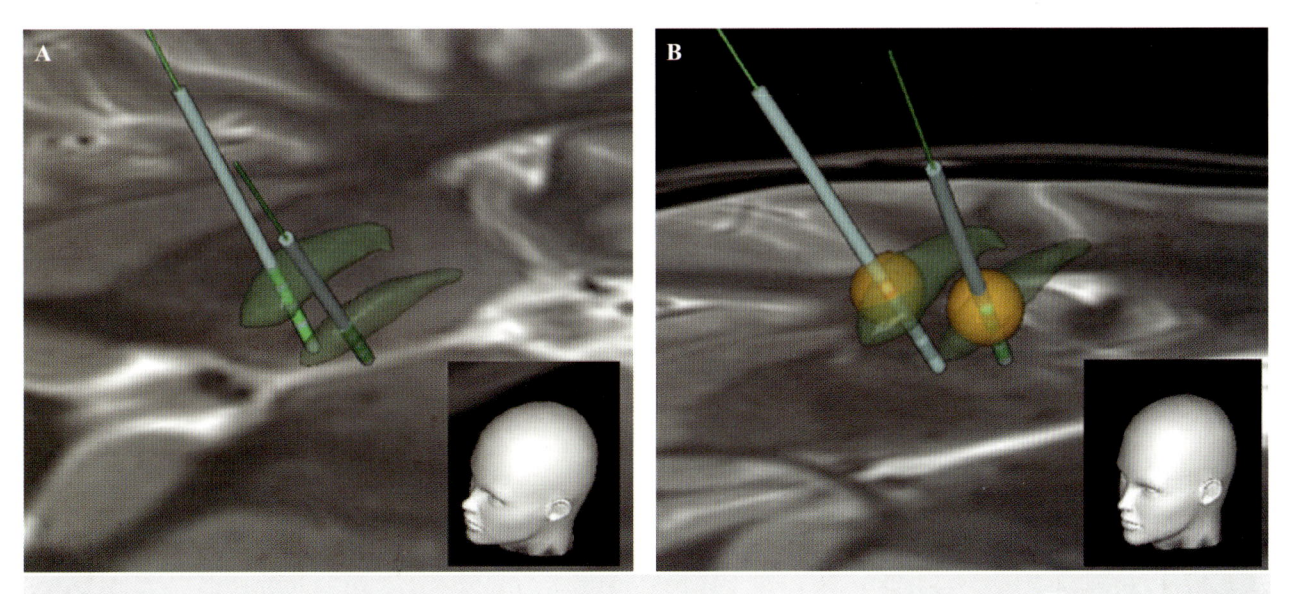

▲ 图 15-5 美敦力 3389 电极成功植入 ANT，最上面的 2 个触点在 ANT 内，深部的 2 个触点在 ANT 下方。利用美敦力 SureTune 3 软件，以最靠颅骨的触点为负极，可视化激活组织体积

185

脑室进入 ANT 后出现神经元放电，沿路径继续向前，进入丘脑背内侧核后，信号特征进一步改变。最近对这一技术重新审视，根据最终的 DBS 电极位置调整计划路径后，对 MER 信号进行重新评估。记录到的 MER 信号与显示 ANT 边界的 3T MRI 成像信息相关性较强（图 15-6）。使用 3T 磁共振更好地显示 ANT 边界，追踪原始记录点的可靠性更强。有趣的是，与 ANT 相比，在腹前核（ventral anterior nucleus，VA）似乎记录到了更多的神经元放电。重要的是，由于白质中缺少神经元放电，可以确定出 ANT 和邻近核团（VA、DM）间的薄层白质纤维。

最近，另一个研究小组报告了类似的发现。Schaper 等报道，当通过侧脑室外入路进入 ANT 时，在 ANT 内记录到了双相模式的神经元放电。与 Möttönen 等的研究结果相反，他们在 ANT 记录到比邻近的丘脑核团更频繁的突发信号。在 ANT 和外侧核团的边界处记录到神经元放电减少。他们未能发现 MER 模式和临床结果之间的关联性。

总之，微电极记录 ANT 具有一定的定位价值。首先，可以很容易地发现从侧脑室到 ANT 的入点，可以明确脑脊液（CSF）-丘脑边界。如果实际路径在 ANT 外侧的薄层白质纤维中走行，则无法检测到神经元放电（图 15-7）。从这一区域记录到的信号可能会被误认为是脑脊液。因此，短暂的放电模式确实也有定位价值，如果神经元的放电出现的比预期要晚，则表明该路径沿 ANT 的外侧走行。成功记录到 ANT 信号后，神经元放电停止，则提示进入丘脑板内核群。如果通过侧脑室外入路到达 ANT，在到达 ANT 之前，记录到 VA 信号后，应该会有一段区域无法记录到放电。由于 ANT 的前表面和上表面有时

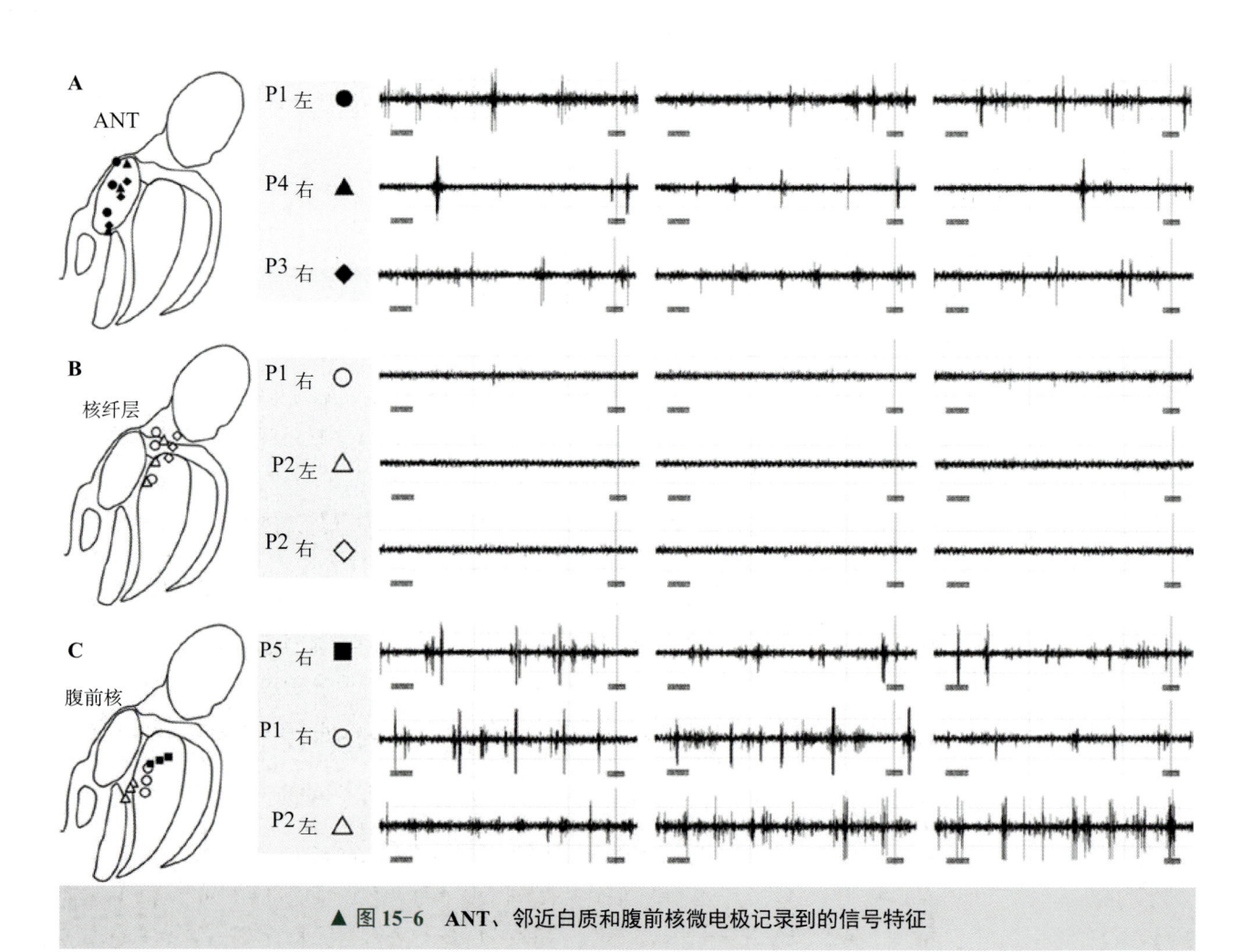

▲ 图 15-6 ANT、邻近白质和腹前核微电极记录到的信号特征

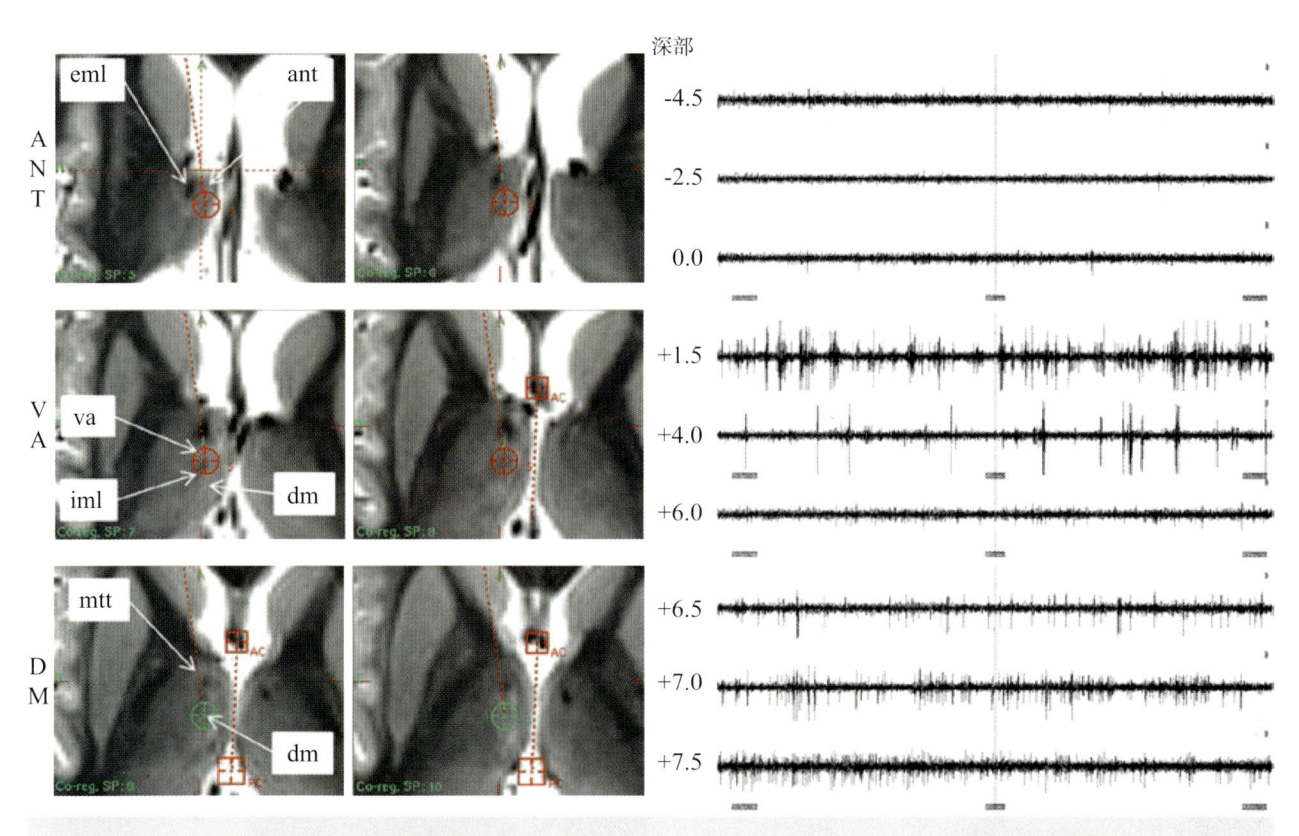

▲ 图 15-7 沿 ANT 核略偏外侧的路径记录到的信号特征。在预期 ANT 水平上观察不到典型的神经元放电。相反，由于形态相似，来自 VA 的神经元放电活动可能会被误认为来自 ANT
ANT. 丘脑前核；VA. 前腹核；DM. 背腹核

会附有较多血管，所以应当仔细权衡微电极记录的优点。

四、DBS 结果

根据 SANTE 试验，在 2 年后的非盲阶段，癫痫发作的中位数减少了 56%。有趣的是，少数患者简单部分性发作次数增加，而发作期伴意识障碍的癫痫发作次数明显减少。这提示，ANT-DBS 可能存在特别作用于癫痫扩散导致意识障碍的机制。与 VNS 效果类似，随着时间的推移，结果有所改善，5 年时癫痫发作的中位数减少了 69%，68% 的患者癫痫发作的中位数减少了 50% 或更多。重要的是，这一结果是在一组接受积极治疗的患者中观察到的，随访时间整整 5 年。目前尚不清楚患者预后的改善是由于成功调整程控参数，还是由于慢性 ANT 刺激的疾病修饰效应。

几项单中心研究报告了与 SANTE 试验相当的预后结局。Lee 等报道，在 16 名患者中，使用低电压（1.5～3.1V）持续刺激，患者癫痫发作平均减少 70%。我们观察到 15 名患者有 67% 的有效率。多伦多报道 15 名患者的应答率为 68.8%，但在长期随访期间有效率大幅下降。Krishna 等的研究与其他研究的主要区别在于他们的研究包括了全身性癫痫患者。作者推测，这可能可以解释较差的长期结果。多个中心使用相似的外科手术方法重复出 SANTE 试验的结果，并且结果具有可比性。约 2/3 的患者对 ANT-DBS 有效，而 1/3 的患者对 ANT-DBS 仍无效。

五、程控

癫痫患者程控面临着不同于运动障碍患者程控的挑战。第一，无法直接观察到刺激效果（如静止性震颤或动作性震颤停止）。相反，需要几个月的随访来评估选定刺激部位和参数是否成功。第二，在运动障碍疾病中 DBS 的目的是使持续的异常神经网络活动正常化，而在癫痫中刺激的目的是防止癫痫发生或在大脑中更广泛的传播。因此，其基本作用机制不同于传统的运动障碍疾病。

ANT-DBS 刺激参数也与其他 DBS 不同。由于 ANT 体积较大，在初步研究和最终的 SANTE 试验中，选择了相对较高的刺激电压（5V）。为了使刺激达到抑制作用，刺激频率选择为 145Hz 的高频刺激。由于上述参数能耗较高，模仿 VNS 循环刺激模式，ANF-DBS 采用了一种独特的刺激模式，即刺激 1min，关闭 5min。有趣的是，后来进行的大型动物研究提供了支持这些刺激参数的电生理学证据，研究表明超过 80Hz 的刺激频率与青霉素致痫海马的持续癫痫活动的抑制相关。这一研究还表明，持续 10～40s 的刺激与持续几分钟的癫痫活动抑制相关。

根据已发表的临床资料，ANT-DBS 治疗成果的关键是选择的触点在 ANT 中的位置（图 15-3）。如果在刺激 2～3 个月后没有观察到效果，应重新评估刺激触点。治疗的初期也有可能观察到诱发性癫痫或类似癫痫的症状。与 SANTE 试验中的 2 名患者相似，我们最近报告了 1 名患者，他在开始 ANT-DBS 治疗时出现了新的视觉症状和非典型性癫痫发作。视频脑电证实降低刺激电压可以缓解这些症状。随后的初始电压值刺激既没有引起视觉症状的复发，也没有导致新的发作类型，在长期的随访中，患者的发作似乎得到了缓解。因此，DBS 治疗初期出现的刺激诱发发作不应被认为是失败，治疗有效的可能性仍然存在。

Papez 环路最初被描述为情感和记忆网络的环路，ANT 是其中的关键节点。很少有 ANT-DBS 术后导致严重抑郁症的报道。在我们的病例中，包括 22 名连续的植入 ANT-DBS 的患者，精神方面的不良反应与刺激 ANT 核下部有关，通过重新程控刺激触点，以更好地刺激 ANT 而不是丘脑深部核团，如背内侧核，可以改善精神方面不良反应。

一系列病例表明，刺激 ANT 也会影响睡眠质量。在 9 名接受 ANT-DBS 默认刺激参数治疗的患者中，多导睡眠图发现 14%～67% 的深部电刺激导致了患者电临床唤醒。当 8 名患者夜间的 DBS 电压调低时，未见癫痫发作恶化，4 名患者先前观察到的神经精神症状也得到缓解。对于有神经精神症状的患者，在夜间应考虑使用与白天刺激不同的一组单独的刺激参数，降低电压。对所有 ANT-DBS 的患者应进行睡眠质量评估。

六、讨论

如本书前几章所示，DBS 在运动障碍疾病领域有着悠久而成功的历史。DBS 在治疗精神疾病尤其是强迫症方面的成功表明，DBS 也可以用于调节非运动神经元网络。扩大 DBS 对难治性癫痫的适应证具有深远的影响。除了癫痫外，ANT 还是情绪、记忆和意识的神经网络中的一个关键节点。DBS 不仅是一种强大、安全的治疗方法，还是一种精密的研究工具，研究人员还可以设置任何期望的参数进行刺激或关闭。因此，我们现在可以利用各种研究范式研究各种新的神经过程。在未来几年内，传感技术将使我们能够更可靠地检测难治性癫痫患者的癫痫发作。

与以前的适应证相比，DBS 治疗癫痫在许多方面有所不同。首先，在运动障碍疾病（特发性震颤、帕金森病和肌张力障碍）中，刺激使持续的异常神经元活动正常化，并且可以相对迅速地（特发性震颤和帕金森症）或在短暂的延迟后（肌张力障碍）观察到治疗效果。DBS 治疗强迫症虽可能立即改善情绪，但改善强迫症和强迫行为通常也需要时间。相反，在癫痫中，刺激的目的是防止癫痫活动的发生和扩散，但在理论上，神经网络在癫痫发作间期时的功能是正常的。因此，我们的目标不是减少持续性的神经症状，而是预防阵发性症状。此外，在运动障碍疾病和强迫症中，神经网络的异常信号在生理范围内。然而，在癫痫发作期间，与生理性兴奋和抑制信号相比，神经元过度兴奋，神经递质释放过量。脑电图上可以观察到病理性放电的扩散。事实上，在临床应用中使用 DBS 装置刺激 ANT 可以抑制海马等较远脑区的病理性神经元兴奋，这一点非常重要。

在难治性癫痫治疗方案中，ANT–DBS 疗效介于迷走神经刺激和切除性手术两者之间。最近新出现了一种类似的疗法，即反应性神经电刺激（responsive neurostimulation，RNS），它结合了切除性手术和 DBS 的某些特点。这一疗法从大脑皮质或深部病灶检测癫痫发作，然后对癫痫病灶进行电刺激。切除性手术和 RNS 都需要基于有创性检查获取的癫痫病灶的详细信息。传统上，VNS 疗法用于治疗没有明显致痫灶或多发致痫灶的难治性癫痫患者。ANT–DBS 与 VNS 相似，它们都不依赖致痫灶的明确信息。这一特点可能具有深远意义，ANT–DBS 潜在适应患者群体可能更广泛。然而，它比 VNS 侵入性更强，在技术上也更具挑战性。DBS 也对患者提出了更高的要求，因为合作和对治疗的依从性是必不可少的。

七、结论

对于早先治疗选择有限的患者，ANT–DBS 是一种新颖的极有吸引力的疗法。这种疗法的有效性和安全性介于 VNS 和更具侵袭性的手术（如 RNS 和切除性手术）之间。这种疗法仍处于起步阶段，最理想的患者选择、癫痫类型和手术方法需要进一步研究。很明显，手术靶点的高质量成像是治疗成功的关键因素。从基础科学角度来看，ANT–DBS 为更详细地研究记忆和情绪等神经现象开辟了道路。

参考文献

[1] Aggleton JP, O'Mara SM, Vann SD, et al. Hippocampal-anterior thalamic pathways for memory: uncovering a network of direct and indirect actions. Eur J Neurosci. 2010;12:2292–307.

[2] Andrade DM, Zumsteg D, Hamani C, et al. Long-term follow-up of patients with thalamic deep brain stimulation for epilepsy. Neurology. 2006;66:1571–3.

[3] Buentjen L, Kopitzki K, Schmitt FC, et al. Direct targeting of the thalamic anteroventral nucleus for deep brain stimulation by T1-weighted magnetic resonance imaging at 3 T. Stereotact Funct Neurosurg. 2014;92:25–30.

[4] Coenen VA, Panksepp J, Hurwitz TA, et al. Human medial forebrain bundle (MFB) and anterior thalamic radiation (ATR): imaging of two major subcortical pathways and the dynamic balance of opposite affects in understanding depression. J Neuropsychiatry Clin Neurosci. 2012;2:223–36.

[5] Cukiert A, Lehtimäki K. Deep brain stimulation targeting in refractory epilepsy. Epilepsia. 2017;58:80–4.

[6] de Tisi J, Bell GS, Peacock JL, et al. The long-term outcome of adult epilepsy surgery, patterns of seizure remission, and relapse: a cohort study. Lancet. 2011;378:1388–95.

[7] Engel J Jr, Wiebe S, French J, et al. Practice parameter: temporal lobe and localized neocortical resections for epilepsy: report of the Quality Standards Subcommittee of the American Academy of Neurology, in association with the American Epilepsy Society and the American Association of Neurological Surgeons. Neurology. 2003;60:538–47.

[8] Fisher R, Salanova V, Witt T, et al. Electrical stimulation of the anterior nucleus of thalamus for treatment of refractory epilepsy. Epilepsia. 2010;51:899–908.

[9] Fisher RS, Cross JH, French JA, et al. Operational classification of seizure types by the International League Against Epilepsy: Position Paper of the ILAE Commission for Classification and Terminology. Epilepsia. 2017;58:522–30.

[10] Gooneratne IK, Green AL, Dugan P, et al. Comparing neurostimulation technologies in refractory focal-onset epilepsy. J Neurol Neurosurg Psychiatry. 2016;87:1174–82.

[11] Heck CN, King-Stephens D, Massey AD, et al. Two-year seizure reduction in adults with medically intractable partial onset epilepsy treated with responsive neurostimulation: final results of the RNS System Pivotal trial. Epilepsia. 2014;55:432–41.

[12] Heilbronner SR, Haber SN. Frontal cortical and subcortical projections provide a basis for segmenting the cingulum bundle: implications for neuroimaging and psychiatric disorders. J Neurosci. 2014;34:10041–54.

[13] Hodaie M, Wennberg RA, Dostrovsky JO, Lozano AM. Chronic anterior thalamus stimulation for intractable epilepsy. Epilepsia. 2002;43:603–8.

[14] Jankowski MM, Ronnqvist KC, Tsanov M, et al. The anterior thalamus provides a subcortical circuit supporting memory and spatial navigation. Front Syst Neurosci. 2013;7:45.

[15] Järvenpää S, Rosti-Otajärvi E, Rainesalo S, et al. Executive functions may predict outcome in deep brain stimulation of anterior nucleus of thalamus for treatment of refractory epilepsy. Front Neurol. 2018;9:324.

[16] Jiltsova E, Möttönen T, Fahlström M, et al. Imaging of anterior nucleus of thalamus using 1.5T MRI for deep brain stimulation targeting in refractory epilepsy. Neuromodulation. 2016;19:812–7.

[17] Jones EG. Anterior nuclei and lateral dorsal nucleus. In: The thalamus. 2nd ed. Cambridge: Cambridge University Press; 2007.

[18] Kerrigan JF, Litt B, Fisher RS, et al. Electrical stimulation of the anterior nucleus of the thalamus for the treatment of intractable epilepsy. Epilepsia. 2004;45:346–54.

[19] Krishna V, King NK, Sammartino F, et al. Anterior nucleus deep brain stimulation for refractory epilepsy: insights into patterns of seizure control and efficacious target. Neurosurgery. 2016;78:802–11.

[20] Kulju T, Haapasalo J, Lehtimäki K, et al. Similarities between the responses to ANT-DBS and prior VNS in refractory epilepsy. Brain Behav. 2018;8:e00983. Kwan P, Brodie MJ. Early identification of refractory epilepsy. N Engl J Med. 2000;342:314–9.

[21] Kwan P, Arzimanoglou A, Berg AT, et al. Definition of drug resistant epilepsy: consensus proposal by the ad hoc Task Force of the ILAE Commission on Therapeutic Strategies. Epilepsia. 2010;51:1069–77.

[22] Lee KJ, Jang KS, Shon YM. Chronic deep brain stimulation of subthalamic and anterior thalamic nuclei for controlling refractory partial epilepsy. Acta Neurochir Suppl. 2006;99:87–91.

[23] Lee KJ, Shon YM, Cho CB. Long-term outcome of anterior thalamic nucleus stimulation for intractable epilepsy. Stereotact Funct Neurosurg. 2012;90:379–85.

[24] Lehtimäki K, Möttönen T, Järventausta K, et al. Outcome based definition of the anterior thalamic deep brain stimulation target in refractory epilepsy. Brain Stimul. 2016;9:268–75.

[25] Lehtimäki K, Coenen VA, Gonçalves Ferreira A, et al. The surgical approach to the anterior nucleus of thalamus in patients with refractory epilepsy: experience from the International Multicenter Registry (MORE). Neurosurgery. 2019;84:141–50.

[26] Lim SN, Lee ST, Tsai YT, et al. Electrical stimulation of the anterior nucleus of the thalamus for intractable epilepsy: a long-term follow-up study. Epilepsia. 2007;48:342–7.

[27] Mai J, Majtanik M, Paxinos G. Atlas of the human brain. 4th ed. New York: Academic; 2015.

[28] Mohanraj R, Brodie MJ. Diagnosing refractory epilepsy: response to sequential treatment schedules. Eur J Neurol. 2006;13:277–82.

[29] Morris GL 3rd, Mueller WM. Long-term treatment with vagus nerve stimulation in patients with refractory epilepsy. Neurology. 1999;53:1731–5.

[30] Möttönen T, Katisko J, Haapasalo J, et al. Defining the anterior nucleus of the thalamus (ANT) as a deep brain stimulation target in refractory epilepsy: delineation using 3 T MRI and intraoperative microelectrode recording. Neuroimage Clin. 2015;7:823–9.

[31] Möttönen T, Katisko J, Haapasalo J, et al. The correlation between intraoperative microelectrode recording and 3-Tesla MRI in patients undergoing ANT-DBS for refractory epilepsy. Stereotact Funct Neurosurg. 2016;94:86–92.

[32] Murray CJL, Lopez AD. Global comparative assessment in the health sector; disease burden, expenditures, and intervention packages. Geneva: World Health Organization; 1994.

[33] Nora T, Heinonen H, Tenhunen M, et al. Stimulation induced electrographic seizures in deep brain stimulation of the anterior nucleus of the thalamus do not preclude a subsequent favorable treatment response. Front Neurol. 2018;9:66.

[34] Osorio I, Overman J, Giftakis J, Wilkinson SB. High frequency thalamic stimulation for inoperable mesial temporal epilepsy. Epilepsia. 2007;48:1561–71.

[35] Papez JW. A proposed mechanism of emotion. 1937. J Neuropsychiatry Clin Neurosci. 1995;7:103–12.

[36] Salanova V, Witt T, Worth R, et al. Long-term efficacy and safety of thalamic stimulation for drug-resistant partial epilepsy. Neurology. 2015;84:1017–25.

[37] Schaltenbrand G, Wahren W. Atlas for sterotaxy of the human brain. 2nd ed. Stuttgart: Thieme; 1998.

[38] Schaper FLWVJ, Zhao Y, Janssen MLF, et al. Single-cell recordings to target the anterior nucleus of the thalamus in deep brain stimulation for patients with refractory epilepsy. Int J Neural Syst. 2018;29:1850012.

[39] Shibata H, Naito J. Organization of anterior cingulate and frontal cortical projections to the anterior and laterodorsal thalamic nuclei in the rat. Brain Res. 2005;1059:93–103.

[40] Stypulkowski PH, Giftakis JE, Billstrom TM. Development of a large animal model for investigation of deep brain stimulation for epilepsy. Stereotact Funct Neurosurg. 2011;89:111–22.

[41] Stypulkowski PH, Stanslaski SR, Denison TJ, Giftakis JE. Chronic evaluation of a clinical system for deep brain stimulation and recording of neural network activity. Stereotact Funct Neurosurg. 2013;91:220–32.

[42] van Buren JM, Borke RC. The nuclei and cerebral connections of the human thalamus. In: Variations and connections of the human thalamus. Berlin: Springer; 1972.

[43] Van Gompel JJ, Klassen BT, Worrell GA, et al. Anterior nuclear deep brain stimulation guided by concordant hippocampal recording. Neurosurg Focus. 2015;38:E9.

[44] van Groen T, Kadish I, Wyss JM. Efferent connections of the anteromedial nucleus of the thalamus of the rat. Brain Res Brain Res Rev. 1999;30:1–26.

[45] Voges B, Schmitt F, Hamel W, et al. Deep brain stimulation of anterior nucleus thalami disrupts sleep in epilepsy patients. Epilepsia. 2015;56:99–103.

第 16 章 抽动秽语综合征
Gilles de la Tourette Syndrome

Anouk Y. M. Smeets　Albert F. G. Leentjens　Linda Ackermans　著
刘德峰　刘焕光　译　张弨　杨岸超　张建国　校

摘要：抽动秽语综合征（Tourette syndrome，TS）是一种儿童时期起病的复杂性神经精神障碍，其特征是多个部位运动性抽动，加上一个或多个发声性抽动，且持续时间＞1年。儿童TS的患病率为0.3%~0.9%，总体预后良好。1/3患有TS的儿童在青春期会经历显著的抽动症状减轻，另外1/3的儿童将完全缓解。然而，其余的TS患者无法缓解。当前TS没有临床治愈的方法，治疗的目的是减少或缓解抽动和其他共病症状。行为疗法和药物治疗可能会起到缓解作用，但一些患者仍然难以治愈或出现无法忍受的不良反应。对于这一类患者，可以考虑脑深部电刺激（DBS）手术。1999年，第1例TS患者接受了丘脑DBS手术治疗；从那时起，有270名患者陆续接受了该手术。获得最佳手术预后的一个关键因素是靶点选择，但由于TS患者表现出复杂的临床特征，这一话题仍存在争论。到目前为止，已有9个不同的大脑区域成为靶点，包括丘脑内侧部分（3个不同区域）、苍白球内侧部（internal globus pallidus，GPI）（前部和后部）、苍白球外侧部（external globus pallidus，GPE）、伏隔核（nucleus accumbens，NA）、内囊前肢（anterior limb of the internal capsule，ALIC）和底丘脑核（subthalamic nucleus，STN）。在基底神经节的主要输出站或中继站之一的层面上进行DBS可能对难治性TS患者有临床益处。总体而言，以耶鲁综合抽动严重程度量表（Yale Global Tic Severity Scale，YGTSS）为评估指标，所有靶点的DBS在短期内症状均显著改善，平均达53%。丘脑和GPI靶点的DBS对抽动症状改善的程度可能是最好的。进一步的研究应该在最佳靶点的选择、刺激参数的选择，以及该疗法的有效性方面提供更多的证据。

一、背景

（一）流行病学

1885年，一位法国神经学家，夏科特医生的学生，乔治·吉勒·德拉图雷特（George Gilles de la Tourette）描述了一种临床综合征，其特征是多发性抽动、污秽言语和模仿言语的临床三联征（Gilles de la Tourette，1885；Kramer和Daniels，2004）。夏科特后来为这种综合征命名为"抽动秽语综合征"。然而，记录抽动障碍患者的早期病历（现在被认为是抽动秽语综合征）早于该时期便已经公布。早在1825年，法国医生伊塔德就描述了丹皮埃尔侯爵的离奇行为，他从7岁起就表现出奇怪的身体动作、奇特的发声和淫秽的言论（Kramer和Daniels，2004；Itard，1825）。

儿童 TS 的患病率（这里定义为年龄＜18 岁）为 0.3%～0.9%，男性的患病率是女性的 2～4 倍。平均而言，抽动症状开始出现于 4—6 岁；症状最严重的时期一般是第二个 10 年的早期，8—12 岁；其后严重程度稳步下降。在 TS 的自然发生过程中，抽动每天可发生多次，随着时间的推移，抽动的严重程度会逐渐降低。总体而言，TS 预后良好。1/3 患有 TS 的儿童在青春期将经历抽动严重程度和频率的显著下降，最终只有轻微的抽动，不需要临床治疗，另外 1/3 的儿童将完全缓解。然而，另一小部分患者仍然无法缓解，在这一群体中，有部分患者不仅在青春期经历抽动症状恶化，而且还发展为最严重的 TS 类型。在 5% 的患者中，TS 症状严重甚至危及生命，并被称为"恶性"TS，其特征是抽动相关的伤害、自残行为、无法控制的暴力行为和自杀企图（Bloch 和 Leckman，2009）。

（二）症状学

抽动秽语综合征（TS）是一种儿童时期起病的复杂性神经精神障碍，以抽动为主要临床症状（Robertson，2000）。抽动被定义为突然的、快速的、反复的、非节律性的肌肉收缩，产生刻板印象的动作（运动性抽动）或声音（声音或语音抽动）。抽动可以是突然发作、快速而短暂的（阵挛性抽动），也可以是缓慢而持续的（肌张力性或强直性抽动）（Leckman，2002）。TS 的诊断一般以第 5 版《精神疾病诊断与统计手册》（DSM-5）的诊断标准为依据（American Psychiatric Association，2013）。根据诊断标准，多发运动性抽动和一种或多种发声性抽动必须存在 1 年以上，并且需要在 18 岁之前发病。除了 TS（DSM-5 编码 307.23），DSM-5 还列出了另外两种抽动障碍，即"持续性运动或发声抽动障碍"（307.22）和"暂时性抽动障碍"（307.21）。持续性运动或发声抽动障碍的诊断标准与 TS 相同，只是诊断时需要运动或发声抽动障碍中的一种，而不是两者都需要。在"暂时性抽动障碍"中，符合 TS 的其他诊断标准，除了这种症状持续超过 1 年。表 16-1 列出了 TS 的 DSM-5 诊断标准。

TS 的抽动症状通常在 4—6 岁出现，开始为简单运动性抽动（如眨眼、面部做鬼脸等），然后是 1～2 年后出现简单发声抽动（如清嗓、嗅闻等）。抽动发作后，往往有一个进行性的恶化过程，使得抽动症状变得更加复杂（Robertson 等，2000）。污言秽语是最使患者衰弱的症状之一，14%～20% 的患者会出现这种症状（Robertson，2008）。许多患者描述了先兆感觉，即抽动前紧张感的增强，这些感觉往往比抽动本身更痛苦。抽动症状发生后，会有短暂的缓解过程（Leckman，2002）。大多数患者可以暂时抑制抽动，但是会使得抽动症状反弹并且加剧。尽管许多患者描述了这样的反弹，但这一现象尚未在研究中得到证实（Verdellen 等，2007；Müller-Vahl 等，2014）。抽动的严重程度也会受到环境的影响；随着压力、焦虑和疲劳的增加，抽动的严重程度可能会增加，而集中精力的活动和饮酒可能会降低抽动的强度（Leckman，2002）。

表 16-1 抽动秽语综合征的 DSM-5 诊断标准

标 准	描 述
A	病程中具有多种运动性抽动及一种或多种发生性抽动，而不必在同一时间出现
B	抽动的频率可能会起伏不定，但抽动病程在 1 年以上
C	18 岁以前起病
D	抽动症状不是直接由某些药物（如可卡因）或内科疾病（如亨廷顿舞蹈病或者病毒性脑炎）所致

对于抽动秽语综合征的诊断，患者应符合以下所有标准：DSM-5：第 5 版《精神疾病诊断和统计手册》（APA，2013）

50%～90% 的 TS 患者合并精神疾病，导致该疾病出现异质表型（Robertson 等，2000；Leckman 等，2006）。在一些患者中，这些并存的疾病造成的伤害甚至比抽动本身更严重。

注意力缺陷和多动障碍（attention deficit and hyperactivity disorder，ADHD）出现在 50% 的 TS 患者中，而强迫症行为出现在 50%～75% 的 TS 患者中。强迫症可能涉及暴力、攻击、性行为等。强迫行为通常与检查、计数、强行触摸和自我伤害有关。除了上述两种精神疾病外，TS 患者的情绪障碍和焦虑症以及破坏性行为的患病率也有所增加，每种疾病发生在 30% 的患者中（Hirschtritt 等，2015）。超过 1/3 的 TS 患者表现出自残行为，最常见的是撞击头部（Leckman 等，2006）。

（三）常规治疗

1. 社会心理或行为治疗

对于许多症状较轻的患者来说，社会心理或行为干预可能会有效地缓解症状。社会心理干预措施包括旨在提高症状耐受性和减轻压力的心理教育（Verdellen 等，2011）。行为方法包括习惯逆转治疗，暴露和反应预防，放松训练，应急管理，自我监控，生物（神经）反馈和认知行为治疗（Shprecher 和 Kurlan，2009；Verdellen 等，2011）。在习惯逆转疗法中，训练患者识别先兆冲动，并对这些冲动做出自主的竞争性或不相容性反应，例如"反抽动"收缩的肌肉或放松"抽动肌肉"。习惯逆转疗法也可能与放松训练和应急管理相冲突。暴露和反应预防包括在长时间抽动抑制和刺激适应过程中暴露于先兆感觉冲动。放松训练一般集中在肌肉放松和对先兆冲动的反应上。应急管理包括对环境突发事件的处理，以便积极增加无抽动间隔而减少抽动行为。

2. 药物治疗

如果患者的抽动症状引起主观不适（如疼痛或受伤害）、持续的社会问题（如社会暴露或欺凌）、情绪问题（例如反应性抑郁症状）或功能障碍（如学业成绩受损），并且社会心理或行为干预无效，那么药物治疗是一种选择。重要的是要认识到，药物治疗对 TS 的长期自然病程有何影响以及它如何影响大脑发育仍是未知的（Roessner 等，2011）。临床上使用最广泛的药物是典型抗精神病药物，如吡莫齐特和氟哌啶醇，它们可以阻断突触后多巴胺 $-D_2$ 受体。对于成人 TS 患者，这些是首选药物。另一种选择是非典型抗精神病药物，如利培酮、奥氮平、喹硫平、齐拉西酮和阿立哌唑，它们有更强的 5- 羟色胺能和去甲肾上腺素能作用。另一种用于治疗抽动症状的去甲肾上腺素药物是可乐定，它经常被用作治疗儿童 TS 的首选药物。苯甲酰胺类药物，如硫必利和舒必利，也通过多巴胺能系统起作用，并且同样有治疗效果。许多其他的药理干预也显示出在缓解 TS 患者抽动症状方面的效果，包括囊泡单胺转运蛋白 2（vesicular monoamine transporter 2, VMAT2）抑制药，如四苯嗪和利血平，去甲肾上腺素能药物和四氢大麻酚（Robertson 等，2000；Leckman 等，2002；Roessner 等，2011）。据报道，所有上述类型的药物都有轻微的不良反应，如镇静和过敏。抗精神病药物有更严重的不良反应，如锥体外系症状（如迟发性运动障碍或帕金森症）、体重增加、糖耐量减退和抑郁。对于典型抗精神病药来说，类似帕金森症的不良反应最为明显（Roessner，2011）。在使用 VMAT2 抑制药治疗 TS 期间，抑郁症尤其容易发生。如果抽动仅限于一块肌肉或一组肌肉，注射肉毒杆菌毒素也是一种选择。推荐使用选择性 5- 羟色胺再摄取抑制药和氯丙咪嗪来治疗强迫症和抑郁症。精神兴奋剂，如哌甲酯，可用于治疗并发 ADHD（Robertson 等，2000；Leckman，2002；Roessner 等，2011）。

（四）病理生理学

TS 的病理生理学仍然是未知的。在过去的几年中，大量的研究已经指向遗传和自身免疫性因素。功能和结构影像研究显示抽动时 TS 患者大脑的几个皮质和皮质下区域出现异常，其中包括基底神经节（basal ganglia, BG）（Mink, 2001；Singer 等, 2003）。BG 调节行为的机制包括通过不同的 BG 环路改变皮质兴奋性（图 16-1；见第 2 章）。

直接环路从纹状体延伸到苍白球内侧部（GPI）和黑质网状部（SNr），通过去抑制丘脑来兴奋皮质。从纹状体延伸到苍白球外侧部（GPE）再到底丘脑核（STN）的间接通路抑制了丘脑的投射。超直接通路绕过纹状体，将皮质信号直接投射到 STN，再投射到 GPI/SNr。通常，直接通路激活预期程序，而超直接和间接通路抑制非必需的竞争程序（Mink, 2001）。有假说认为，在 TS 中，由于多巴胺能功能障碍，纹状体中的局灶性畸变导致直接通路中 GPI/SNR 的过度抑制，从而由于过度的去抑制而导致皮质执行不自主的运动命令（Singer 和 Minzer, 2003；Gundus 和 Okun, 2016）。皮质 - 基底神经节 - 丘脑皮质（cortico-basal-ganglia-thalamocortical, CBGT）投射可以分为 5 个重要的功能环路，根据它们的皮质起源和作用区域命名，通过 BG 核的不同部分，包括运动、联合、边缘、动眼和眶额回环路。

二、手术治疗

TS 是无法治愈的。因此，治疗目的旨在减轻或缓解抽动症状，并治疗合并的精神症状。做出治疗决定的关键步骤是选择最合适的目标症状，这些症状会在患者的日常工作中造成最多的困扰（Shprecher 和 Kurlan, 2009）。在一些患者中，这个症状可能是抽动本身，但在另一些患者中，这可能是共病的精神障碍，如 ADHD，或两者兼而有之。

（一）手术的选择

尽管进行了社会心理和行为治疗以及药物治疗，但仍有一小部分患者对治疗无反应或出现了无法忍受的不良反应，并在整个青少年和成年生活中继续存在严重的症状（Verdellen 等, 2011；Roessner 等, 2011）。对于这一类患者，可以考虑脑深部电刺激（DBS）手术。抽动秽语综合征协会（Tourette Syndrome Association, TSA）已经提出了适应证指南（Schrock 等, 2015）（表 16-2）。

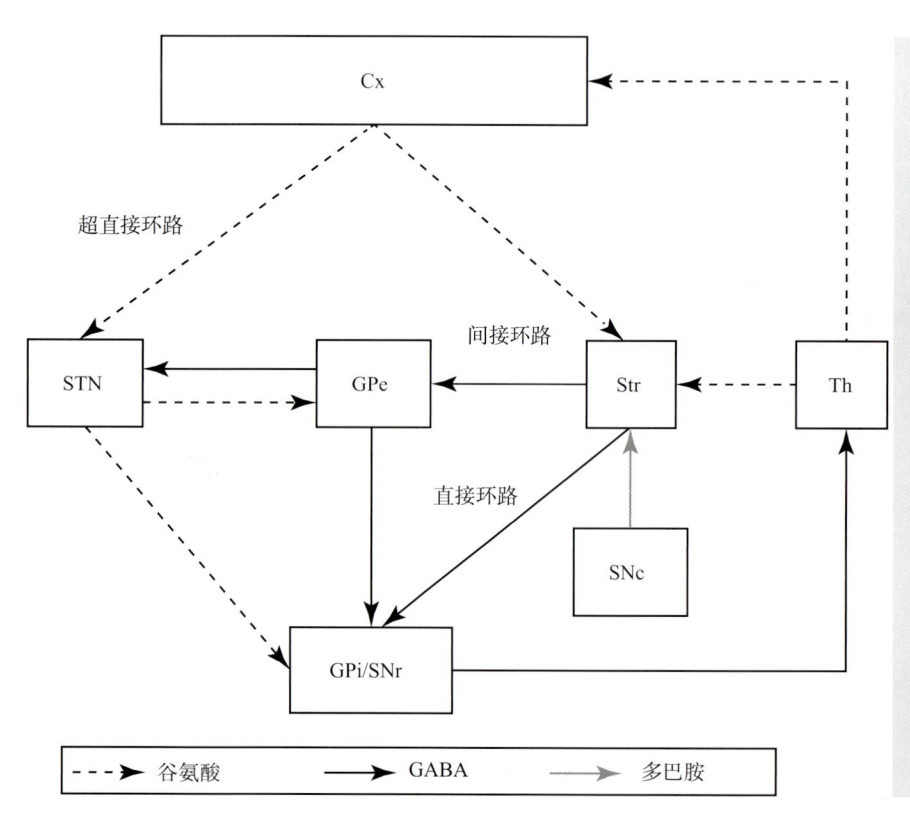

◀ 图 16-1 皮质 - 基底节 - 丘脑皮质通路的示意图

Cx. 大脑皮质；STN. 底丘脑核；GPE. 苍白球外侧部；Str. 纹状体；Th. 丘脑；GPI. 苍白球内侧部；SNr. 黑质网状部；SNc. 黑质致密部；GABA. γ- 氨基丁酸

表 16-2　脑深部电刺激治疗抽动秽语综合征患者的指征

	指　征
诊断	根据 DSM-5 标准确诊抽动秽语综合征
年龄	>18 岁
严重程度	YGTSS>35/50
神经精神共病	• 抽动肯定是最主要的症状。如果存在神经精神疾病并发症，则不应占主导地位 • 过去 6 个月并无自杀意念或企图自杀 • 共病的神经精神障碍必须稳定至少 6 个月 • 应使用有效的评分量表对合并神经精神疾病的发病率进行评分，以便术后能够监测这些症状
既往治疗	• 至少使用 3 种药物进行治疗后没有效果或患者无法耐受 　　－ D_2 受体拮抗药 　　－ 非典型抗精神病药物 　　－ α 肾上腺素激动药 　　－ 其他 　　－ 反转疗法 　　－ 暴露和反应预防 • 行为治疗无效
社会心理因素	• 充分的社会支持，没有任何急性或亚急性压力来源 • 如有必要，愿意接受术后心理治疗 • 照顾者对参与术后咨询的准备

DSM-5. 第 5 版《精神疾病诊断和统计手册》（APA，2013）；YGTSS. 耶鲁综合抽动严重程度量表；D_2. 多巴胺 2 型

在严重的 TS 病例中，例如 YGTSS 评分>35 分，可以考虑应用 DBS。抽动应该对患者的个人、职业和社会功能有明显的影响。TS 的诊断必须是肯定的，并且症状必须至少存在 5 年。即使存在精神共病，它也不应该是主要的主诉。选择手术前必须进行充分的药物治疗。患者至少应该尝试过 3 种不同的药物。这些药物没有显示出显著疗效，或者导致了严重的不良反应，以至于治疗无法继续下去。此外，患者至少应该接受一种形式的行为治疗且同样没有取得满意疗效。2006 年，第一个版本的治疗指南里建议接受手术的患者最低年龄为 25 岁，因为 TS 具有自限性，青春期后往往会出现改善。最近的一份指南提到可以接受手术的患者最低年龄为 18 岁。然而，其他学者指出，由于抽动症状的破坏性，在严重 TS 的情况下对在更低年龄的患者应用 DBS 手术可能会带来更多的益处。较年轻的患者通常无法上学，接受培训或保持工作；他们倾向于避免参加社交活动，或者不能够发展友谊或情感关系，并且通常自卑。这可能会在以后的生活中产生长期的影响（Smeets 等，2018b）。拥有一个在手术前后提供充足支持的社交网络也是非常重要的。DBS 手术的禁忌证包括严重的系统疾病或大脑磁共振成像（magnetic resonance imaging，MRI）上的结构异常，这会干扰放置电极的安全性及最佳位置。进行 DBS 手术的最终决定应该在一个多学科团队中达成共识，其中有神经外科医生、精神病学家，最好还有心理学家参与。

（二）手术入路

在 TS 患者中实施 DBS 的外科医生应该在 DBS 治疗运动障碍方面有丰富的经验，以提高疗效并将并发症发生率降至最低。应用于 TS 的 DBS 技术与用于更经典适应证的技术相似。TS 的靶点（如丘脑内侧部分的核团）在当前的成像技术中几乎是不可见的。此外，由于头部区域中发生运动抽动的比例很高，TS 患者可能会位移出立体定向框架。一种解决方案是在患者全身麻醉的情况下进行手术。由于理想靶点的不确定

性和术中定位的重要性，因此患者在手术期间应保持合作。最好是在保持与患者沟通的情况下使患者镇静以获得抽动抑制。患者可以联合使用氯美西泮和可乐定，使用异丙酚靶控输注，或使用右美托咪啶，充分减少抽动对立体定向手术的影响。这样手术的同时可以保留与患者的沟通，术中观察到急性负极刺激引起的不良反应，继而调整电极的位置。

内侧丘脑和苍白球是最常用的靶点。使用 Leksell 立体定向架进行手术。丘脑靶点是丘脑的中央中核、脑室旁灰质和腹嘴侧核（centromedian nucleus, substantia periventricularis, and nucleus ventrooralis internus, Cm-Spv-Voi），使用以下标准坐标：x= 前－后连合中线外侧（anterior commissure–posterior commissure, AC-PC）5mm，y=AC-PC 平面上距中连合点后方 4mm，z= 在 AC-PC 平面的位置。苍白球靶点是苍白球（GPI）的内侧部，使用以下标准坐标：x=AC-PC 中线外侧 12mm，y=AC-PC 平面上连合点中部前 6～9mm，z=AC-PC 平面上方 0～3mm（图 16-2）。靶点坐标可以根据第三脑室的宽度和 AC-PC 长度在高场强 T_2 加权 MRI 图像上进行可视化和调整。

按照计划的路径放置导管，并进行微电极记录（multiple-electrode extracellular single-unit recordings，MER）。记录 0.5～1.0mm 的步长从靶点上方 10mm 到靶点下方 4mm 进行。随后，沿着具有最佳 MER 记录的路径执行测试刺激，以评估刺激引起的不良反应。最后，四触点电极取代测试电极，电极的第二深度触点（触点 1）在靶点的水平上，该触点没有不良反应或仅在最高刺激强度下产生。随后，在全身麻醉下，植入脉冲发生器。术后第一天，进行 CT 扫描以发现无症状的出血并评估电极的位置。术后调整刺激参数，以获得最有效的刺激参数。

三、DBS 的预后

自 1955 年以来，外科医生一直在尝试应

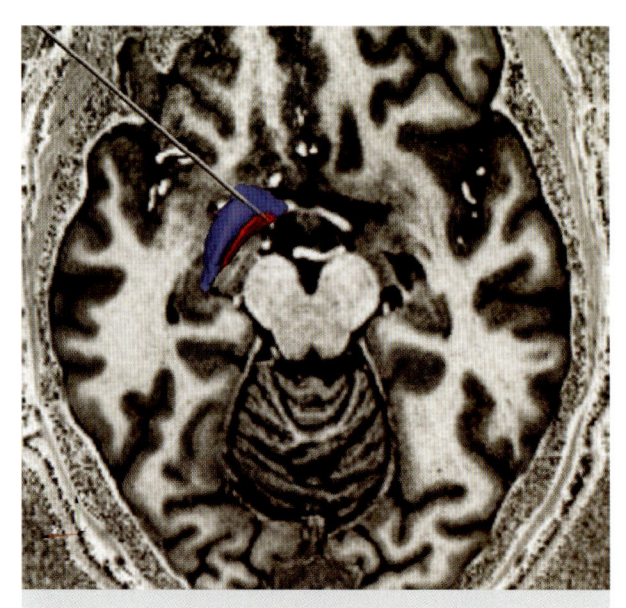

▲ 图 16-2　电极放置在右侧苍白球的内侧
图片由 Israelashvili 等提供，2017

用外科手术治疗 TS。期间共有 65 名患者接受了针对不同脑区的消融手术，其中包括额叶皮质、丘脑、苍白球和小脑（Temel 和 Visser-Vandewalle，2004）。但这些干预措施没有得到理想的疗效，并出现了严重的并发症，如偏瘫和肌张力障碍。随着外科手段治疗运动障碍疾病的研究取得进展，丘脑 DBS 在 1999 年首次用于治疗顽固性 TS（Vandewalle 等，1999）。这一过程需要通过双侧大脑深部结构植入电极并进行电刺激，这些电极从皮下植入的脉冲发生器接收高频脉冲。DBS 的主要目的是改变神经元的放电模式，影响 CBGT 环路中节点的信息传递，从而改善 TS 的症状。这对症状的影响与消融手术相同，但却是可逆的。有证据表明，DBS 通过引起功能性消融来发挥作用，从而减少了通过刺激靶点的信息流（Israelashvili 等，2015）。

自 1999 年以来，全世界已经发表了 57 项关于 DBS 治疗 TS 的研究，这些研究总共包括来自 13 个国家 23 个中心的 156 名患者（Baldermann 等，2016）。获得最佳手术预后的一个关键因素是靶点选择，但由于 TS 患者表现出复杂的临床特征，这一话题仍存在争论。

到目前为止，已有 9 个独立的大脑区域成为刺激靶点，具体如下。

- 丘脑的内侧部分。
  - 丘脑的中央正中核、脑室旁灰质和腹嘴侧核的交叉点（Cm-Spv-Voi）。
  - 丘脑中央正中核-束旁复合体（centromedian nucleus–parafascicular complex，CM-PF）。
  - 丘脑背内侧核-束旁复合体（dorsomedian nucleus–parafascicular complex，DM-PF）。
- 苍白球内侧部（GPI）。
  - 后外侧运动部（后 GPI）。
  - 前内侧边缘部（GPI 前部）。
- 苍白球外侧部（GPE）。
- 伏隔核（NA）。
- 内囊前肢（ALIC）。
- 底丘脑核（STN）。

此外，有学者还分别或同时进行了针对多个大脑区域的研究。在基底神经节的主要输出站或中继站之一的层面上进行 DBS 可能对难治性 TS 患者有临床益处。总体而言，以 YGTSS 为评估指标，所有靶点的 DBS 的短期内症状显著改善，平均达 53%。

对照研究的分析表明，与关闭 DBS 刺激相比，开启刺激时患者抽动症状有显著改善。总体而言，对于丘脑和 GPI 靶点进行 DBS，患者的抽动症状改善的程度可能是最好的（Baldermann 等，2016）。

（一）内侧丘脑 DBS

文献报道有 3 例患者内侧丘脑进行 DBS 治疗 TS，靶点是丘脑的 Cm-Spv-Voi 交叉点，其结果是 YGTSS 术后评分分别减少了 72%、83% 和 90%（Visser-Vandewalle 等，2003）。这个靶点的选择是基于 Hassler 和 Dieckmann 报道的一个应用立体定向毁损手术成功改善患者症状的病例（1970）。其假说是刺激 Cm 和 Spv 会抑制兴奋性反馈投射到纹状体的运动和边缘部分，减轻抽动症状，改善行为障碍。对 Voi 的刺激应该包括前运动皮质的面部部分的投射，从而可以调节口面部抽动的症状。自那以来，已有 22 项研究报告了 78 名丘脑 DBS 患者（Baldermann 等，2016）。YGTSS 评分的平均改善百分比为 53%，其中 52% 的患者在最后一次随访中报告至少 50% 的改善。随访结果差异较大，只有 20% 的纳入患者的随访时间＞1 年。文献报道的不良反应包括性欲减退、嗜睡、视力障碍和体重减轻。另外也有精神病、抑郁和轻躁狂症病例的报道，但通过调整刺激参数，这些情况可能会被逆转（Fraint 和 Pal，2015）。

（二）苍白球 DBS

苍白球由内侧部分和外侧部分（GPI 和 GPE）组成，大多数研究都针对 GPI。只有 1 例病例报告了刺激 GPE 对 TS 的影响，结果是刺激 6 个月后 YGTSS 评分改善了 70%（Piedimonte 等，2013）。GPI 由后外侧运动部（后 GPI）和前内侧边缘部（前 GPI）组成。这两个区域都是 DBS 治疗 TS 的靶点。一些研究没有具体报告 GPI 的哪个部分是刺激靶点。后 GPi 的 DBS 于 2002 年首次进行，并取得了良好的疗效（van der Linden 等，2002），此后已有 20 名患者被文献报道（Baldermann 等，2016）。据报道，YGTSS 评分平均改善了 57%，61% 的患者在最后一次随访中至少报告了 50% 的改善（表 16-3）。到目前为止，更多的患者接受了前 GPI 的 DBS。这些患者的 YGTSS 评分平均改善 52%，其中 66% 的患者报告至少 50% 的改善（表 16-3）。已知的苍白球 DBS 的不良反应有焦虑、烦躁、体重减轻、恶心、眩晕和感觉异常，其中大部分可能是短暂的（Fraint 和 Pal，2015）。

在 2 项随机对照试验（randomized controlled trials, RCT）中，前 GPi DBS 的临床疗效并不显著。Kefalopoulou 等（2015）分析了 15 名 TS 患者的前 GPI DBS 的结果。他们比较了盲法刺激的刺激开期和刺激关期，结果显示，尽管各组之间患者症状改善程度存在很大差异（-3%～57%），但在小组水平上 YGTSS 评分平均改善仅为 15%。未观察到对强迫行为有显著影

表 16-3　脑深部电刺激治疗抽动秽语综合征的疗效

靶　点	N	平均改善（%）[a]	≥25% 响应（%）[a]	≥50% 响应（%）[a]
丘脑	78	53（26）	82	52
后 GPi	20	57（35）	78	61
前 GPi	44	52（55）	77	66
GPe/STN	2	-	-	-
NA/ALIC	9	44（15）	75	38
其他[b]	3	45（27）	67	67
总数	156	53（27）	81	54

N. 数量；GPi. 苍白球内侧部；NA. 伏隔核；ALIC. 内囊前肢；GPe. 苍白球外侧部；STN. 底丘脑核
a. YGTSS 得分和反应百分比的平均变化；b.GPI 靶点不明（n=2），GPI 前后部均有刺激（n=1）
（经许可转载，引自 Baldermann 等，2016）

响。在 8~36 个月的揭盲刺激期中，患者的抽动症状改善了 40%。这种显著的抽动改善在长期随访中保持不变。Welter 等进行了一项双盲 RCT 试验，其中招募了 16 例接受前 GPi DBS 的难治性 TS 患者（Welter 等，2017）。3 个月后，所有患者被随机分配，在接下来的 3 个月里接受刺激或假刺激。之后，所有患者在接下来的 6 个月内接受非盲的刺激。3 个月双盲期前后 YGTSS 评分差异无显著性，刺激组 YGTSS 评分平均改善 10%，假刺激组 YGTSS 平均改善 4%。2 组所有患者的 YGTSS 评分都有改善，非盲期结束时 YGTSS 评分改善了 40%。

（三）伏隔核和内囊前肢 DBS

只有 9 名患者接受了 NA/ALIC DBS 治疗，YGTSS 平均改善了 44%，38% 的患者报告了 50% 以上的改善（表 16-3）。尽管证据不充分，但对这一靶点的刺激可能没有其他靶点那么有效。NA DBS 的潜在不良反应包括脸红、焦虑、出汗、轻躁狂、烦躁不安和精神错乱。ALIC DBS 的潜在不良反应是欣快感、头晕、焦虑、惊慌和恐惧（Fraint 和 Pal，2015）。

（四）底丘脑核 DBS

有文献报道 1 例 38 岁的帕金森病（Parkinson disease，PD）的男子同时患有 TS。在进行 STN DBS 治疗他的帕金森病后，不仅患者的运动症状有所改善，而且抽动频率在 1 年时也减少了 97%（Martinez-Torres 等，2009）。

（五）并发症和不良事件

Saleh 和 Fontaine（2015）分析了治疗 TS 和其他精神疾病的 DBS 术后的所有报道的并发症和不良事件。16%~5% 的病例报告了长期存在并发症和不良事件，其中 6.2% 与手术或硬件有关，10.2% 与慢性刺激有关。一些研究表明，由于 TS 患者的特殊行为特征，TS 患者比其他接受 DBS 的患者有更高的炎症并发症发生率（Servello 等，2011）。TS 患者 DBS 术后与刺激相关的不良反应包括焦虑（n=7）、情绪改变（n=2）、精神错乱（n=1）、冷漠（n=13）和性功能改变（n=6）（Saleh 和 Fontaine，2015）。值得注意的是，冷漠只在丘脑 DBS 患者中观察到。大多数报道的不良反应可能是暂时的，或者可以通过调整刺激参数来解决。但这与我们在丘脑 DBS 的患者的长期随访中的经验不符，在丘脑 DBS 的长期随访中（Smeets 等，2018a），不良反应往往对刺激参数的调整没有反应，并且随着治疗时间的延长变得更加明显。

四、讨论

非盲序列和小型双盲试验报告了针对几个大脑靶点的 DBS 对 TS 患者抽动症状的积极效果，主要是内侧丘脑和前部 GPi。由于缺乏证据，用于 TS 的 DBS 没有得到欧盟委员会（European Commission，EC）和美国食品药品管理局（U.S. Food and Drug Administration，FDA）的批准。缺乏证据的主要原因是难以以随机对照的方式进行高质量的研究，加上手术效果不一，靶点数量众多，以及全球范围内患有 TS 并适合进行 DBS 的患者总数很少。因此，必须将其视为一种试验性治疗，这意味着只有那些症状最严重且已被证明对保守治疗无效的患者才可以被视为 DBS 的候选。应告知患者该疗法相对缺乏证据，并应特别注意避免患者发生所谓的治疗误解。对治疗的误解意味着患者期望获得明显的个人利益，但却无法意识到治疗的试验特征，并且低估了个体治疗反应不确定，长期认知，情感和行为影响在很大程度上未知的事实。进一步研究 DBS 用于该适应证的安全性和有效性是必要的。然而，目前大规模的 RCT 是不可行的，因为即使在经验丰富的 DBS 中心，每年也只对 TS 患者进行少量 DBS 手术。此外，不同的临床中心使用不同的手术技术和靶点，这使得获得和解释大规模序列的结果变得困难。从理论上讲，多中心 RCT 是可取的，但由于实际原因，该研究方案未来持续多年都很难实现。目前，纳入过程、手术技术、靶点、规划和术后护理在不同的机构和国家之间差别很大。此外，在这样的研究过程中，可能会获得新的见解，例如，研究发现不同的手术靶点的效果或手术中的其他变化，这对于后来的参与者而言是不道德的（Smeets 等，2018b）。为了从临床经验中获得最大收益，我们建议应将所有进行 DBS 手术的 TS 病例注册在一个中央数据库中，数据库涵盖一系列标准化的信息。这样的数据库目前已经在运行（Deeb 等，2016）。一场围绕 DBS 可治疗最低年龄伦理争论也在进行之中。鉴于抽动可能对儿童的社会、心理和智力发展造成严重的、有时是无法弥补的伤害，越来越多的人考虑在更小的年龄进行手术。但是，考虑到 TS 的自限性，即青春期后会有所改善，这可能会导致 DBS 装置在植入数年后随着患者抽动症状自发停止而被停用。另外，青春期的行为障碍可能会干扰治疗过程（Smeets 等，2018b）。持续的和积极主动的伦理思考应该在未来的临床实践继续进行，而不仅是在当前的试验治疗案例中。其中不仅涵盖理论思想，还包括对相关人员（即患者、家庭成员和专业人员）的观点提供解释。

五、结论

根据已发表的样本量有限的病例研究结果，DBS 可以安全有效地治疗经过严格筛选的难治性 TS 患者。然而，对于纳入标准、刺激靶点、刺激参数设置和长期疗效，目前还没有达成一致意见。进一步的研究应该会在上述领域提供更多的证据。在实现这一目标之前，DBS 被认为是治疗 TS 的"最后手段"，且只能在特定的治疗中心进行。当前和未来的临床实践应伴随着伦理思考。

参考文献

[1] American Psychiatric Association. Diagnostic and statistical manual of mental disorders, Five Edition Text Revision (DSM-V) Washington, DC, USA. Washington, DC: American Psychiatric Association Press; 2013.

[2] Baldermann JC, Schuller T, Huys D, et al. Deep brain stimulation for Tourette-syndrome: a systematic review and meta-analysis. Brain Stimul. 2016;9:296–304.

[3] Bloch MH, Leckman JF. Clinical course of Tourette syndrome. J Psychosom Res. 2009;67:497–501.

[4] Deeb W, Rossi PJ, Porta M, et al. The International Deep Brain Stimulation Registry and Database for Gilles de la Tourette syndrome: how does it work? Front Neurosci. 2016;10:170.

[5] Fraint A, Pal G. Deep brain stimulation in Tourette's syndrome. Front Neurol. 2015;6:170.

[6] Gilles de la Tourette G. Etude sur un affection nerveuse caractérisée par l'incoordination motrice accompagnée d'echolalie et de coprolalie. Arch Neural. 1885;9:19–42, 158–200.

[7] Gundus A, Okun MS. A review and update on Tourette syndrome: where is the field headed? Curr Neurol Neurosci Rep. 2016;16:37.

[8] Hassler R, Dieckmann G. Stereotaxic treatment of tics and inarticulate cries or coprolalia considered as motor obsessional phenomena in Gilles de la Tourette's disease. Rev Neurol.

1970;123:89–100.

[9] Hirschtritt ME, Lee PC, Pauls DL, et al. Lifetime prevalence, age of risk, and aetiology of comorbid psychiatric disorders in Tourette syndrome. JAMA Psychiat. 2015;72:325–33.

[10] Israeleashvilli M, Smeets AYJM, Bronfeld M, et al. Functional derivatives of tonic and phasic changes in pallidal activity during Tourette syndrome. Mov Disord 2017;32:1091–6.

[11] Israelashvili M, Loewenstern Y, Bar-Gad I. Abnormal neuronal activity in Tourette syndrome and its modulation using deep brain stimulation. J Neurophysiol. 2015;114:6–20.

[12] Itard JEE. Memoire sur quelques fonctions involuntaires des appareils de la locomotion, de la prehension et de la voix. Arch Gen Med. 1825;8:385–407.

[13] Kefalopoulou Z, Zrinzo L, Jahanshahi M, et al. Bilateral globus pallidus stimulation for severe Tourette's syndrome: a double-blind, randomised crossover trial. Lancet Neurol. 2015;14:595–605.

[14] Kramer H, Daniels C. Pioneers of movement disorders: Georges Gilles de la Tourette. J Neural Transm. 2004;111:691–701.

[15] Leckman JF. Tourette's syndrome. Lancet. 2002;360(9345):1577–86.

[16] Leckman JF, Bloch MH, Scahill L, King RA. Tourette syndrome: the self under siege. J Child Neurol. 2006;21:642–9.

[17] Martinez-Torres I, Hariz MI, Zrinzo L, et al. Improvement of tics after subthalamic nucleus deep brain stimulation. Neurology. 2009;72:1787–9.

[18] Mink JW. Basal ganglia dysfunction in Tourette's syndrome: a new hypothesis. Pediatr Neurol. 2001;25:190–8.

[19] Müller-Vahl KR, Riemann L, Bokemeyer S. Tourette patients' misbelief of a tic rebound is due to overall difficulties in reliable tic rating. J Psychosom Res. 2014;76:472–6.

[20] Piedimonte F, Andreani JC, Piedimonte L, et al. Behavioral and motor improvement after deep brain stimulation of the globus pallidus externus in a case of Tourette's syndrome. Neuromodulation. 2013;16:55–8.

[21] Robertson MM. Tourette syndrome, associated conditions and the complexities of treatment. Brain. 2000;123(Pt 3):425–62.

[22] Robertson MM. The prevalence and epidemiology of Gilles de la Tourette syndrome. Part 1: the epidemiological and prevalence studies. J Psychosom Res. 2008;65:461–72.

[23] Roessner V, Plessen KJ, Rothenberger A, et al. European clinical guidelines for Tourette syndrome and other tic disorders. Part II: pharmacological treatment. Eur Child Adolesc Psychiatry. 2011;20:173–96.

[24] Saleh C, Fontaine D. Deep brain stimulation for psychiatric diseases: what are the risks? Curr Psychiatry Rep. 2015;17:33.

[25] Schrock LE, Mink JW, Woods DW, et al. Tourette syndrome deep brain stimulation: a review and updated recommendations. Mov Disord. 2015;30:448–71.

[26] Servello D, Sassi M, Gaeta M, et al. Tourette syndrome (TS) bears a higher rate of inflammatory complications at the implanted hardware in deep brain stimulation (DBS). Acta Neurochir. 2011;153:629–32.

[27] Shprecher D, Kurlan R. The management of tics. Mov Disord. 2009;24:15–24.

[28] Singer HS, Minzer K. Neurobiology of Tourette's syndrome: concepts of neuroanatomic localization and neurochemical abnormalities. Brain Dev. 2003;25(Suppl 1):S70–84.

[29] Smeets AY, Duits AA, Leentjens AFG, et al. Thalamic deep brain simulation for refractory Tourette syndrome: clinical evidence for increasing disbalance of therapeutic effects and side effects at long-term follow-up. Neuromodulation. 2018a;21:197–202.

[30] Smeets AYJM, Duits AA, Verdellen C, et al. Ethics of deep brain stimulation in adolescent patients with refractory Tourette syndrome: a systematic review and two case discussions. Neuroethics. 2018b;11:143–55.

[31] Temel Y, Visser-Vandewalle V. Surgery in Tourette syndrome. Mov Disord. 2004;19:3–14.

[32] van der Linden C, Colle H, Vandewalle V, et al. Successful treatment of tics with bilateral internal pallidum stimulation in a 27-year old male patient with Gilles de la Tourette syndrome. Mov Disord. 2002; 17:341.

[33] Vandewalle V, van der Linden C, Groenewegen HJ, Caemaert J. Stereotactic treatment of Gilles de la Tourette syndrome by high frequency stimulation of thalamus. Lancet. 1999;353(9154):724.

[34] Verdellen CW, Hoogduin CA, Keijsers GP. Tic suppression in the treatment of Tourette's syndrome with exposure therapy: the rebound phenomenon reconsidered. Mov Disord. 2007;22:1601–6.

[35] Verdellen C, van de Griendt J, Hartmann A, et al. European clinical guidelines for Tourette syndrome and other tic disorders. Part III: behavioural and psychosocial interventions. Eur Child Adolesc Psychiatry. 2011;20:197–207.

[36] Visser-Vandewalle V, Temel Y, Boon P, et al. Chronic bilateral thalamic stimulation: a new therapeutic approach in intractable Tourette syndrome. Report of three cases. J Neurosurg 2003;99:1094–100.

[37] Welter ML, Houeto JL, Thobois S, et al. Anterior pallidal deep brain stimulation for Tourette's syndrome: a randomised, double-blind, controlled trial. Lancet Neurol. 2017;16:610–9.

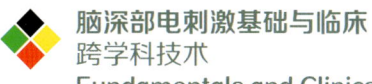

第三篇

精神病学
Psychiatry

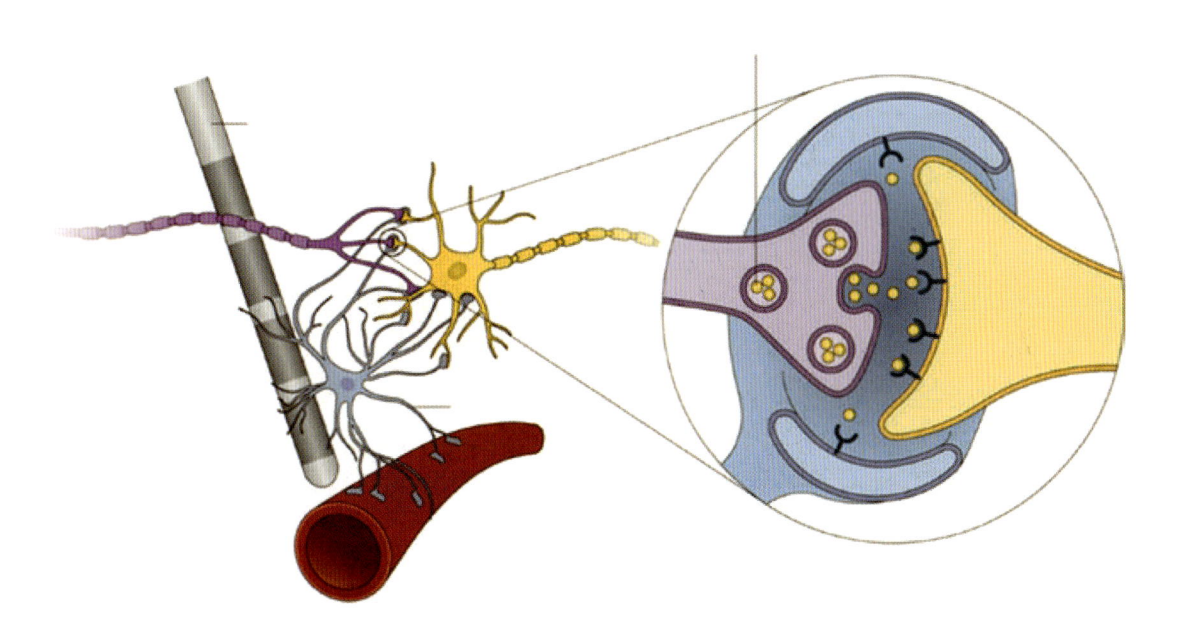

第17章 强迫症的脑深部电刺激治疗
Deep Brain Stimulation in Obsessive-Compulsive Disorder

Mircea Polosan　Albert F. G. Leentjens　著
刘德峰　刘焕光　译　张�　杨岸超　张建国　校

> **摘要：** 严重的强迫症（OCD）患者可能对传统的心理治疗和药物治疗无效，而脑深部电刺激术（DBS）对其来说是一种十分有前景的治疗方法。DBS既能改善OCD患者功能，又能提高生活质量，其症状平均改善约为45%。尽管应用了许多不同的解剖学靶点，但是就有效性或不良反应而言，目前可用的证据尚不支持某一特定靶点优于另一特定靶点。缺乏对OCD各种症状背后的神经解剖学差异的认识，以及可靠的生物标志物，造成了DBS的指征建立、靶点选择和有效路径规划的障碍。然而，迄今为止临床试验的良好结果，以及潜在的神经环路和技术发展方面的重大研究进展，都支持DBS针对这一适应证进一步应用和研究。技术发展应该伴随着持续的、积极主动的伦理思考。因此，进一步研究有助于确定DBS在OCD治疗选择中的定位，并通过进一步降低治疗难度，为OCD患者打开一个新的视角。

一、背景

（一）流行病学

强迫症（OCD）是一种以强迫观念和（或）强迫行为为特征的慢性精神障碍 [American Psychiatric Association（APA），2013]。世界卫生组织（World Health Organization, WHO）将OCD列为继发性残疾的第11大最常见原因，约占失能生存年（years lived with disability, YLD）总数的2.2%（Vos等，2012）。在成人中的患病率为0.8%～3%（Heyman等，2006）。发病年龄通常在青春期后期（18岁），且男性的发病年龄比女性早（Brakoulias等，2017）。OCD的病程通常是慢性的，并且症状会随时间波动（Ruscio等，2010）。在儿童期或青春期发病的OCD患者中，高达40%的人在成年初期可能会得到缓解。当患者将他们的强迫性规则强加给家人时，与OCD相关的功能障碍可能会扩散到周围环境中，从而导致家庭功能障碍。据报道，多达一半的OCD患者存在自杀念头，并且与普通人群相比，OCD患者自杀未遂（OR=5.5）和实际自杀（OR=9.8）的风险明显更高（De La Cruz等，2017）。

（二）临床表现

OCD的特征是存在导致严重痛苦和伤害的强迫观念和（或）强迫行为。强迫观念被定义为不想要的和侵入性的想法、影响或冲动，而强迫行为则表现为重复的行为，由患者以刻板的方式进行，试图压制不想要的强迫行为，减少相关的焦虑或不适，或者防止在不执行强迫症的情况下可能经历的焦虑或不适。然而，OCD并不总是与焦虑联系在一起，例如在"恰到好处"的强迫观念和（或）强迫行为的情况下。尽管OCD有一些特殊的表现，但可以确定一些常见的主要症状，如害怕污染或强迫性清洁、需要对称、重复、命令或计数、不可接受或被禁止的想法（通常是攻击性的、性的或宗教性质的）和伤害（如担心对自己或他人的伤害负责），以及"恰到好处"的强迫观念。这些不同的症状可能由不同的神经元环路支撑，因此也可能与治疗选择相关（APA，2013；Mataix-Cols等，2004）。

OCD的一个共同特征是患者主观上感觉到失去了自由意志，以及强加在精神上的一种缺乏控制感，尽管患者意识到这些症状是由于自己的心理造成的。OCD的这种自我紧张性特征反映了一个人的强迫症和他/她的自我形象之间的冲突。这对于区分强迫症和强迫症人格障碍有特别重要的意义（Denys，2011）。

在DSM-5分类中，OCD不再被认为是焦虑症，焦虑也不再被认为是OCD的核心症状。相反，OCD被归入新的更广泛的"强迫症和相关障碍"类别，其中还包括躯体变形障碍、囤积症、拔毛症和抠抓皮肤（APA，2013）。

（三）常规治疗

OCD的常规治疗包括心理干预治疗和药物治疗，两者经常结合使用。

心理干预治疗主要基于认知行为疗法（cognitive behavioral therapy, CBT）的原则，涉及对适应不良认知和信念的认知重新评价和重构。一种特定类型的CBT，暴露和反应预防（exposure in vivo and response prevention, ERP）被认为是最有效的治疗方法，在接受药物治疗和不接受药物治疗的患者中，应答率都在50%。然而，暴露可能会导致高度焦虑，从而导致过早终止治疗。此外，ERP对主要经历强迫观念而不是强迫行为的患者可能疗效较差。CBT疗程的可接受性和依从性不高：在非抗药性强迫症队列中，只有24%的患者完成了计划的全程疗程（Mancebo等，2006）。

大量证据支持血清素抗抑郁药的疗效，包括选择性5-羟色胺再摄取抑制药（selective serotonin reuptake inhibitors, SSRI）和三环类抗抑郁药（氯丙咪嗪）。然而，40%～60%的患者在药物治疗后没有得到缓解，仍然会出现致残症状。虽然缺乏足够的证据，但这将证明OCD的强化治疗策略是合理的，例如高剂量血清素能药物的组合，抗精神病药的添加，以及其他药物的使用（如米氮平、利鲁唑、氯胺酮、美金刚、N-乙酰半胱氨酸、拉莫三嗪、恩丹西酮、d-环丝氨酸等）（Hirschtritt等，2017）。

尽管采取了这些常规治疗方法，但治疗耐药性仍然很高，平均有25%的患者没有从治疗中受益。对于这些患者，可以考虑脑深部电刺激术（DBS）。目前的治疗指南建议将DBS作为治疗方法的最后一步，与其他神经调节方法，如重复经颅磁刺激（repetitive transcranial magnetic stimulation, rTMS），以及神经外科手术（如内囊切开术和扣带回切开术）处于同一水平（Hirschtritt等，2017）。OCD是DBS唯一确定的精神疾病适应证，它于2008年获得FDA批准（作为人道主义设备豁免），并于2009年获得CE批准。

（四）病理生理学

虽然OCD的典型症状强调强迫行为的作用，认为强迫行为可以中和与强迫观念有关的焦虑，但最近的数据表明，强迫行为与养成习惯的特定脆弱性有关，主要是回避习惯（Gillan等，2014）。这是以目标为导向的行为及某些机制的功能障碍为代价的，例如监测不确定性和偏执，决策及反应抑制的机制。

脑损伤诱发强迫行为的病例报告支持了OCD涉及皮质-纹状体-丘脑回路，顶叶和颞叶皮质，小脑和脑干的假说（Figee等，2013）。有研究报道在壳核、内囊和额顶叶损伤后，OCD症状出现改善或缓解，这也提供了腹侧纹状体和内囊 DBS 治疗 OCD 的理论基础的证据（Figee 等，2013）。

神经影像学研究一致发现 OCD 患者眶额叶皮质、前扣带皮质和基底神经节（主要是纹状体）代谢活动亢进，这支持了 OCD 中皮质 - 基底神经节 - 丘脑 - 皮质环路异常与非运动环路中直接和间接通路失衡的因果关系（Maia 等，2008）。最初认为是运动环路的一部分皮质 - 底丘脑核的超直接联系可能也十分重要，因为在灵长类动物中，该通路被证明涉及认知 / 联想和动机 / 边缘环路（Haynes 和 Haber，2013）。这种功能性分布与来自不同皮质区域向皮质下水平的投射的高度汇聚有关，因此提示多模态信息在底丘脑核（subthalamic nucleus，STN）水平上的整合（Haynes 和 Haber，2013）。STN 是皮质 - 基底神经节间接和超直接通路中的重要中继站。STN-DBS 治疗帕金森病（Parkinson disease，PD）的有效性为 STN 在复杂运动和非运动症状中的作用提供了证据（Krack 等，2001；Castrioto 等，2014）。

尽管大脑网络抑制过程的减弱与 OCD 尤为相关，但影像学研究揭示了 STN 与不恰当响应的抑制性大脑网络的关系，其中伴有辅助运动区（presupplementary motor area，preSMA）和下额叶皮质的参与（Chamberlain 等，2005；Aron，2011）。电生理学研究为 STN 在抑制功能中的作用提供了更具体的信息，即有助于从自动行为切换到受控行为，这对于将 OCD 患者的强迫习惯转变为更具目标导向的动作具有潜在的好处。此外，STN-DBS 在 PD 患者的研究表明，STN 在执行控制中起主动和反应性抑制作用（Hikosaka 和 Isoda，2010；Benis 等，2013；Jahanshahi 等，2015）。

与 STN 相似，内囊前肢（anterior limb of internal capsule，ALIC）腹侧的纤维束与广泛的脑网状区域相连。腹侧内囊 / 腹侧纹状体（ventral capsule/ventral striatum，VC/VS）区域的 DBS 针对的是眶额叶皮质（orbitofrontal cortex，OFC）与丘脑之间的相互兴奋性连接，从而降低了眶额及尾 - 苍白球 - 丘脑环路内的异常反射活动（Makris 等，2016）。刺激在 VC/VS 内不同的电极触点可以交替刺激内侧和（或）外侧眶前丘脑纤维，它们在功能上是不同的（Karas 等，2019）。

二、DBS 手术筛选

筛选符合 DBS 指征的 OCD 患者对于治疗预后至关重要。在 OCD 患者中应用 DBS 治疗的主要筛选标准是选择慢性、重度和残疾及难治的病例（表 17-1）。

OCD 应由精神病学专家按照 DSM-5 OCD 诊断标准进行诊断（APA，2013）。不同的精神病学表现或并发症提示潜在的神经生物学功能障碍存在异质性，因此这形成了特定靶点 DBS 响应变异性的潜在来源。囤积已经被认为是 OCD 的一种特殊形式，它对常规治疗的反应较小，并且可能有与典型 OCD 相比具有不同的神经生物学底物支持。因此，如果囤积是患者的主要症状表现，这通常被认为不是应用 DBS 治疗的指征。其他与 OCD 相关的疾病，如拔毛症和抠抓皮肤，通常不被认为是禁忌证，但这些疾病临床治疗反应较差。OCD 患者常常伴有精神疾病。78% 的患者经历终生并发症，这些问题应该在 DBS 适应证的筛查过程中予以处理（Hofmeijer-Sevink 等，2013）。在 OCD 患者中，重度抑郁障碍是最常见的共病，终生患病率为 51%（Brakoulias 等，2017）。到目前为止，情绪障碍还没有被认为是 DBS 的禁忌证，主要是因为 DBS 可能会对情绪产生积极影响。然而，自杀意向和行为应在纳入 DBS 治疗之前予以处理。其他共病，如焦虑症，其中广泛性焦虑症和特殊恐惧症或抽搐不被认为是 DBS 的禁忌证。OCD 患者合并成瘾症占 14%，评估时实际的药物滥用或尚未稳定缓解药物滥用或依赖的应视为 DBS 禁忌证，因为药物滥用可能会影响治疗依从性和结果。

自闭症和精神障碍同样也不是适应证，尽管有极少的数据报告表明残留精神分裂症患者的强

表 17-1 DBS 治疗 OCD 的纳入和排除标准概况

	纳入标准	排除标准
精神病学诊断	• 符合 DSM-5 中 OCD 的诊断	• 囤积是主要症状 • 双相情感障碍 • 终生精神病诊断 • 在过去 12 个月内存在滥用或依赖药物的情况 • 严重 A 类或 B 类人格障碍 • 自杀倾向
年龄	• 20—70 岁	
严重程度	• Y-BOCS 评分>25～30 • GAF 评分<45	• Y-BOCS 评分<25 • GAF 评分>45
抗药性	• 至少使用两种 SSRI（其中一种是氯丙咪嗪）治疗无效，以及认知行为疗法的充分治疗后效果不佳	• 不符合治疗抵抗的标准
认知	• 能够提供知情同意	• 无法提供知情同意 • 认知能力下降 • 理解能力差
躯体诊断		• 脑部病变（包括脑卒中、肿瘤等） • 神经外科手术病史（例如内囊切开术） • 妊娠 • 任何手术、麻醉或 MRI 扫描的一般禁忌证

Y-BOCS. 耶鲁 – 布朗强迫量表；GAF. 功能大体评定量表

迫症有所改善（Plewnia 等，2008）。洞察力评估对于排除精神障碍和坚持治疗可能是有用的，因此一些 DBS 临床中心认为患者缺乏洞察力［如布朗信念评估量表（Brown assessment of beliefs scale, BABS）评分>12］是 DBS 手术的排除标准（Eisen 等，1998）。

DBS 纳入标准中需要包含最低病情严重程度和最低程度的功能损伤。大多数临床中心要求耶鲁 – 布朗强迫量表（Yale–Brown obsessive-compulsive scale, Y-BOCS）的最低分数为 25～30/40（Goodman 等，1989）。功能大体评定量表（global assessment of function, GAF）可以用来量化残疾程度，临床中心可能需要 GAF 评分<40 或 45 才能纳入 DBS（APA 1994）。

至少 5 年的 OCD 病程才能确认慢性化和治疗难治性，特别是因为 OCD 的特征是症状严重程度可能随时间波动，存在消长。

应记录治疗难治性，其通常定义为初始 Y-BOCS 评分降低<25% 或（临床医师评分）临床疗效总评量表（clinical global impression, CGI）小于"最小改善"。通常情况下，难治性的标准是使用至少 2 个足量的血清素能抗抑郁药的治疗，其中一个是氯丙咪嗪，至少一项非典型抗精神病药物的强化策略，以及在 1 年内至少 20 个疗程的认知行为疗法或暴露和反应预防（Pallanti and Hollander，2014；Nuttin 等，2003）。药物治疗应给予足够大的剂量，并持续足够长的时间。心理治疗应该以"最先进的"方式进行。

另一个重要的纳入标准是患者理解 DBS 手术过程并给予知情同意的能力。患者需要严格遵守该程序及医疗建议。优化 DBS 的益处/不良反应比率可能需要时间，患者应坚持评估和此类治疗所需的长期随访。因此，A 类人格障碍（如偏执型或分裂型人格障碍）或 B 类人格障碍（如边缘型或反社会人格障碍），包括患者行为失控和依从性差的可能，一般应被视为禁忌证。神经认知评估显示的认知障碍也是一种禁忌证。

任何大脑组织病变，如中度或明显的脑萎缩、脑卒中、肿瘤或以前的神经外科手术（即内囊切开术），都可能影响强迫症的神经生物学基础，从而影响DBS的疗效。因此，通常应将上述病变视为禁忌证。此外，还应考虑麻醉，手术或进行MRI扫描的一般禁忌证。

出于多方面的考虑，DBS手术需要由经验丰富的精神科医生、神经心理学家、神经外科医生和麻醉科医生组成的多学科团队进行评估。通常，出于伦理原因，由不参与患者治疗的独立的精神科医生参与手术纳入与排除过程。

我们在OCD中应用DBS的临床经验强调了尽早评估患者期望的重要性。事实上，当患者感到缺乏其他治疗选择时，他们可能会表达出对个人获益的不切实际的期望，或期望将手术的风险降到最低（Christopher等，2011；Maier等，2013）。患者可能会突出自己的缺陷，但是评估患者的主诉，缺陷和OCD之间的关系至关重要。让患者准备好面对潜在的结果需要解决侵入性治疗（如脑外科手术）的潜在理想化问题。

手术路径

患者需要做术前准备。特别是如果在局部麻醉下以"清醒手术"方式进行植入（请参见第7章"麻醉学"），应对其进行术前压力管理培训和完整手术流程的详细说明，以使其受益。根据一些学者的观点，"清醒手术"有一些明显的优点，因为它允许在短暂的手术刺激期间评估潜在的积极影响和不良反应。除了获得电生理数据之外，还可以确认植入电极轨迹的准确性。术中微电极记录（micro-electrode recording, MER）有助于确定正确的电极位置。例如，在STN-DBS手术中，运动动作（如肢体运动）过程中未记录到神经元放电，就可以确认电极处于STN的非运动分区中的位置。需要注意的是，术中刺激诱导的情绪行为可能是OCD对DBS后期反应的预测因素。这些效应表现在STN-DBS术中可能是一种缓解焦虑的"苯二氮䓬类"效应，或者在ALIC-NA DBS术中可能是一种无法控制的微笑或大笑（Polosan等，2016；Haq等，2011）。STN-DBS术中引起的笑声也可确认电极的触点

位置在STN腹内侧缘内（Huang等，2018）。

DBS手术的最后步骤是将神经刺激器/植入式脉冲发生器（implantable pulse generator, IPG）植入到胸部区域或腹部区域，并通过皮下导线连接到颅内刺激电极。

根据已发表的PD合并OCD的病例报道和临床研究，对于STN-DBS，OCD的手术靶点应该是STN的前腹内侧部，它被认为是STN的非运动性、认知性/边缘性部分（Fontaine等，2004；Mallet等，2002,，2008；Chabardès等，2013）。靶点坐标为中连合点前方1 mm，中线外侧10 mm，AC-PC线下方4 mm（Chabardès等，2013）（图17-1）。当VC/VS是刺激靶点时，电极被植入到靠近前连合且Talairach坐标平均为X（左右径）=6.5mm、Y（前后径）=0mm和Z（背腹侧）=3.5mm的位置（Greenberg等，2010）。

三、DBS的疗效和不良反应

（一）治疗效果

自Nuttin等（1999）的开创性工作以来，随着对内囊前肢（ALIC）的DBS手术的开展，许多其他靶点也被使用，其中一些与ALIC有关，如腹侧内囊/腹侧纹状体（VC/VS）和伏隔核（NA）（Greenberg等，2010；Goodman等，2010；Sturm等，2003；Huff等，2010；Van Den Munckhof等，2013）。另一个主要靶点是STN。在2项分别对5名和6名患者进行的小型研究中，报道了STN-DBS的阳性结果（Jiménez等，2013；Jimenez-Ponce等，2009）。最近提出的靶点，即终纹床核（bed nucleus of stria terminalis, BNST）也显示出令人振奋的结果（Luyten等，2016）。根据以往的2个病例，最初在难治性重度抑郁症中评估的内侧前脑束（superolateral branch of the medial forebrain bundle, slMFB）的上外侧分支也是DBS治疗OCD潜在的靶点（Coenen等，2017；Liebrand等，2019）。

▲ 图 17-1 OCD 患者左侧大脑半球 STN 植入电极的矢状位视图

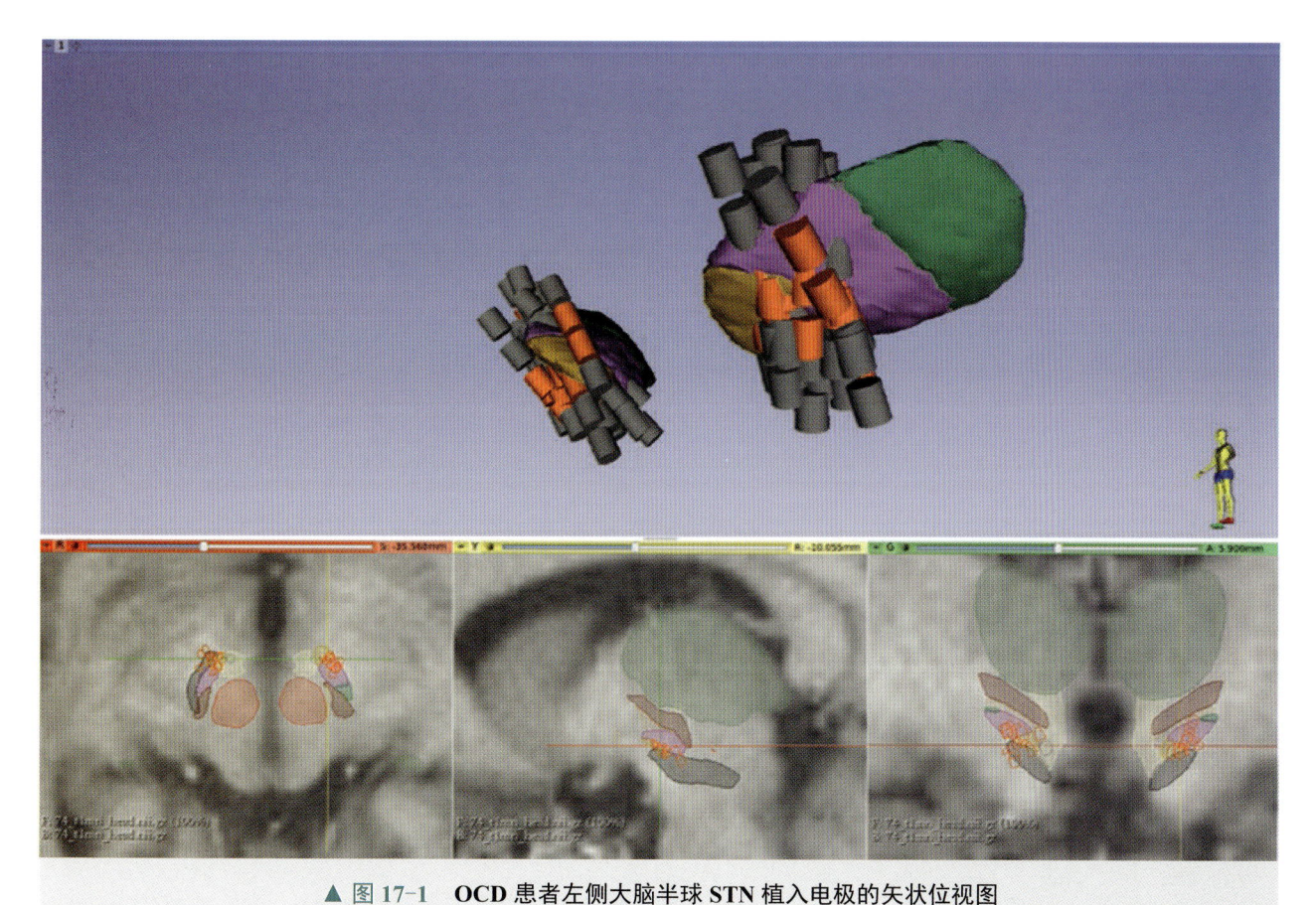

YeB 图谱所划定的 STN 的功能区域（http://pf-stim.cricm.upmc.fr/les-outils-2/ latlas-yeb/）：运动（绿色），联合（紫色），边缘（黄色）（图片由 S. Fernandez，J. Yelnik，Polosan 和 Chabardes 提供）

最近的 Meta 分析显示，无论采用何种靶点，DBS 均可使 OCD 严重程度的总体改善 Y-BOCS 评分降低约 45%，约 60% 的患者可被视为有反应（这里的定义是 Y-BOCS 评分下降 35%）（Alonso 等，2015；Kisely 等，2014）。表 17-2 概述了关于 DBS 治疗 OCD 疗效的研究报道（BATION，2018）。

DBS 治疗 OCD 的临床研究多采用双侧植入刺激电极的方法。然而，单侧刺激效应的问题也已经被提出，有文献报道刺激右 ALIC、右 NA，以及左 STN 和左 NA 对 OCD 患者有一定疗效（Barcia 等，2014）。也有文献报道的电生理数据支持左侧 STN 的单侧刺激效应（Piallat 等，2011）。因此，一些证据表明 OCD 在皮质和基底神经节水平存在不对称的神经基础。他们相关的功能偏侧化可能因每个患者而异。

（二）不良反应和并发症

人们特别注意与 DBS 相关的不良反应，其中不良事件发生率高达 1/3（Kisely 等，2014）。这些可能与手术过程，DBS 设备或刺激参数设置有关。大多数不良反应是由刺激参数设置引起的，并且可以通过重新调整这些参数设置来缓解。在对电极触点进行测试或调整刺激参数期间，患者可能会感受到一些强烈的不良反应，包括灼热感、出汗和瞳孔放大等自主神经症状。在慢性刺激期间，这些症状通常不会持续存在。耐受期可能伴随着其他潜在的不良反应，如感觉异常和眼球偏斜。刺激依赖效应包括轻度躁狂、焦虑、运动障碍、感觉异常、冲动、构音障碍、吞

表 17-2 DBS 治疗 OCD 临床试验及反应率概况

作者	年份	数量	持续时间（个月）	靶点	设计	Y-BOCS 减少（%）	应答者（完成,%）	应答者（部分和全部,%）
Mallet	2008	16	3	STN	交叉	37.8	44	75
Chabardes	2013	2	6	STN	开放	56.0	50	100
Mallet	2002	2	6	STN	开放	81.7	100	100
Polosan	2019	12	5~71	STN	开放	41.4	58	66.7
STN 的全部数量		32						
Greenberg	2006	10	24~36	VC/VS	开放	35.5	50	70
Goodman	2010	6	12	VC/VS	交错起效	47.9	67	67
Fayad[a]	2016	6[a]	73~112	VC/VS	开放	56.6	67	83
Abelson	2005	4	4~23	VC/VS	交叉	30.3	50	50
Tsai	2014	4	15	VC/VS	开放	33.0	50	75
Roh	2012	4	24	VC/VS	开放	59.7	100	100
Anderson	2003	1	3	VC/VS（ALIC）	开放	79.4	100	100
Burdick	2010	1	30	VC/VS	开放	0	0	0
Chang	2013	3	24	VC/VS+CIN	开放	45.2	100	100
Real	2016	1	12	VC/VS	开放	42.0	100	100
Luyten	2016	24	12~171	BNST	交叉（n=17）	45	67	75
Islam[b]	2015	4	6~12	BNST	开放	43.8	100	100
	2015	4	60	NA	开放	41.3	50	75
Denys	2010	16	21	NA	交叉	46	56	NA
Huff	2010	10		rNA	交叉	21.1	10	50
Sturm	2003	4	24~30	rNA	开放	NA	75	75
Plewia	2008	1	12	NA	开放	25.0	0	100
Guehl	2008	3	12	NA NC	开放	51.7	100	100
VC/VS 的全部数量		102						
Coenen	2016	2	12	slMFB	开放	41.5	50	100
Maarouf	2016	4		丘脑	开放		0	25
Jimenez-Pon	2012	6	36	ITP	开放	51.0	100	100

STN. 底丘脑核；VC/VS. 腹侧内囊/腹侧纹状体；ALIC. 内囊前肢；CIN. 扣带回；BNST. 终纹床核；NA. 伏隔核；rNA. 右侧伏隔核；slMFB. 内侧前脑束上外侧支；ITP. 丘脑下脚

a. Goodman 等的长期随访（2010）；b. 一篇论文报道了 2 个案例

咽困难、颜面部不对称、无力、易怒和下肢不宁综合征。

DBS临床试验中不良反应的出现频率应该与基于心理疗法和精神药理学的相关传统治疗进行比较（Staudt等，2019）。用药必须谨慎并避免突然停药，因为这也可能引起不良反应，在STN-DBS的情况下，刺激该靶点对5-羟色胺能系统的影响可能会促进不良反应，即抑制中缝背核中5-羟色胺能神经元的放电（Temel等，2007）。总体而言，在DBS临床研究中报道的一些神经和精神障碍的不良事件在52%的病例中与刺激无关，如果存在，这些不良事件似乎与较差的功能和较低的生活质量无关（Burdick等，2010）。表17-3总结了已发表研究中报道的不良反应。

（三）DBS刺激参数编程

DBS的刺激参数编程是决定疗效的关键一步。考虑到DBS的不同作用机制，需要强调的是经典精神药理学研究的方案设计不能应用于DBS研究的方案设计（Lozano and Lipsman 2013）。与增加精神药物剂量相比，优化DBS参数需要更多的时间才能见效。此外，尚无研究得出有关每个患者最佳参数的结论。不同临床中心可能会提出不同的算法，但目前DBS的参数管理主要是通过试错策略来实现。神经影像可能有助于发现电极的不同触点位于大脑靶点内的位置并显示连接模式，这可能有助于预测效果（Barcia等，2019）。模拟激活的组织体积可为DBS的刺激参数的管理提供宝贵的帮助，该模拟可显示被刺激的大脑区域，并提示其对邻近靶点的大脑结构的潜在影响和不良反应（Chaturvedi等，2012）。

DBS参数设置的优化是基于下列假设，即通过增加解剖靶区神经元的激活使DBS疗效最大化的同时减少相邻脑结构的激活使不良反应最小化。然而，也有学者认为间接激活其他一些与靶点功能相关的、距离更远的大脑结构也可能有助于临床反应（图17-2）。

在记录刺激电极上每个触点的刺激直接效应和不良反应的之后，刺激通常从双侧单极刺激开始。通常建议采用"从低参数开始，缓慢提高"的策略来优化刺激参数。为了扩大DBS的治疗窗，在出现不良反应的情况下，建议可以使用更短的脉冲宽度，而频率也可以根据算法进行调整（Reich等，2015；Karamintziou等，2015）。如果是在常规的参数下影响与靶点相邻的结构而发生不良反应，则可以考虑双极电极配置，因为这将在空间上限制电流继而减小不良反应。双单极配置也可能导致刺激更大体积的区

表17-3 已报道的DBS治疗OCD的不良反应

不良反应	注　释
手术相关	
脑出血[无症状和（或）有症状]	• 患者在手术前已被告知了这种风险。传统的难治性OCD患者必须面对这种情况，在9%~15%的病例中会导致严重的功能障碍和自杀未遂 • 脑出血可无症状（1.2%~4.2%）或导致运动症状；其症状与先前在STN DBS治疗PD患者和DBS治疗OCD患者的研究中报道的相似；对于难治性强迫症患者，接受损伤性手术（如扣带回切开术、内囊切开术）后也可能会出现这些症状 • 已经有过颅内出血导致死亡的病例报道，但这种情况很罕见（121名PD患者中有1名；在200名植入STN和GPI的队列中有2名），但这在DBS治疗OCD的研究中尚未报道，无论靶点是什么
癫痫	• DBS治疗OCD的研究中的报道有2名（共109名患者），与靶点无关；但在STN-DBS治疗OCD的研究中未见报道。手术后，可以通过药物治疗来控制潜在的癫痫发作风险，从而可以继续进行DBS治疗。通常风险很低，很容易被DBS的预期收益所抵消
无力	• 通常仅在术后即刻短暂的出现
过敏反应	• 罕见，仅在VC/VS DBS的研究中报道1名

(续表)

不良反应	注　释
伴有电极周围水肿的笨拙和复视	• 与电极植入有关的暂时性效应，在术后几天内可恢复；相关的不适并不持久
感染（需要移除IPG）	• 感染率1%~15%（在法国STOC OCD DBS队列研究中）；在不同的研究中报道：11.8%（17名患者中有2名）和4.3%（116名患者中有5名）
发炎	• 在DBS治疗OCD患者的文献中仅报道有1名。在术后仔细监测瘢痕可以预防炎症，并及早治疗病因
遗尿、排尿、多尿	• 17名STN-DBS治疗OCD患者中有1名；44名其他靶点DBS治疗OCD患者中有4名。如果有任何功能障碍，适当的药物治疗可能会降低这种风险。该症状大多是短暂的，但如果有持续残留的风险，可以药物控制
头痛	• 44名DBS治疗OCD患者中有6名，无论靶点是什么
疼痛（局部）	• 17名患者中有1名，大部分是暂时性的
眩晕或头晕	• 文献报道了2/44~1/17名患者
视力障碍	• DBS参数调整可以减轻不良反应
设备相关	
导线或延长线断裂	• 罕见（在VC/VS和ALIC DBS研究中报道为109名患者中有5名）
感觉异常	• 1%~12.5%，短暂的
不适	• 1.7%~8.6%，与靶点无关
电池故障	• 曾有报道（109名患者中有6名），通常伴有临床状态恶化（焦虑、情绪障碍、自杀倾向、疲劳和不安感增加）
刺激相关	
自杀	• 1名患者术后自杀，与本研究无关。将自杀归咎于DBS是有争议的
轻度躁狂/躁狂	• 24%~38%的患者；调整刺激参数可缓解
焦虑	• 短暂的，可以通过调整刺激参数缓解
抑郁和自杀倾向	• 5%的患者，与靶点无关；这一风险必须被彻底监测，因为据估计，OCD患者一生中有自杀念头的比例为52%~97%
运动障碍和舞蹈病	• 17名患者中有1名被报道，以及1名使用STN-DBS治疗的患者
冲动控制障碍	• 6%的患者，可以通过循序渐进的DBS刺激参数管理和调整来缓解
构音障碍，吞咽困难，步态和平衡障碍，面部感觉不对称	• 短暂性，见于17名患者中的1~3名STN-DBS患者
体重增加/减少	• 不论靶点，在OCD的DBS研究中占0.9%~4.3%；长期STN-DBS对OCD患者体重无显著影响
认知衰退（语言流畅性障碍、冷漠；健忘；找词困难）	• 44名患者中有3~6名DBS治疗OCD患者，与靶点无关，但长期STN-DBS患者未见报道该症状
胃痛	• 44名患者中有4名被报道；大多是短暂的，有症状的可以药物治疗
性欲增加	• 44名患者中有8名被报道，与靶点无关
失眠	• 3.4%（116名患者，与靶点无关）

改编自Dougherty等，2002；Krack等，2003；Rezai等，2006；Greenberg等，2006；Lipsman等，2007；Mallet等，2008；Vora等，2012；Kohl等，2014；Kisely等，2014；Alonso等，2015；De La Cruz等，2017；Brakoulias等，2017；Mulders等，2016；Mulders等，2017

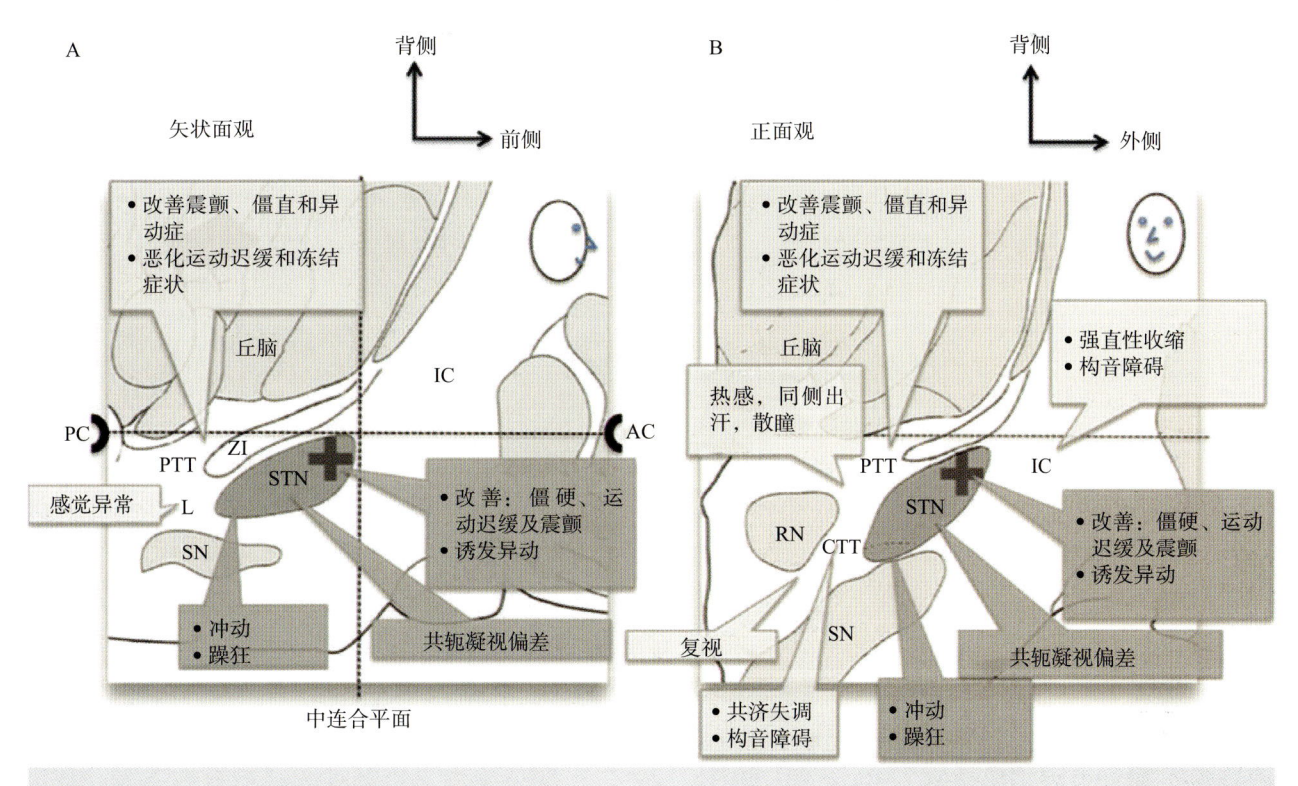

▲ 图 17-2　A. 丘脑底的矢状面（中线外侧 12mm）；B. 正面（中连合平面后 3mm）部分，显示了底丘脑核（STN）背外侧区域和周围结构对高频刺激的行为反应

AC. 前连合；CTT. 小脑丘脑束；IC. 内囊；L. 丘系；PC. 后连合；PTT. 苍白丘脑束；RN. 红核；SN. 黑质；ZI. 未定带（经许可转载，引自 Castrioto 等，2013）

域。这一策略必须单独评估以便进一步改善症状，因为激活相邻的电极触点可能不会每次都起作用。

DBS 治疗 OCD 的全部疗效是需要通过长期刺激获得的，至少在第 1 年中可能会有所改善。DBS 的急性停止（如 IPG 失效或电池耗尽时可能发生）通常会导致 OCD 症状的复发，尽管程度通常比手术前要轻。还可能伴随着情感症状的反弹（Vora 等，2012；Ooms 等，2014a）。因此，为了避免这种情况，监测电池寿命和预测电池电量的变化是很重要的。在 DBS 无反应的情况下，评估电极在靶点内的位置是要考虑的第一步，因为可能需要电极调控和再植入。实际上，应该考虑定位不同的大脑区域并使用较大的电极（旨在覆盖更大的解剖区域），因为它可能会优化预后（Real 等，2016）。然而，就改善率而言，目前还没有有力的证据支持某个特定的大脑靶点，也没有某个针对特定的 OCD 症状的靶点。

四、讨论

DBS 是治疗重度难治性 OCD 的一种很有前景的治疗方法。除了症状改善（总体约为 45%）之外，DBS 还可以改善功能并提高生活质量（Alonso 等，2015；Ooms 等，2014b）。尽管已获得 FDA 和 EC 的批准，但显然该治疗方式仍在发展中，存在许多不确定性，并且在各个关键方面缺乏共识。更好地了解特定的 OCD 症状对不同靶点刺激的差异反应以及识别反应的生物标志物，有助于筛选 DBS 患者，选择刺激靶点并确定 DBS 在治疗 OCD 的选择中的定位。当前可用的研究数据并不支持所讨论的任何特定的大脑靶点。

临床实践中用于评估 OCD 严重程度的心理评估量表可以进一步改进。例如，在患有严重 OCD 的患者中，OCD 的持续时间从 7h 减少到 3.5h 不会导致 Y-BOCS 评分的降低，尽管患者的 OCD 的持续时间得到 50% 的积极改善，并且在改善生活质量方面可能具有重要意义。结合主观与客观的心理测量评估，以及使用与神经生理病理基础相关的神经行为测试评估 OCD 特定症状，对于制定最佳的评估方式和了解症状严重程度的临床相关变化十分重要。

在设计未来的研究方案时，有必要利用在 DBS 研究中收集到的病理生理学知识。事实上，DBS 的研究极大地拓展了对病理生理学的认识。DBS 手术过程中的电生理记录突出了 STN 神经元的电生理特性（放电率、频率、脉冲、振荡活动等）与 OCD 症状严重程度之间的关系，以及潜在的左侧为主的功能障碍（Welter 等，2011；Piallat 等，2011）。此外，STN 的前-腹联合-边缘区域的 DBS 增加了认知（决策）冲动，但是以一种适应性的方式，即倾向于不太谨慎的风格，更接近于健康受试者（Voon 等，2017）。此外，STN 的联合-边缘部分可能影响 OCD 患者的负性认知偏差，降低对情绪刺激的负性评价，继而有助于长期 DBS 的情绪改善效应（Polosan 等，2019）。在神经环路方面，STN-DBS 已被证明可调节特定的皮质-皮质下回路的活动，减少从基底节到具有抑制性控制作用的右额下回的连接，并减少前扣带回和内侧额/眶额皮质的代谢活动（Kibleur 等，2016；Le Jeune 等，2008）。

神经影像学方法如纤维跟踪成像，可改善和个体化解剖定位，并将为改进临床应用提供具有潜在预测价值的生物标志物。因此，在 ALIC-NA DBS 中，对额丘脑束的刺激被认为对阳性结果至关重要，并且刺激部位与内侧和外侧前额叶皮质之间的连通程度可显著预示临床改善（Baldermann 等，2019）。模拟纤维束激活的计算机模型将进一步改善靶点定位和 DBS 疗效。例如，连接右前额中回至 ALIC-NA 的纤维的激活与 DBS 的良好预后相关（Hartmann 等，2016）。将 DBS 诱发的轴突激活的估值与人脑的结构连接相结合，可以更准确地评估 DBS 的反应（Gunalan 等，2018）。

其他有前景的技术发展与 DBS 设备有关。具有方向性的刺激电极可将刺激集中在目标区域和纤维上，并避开那些可能引起不良反应的结构（Chaturvedi 等，2012）。闭环 DBS 系统的开发是 DBS 临床应用的另一个具有挑战性的领域，需要识别与疾病相关的特定生物标记。在 PD 中，这种闭环 DBS 正在研发，而在 OCD 中，尚不清楚可用于反馈和适应的特定电生理参数。最近的研究强调了 θ 振荡在 OCD 某些特定症状，以及 δ 振荡在静息状态中的作用，这对于开发用于在 OCD 中传递自适应神经调节作用的闭环 DBS 系统可能具有潜在的意义（Bastin 等，2014；Rappel 等，2018）。

DBS 作为全新的神经技术干预措施，引发了一些伦理方面的担忧。其中一个经常争论的问题是 DBS 是否会造成人格变化，这可能改变人格同一性。人格结构包括构成一个人身份的认知，情感和行为。这些代表着一个动态的概念，其中包括生物和环境的决定因素，即所谓的"气质"和"性格"。定义患有长期影响认知和情感过程的慢性病的患者的发病前人格是相当具有挑战性的。这种情况在人格被认为还没有完全形成的青春期之前的早发型 OCD 中更是如此。因此，在 OCD 中，患者的人格变化和慢性疾病是交织在一起的。诱导一些有助于 DBS 临床疗效的基本认知和情绪过程的改变实际上可能代表了患者所期望的效果，而不一定被认为对自己是陌生的。而且患者通常表示 DBS 系统在日常生活中不是问题。在某些技术或躯体问题提醒他们身上有设备之前，它一直被"遗忘"（De Haan 等，2017）。尽管在使用 DBS 治疗的患者中应彻底仔细的进行不良反应评估，但人格特质的变化不应被视为 DBS 特有的潜在不良反应，因为 OCD 和常规治疗（包括药物）都可能具有对人格的影响（Lyoo 等，2003）。DBS 研究不仅应该评估患者及其家人所认识到的风险、收益，以及人格的潜在变化，而且还应评估患者是否经历了这些不良反应。

新的神经影像技术，例如连接组方法，以及对各种 OCD 亚型的不同认知和情感症状的评估，以及国际 DBS 登记和 DBS 设备开发中的大量数据收集，将有助于使这些反应标记物和大脑靶点的特异性个性化，并可以给予更具体、更适合的刺激，同时最大限度地降低手术过程的风险。最后，制订针对 DBS 的术后康复计划将改善这些患者的功能预后和生活质量。

五、结论

尽管难治性 OCD 是 DBS 的公认适应证，但这种治疗方法仍在进一步研究中。迄今为止，研究人员在临床试验中取得了可喜的成果，在理解潜在的神经环路方面取得了重大进展，以及技术发展的进步，这些都鼓励研究人员针对该适应证的 DBS 进行进一步研究。未来的 DBS 试验设计将以更好定义的新的生物标记物为基础，以更加个性化和优化的方式改善患者日常功能和生活质量。技术发展应伴随着持续和积极的道德反思。因此，未来的研究将有助于确定 DBS 在治疗选择中的定位，并通过进一步降低治疗难度，为 OCD 患者打开一个新的视角。

参考文献

[1] Abelson JL, Curtis GC, Sagher O, et al. Deep brain stimulation for refractory obsessive-compulsive disorder. Biol Psychiatry. 2005;57:510–6.

[2] Alonso P, Cuadras D, Gabriëls L, et al. Deep brain stimulation for obsessive-compulsive disorder: a meta-analysis of treatment outcome and predictors of response. PLoS One. 2015;10:e0133591.

[3] American Psychiatric Association (APA). Diagnostic and statistical manual of mental disorders. 4th ed. Washington, DC: American Psychiatric Publishing; 1994.

[4] American Psychiatric Association (APA). Diagnostic and statistical manual of mental disorders. 5th ed. Washington, DC: American Psychiatric Publishing; 2013.

[5] Anderson D, Ahmed A. Treatment of patients with intractable obsessive-compulsive disorder with anterior capsular stimulation. Case report. J Neurosurg. 2003;98:1104–8.

[6] Aron AR. From reactive to proactive and selective control: developing a richer model for stopping inappropriate responses. Biol Psychiatry. 2011;69:e55–68.

[7] Baldermann JC, Melzer C, Zapf A, et al. Connectivity profile predictive of effective deep brain stimulation in obsessive-compulsive disorder. Biol Psychiatry. 2019;85:735–43.

[8] Barcia JA, Reyes L, Arza R, et al. Deep brain stimulation for obsessive-compulsive disorder: is the side relevant. Stereotact Funct Neurosurg. 2014;92:31–6.

[9] Barcia JA, Avecillas-Chasín JM, Nombela C, et al. Personalized striatal targets for deep brain stimulation in obsessive-compulsive disorder. Brain Stimul. 2019;12:724–34.

[10] Bastin J, Polosan M, Piallat B, Krack P, Bougerol T, Chabardes S, et al. Changes of oscillatory activity in the subthalamic nucleus during obsessive-compulsive disorder symptoms: two case reports. Cortex. 2014;60:145–50.

[11] Bation R. Stimulation électrique par courant continu (tDCS) dans les troubles obsessionnels et compulsifs résistants: effets cliniques et électrophysiologiques. 2018, thèse d'université, Université Claude Bernard Lyon 1, Lyon. p. 51.

[12] Benis D, David O, Lachaux J-P, Seigneuret E, Krack P, Fraix V et al. Subthalamic nucleus activity dissociates proactive and reactive inhibition in patients with Parkinson's disease. NeuroImage. 2013;91:1–9.

[13] Brakoulias V, Starcevic V, Belloch A, et al. Comorbidity, age of onset and suicidality in obsessive-compulsive disorder (OCD): An international collaboration. Compr Psychiatry. 2017;76:79–86.

[14] Burdick AP, Fernandez HH, Okun MS, et al. Relationship between higher rates of adverse events in deep brain stimulation using standardized prospective recording and patient outcomes. Neurosurg Focus. 2010;29:E4.

[15] Castrioto A, Volkmann J, Krack P. Postoperative management of deep brain stimulation in Parkinson's disease. In: Handbook of clinical neurology, vol. 116 (3rd series); 2013. pp. 129–46.

[16] Castrioto A, Lhommée E, Moro E, Krack P. Mood and behavioural effects of subthalamic stimulation in Parkinson's disease. Lancet Neurol. 2014;13:287–305.

[17] Chabardès S, Polosan M, Krack P, et al. Deep brain stimulation for obsessive-compulsive disorder: subthalamic nucleus target. World Neurosurg. 2013;80:S31.e1.

[18] Chamberlain SR, Blackwell AD, Fineberg NA, et al. The neuropsychology of obsessive compulsive disorder: the importance of failures in cognitive and behavioral inhibition as candidate endophenotypic markers. Neurosci Biobehav Rev. 2005;29:399–419.

[19] Chang WS, Roh D, Kim CH, Chang JW. Combined bilateral anterior cingulotomy and ventral capsule/ventral striatum deep brain stimulation for refractory obsessive-compulsive disorder with major depression: do combined procedures have a long-term benefit? Restor Neurol Neurosci. 2013;31:723–32.

[20] Chaturvedi A, Foutz TJ, McIntyre CC. Current steering to activate targeted neural pathways during deep brain stimulation of the subthalamic region. Brain Stimul. 2012;5:369–77.

[21] Christopher PP, Leykin Y, Appelbaum PS, et al. Enrolling in deep brain stimulation research for depression: influences on potential subjects' decision making. Depress Anxiety. 2011;29:139–46.

[22] Coenen VA, Schlaepfer TE, Goll P, et al. The medial forebrain bundle as a target for deep brain stimulation for obsessive-compulsive disorder. CNS Spectr. 2017;22:282–9.

[23] de Haan S, Rietveld E, Stokhof M, Denys D. Becoming more oneself? Changes in personality following DBS treatment for psychiatric disorders: experiences of OCD patients and general considerations. PLoS One. 2017;12:e0175748.

[24] de la Cruz LF, Rydell M, Runeson B, et al. Suicide in obsessive–compulsive disorder: a population-based study of 36.788 Swedish patients. Mol Psychiatry. 2017;22:1626–32.

[25] Denys D. Obsessionality and compulsivity: a phenomenology of obsessive-compulsive disorder. Philos Ethics Humanit Med. 2011;6:3.

[26] Denys D, Mantione M, Figee M, et al. Deep brain stimulation of the nucleus accumbens for treatment-refractory obsessive-compulsive disorder. Arch Gen Psychiatry. 2010;67:1061–8.

[27] Dougherty DD, Baer L, Cosgrove GR, et al. Prospective long-term follow-up of 44 patients who received cingulotomy for treatment-refractory obsessive-compulsive disorder. Am J Psychiatry. 2002;159:269–75.

[28] Eisen JL, Phillips KA, Baer L, et al. The Brown Assessment of Beliefs Scale: reliability and validity. Am J Psychiatry. 1998;155:102–8.
[29] Fayad SM, Guzick AG, Reid AM, et al. Six-nine year follow-up of deep brain stimulation for obsessive-compulsive disorder. PLoS One. 2016;11:e0167875.
[30] Figee M, Wielaard I, Mazaheri A, Denys D. Neurosurgical targets for compulsivity: what can we learn from acquired brain lesions? Neurosci Biobehav Rev. 2013;37:328–39.
[31] Fontaine D, Mattei V, Borg M, et al. Effect of subthalamic nucleus stimulation on obsessive-compulsive disorder in a patient with Parkinson disease. Case report. J Neurosurg. 2004;100:1084–6.
[32] Gillan CM, Morein-Zamir S, Urcelay GP, et al. Enhanced avoidance habits in obsessive-compulsive disorder. Biol Psychiatry. 2014;75:631–8.
[33] Goodman WK, Price HL, Rasmussen SA, et al. The Yale-Brown Obsessive Compulsive Scale: I. Development, use, and reliability. Arch Gen Psychiatry. 1989;46:1006–11.
[34] Goodman WK, Foote KD, Greenberg BD, et al. Deep brain stimulation for intractable obsessive compulsive disorder: pilot study using a blinded, staggered-onset design. Biol Psychiatry. 2010;67:535–42.
[35] Greenberg BD, Malone DA, Friehs GM, et al. Three-year outcomes in deep brain stimulation for highly resistant obsessive–compulsive disorder. Neuropsychopharmacology. 2006;31:2394.
[36] Greenberg BD, Rauch SL, Haber SN. Invasive circuitry-based neurotherapeutics: stereotactic ablation and deep brain stimulation for OCD. Neuropsychopharmacology. 2010;35:317–36.
[37] Guehl D, Benazzouz A, Aouizerate B, et al. Neuronal correlates of obsessions in the caudate nucleus. Biol Psychiatry. 2008;63(6):557–62. Epub 2007 Oct 22.
[38] Gunalan K, Howell B, McIntyre CC. Quantifying axonal responses in patient-specific models of subthalamic deep brain stimulation. Neuroimage. 2018;172:263–77.
[39] Haq IU, Foote KD, Goodman WG, et al. Smile and laughter induction and intraoperative predictors of response to deep brain stimulation for obsessive-compulsive disorder. Neuroimage. 2011;54:S247–55.
[40] Hartmann CJ, Lujan JL, Chaturvedi A, et al. Tractography activation patterns in dorsolateral prefrontal cortex suggest better clinical responses in OCD DBS. Front Neurosci. 2016;9:1104–10.
[41] Haynes WI, Haber SN. The organization of prefrontal-subthalamic inputs in primates provides an anatomical substrate for both functional specificity and integration: implications for basal ganglia models and deep brain stimulation. J Neurosci. 2013;33:4804–14.
[42] Heyman I, Mataix-Cols D, Fineberg NA. Obsessive-compulsive disorder. BMJ. 2006;333:424–9.
[43] Hikosaka O, Isoda M. Switching from automatic to controlled behavior: cortico-basal ganglia mechanisms. Trends Cogn Sci. 2010;14:154–61.
[44] Hirschtritt ME, Bloch MH, Mathews CA. Obsessive-compulsive disorder: advances in diagnosis and treatment. JAMA. 2017;317:1358–67.
[45] Hofmeijer-Sevink MK, van Oppen P, van Megen HJ, et al. Clinical relevance of comorbidity in obsessive com-pulsive disorder. The Netherlands OCD Association Study. J Affect Disord. 2013;150:847–54.
[46] Huang Y, Aronson JP, Pilitsis JG, et al. Anatomical correlates of uncontrollable laughter with unilateral subthalamic deep brain stimulation in Parkinson's sisease. Front Neurol. 2018;9:569–6.
[47] Huff W, Lenartz D, Schormann M, et al. Unilateral deep brain stimulation of the nucleus accumbens in patients with treatment-resistant obsessive-compulsive disorder: outcomes after one year. Clin Neurol Neurosurg. 2010;112:137–43.
[48] Islam L, Franzini A, Messina G, et al. Deep brain stimulation of the nucleus accumbens and bed nucleus of stria terminalis for obsessive-compulsive disorder: a case series. World Neurosurg. 2015;83:657–63.
[49] Jahanshahi M, Obeso I, Rothwell JC, Obeso JA. A fronto-striato-subthalamic-pallidal network for goal-directed and habitual inhibition. Nat Rev Neurosci. 2015;16:719–32.
[50] Jiménez F, Nicolini H, Lozano AM, et al. Electrical stimulation of the inferior thalamic peduncle in the treatment of major depression and obsessive compulsive disorders. World Neurosurg. 2013;80(S30):e17–25.
[51] Jimenez-Ponce F, Velasco-Campos F, Castro-Farfan G, et al. Preliminary study in patients with obsessive-compulsive disorder treated with electrical stimulation in the inferior thalamic peduncle. Neurosurgery. 2009;65:203–9.
[52] Karamintziou SD, Deligiannis NG, Piallat B, et al. Dominant efficiency of nonregular patterns of subthalamic nucleus deep brain stimulation for Parkinson's disease and obsessive-compulsive disorder in a data-driven computational model. J Neural Eng. 2015;13:1–20.
[53] Karas PJ, Lee S, Jimenez-Shahed J, Goodman WK, Viswanathan A, Sheth SA. Deep Brain Stimulation for Obsessive Compulsive Disorder: Evolution of Surgical Stimulation Target Parallels Changing Model of Dysfunctional Brain Circuits. Front Neurosci. 2019;12:998.
[54] Kibleur A, Gras-Combe G, Benis D, et al. Modulation of motor inhibition by subthalamic stimulation in obsessive-compulsive disorder. Transl Psychiatry. 2016;6:e922.
[55] Kisely S, Hall K, Siskind D, et al. Deep brain stimulation for obsessive–compulsive disorder: a systematic review and meta-analysis. Psychol Med. 2014;44:3533–42.
[56] Kohl S, Schönherr DM, Luigjes J, et al. Deep brain stimulation for treatment-refractory obsessive compulsive disorder: a systematic review. BMC Psychiatry. 2014;14:214.
[57] Krack P, Kumar R, Ardouin C, et al. Mirthful laughter induced by subthalamic nucleus stimulation. Mov Disord. 2001;16:867–75.
[58] Krack P, Batir A, Van Blercom N, et al. Five-year follow-up of bilateral stimulation of the subthalamic nucleus in advanced Parkinson's disease. N Engl J Med. 2003;349:1925–34.
[59] Le Jeune F, Péron J, Biseul I, et al. Subthalamic nucleus stimulation affects orbitofrontal cortex in facial emotion recognition: a PET study. Brain. 2008;131:1599–608.
[60] Liebrand LC, Caan MWA, Schuurman PR, et al. Individual white matter bundle trajectories are associated with deep brain stimulation response in obsessive-compulsive disorder. Brain Stimul. 2019;12:353–60.
[61] Lipsman N, Neimat JS, Lozano AM. Deep brain stimulation for treatment-refractory obsessive-compulsive disorder: the search for a valid target. Neurosurgery. 2007;61:1–11.
[62] Lozano AM, Lipsman N. Probing and regulating dysfunctional circuits using deep brain stimulation. Neuron. 2013;77:406–24.
[63] Luyten L, Hendrickx S, Raymaekers S, et al. Electrical stimulation in the bed nucleus of the stria terminalis alleviates severe obsessive-compulsive disorder. Mol Psychiatry. 2016;21:1272–80.
[64] Lyoo IK, Yoon T, Kang DH, Kwon JS. Patterns of changes in temperament and character inventory scales in subjects with obsessive-compulsive disorder following a 4-month treatment. Acta Psychiatr Scand. 2003;107:298–304.
[65] Maarouf M, Neudorfer C, El Majdoub F, et al. Deep brain stimulation of medial dorsal and ventral anterior nucleus of the thalamus in OCD: a retrospective case series. PLoS One. 2016;11:e0160750.
[66] Maia TV, Cooney RE, Peterson BS. The neural bases of obsessive–compulsive disorder in children and adults. Dev Psychopathol. 2008;20:1251–83.
[67] Maier F, Lewis CJ, Horstkoetter N, Eggers C, Kalbe E, Maarouf M, et al. Patients' expectations of deep brain stimulation, and subjective perceived outcome related to clinical measures in Parkinson's disease: a mixed-method approach. J Neurol Neurosurg Psychiatry. 2013;84:1273–81.
[68] Makris N, Rathi Y, Mouradian P, et al. Variability and anatomical specificity of the orbitofrontothalamic fibers of passage in the ventral capsule/ventral striatum (VC/ VS): precision care for patient-specific tractography-guided targeting of deep brain stimulation (DBS) in obsessive compulsive disorder (OCD). Brain Imaging Behav. 2016;10:1054–67.
[69] Mallet L, Mesnage V, Houeto J-L, et al. Compulsions, Parkinson's disease, and stimulation. Lancet. 2002;360:1302–4.
[70] Mallet L, Polosan M, Jaafari N, et al. Subthalamic nucleus stimulation in severe obsessive-compulsive disorder. N Engl J Med. 2008;359:2121–34.
[71] Mancebo MC, Eisen JL, Pinto A, et al. The Brown Longitudinal

Obsessive Compulsive study: treatments received and patient impressions of improvement. J Clin Psychiatry. 2006;67:1713–20.
[72] Mataix-Cols D, Wooderson S, Lawrence N, et al. Distinct neural correlates of washing, checking, and hoarding symptom dimensions in obsessive-compulsive disorder. Arch Gen Psychiatry. 2004;61:564–76.
[73] Mulders AEP, Plantinga BR, Schruers K, et al. Deep brain stimulation of the subthalamic nucleus in obsessive-compulsive disorder. Neuroanatomical and pathophysiological considerations. Eur Neuropsychopharmacol. 2016;26:1909–19.
[74] Mulders A, Leentjens AFG, Plantinga B, et al. Choreatic side effects of deep brain stimulation of the subthalamic nucleus for treatment-resistant obsessive- compulsive disorder: a case report. World Neurosurg. 2017;104:1048.e9–1048.e13.
[75] Nuttin B, Cosyns P, Demeulemeester H, et al. Electrical stimulation in anterior limbs of internal capsules in patients with obsessive-compulsive disorder. Lancet. 1999;354:1526.
[76] Nuttin BJ, Gabriëls LA, Cosyns PR, et al. Long-term electrical capsular stimulation in patients with obsessive-compulsive disorder. Neurosurgery. 2003;52:1263–72.
[77] Ooms P, Blankers M, Figee M, et al. Rebound of affective symptoms following acute cessation of deep brain stimulation in obsessive-compulsive disorder. Brain Stimul. 2014a;7:727–31.
[78] Ooms P, Mantione M, Figee M, et al. Deep brain stimulation for obsessive-compulsive disorders: long-term analysis of quality of life. J Neurol Neurosurg Psychiatry. 2014b;85:153–8.
[79] Pallanti S, Hollander E. Pharmacological, experimental therapeutic, and transcranial magnetic stimulation treatments for compulsivity and impulsivity. CNS Spectr. 2014;19:50–61.
[80] Piallat B, Polosan M, Fraix V, et al. Subthalamic neuronal firing in obsessive-compulsive disorder and Parkinson disease. Ann Neurol. 2011;69:793–802.
[81] Plewnia C, Schober F, Rilk A, et al. Sustained improvement of obsessive–compulsive disorder by deep brain stimulation in a woman with residual schizophrenia. Int J Neuropsychopharmacol. 2008;11:1181–3.
[82] Polosan M, Chabardes S, Bougerol T, et al. Long-term improvement in obsessions and compulsions with subthalamic stimulation. Neurology. 2016;87:1843–4.
[83] Polosan M, Droux F, Kibleur A, et al. Affective modulation of the associative-limbic subthalamic nucleus: deep brain stimulation in obsessive–compulsive disorder. Transl Psychiatry. 2019;9:73.
[84] Rappel P, Marmor O, Bick AS, et al. Subthalamic theta activity: a novel human subcortical biomarker for obsessive compulsive disorder. Transl Psychiatry. 2018;8:118.
[85] Real E, Plans G, Alonso P, et al. Removing and reimplanting deep brain stimulation therapy devices in resistant OCD (when the patient does not respond): case report. BMC Psychiatry. 2016;16:26.
[86] Reich MM, Steigerwald F, Sawalhe AD, et al. Short pulse width widens the therapeutic window of subthalamic neurostimulation. Ann Clin Transl Neurol. 2015;2:427–32.
[87] Rezai AR, Kopell BH, Gross RE, et al. Deep brain stimulation for Parkinson's disease: surgical issues. Mov Disord. 2006;21:S197–218.
[88] Roh D, Chang WS, Chang JW, Kim CH. Long-term follow-up of deep brain stimulation for refractory obsessive-compulsive disorder. Psychiatry Res. 2012;200:1067–70.
[89] Ruscio AM, Stein DJ, Chiu WT, Kessler RC. The epidemiology of obsessive–compulsive disorder in the National Comorbidity Survey Replication. Mol Psychiatry. 2010;15:53–63.
[90] Staudt MD, Herring EZ, Gao K, et al. Evolution in the treatment of psychiatric disorders: from psychosurgery to psychopharmacology to neuromodulation. Front Neurosci. 2019;13:108.
[91] Sturm V, Lenartz D, Koulousakis A, et al. The nucleus accumbens: a target for deep brain stimulation in obsessive-compulsive- and anxiety-disorders. J Chem Neuroanat. 2003;26:293–9.
[92] Temel Y, Boothman LJ, Blokland A, et al. Inhibition of 5-HT neuron activity and induction of depressive-like behavior by high-frequency stimulation of the subthalamic nucleus. Proc Natl Acad Sci U S A. 2007;104:17087–92.
[93] Tsai HC, Chang CH, Pan JI, et al. Acute stimulation effect of the ventral capsule/ventral striatum in patients with refractory obsessive-compulsive disorder—a double-blinded trial. Neuropsychiatr Dis Treat. 2014;10:63–9.
[94] van den Munckhof P, Bosch DA, Mantione MH, et al. Active stimulation site of nucleus accumbens deep brain stimulation in obsessive-compulsive disorder is localized in the ventral internal capsule. Acta Neurochir Suppl. 2013;117:53–9.
[95] Voon V, Droux F, Morris L, et al. Decisional impulsivity and the associative-limbic subthalamic nucleus in obsessive-compulsive disorder: stimulation and connectivity. Brain. 2017;140:442–56.
[96] Vora AK, Ward H, Foote KD, et al. Rebound symptoms following battery depletion in the NIH OCD DBS cohort: clinical and reimbursement issues. Brain Stimul. 2012;5:599–604.
[97] Vos T, Flaxman AD, Naghavi M, et al. Years lived with disability (YLDs) for 1160 sequelae of 289 diseases and injuries 1990–2010: a systematic analysis for the Global Burden of Disease Study 2010. Lancet. 2012;380:2163–96.
[98] Welter ML, Burbaud P, Fernandez-Vidal S, et al. Basal ganglia dysfunction in OCD: subthalamic neuronal activity correlates with symptoms severity and predicts high-frequency stimulation efficacy. Transl Psychiatry. 2011;1:e5–10.

第18章 脑深部电刺激治疗抑郁症
Deep Brain Stimulation for Depression

Isidoor O. Bergfeld　Martijn Figee　著
刘钰晔　王 秀　译　韩春雷　杨岸超　张建国　校

> **摘要**：脑深部电刺激（DBS）治疗难治性抑郁症（treatment-resistant depression，TRD）的开放性研究被认为有很好的前景，40%的患者在胼胝体下扣带皮质（subcallosal cingulate cortex，SCC）或腹侧内囊/腹侧纹状体（ventral capsule and ventral striatum，VC/VS）的DBS治疗后症状至少消失一半。但到目前为止，假刺激对照试验的结果好坏参半，尚有很大的研究空间。70%以上的患者对个体化的SCC束或内侧前脑束（medial forebrain bundle，MFB）靶点的治疗有反应，表明靶向特异性的白质束研究很有价值；同时进行康复和认知行为疗法、优化参数选择，可以增加治疗效果。

一、概述

2005年，Mayberg等发表了第一项对胼胝体下扣带皮质（SCC）进行脑深部电刺激（DBS）治疗慢性抑郁症的研究，研究对象为认知行为疗法、抗抑郁药物治疗、联合用药和电惊厥疗法（ECT）无效的6名患者（Mayberg等，2005）。症状至少减少一半是严重抑郁症试验中常见的指标，在SCC-DBS治疗6个月后，6名患者中有4人达到该指标。考虑到这些患者对DBS以外的干预完全无效，这个结果令人振奋。在那之后的几年里，以腹侧纹状体和邻近腹侧内囊（VC/VS）（Schlaepfer等，2008）和内侧前脑束（MFB）（Schlaepfer等，2013）作为靶点的DBS治疗也显示卓有成效。另外还有DBS作用于丘脑下脚（Jiménez等，2005）和外侧缰核（Sartorius等，2010）的病例报告。在本章中，我们将回顾文献，总结有关SCC、VC/VS和MFB靶点治疗难治性抑郁症（TRD）的有效性、安全性和作用机制。

二、患者选择

目前还没有国家或地区批准DBS用于治疗抑郁症，它只作为临床试验用于治疗药物难治性抑郁症患者。在应用中，患者一般至少4次连续用药无效（如选择性5-羟色胺再摄取抑制药、三环类抗抑郁药、锂剂或单胺氧化酶抑制药），大多数研究受试者同时ECT治疗无效。一般只纳入单相抑郁患者，但一项有6名双相患者的研究显示SCC-DBS治疗也是安全的（Holtzheimer等，2012）。

三、靶点

DBS治疗TRD可选择不同靶点，其中最重要的是SCC、VC/VS和MFB。另外还有DBS

作用于丘脑下脚和外侧缰核的病例报告。

（一）胼胝体下扣带皮质

胼胝体下扣带皮质（SCC）是DBS治疗TRD的第一个靶点（Mayberg等，2005）。该靶点应用的理论基础是，在悲伤急性期膝下扣带回区域（Brodmann区25）的活动增加，临床上对抗抑郁药物、ECT、重复的经颅磁刺激（rTMS）和消融手术有效时，该区域的活动减少（Mayberg 1997）。

SCC靶区由邻近第25区灰质的白质束组成，术前MRI扫描通常将其界定为SCC白质区，约为从前连合到胼胝体膝部灰质边缘所界定平面距离的75%。

1. 疗效

有9项研究共189名TRD患者应用SCC-DBS的治疗结果公开发表（表18-1）（Lozano等，2008，2012；Holtzheimer等，2012，2017；Puigdemont等，2012；Ramasubbu等，2013；Torres等，2013；Riva-Posse等，2017；Merkl等，2017；Eitan等，2018）。治疗12个月后，181名患者中66名（36.5%）完全缓解。两项研究以随机、假刺激对照的方式探讨了SCC-DBS的有效性。一项研究将患者在手术后立即随机分组，60人进入SCC-DBS刺激组和30人进入假刺激组，持续6个月（Holtzheimer等，2017）。60名DBS患者中12名（20%）有效，30名假刺激患者中5名（17%）有效，差异无显著性。该研究原计划纳入201名患者，但中期结果不佳导致了研究暂停。在第二个较小的研究中，8名患者在术后7天被随机分SCC-DBS刺激组和假刺激组，每组4人，持续4周，结果两组抑郁评分没有差异，都没有明显的改善（Merkl等，2017）。在这两项研究的后续开放性试验中，患者可根据症状接受无限制的参数调整，2年后有效率为33%~48%。这表明对DBS的抗抑郁反应可能需要刺激更长的时间。

2. 不良反应

文献已经报道了178名SCC-DBS患者的不良事件（表18-1），一般与手术、设备或刺激相关。手术相关的不良事件最常见的是电极植入后的一过性轻度躁狂（$n=8$，4.5%）、伤口感染（$n=5$，2.8%）和癫痫（$n=2$，1.1%）。最常见的设备相关不良事件是脉冲发生器（IPG）或延伸导线周围的疼痛或不适（$n=13$，7.3%），其中2名患者导致设备移除。此外，3名患者有延伸导线或电极断裂（1.7%），1名患者有设备移位（0.6%）。最常见的刺激相关不良事件为抑郁增加（$n=11$，6.2%）、焦虑增加（$n=6$，3.4%）和激越（$n=3$，1.7%）。与刺激相关的不良事件大多是暂时的，可以通过参数调整来解决。在SCC-DBS之后，178名患者中有6名自杀未遂，1名患者自杀成功。

从目前来看，SCC-DBS对认知没有损害。在小样本、非对照研究中，患者通常在SCC-DBS后的认知测试中与之前持平或有所改善，但不能排除练习效应的影响（McNeely等，2008年；Guinjoan等，2010；Bogove等，2014；Moreines等，2014）。只有一项研究比较了8名SCC-DBS治疗的患者和8名药物治疗患者1年后的认知结果（SerraBlasco等，2015），两组之间没有明显差异，但这个结果也可能因为样本量较小，仅能检测出较大差异。

3. 作用机制

SCC作为DBS靶点的最初理论基础是，难治性抑郁症中调节负面情绪的膝下扣带回区域存在过度活跃，并且在非难治性MDD患者中这种过度活跃可被抗抑郁药物干预下调（Mayberg 1997）。研究表明，最早接受SCC-DBS治疗的4名患者在接受3个月刺激后SCC血液流动下降（Mayberg等，2005）。此外，SCC-DBS还调节了其他参与情绪和动机处理的区域，如岛叶、杏仁核、下丘脑、伏隔核、眶额皮质，以及背外侧和额叶内侧皮质（Mayberg等，2005；Lozano等，2008）。纤维示踪成像显示，对SCC-DBS有反应的患者的刺激位置通过与额钳钩束、扣带束和额纹状体纤维相连的区域（Riva-Posse等，2014年；Choi等，2015）。根据纤维示踪成像，手术

表 18-1 SCC-DBS 治疗的研究汇总

胼胝体下扣带皮质（SCC）

作 者	例 数	效 果	不良反应
• Lozano 等（2008） • Kennedy 2011，3～6 年） • Mayberg 2005，n = 6）	20	• 6 个月：12/20 人有反应（response），7 人缓解（remission） • 12 个月：11/20 人有反应，7 人缓解	• 与手术相关的不良事件（AE）：伤口感染（n=4），头痛（n=4），情绪恶化/易怒（n=2），癫痫发作（n=1） • 与设备相关的 AE：IPG 疼痛（n=1）
• Holtzheimer 等（2012） 备注：10 名严重抑郁障碍，7 名 2 型双相情感障碍	17	• 6 个月：7/17 人有反应，3 人缓解 • 12 个月：5/14 人有反应，5 人缓解	• 与手术相关的严重不良事件（SAE）：感染（n=1） • 其他 SAE：自杀未遂（n=2），焦虑增加（n=2），自杀意念（n=1），抑郁加重（n=1） • 与设备相关的 AE：设备移位（n=1），导线断裂，糜烂，感染（全部 n=1） • 与刺激相关的 AE：恶心（n=1）
• Lozano 等（2012）	21	• 6 个月：10/21 人有反应，缓解人数未报道 • 12 个月：6/21 人有反应	• 与手术相关的 SAE：皮肤糜烂（n=1） • 与设备相关的 SAE：导线断裂（n=2） • 其他 SAE：自杀（n=1），自杀未遂（n=1），感染（n=1），肺炎（n=1），胸痛（n=1） • 与刺激相关的 AE：激惹（n=3）
• Puigdemont 等（2012）	8	• 6 个月：7/8 人有反应，3 人缓解 • 12 个月：5/8 人有反应，3 人缓解	• 其他 SAE：自杀未遂（n=1） • 与设备相关的 AE：皮下导线部位疼痛（n=3），头痛（n=2）
• Torres 等（2013） 备注：1 型双相情感障碍	1	• 6 个月：1/1 人有反应，0 人缓解 • 最后随访时间为 9 个月：1/1 人有反应，1 人缓解	• 与刺激相关的 AE：强直-阵挛发作（n=1）
• Ramasubbu 等（2013）	4	• 6 个月：1/4 人有反应，0 人缓解 • 最后随访时间为 36 个月：2/4 人有反应，0 人缓解	• 与刺激相关的 AE：焦虑增加（n=1），失眠（n=1）
• Merkl 等（2017） 备注：1 型双相情感障碍	8	• 6 个月：3/8 人有反应，1 人缓解 • 12 个月：3/8 人有反应，1 人缓解	• 与设备相关的 SAE：移动不便需要移除（n=2） • 与手术相关的 AE：一过性低躁狂症（n=1），踝扭（n=1），多个未指明的 AE 通过调整参数好转 • 与刺激相关的 AE：
• Holtzheimer 等（2017）	90	• 6 个月：17/90 人有反应，8 人缓解 • 12 个月：27/90 人有反应，6 人缓解	• 刺激组比假刺激组更突出的 SAE：抑郁增加 12% vs. 3%，感染 8% vs. 3%，焦虑 5% vs. 0%，自杀念头，术后不适，听力和视觉障碍，局部皮肤糜烂，择期住院（均为 2% vs. 0%） • 刺激组比假刺激组更突出的 AE：沿导线部位的牵拉感（10% vs. 3%），听力和视觉障碍（8% vs. 0%），抑郁加重（5% vs. 3%），神经痛（2% vs. 0%）
• Eitan 等（2018）	9	• 6 个月：1/9 人有反应，0 人缓解 • 12 个月：3/9 人有反应，0 人缓解	• 可能与刺激相关的 SAE：自杀未遂（n=1） • 与手术相关的 AE：切口疼痛和（或）压痛（n=5），头皮感觉异常（n=3），切口肿胀（n=2），头痛（n=3），切口出血（n=1），切口周围搏动（n=1），右手中部三指及掌部疼痛（n=1） • 与设备相关的 AE：IPG 周围的振动（n=1） • 与刺激相关的 AE：头痛（n=1），食管刺激（n=1），跌倒（n=1），颈部僵硬（n=1），近期记忆力差（n=1），神经痛（n=1）

(续表)

作 者	例数	效 果	不良反应
Riva-Posse 等（2017）	11	• 6 个月：8/11 人有反应，5 人缓解 • 12 个月：9/11 人有反应，6 人缓解	• 未报道

腹侧内囊/腹侧纹状体（VC/VS）

作 者	例数	效 果	不良反应
Malone 等（2009）	15	• 6 个月：7/15 人有反应，3 人缓解 • 12 个月：8/15 人有反应，6 人缓解	• 与手术相关的 SAE：切口疼痛（n=1） • 与设备相关的 SAE：导线断裂（n=1） • 与刺激相关的 SAE：混合性双相情感障碍（n=1），晕厥（n=1） • 其他 SAE：自杀意念增加或抑郁（n=5），晕厥，癌症，肺钙化，气短（全部 n=1） • 与刺激相关的 AE：轻躁狂（n=2）
Dougherty 等（2015）（Kubu 2017 cogn 成果报道）	29	• 12 个月：6/29 人有反应，5 人缓解 备注：14 名患者在 12 个月随访时只接受了 8 个月的刺激	• 与手术相关的 SAE：植入部位感染（n=5） • 其他 SAE：抑郁加重（n=8），自杀意念（n=5），自杀未遂（n=4），自杀（n=1） 刺激组比假刺激组更突出的 AE：抑郁加重（33.3% vs. 21.4%），失眠（26.7% vs. 21.4%），易怒，自杀意念，轻躁狂，脱抑制（均为 20.0% vs. 0%），狂躁（6.7% vs. 0%）
Bewernick 等（2010）（n=10） Bewernick 等（2012）	11	• 12 个月：5/11 人有反应，3 人缓解	• 其他 SAE：自杀（n=1），自杀未遂（n=1） • 与刺激相关的 AE：眼球肿胀（n=6），疼痛（n=4），电极脱出（n=3），吞咽困难（n=4），平衡失调（n=3），激越（n=3），出汗增加，一过性焦虑增加，红斑（全部 n=4），平衡失调（n=3），激越（n=3），一过性情绪高涨（n=1）
Bergfeld 等（2016）	25	• 6 个月：8/25 人有反应，5 人缓解 • 12 个月：10/25 人有反应，5 人缓解	• 其他相关的 SAE：恶心（n=1） • 其他 SAE：自杀未遂（n=4），自杀意念（n=2） • 与刺激相关的 AE：眼睛肿胀（n=6），切口周围疼痛（n=6），头痛或非特异性躯体症状（n=2），出血，伸展周围刺激，颈部疼痛，木后妄想（全部 n=1） • 与设备相关的 AE：IPG 周围疼痛（n=3），导线周围疼痛（n=2），切口周围疼痛（n=2），头痛（n=6），多汗（n=5），躁狂， • 与刺激相关的 AE：激越（n=7），脱抑制（n=6），头痛（n=5），多汗（n=3），躁狂，平衡障碍，味觉改变，颈部疼痛，睡眠障碍（全部 n=2），夜尿症，尿频，思维奔逸，幻觉，轻躁狂，恶心（全部 n=1） 刺激组比假刺激组更突出的 AE：视力模糊（3 vs. 0），睡眠障碍（3 vs. 0），脱抑制（2 vs. 0），非特异性躯体症状（2 vs. 1），注意力障碍，中毒，腹泻，思维奔逸，性欲增强，尿路感染，IPG 周围颤动（全部 n=1），自发中断刺激 1 vs. 0
Millet 等（2014）	4	• 6 个月：0/4 人有反应，0 人缓解 • 12 个月：3/4 人有反应，1 人缓解	• 其他 SAE：自杀未遂（n=1），自杀意念（n=1） • 与刺激相关的 AE：头痛（n=1），疼痛（n=1） • 与设备相关的 AE：自发中断刺激（n=1）

内侧前脑束（MFB）

作 者	例数	效 果	不良反应
Bewernick 等（2017）	8	• 12 个月：6/8 人有反应，3 人缓解	• 与手术相关的 SAE：颅内出血（n=1） • 与设备相关的 SAE：构音障碍，高血压，部分性偏瘫（全部 n=1） • 与刺激相关的 SAE：接触不良 • 与刺激相关的 AE：视力/眼动障碍（n=8），视物模糊（n=5），头晕（n=4），出汗增加，IPG 感染，眼压高（全部 n=2），低血压，运动障碍，烦躁（n=1）

(续表)

作 者	例数	效 果	不良反应
Coenen 等（2019）	16	• 12个月：16/16人有反应，10人缓解	• 与手术相关的 SAE (n=2)：设备移除 (n=1) • 与刺激相关的 SAE：运动亢进 (n=1) • 其他 SAE：自杀未遂 (n=1)、药物滥用 (n=1) • 与刺激相关的 AE：视力障碍 (n=16)、轻躁狂 (n=1)、躁动 (n=1)、说话含糊 (n=1)
Bewernick 等（2018）	21	• 6个月：9/21人有反应，8人缓解 • 5年：8/11人有反应，8人缓解 • 备注：本样本由 Bewernick 等（2017）和 Coenen 等（2019）的子样本组成；12个月结果见上文	备注：本样本由 Bewernick 等（2017）和 Coenen 等（2019）的子样本组成，不良反应见上文
Fenoy 等（2016, 2018）	6	• 6个月：4/5人有反应，4人缓解 • 12个月：4/5人有反应，3人缓解 • 备注：1名患者在刺激1周后退出试验，该患者退出时刺激有效	• 与手术相关的 AE：术后头痛 (n=4) • 与刺激相关的 AE：垂直复视 (n=4)
Sani 等（2017）	1	• 6个月：0/1人有反应	• 与刺激相关的 AE：焦虑增加，步态改变伴僵硬增加（全部 n=1）
Blomstedt 等（2017）	1	• 12个月：0/1人有反应	• 视物模糊（因此电极重新植入 BNST，反应良好）
丘脑下脚			
Jiménez 等（2005）	1	• 6个月：1/1人有反应，1人缓解 • 12个月：1/1人有反应，1人缓解	• 未报道
缰核			
Sartorius 等（2010）	1	• 6个月：1/1人有反应，1人缓解 • 12个月：1/1人有反应，1人缓解	• 未报道

除非另有说明，否则有反应（response）定义为症状评分比基线降低≥50%。缓解（remission）定义为汉密尔顿抑郁评定量表（Hamilton depression rating scale，HAM–D），17 项≤7，HAM–D，28 项≤10，或蒙哥马利－阿斯伯格抑郁评定量表（Montgomery–Asberg Depression Rating Scale）≤10。所有报告的严重不良事件（SAE）汇总，不考虑与 DBS 的关联，以及所有可能或肯定与 DBS 相关的不良事件（AE）。不良事件的数量考虑了报告事件的患者的数量

AE. 不良事件；SAE. 严重不良事件；IPG. 脉冲发生器；BNST. 终纹床核

经许可转载，引自 Van Laere K, Nuttin B, Gabriels L 等，JNucl Med., 2006; 47:740–7

靶点显示为这些区域之间最大的连接时，11名患者中有9名（82%）在1年后对SCC-DBS有反应（Riva-Posse等，2017）。综上，SCC-DBS的抗抑郁作用似乎依赖于局部对SCC过度活动的下调，以及对分布在边缘、额叶和内脏运动网络的调节。

SCC-DBS是否仍然需要抗抑郁药物治疗，目前还没有系统的研究。在1名抑郁症患者的病例报告中，以及类似抑郁症的动物模型中，SCC-DBS与单胺氧化酶抑制药联合使用时更有效，但与其他抗抑郁药物联合使用时没有这种现象（Hamani等，2012）。

电生理研究中尚未得到明确的抗抑郁生物标志物，但一些研究表明，SCC-DBS的抗抑郁作用与额叶皮质θ频段脑电同步化活动的变化和有效触点处θ频段功率的变化有关（Sun等，2015）。

（二）腹侧内囊/腹侧纹状体

TRD的另一个常用的靶点是腹侧纹状体（主要是伏隔核）和邻近的腹侧内囊。这一靶点的选择是基于其在奖励回路中的核心作用，并基于该区域切开术和DBS治疗强迫症（OCD）的抗抑郁效果（Russo和Nestler，2013；Salgado和Kaplitt，2015）。这个靶区有不同的名称，如伏隔核（NAC）、腹侧内囊/腹侧纹状体（VC/VS）或内囊腹侧前肢（vALIC）。尽管确切的位置在这些靶点之间略有不同，但它们都共享一条穿过内囊前肢的路径，其中最深的1~2个触点在伏隔核中，其余触点在内囊中。

1. 疗效

目前有5项开放性研究的结果发表，共84名患者（表18-1）（Malone等，2009；Bewernick等，2012；Millet等，2014；Dougherty等，2015；Bergfeld等，2016）。DBS治疗6个月后，44名中有21名完全缓解（47.7%）；12个月后，84名患者中有32名有效（38.1%）。

有两项随机对照研究发表，但结果相反。Dougherty等将29名患者随机分为VC/VS DBS刺激组和假刺激组，持续4个月，结果没有显著差异，15名患者中有3名（20.0%）在DBS刺激后有反应；14名患者中有2名（14.3%）在假刺激后有反应（Dougherty等，2015）。另一项研究中，Bergfeld等将内囊腹侧前肢（vALIC）DBS术后患者随机分为2组，其中DBS刺激组25名，假刺激组16名，12个月后发现2组在症状上有很大且显著的差异，假刺激组没有患者有反应（0%），但有7名DBS刺激组患者有反应（43.8%）（Bergfeld等，2016）。

2. 不良反应

在84名患者中，与手术相关的不良事件最常见的是眼球肿胀（$n=12$，14.3%）、伤口感染（$n=5$，5.9%）和吞咽困难（$n=3$，3.6%）。其他报道的不良事件包括导线移位、癫痫发作、出血和术后精神错乱（均为1名，1.2%）。有7名患者（8.3%）报告IPG周围疼痛或不适，2名患者（2.4%）延长导线断裂。最常见的可逆性刺激相关不良事件有激越（$n=13$，15.5%）、脱抑制（$n=9$，10.7%）、轻度躁狂（$n=5$，6.0%）、躁狂（$n=2$，2.4%）或混合双相状态（$n=1$，1.2%）。其他不良事件有躁动或多汗（$n=6$，7.1%）、情绪失衡或抑郁增加（$n=5$，6.0%）、焦虑（$n=4$，4.8%）、自杀意念（$n=3$，3.6%）、精神病性症状（$n=2$，2.4%）。VC/VS DBS后，84名患者中有10名自杀未遂，1名自杀成功。

非对照研究结果显示VC/VS DBS后认知功能有部分改善（Grubert等，2011年；Kubu等，2013）。与健康对照组相比，VC/VS DBS后的练习效应并没有改善，并有近期自传性记忆的加速下降，但优于ECT治疗后的记忆下降（Bergfeld等，2017a，2017b）。此外，与假刺激相比，接受VC/VS DBS的患者在认知抑制方面表现更差（Kubu等，2017）。

3. 作用机制

VC/VS区域在结构和功能上与SCC和MFB相关（Salgado和Kaplitt，2015）。SCC DBS调节NAC的活动，而NAC-DBS调节SCC的活动，其他受影响的区域还包括杏仁核和眶额叶皮质（orbito frontal cortex，OFC）（Bewernick 等，2010）。在患有强迫症的抑郁症患者中，观察到了 VC/VS DBS 对 SCC 过度活动的下调（Rauch 等，2006；Van Laere 等，2006）。综上，VC/VS DBS 可能会对类似边缘激励的神经回路进行"自下而上"的调节，而 SCC-DBS 则以相反的"自上而下"的方式进行调节。这些同一回路的不同调节可能会导致不同但彼此相关的抗抑郁效果（Eggers 等，2014）。根据情绪调节功能，SCC-DBS 起效的第一个表现通常是负面情绪的缓解（Choi 等，2015）；而 NAC-DBS 有效的患者，由于其与奖励和积极情感更相关，兴趣缺失可能得到明显改善（Schlaepfer 等，2008）；vALIC DBS 改善了原发性强迫症患者的情绪，并与纹状体奖励增强和多巴胺释放有关，这可能是逆转重度抑郁症患者快感减退和缺乏积极情绪的重要机制（Denys 等，2010 年；Figee 等，2013，2014）。

（三）内侧前脑束

通过模拟由 SCC 和 VC/VS 激活的共同区域，Coenen 等发现内侧前脑束（MFB）是一个连接枢纽（Coenen 等，2011），并由此假设在 MFB 的根部（上外侧支）刺激比其他靶点更有效地缓解抑郁（Schlaepfer 等，2013）。到目前为止，已有 6 项研究中 32 名患者的结果发表（表 18-1）（Fenoy 等，2016 年，2018 年；Bewernick 等，2017，2018；Sani 等，2017；Coenen 等，2019）。6 个月后，27 名患者中有 13 名（48.1%）有反应；治疗 12 个月后，30 名患者中有 26 名有反应（86.6%）；随访 5 年后，11 名患者中有 8 名（72.7%）有反应（Bewernick 等，2018）。虽然这些结果是基于小样本和非对照研究，但这些结果表明，与其他靶点相比 MFB DBS 的有效率相对较高。此外，第一个随机对照假刺激研究将 16 名患者随机分为假刺激组或 MFB DBS 刺激组，2 个月后结果表明，MFB DBS 比假刺激能更好地减轻症状。

1. 不良反应

32 名患者中，2 名因伤口愈合障碍取出了刺激器（6.3%），1 名术后出血（3.1%）。其他与手术相关的不良事件包括术后头痛（n=4，12.5%）、构音障碍、高血压和部分偏瘫（均为 1 名，3.1%）。设备相关不良反应，目前报告了 1 名 IPG 接触故障和 1 名感染。最常见的刺激相关不良事件是高电压下的视力障碍（n=29，93.5%）。其他报道的事件包括头晕（n=4，12.9%）、躁动、出汗和高眼压（n=2，6.5%），以及轻度躁狂、口齿不清、低血压、运动障碍、烦躁、焦虑和运动僵直（n=1，3.2%），另有 1 名运动亢进（3.2%）。在 MFB DBS 之后，有一起自杀未遂事件，但没有完整的报告。初步结果表明，MFB DBS 之后神经心理测试中认知表现与之前持平（Schlaepfer 等，2013 年；Fenoy 等，2018 年；Coenen 等，2019）。

2. 作用机制

MFB 是第一个基于白质纤维神经成像的靶点，该靶点抗抑郁作用的最初原理，是发现 STN-DBS 治疗的帕金森病患者的轻躁狂与 MFB 有关，纤维示踪成像显示刺激触点与 MFB 有直接联系，而没有轻躁狂的患者触点离 MFB 距离更远（Coenen 等，2009）。健康个体的纤维示踪成像研究显示，MFB 的上外侧分支通过 vALIC 和 NAC，连接腹侧被盖区（VTA）与 OFC 及内侧和背外侧前额叶皮质，共同构成参与奖励、动机和情绪处理的神经环路（Coenen 等，2018）。在之后的 DBS 试验中，靶点定位一直是基于这种超外侧 MFB 的个体纤维示踪成像。MFB DBS 在患者中可能的抗抑郁机制尚不明确，但动物研究表明 MFB DBS 与前额叶皮质（而不是伏隔核）的多巴胺能变化有关（Bregman 等，2015 年；Dandekar 等，2018）。

（四）其他靶点

在 2 个病例报告中，用到了另外 2 个靶点，包括丘脑下脚（inferior thalamic peduncle）（Jiménez 等，2005）和外侧缰核（lateral habenula）（Sartorius 等，2010）。这 2 名患者在 12 个月的刺激后都有症状缓解，但还需要大样本研究。2 名患者均没有报告不良反应，且认知功能稳定。

四、展望

基于解剖标志的 DBS 靶点刺激显示出治疗 TRD 的良好前景，但应用个体化白质束作为靶点产生的抗抑郁效果明显，说明 DBS 治疗可能有相当大的优化空间。传统医疗中，靶点选择一直集中在抑郁症患者中异常神经活动的特定灰质核团，如 SCC 和纹状体（Mayberg，1997；Price and Drists，2010）。较新的技术已经将焦点转移到与抑郁症有关的大脑回路中特定的白质束（Schlaepfer 等，2014；Riva-Posse 等，2017）。该方法的电生理学证据表明 DBS 在轴突中发挥了大部分作用（Brocker 和 Grill 2013），神经生物学证据表明，DBS 的临床效果来源于受影响回路中的振荡去同步和过度活跃的减少（Eusebio 等，2012；Figee 等，2013；Bahramisharif 等，2015；Sun 等，2015；Steiner 等，2017）。因此，根据不同患者，明确个体化最佳抗抑郁效果的特异性白质束，有希望取得更好的 DBS 抗抑郁疗效。

另一种优化方法在于参数选择，目前这主要是一个试错过程。对帕金森病患者的研究表明，不同的频率可能对不同的症状有不同的影响，较低的脉冲宽度可能会导致更宽的治疗窗（DiBiase 和 Fasano，2016；Steigerwald 等，2018；Bouthour 等，2018）。但到目前为止，还缺乏对抑郁症患者不同参数设置的系统性探索。

最后，其他治疗方法可以辅助提高抑郁症患者的 DBS 疗效。许多耐药患者有其他问题，如失业、社会支持有限，以及无法继续进行爱好和体育运动。这些患者通常有极长的病程，许多继发性问题在症状减轻后可能仍然存在（Crowell 等，2015）。因此增加康复和行为疗法很重要，并已经证实在 DBS 治疗强迫症中有疗效加成（Mantione 等，2014）。

五、结论

基于解剖学标志的传统 DBS 靶点（SCC 和 VC/VS）的研究显示，该疗法在缓解抑郁症状方面很有希望，40% 的严重耐药患者在刺激 1 年后有反应，但随机对照研究的结果好坏参半。

限制 DBS 调节节点的 3 项对照研究均未能发现 DBS 刺激和假刺激之间的差异（Dougherty 等，2015；Holtzheimer 等，2017）。但一项在 DBS 调整参数 1 年的对照试验中，两组疗效有显著差异（Bergfeld 等，2016）。此外，从发表的研究看，根据患者特定的白质束轨迹设计电极植入路径的有效率为 75%，但尚未有安慰剂对照研究。

参考文献

[1] Bahramisharif A, Mazaheri A, Levar N, et al. Deep brain stimulation diminishes cross-frequency coupling in obsessive-compulsive disorder. Biol Psychiatry. 2015;80(7):e57–8.
[2] Bergfeld IO, Mantione M, Hoogendoorn MLC, et al. Deep brain stimulation of the ventral anterior limb of the internal capsule for treatment-resistant depression: a randomized clinical trial. JAMA Psychiat. 2016;73:456–64.
[3] Bergfeld IO, Mantione M, Hoogendoorn MLC, et al. Impact of deep brain stimulation of the ventral anterior limb of the internal capsule on cognition in depression. Psychol Med. 2017a;47:1647–58.
[4] Bergfeld IO, Mantione M, Hoogendoorn MLC, et al. Episodic memory following deep brain stimulation of the ventral anterior limb of the internal capsule and electroconvulsive therapy. Brain Stimul. 2017b;10:959–66.
[5] Bewernick BH, Hurlemann R, Matusch A, et al. Nucleus accumbens deep brain stimulation decreases ratings of depression and anxiety in treatment-resistant depression. Biol Psychiatry. 2010;67:110–6.
[6] Bewernick BH, Kayser S, Sturm V, Schlaepfer TE. Long-term effects of nucleus accumbens deep brain stimulation in treatment-resistant depression: evidence for sustained efficacy. Neuropsychopharmacology. 2012;37:1975–85.
[7] Bewernick BH, Kayser S, Gippert SM, et al. Deep brain stimulation to the medial forebrain bundle for depression—long-term outcomes and a novel data analysis strategy. Brain Stimul. 2017;10:664–71.
[8] Bewernick BH, Kilian HM, Schmidt K, et al. Deep brain stimulation of the supero-lateral branch of the medial forebrain bundle does not lead to changes in person-ality in patients suffering from severe depression. Psychol Med. 2018;48:2684–92.
[9] Blomstedt P, Naesström M, Bodlund O. Deep brain stimulation in the bed nucleus of the stria terminalis and medial forebrain bundle in a patient with major depressive disorder and anorexia nervosa. Clin case reports. 2017;5:679–84. https://doi.org/10.1002/ccr3.856.
[10] Bogod NM, Sinden M, Woo C, et al. Long-term neuropsychological safety of subgenual cingulate gyrus deep brain stimulation for treatment-resistant depression. J Neuropsychiatry Clin Neurosci. 2014;26:126–33.

[11] Bouthour W, Wegrzyk J, Momjian S, et al. Short pulse width in subthalamic stimulation in Parkinson's disease: a randomized, double-blind study. Mov Disord. 2018;33:169–73.

[12] Bregman T, Reznikov R, Diwan M, et al. Antidepressant-like effects of medial forebrain bundle deep brain stimulation in rats are not associated with accumbens dopamine release. Brain Stimul. 2015;8:708–13.

[13] Brocker DT, Grill WM. Principles of electrical stimulation of neural tissue. In: Handbook of clinical neurology. New York: Elsevier; 2013. p. 3–18.

[14] Choi KS, Riva-Posse P, Gross RE, Mayberg HS. Mapping the "depression switch" during intraoperative testing of subcallosal cingulate deep brain stimulation. JAMA Neurol. 2015;72:1252.

[15] Coenen VA, Honey CR, Hurwitz T, et al. Medial forebrain bundle stimulation as a pathophysiological mechanism for hypomania in subthalamic nucleus deep brain stimulation for Parkinson's disease. Neurosurgery. 2009;64:1106–14.

[16] Coenen VA, Schlaepfer TE, Maedler B, Panksepp J. Cross-species affective functions of the medial forebrain bundle - implications for the treatment of affective pain and depression in humans. Neurosci Biobehav Rev. 2011;35:1971–81.

[17] Coenen VA, Schumacher LV, Kaller C, et al. The anatomy of the human medial forebrain bundle: ventral tegmental area connections to reward-associated subcortical and frontal lobe regions. NeuroImage Clin. 2018;18:770–83.

[18] Coenen VA, Bewernick BH, Kayser S, et al. Superolateral medial forebrain bundle deep brain stimulation in major depression: a gateway trial. Neuropsychopharmacology. 2019;44:1224–32.

[19] Crowell AL, Garlow SJ, Riva-Posse P, Mayberg HS. Characterizing the therapeutic response to deep brain stimulation for treatment-resistant depression: a single center long-term perspective. Front Integr Neurosci. 2015;9:1–6.

[20] Dandekar MP, Fenoy AJ, Carvalho AF, et al. Deep brain stimulation for treatment-resistant depression: an integrative review of preclinical and clinical findings and translational implications. Mol Psychiatry. 2018;23:1094–112.

[21] Denys D, Mantione M, Figee M, et al. Deep brain stimulation of the nucleus accumbens for treatment-refractory obsessive-compulsive disorder. Arch Gen Psychiatry. 2010;67:1061–8.

[22] di Biase L, Fasano A. Low-frequency deep brain stimulation for Parkinson's disease: great expectation or false hope? Mov Disord. 2016;31:962–7.

[23] Dougherty DD, Rezai AR, Carpenter LL, et al. A randomized sham-controlled trial of deep Brain stimulation of the ventral capsule/ventral striatum for chronic treatment-resistant depression. Biol Psychiatry. 2015;78:240–8.

[24] Eggers AE. Treatment of depression with deep brain stimulation works by altering in specific ways the conscious perception of the core symptoms of sadness or anhedonia, not by modulating network circuitry. Med Hypotheses. 2014;83:62–4.

[25] Eitan R, Fontaine D, Benoît M, et al. One year double blind study of high vs low frequency subcallosal cingulate stimulation for depression. J Psychiatr Res. 2018;96:124–34.

[26] Eusebio A, Cagnan H, Brown P. Does suppression of oscillatory synchronisation mediate some of the therapeutic effects of DBS in patients with Parkinson's disease? Front Integr Neurosci. 2012;6:47.

[27] Fenoy AJ, Schulz P, Selvaraj S, et al. Deep brain stimulation of the medial forebrain bundle: distinctive responses in resistant depression. J Affect Disord. 2016;203:143–51.

[28] Fenoy AJ, Schulz PE, Selvaraj S, et al. A longitudinal study on deep brain stimulation of the medial forebrain bundle for treatment-resistant depression. Transl Psychiatry. 2018;8:111.

[29] Figee M, Luigjes J, Smolders R, et al. Deep brain stimulation restores frontostriatal network activity in obsessive-compulsive disorder. Nat Neurosci. 2013;16:386–7.

[30] Figee M, de Koning P, Klaassen S, et al. Deep brain stimulation induces striatal dopamine release in obsessive-compulsive disorder. Biol Psychiatry. 2014;75:647–52.

[31] Grubert C, Hurlemann R, Bewernick BH, et al. Neuropsychological safety of nucleus accumbens deep brain stimulation for major depression: effects of 12-month stimulation. World J Biol Psychiatry. 2011;12:516–27.

[32] Guinjoan SM, Mayberg HS, Costanzo EY, et al. Asymmetrical contribution of brain structures to treatment-resistant depression as illustrated by effects of right subgenual cingulum stimulation. J Neuropsychiatry Clin Neurosci. 2010;22:265–77.

[33] Hamani C, Giacobbe P, Diwan M, et al. Monoamine oxidase inhibitors potentiate the effects of deep brain stimulation. Am J Psychiatry. 2012;169:1320–1.

[34] Holtzheimer PE, Kelley ME, Gross RE, et al. Subcallosal cingulate deep brain stimulation for treatment-resistant unipolar and bipolar depression. Arch Gen Psychiatry. 2012;69:150–8.

[35] Holtzheimer PE, Husain MM, Lisanby SH, et al. Subcallosal cingulate deep brain stimulation for treatment-resistant depression: a multisite, randomised, sham-controlled trial. Lancet Psychiatry. 2017;4:839–49.

[36] Jiménez F, Velasco F, Salin-Pascual R, et al. A patient with a resistant major depression disorder treated with deep brain stimulation in the inferior thalamic peduncle. Neurosurgery. 2005;57:585–93.

[37] Kennedy SH, Giacobbe P, Rizvi SJ, et al. Deep brain stimulation for treatment-resistant depression: follow-up after 3 to 6 years. Am J Psychiatry. 2011;168:502–10.

[38] https://doi.org/10.1176/appi.ajp.2010.10081187. Kubu CS, Malone DA, Chelune G, et al. Neuropsychological outcome after deep brain stimulation in the ventral capsule/ventral striatum for highly refractory obsessive-compulsive disorder or major depression. Stereotact Funct Neurosurg. 2013;91:374–8.

[39] Kubu CS, Brelje T, Butters MA, et al. Cognitive outcome after ventral capsule/ventral striatum stimulation for treatment-resistant major depression. J Neurol Neurosurg Psychiatry. 2017;88:262–5.

[40] Lozano AM, Mayberg HS, Giacobbe P, et al. Subcallosal cingulate gyrus deep brain stimulation for treatment-resistant depression. Biol Psychiatry. 2008;64:461–7.

[41] Lozano AM, Giacobbe P, Hamani C, et al. A multicenter pilot study of subcallosal cingulate area deep brain stimulation for treatment-resistant depression. J Neurosurg. 2012;116:315–22.

[42] Malone DA, Dougherty DD, Rezai AR, et al. Deep brain stimulation of the ventral capsule/ventral striatum for treatment-resistant depression. Biol Psychiatry. 2009;65:267–75.

[43] Mantione M, Nieman DDH, Figee M, Denys D. Cognitive–behavioural therapy augments the effects of deep brain stimulation in obsessive–compulsive disorder. Psychol Med. 2014;44:3515–22.

[44] Mayberg HS. Limbic-cortical dysregulation: a proposed model of depression. J Neuropsychiatry Clin Neurosci. 1997;9:471–81.

[45] Mayberg HS, Lozano AM, Voon V, et al. Deep brain stimulation for treatment-resistant depression. Neuron. 2005;45:651–60.

[46] McNeely HE, Mayberg HS, Lozano AM, Kennedy SH. Neuropsychological impact of Cg25 deep brain stimulation for treatment-resistant depression: preliminary results over 12 months. J Nerv Ment Dis. 2008;196:405–10.

[47] Merkl A, Aust S, Schneider G-H, et al. Deep brain stimulation of the subcallosal cingulate gyrus in patients with treatment-resistant depression: a double-blinded randomized controlled study and long-term follow-up in eight patients. J Affect Disord. 2017;227:521–9.

[48] Millet B, Jaafari N, Polosan M, et al. Limbic versus cognitive target for deep brain stimulation in treatment-resistant depression: accumbens more promising than caudate. Eur Neuropsychopharmacol. 2014;24:1229–39.

[49] Moreines JL, McClintock SM, Kelley ME, et al. Neuropsychological function before and after subcallosal cingulate deep brain stimulation in patients with treatment-resistant depression. Depress Anxiety. 2014;31:690–8.

[50] Price JL, Drevets WC. Neurocircuitry of mood disorders. Neuropsychopharmacology. 2010;35:192–216.

[51] Puigdemont D, Pérez-Egea R, Portella MJ, et al. Deep brain stimulation of the subcallosal cingulate gyrus: further evidence in treatment-resistant major depression. Int J Neuropsychopharmacol. 2012;15:121–33.

[52] Ramasubbu R, Anderson S, Haffenden A, et al. Double-blind optimization of subcallosal cingulate deep brain stimulation for treatment-resistant depression: a pilot study. J Psychiatry Neurosci. 2013;38:325–32.

[53] Rauch SL, Dougherty DD, Malone D, et al. A functional neuroimaging investigation of deep brain stimulation in patients with obsessive-compulsive disorder. J Neurosurg. 2006;104:558–65.

[54] Riva-Posse P, Choi KS, Holtzheimer PE, et al. Defining critical white matter pathways mediating successful subcallosal cingulate deep brain stimulation for treatment-resistant depression. Biol Psychiatry. 2014;76:963–9.

[55] Riva-Posse P, Choi KS, Holtzheimer PE, et al. A connectomic approach for subcallosal cingulate deep brain stimulation surgery: prospective targeting in treatment-resistant depression. Mol Psychiatry. 2017;23:843–9.

[56] Russo SJ, Nestler EJ. The brain reward circuitry in mood disorders. Nat Rev Neurosci. 2013;14:609–25.

[57] Salgado S, Kaplitt MG. The nucleus accumbens: a comprehensive review. Stereotact Funct Neurosurg. 2015;93:75–93.

[58] Sani S, Busnello J, Kochanski R, et al. High-frequency measurement of depressive severity in a patient treated for severe treatment-resistant depression with deep-brain stimulation. Transl Psychiatry. 2017;7:e1207.

[59] Sartorius A, Kiening KL, Kirsch P, et al. Remission of major depression under deep brain stimulation of the lateral habenula in a therapy-refractory patient. Biol Psychiatry. 2010;67:e9–e11.

[60] Schlaepfer TE, Cohen MX, Frick C, et al. Deep brain stimulation to reward circuitry alleviates anhedonia in refractory major depression. Neuropsychopharmacology. 2008;33:368–77.

[61] Schlaepfer TE, Bewernick BH, Kayser S, et al. Rapid effects of deep brain stimulation for treatment-resistant major depression. Biol Psychiatry. 2013;73:1204–12.

[62] Schlaepfer TE, Bewernick BH, Kayser S, et al. Deep brain stimulation of the human reward system for major depression—rationale, outcomes and outlook. Neuropsychopharmacology. 2014;39:1303–14.

[63] Serra-Blasco M, de Vita S, Rodriguez MR, et al. Cognitive functioning after deep brain stimulation in subcallosal cingulate gyrus for treatment-resistant depression: an exploratory study. Psychiatry Res. 2015;225:341–6.

[64] Steigerwald F, Timmermann L, Kühn A, et al. Pulse duration settings in subthalamic stimulation for Parkinson's disease. Mov Disord. 2018;33:165–9.

[65] Steiner LA, Neumann W-J, Staub-Bartelt F, et al. Subthalamic beta dynamics mirror Parkinsonian bradykinesia months after neurostimulator implantation. Mov Disord. 2017;32:1183–90.

[66] Sun Y, Giacobbe P, Tang CW, et al. Deep brain stimulation modulates gamma oscillations and theta–gamma coupling in treatment resistant depression. Brain Stimul. 2015;8:1033–42.

[67] Torres CV, Ezquiaga E, Navas M, de Sola RG. Deep brain stimulation of the subcallosal cingulate for medication-resistant type I bipolar depression: case report. Bipolar Disord. 2013;15:719–21.

[68] Van Laere K, Nuttin B, Gabriels L, et al. Metabolic imaging of anterior capsular stimulation in refractory obsessive-compulsive disorder: a key role for the subgenual anterior cingulate and ventral striatum. J Nucl Med. 2006;47:740–7.

第 19 章 脑深部电刺激的其他适应证
Other Indications for Deep Brain Stimulation

Sarah A. Hescham　Ali Jahanshahi　**著**
王　垚　张　玿　**译**　朱冠宇　杨岸超　张建国　**校**

> **摘要**：除了普遍接受的适应证外，脑深部电刺激（DBS）在试验性病例研究或初步临床试验中已用于治疗成瘾、亨廷顿病、阿尔茨海默病、神经性厌食症、微意识状态和精神分裂症。DBS 应用于这些适应证的基本原理是调节功能障碍的神经结构或环路，而这些功能障碍被认为是导致临床症状的主要原因。在本章中，我们将重点介绍关于 DBS 适应证的最新研究进展。尽管在这些适应证中大多数已经报道了有效的作用，但我们应该考虑到对于 DBS 有效的作用机制和影响的神经环路仍然知之甚少。了解这些机制将有助于 DBS 在治疗这些疾病时取得更好的效果。此外，当在神经退行性疾病中应用 DBS 时应谨慎，因为进行性脑萎缩可能导致意外的不良反应或无效。

一、概述

全球范围来看，神经和精神疾病的负担是巨大的，并且预计在未来几十年仍会增加（Vigo 等，2016；Feigin 等，2017）。尽管这些疾病的确切原因尚待阐明，但神经影像学的最新进展已经提供了证据，证明我们在患者身上看到的许多症状和体征分别来自于负责运动、情绪和认知功能的特定脑网络的功能障碍（Nestler 等，2002；Price 和 Drevets，2009；Krack 等，2010）。这些观察结果使焦点转移到非药物治疗策略上，如脑深部电刺激（DBS）可以调节环路，并有助于提供环路功能障碍的病理生理学的重要细节。我们目前正处于一个积极的研究阶段，以确定哪些环路和疾病可以用 DBS 治疗（Lozano 和 Lipsman，2013）。

在这一章中，我们描述了 DBS 在成瘾、亨廷顿病、神经性厌食症、阿尔茨海默病、微意识状态和精神分裂症的治疗中的试验性应用。对于每个适应证，我们将简要讨论 DBS 的治疗原理和临床数据。由于研究都是试验性的，这些临床资料主要是个案报道和小病例数量的研究。本章的目的不是对文献进行全面的综述，而是对最近的文章进行权衡并做出选择。

二、成瘾

成瘾的特征是强迫性地参与可给予自身奖励的刺激，尽管这种刺激有心理和生理上的不良后果。导致成瘾的刺激可能是产生依赖性的物质（如酒精、尼古丁、非法药物）或强迫行为（如赌博、运动、食物）。其特征包括对物质或行为的自我控制能力受损，在停止使用时可导致戒断综合征。美国成人一生中，非法药物滥用 / 依赖的流行率约为5%（Sussman等，2011），而可卡因和阿片样物质的年龄标准化使用率分别为524.1/10万和1168.3/10万（Degenhardt等，2018）。药物和心理干预治疗的疗效有限，复发率高。研究表明，65%～70%的阿片依赖者在戒断后1年内复发，特别是在戒断的前3个月内（Gossop等，2002）。

由于药物的使用会产生奖赏作用，所以成瘾回路中的一些结构属于多巴胺能边缘系统，因此成瘾被认为是DBS治疗可能的适应证（Pelloux和Baunez，2013；Tony等，2018）。

对于慢性阿片类药物的成瘾，一则报道描述了1名24岁男性海洛因依赖患者通过双侧伏隔核（NAC）DBS治疗（Zhou等，2011）。刺激参数设置为频率145Hz，脉冲宽度90μs，电压0.8～2.5V。心理评估（韦氏记忆量表、韦克斯勒成人智力量表和明尼苏达多相人格问卷）的比较结果表明，记忆力和智商有显著改善。其性格没有明显变化。此外，受试者在多个自我评定症状量表（症状自评量表90、自我评定抑郁量表和自我评定焦虑量表）上也有所改善。患者在手术后完全停止吸毒，没有任何其他辅助治疗。在6年的随访中没有复发。后来他重新开始全职工作。有趣的是，患者的吸烟也减少了。在2.5年后，电刺激被关闭，而手术的效果仍然存在。在另一个2年随访的病例研究中也得到了类似的发现，其中2名海洛因成瘾患者接受了双侧NAC-DBS治疗（Kuhn等，2014）。这2名患者还服用了其他精神类药物（患者1：酒精和苯丙胺；患者2：苯丙胺和苯二氮䓬）。刺激参数分别设置在频率140Hz、脉冲宽度120μs和电压5.0v（患者1）和频率130Hz、脉冲宽度90μs和电压4.5v（患者2）。有趣的是，尽管DBS产生了持续的海洛因戒断效果，但患者的共病药物服用剂量并没有下降。

在最近对1名可卡因依赖患者进行的双盲试验（$n=1$）中，通过客观和主观测量，术后2.5年的随访表明NAC-DBS显著降低了可卡因依赖的严重程度（Gonçalves-Ferreira等，2016）。本研究采用以下范式：第一阶段（9个月），初始DBS植入，优化刺激参数；第二阶段（9个月），6个月双盲刺激，3个月单盲刺激；第三阶段（12个月），持续刺激。患者为36岁男性，无其他精神障碍、自杀意念、器质性脑功能障碍或获得性免疫缺陷综合征等疾病。刺激采用连续刺激，并可进行逐步调整。右侧NAC刺激参数为频率150Hz，脉冲宽度150μs，电压3～4V，左侧NAC刺激参数为频率150Hz，脉冲宽度150μs，电压2.5～3V。在9个月的盲期内，可卡因的需求和使用量有客观的下降，但"关"和"开"的刺激状态之间没有差异，这表明可能存在潜在的安慰剂效应或突触可塑性改变。

然而，由于患者可能暴露在潜在的严重风险中而没有任何治疗效果，因此对双盲研究和假手术提出了伦理上的质疑（Müller等，2013）。此外，DBS治疗成瘾还存在伦理和逻辑方面的问题。DBS可能不太适合正在药物滥用的患者，因为患者在药物影响下给予知情同意的能力有限。此外，迅速戒毒的患者可能仍存在精神状态和（或）执行能力的改变，限制了他们提供知情同意的能力（Müller等，2013）。基于这些原因，有人建议DBS只用于戒断期患者，以防止复发（Tony等，2018）。

三、亨廷顿病

亨廷顿病（Huntington disease，HD）的起病原因是人类第4对常染色体上的HD基因突变，由5'端不稳定的多态性三核苷酸重复序列（CAG）n的异常重复所致。据研究这会导致突变蛋白的毒性增加。纹状体神经元出现明显变性（Vonsattel等，1985；Graybiel 1995；Sieradzan和Mann，2001），苍白球和底丘脑核（STN）神经元活性受损（Vonsattel等，1985；Vlamings等，2012）。神经退行性变导致皮质-基底节-丘脑-皮质回路的功能障碍和失衡，因此HD患者出现多种边缘系统、运动和认知症状（Joel，2001）。基于这一病理生理背景，包括苍白球DBS在内的功能神经外科技术，被认为是对抗皮质-基底节-丘脑-皮质通路功能障碍的一种对症治疗方法。

Moro等（2004）第一次报道了DBS治疗HD。然而，关于苍白球（GPi）DBS治疗HD的疗效，目前报道的资料有限。迄今为止，只有少数的个案研究。因此，人们对这种治疗方法的长期效果知之甚少（Ligot等，2011；Zeef等，2011；Edwards等，2012；Spielberger等，2012）。这些小病例报道主要显示了GPi-DBS后亨廷顿病的短期和长期改善。不幸的是，GPi-DBS对认知和精神的影响还没有准确的报道，而且GPi-DBS似乎并不总能改善运动迟缓或其他少动性症状。苍白球外侧部（GPe）可能也是治疗HD的一个有趣靶点，因为HD中纹状体神经元死亡，GPe被认为是过度激活的。临床前试验研究表明，大鼠的GP（灵长类GPe的同源核团）和STN刺激能改善亨廷顿病和认知功能（Temel等，2006；Vlamings等，2012），但缺乏相关核团DBS的临床数据。但是，Ligot等（2011）显示GPe-DBS后皮质血流量增加。目前尚不清楚HD患者双侧DBS后的变化是否依赖刺激参数，因为低频和高频刺激都对HD患者的运动症状都有有益的影响。Hebb等（2006）报告了180Hz电刺激有效，而其他人则发现40Hz和130Hz刺激也都可以控制亨廷顿病（Moro等，2004）。除了苍白球外，根据动物实验的研究结果，还提出了一些其他的潜在的靶点（Temel等，2006；Vlamings等，2012）。这些靶点的共同特性是它们都是皮质-基底节-丘脑-皮质环路的一部分。另一个有趣的理论提出黑质致密部（SNC）是一个潜在的靶点，基于Bonelli和同事的观察，他们报告了HD患者舞蹈样不自主动作可以自发下降。后来，有报道称亨廷顿病的消失可能是由于SNC的萎缩，并提示该可对该区域行DBS（Bonelli和Gruber，2002）。有趣的是，在人类尸检相关的研究中，HD受试者的脑干和基底节出现了高多巴胺能状态（Bird 1980；Bird等，1980；Jahanshahi等，2013）。

众所周知，在已知脑功能失调区域时，DBS对神经系统疾病的治疗特别有效。在HD中，虽然不同方面的神经退行性变已被很好地描述，但研究表明进行性脑萎缩可影响DBS的长期预后，产生不良反应，并可能使程控更困难（Martens等，2011；Martinez-Ramirez等，2014；VedamMai等，2016）。此外，患者可能会出现疾病进展的症状，并伴有刺激性不良反应，导致复杂症状的产生。

萎缩可能导致邻近结构与GPi的距离增加，或者电极触点位置的改变可能使其更接近主要的纤维束（如内囊），从而产生严重的不良反应。针对这方面，最近在DBS技术上的创新，如电流转向导联，似乎可以更好地应对由于逐渐脑萎缩而引起的解剖结构变化。

总之，由于DBS的最佳靶点仍不确定，DBS治疗HD仍然应该被看作是试验性的。可惜的是，虽然大多数病例报告对运动症状给出了引人关注的结果，但是对患者的生活质量缺乏完整或清晰的描述。此外，在描述术前、术后运动和非运动症状方面的研究也不一致，而且常常缺乏对DBS电极确切位置的描述。从非临床试验推广到临床应用，有几个问题需要解决，比如DBS手术的时间点，HD患者是否可以完全同意手术，以及可以预见的神经心理不良反应等。此外，来自患者关于随着疾病进展导致的手术无效或症状加重的咨询值得认真考量。

四、神经性厌食症

神经性厌食症（anorexia nervosa，AN）是一种饮食失调，其特征是异常低体重，对增重的强烈恐惧，以及对体重的扭曲感知，最终导致进食受限。欧洲和北美年轻女性的神经性厌食症患病率为0.3%（Favaro等，2003；Hoek和van Hoeken，2003）。AN的药物和心理治疗主要针对如体重、食欲、扭曲的思想和行为等主要症状，以及如抑郁和焦虑等次要症状（Bodell和Keel，2010）。在标准治疗流程下，其复发率为30%～50%，由于较高的发病率和死亡率（Guarda，2008），研究人员目前正在研究新的治疗方法，如DBS。考虑到强迫症（OCD）和AN等奖赏相关疾病在症状学和神经环路上有所重叠，故伏隔核（NAC）和其他与奖赏相关的区域，如前扣带回皮质（ACC），成为DBS治疗的潜在靶点（Oudijn等，2013；Lipsman等，2017）。

在最近的一项开放性试验中，16名难治性厌食症患者接受了胼胝体下扣带回的DBS治疗（Lipsman等，2017）。患者平均年龄34岁，平均病程18年。手术时的平均BMI为13.83±1.49，16名患者中有14名（88%）同时患有情绪障碍、焦虑障碍或两者兼有。平均BMI在12个月内显著增加到17.34±3.4。14名患者中有8名（57%）在12个月的随访中BMI＞17.0，其中6名（43%）的BMI≥18.5。术后至少3个月体重才开始变化。DBS还可显著改善抑郁、焦虑和情感调节。事实上，研究人员认为，对情绪紊乱和焦虑的治疗对于获得持续的、长期的益处和减少神经性厌食症的复发至关重要。与此相一致，他们的研究结果显示，与同期抑郁和焦虑评分的下降相比，前3个月的体重变化相对较小。这表明边缘系统功能障碍的改善可能先于体重的变化，也可能和体重的改变相伴随。尽管总体结果令人鼓舞，但该研究的开放式设计（患者和临床医生对电刺激都知情）有一些局限性。这项研究没有包括任何一个阶段的盲法假刺激或盲法评估。因此，结果可能与安慰剂效应有关。

DBS治疗神经性厌食症的进一步挑战是很多的，包括患者经常否认该疾病，随后尽管病情严重但仍未能获得或不愿寻求治疗，以及情绪和焦虑障碍的高共病率。

五、微意识状态

微意识状态被定义为严重改变的意识状态，在这种状态下，患者的意识部分保留，并且可以通过移动手指来交流或响应简单的命令。遭受严重创伤性颅脑损伤（TBI）的患者可以表现出渐进性的意识恢复，通过一系列的临床状况，包括植物状态（VS）和（或）微意识状态（MCS）逐渐进行过渡（Bernat，2009；De Jong，2013）。虽然这些可能是暂时的临床情况（De Jong，2013），但在某些情况下，它们是急性脑事件的稳定结果，患者永远无法恢复完全意识（Bernat，2010）。目前对于微意识状态的患者尚无有效的治疗方法。丘脑网状核DBS作为一种治疗TBI的主要方法已被尝试。将DBS靶点定在丘脑核团和网状系统的理论基础是这些结构在觉醒中起着关键的作用（Moruzzi和Magoun 1949；Purpura和Schiff 1997）。

1名男性患者，38岁，维持MCS状态6年以上，接受了双侧中央丘脑DBS（Schiff等，2007）。尽管患者住院康复治疗了2年，随后在疗养院中度过4年，他也未能恢复连续的执行命令和沟通能力，并且无自主语言能力。功能磁共振显示大范围的双半球仍具有大脑语言网络，表明存在进一步恢复的功能基础。逐渐调节患者DBS的参数设置，最终刺激参数设置为频率100 Hz，右侧双极刺激，左侧单极刺激，电压均为4V。在为期6个月的双盲交替期中，当DBS处于"开启"状态时，患者在对命令的反应、物体的使用、可理解的发声和语言反馈方面均表现出进步。作者的结论是，DBS的作用补偿了正常情况下由大脑额叶控制的觉醒调节功能的丧失。

在最近的一项研究中，我们调查了14名患者应用DBS的治疗情况，其中4名是MCS患者，10名是VS患者（Chudy等，2018）。VS或MCS的病因有4名为TBI，有10名为心搏骤停性缺氧性脑病。DBS的靶点是中央中核-束旁核复合体，随访时间为38～60个月。在白天DBS每隔2h刺激30min，刺激参数设置为单极刺激、频率25Hz、脉冲宽度90μs，患者电压设置范围为2.5～3.5V。随访结束时，2名MCS患者恢复了意识，恢复了行走、语言流利、独立生活的能力。1名MCS患者意识清醒但仍坐在轮椅上。1名VS患者提高了意识水平，目前可对简单的命令做出反应。3名VS患者死于呼吸道感染、败血症或脑血管损伤。其余 7 名患者意识水平无明显提高。本研究中，DBS 的成功率为 29%。尽管观察到一些患者恢复了意识是很鼓舞的，但同时我们也面临着筛选手术适应证的挑战，因为没有明确的神经生理学或神经放射学标准可以准确地预测 VS 或 MCS 患者中谁可能从 DBS 中受益。

六、阿尔茨海默病

阿尔茨海默病（Alzheimer disease，AD）是一种慢性神经退行性疾病，主要表现为慢性、进行性加重的认知功能障碍。随着病情的进一步发展，患者会出现失去方向感、失认、失语、失用，最后出现长期记忆丧失等症状。年平均发病率为 1%~3%，与 65 岁以上人群 10%~30% 的总发病率一致（Masters 等，2015）。目前的药物治疗只会暂时帮助觉醒、提高注意力和记忆力。因此，研究人员正在研究非药物治疗方案，如脑深部电刺激。目前，有两种结构已经成为临床试验的靶点，包括穹窿（Laxton 等，2010；Smith 等，2012；Fontaine 等，2013；Lozano 等，2016）和 Meynert 基底核（NBM）（Turnbull 等，1985；Kuhn 等，2014）。

通过 DBS 刺激 Papez 环路中某些结构的基本原理是拮抗 AD 病理引起的神经元信息处理功能障碍。穹窿作为治疗 AD 的 DBS 的靶点是偶然被发现的（Hamani 等，2008）。NBM 的 DBS 被认为能提高靶区乙酰胆碱的浓度，类似于乙酰胆碱酯酶抑制药的作用，因为胆碱能传递被认为是认知能力的关键（Hescham 等，2013）。

2010 年报道了 DBS 用于治疗 AD 的 Ⅰ 期临床试验结果。6 名轻度 AD 患者接受双侧穹窿/下丘脑 DBS，刺激参数为频率 130Hz，脉冲宽度 90μs，电压 3.0~3.5V（Laxton 等，2010）。经过 12 个月的刺激，PET 扫描显示早期显著的颞叶和顶叶葡萄糖代谢受损得到逆转。此外，AD 评定量表认知分量表（ADAS-cog）和简易精神状态检查量表（MMSE）结果显示，尤其是轻度认知障碍的患者更可能从这种治疗中获益。在这之后，作者又报道了穹窿 DBS 使这些患者的 Papez 环路中的结构得到改变（Sankar 等，2015）。用磁共振成像（MRI）测量 DBS 后 1 年和基线时海马、穹窿和乳头体的体积，作者发现，与年龄、性别和严重程度匹配的 25 名未接受 DBS 治疗的 AD 患者相比，接受穹窿 DBS 治疗的患者海马萎缩的速度较慢（Sankar 等，2015）。有趣的是，2 名对穹窿 DBS 临床反应最好的患者甚至显示双侧海马体积分别增加了 5.6% 和 8.2%。其中 1 名患者在植入 DBS 后，海马体积保持不变 3 年。目前尚不清楚这种体积增加是由于突触可塑性增强、神经再生、胶质增生、海马区血管化增加还是其他原因引起的。

在上述第一阶段试验之后，Lozano 等（2016）启动了第二阶段试验，其中包括来自美国和加拿大不同中心的 42 名年龄在 45—85 岁的 AD 患者，ADAS-cog 评分在 12~24。研究设计为双盲法，21 名患者术后 2 周开始在频率 130Hz，脉冲宽度 90μs，3.0~3.5V 电压下接受双侧穹窿 DBS 电刺激，持续 12 个月。另一组 21 名患者作为假对照组（"关"刺激）。在整个队列中，12 个月时"开"刺激组和"关"刺激组的主要认知结果指标，如 ADAS-cog 和临床痴呆评定量表没有显著差异。接受刺激的患者在开机后 6 个月时大脑的几个区域葡萄糖代谢增加，但在 12 个月时差异并不显著。作者发现，年龄＜65 岁（n=12）的患者行 DBS 可以使疾病进展加剧。而年龄＞65 岁（n=30）的患者使用穹窿 DBS 则显示出有效的临床结果和脑葡萄糖代谢的增加。

NBM-DBS 在 6 名轻中度 AD 患者中的 Ⅰ 期临床试验结果已于 2014 年发表（Kuhn 等，2014）。刺激参数设置为频率 20Hz、电压 2.5v 和脉冲宽度 90μs。研究设计分为 2 个阶段，包括 1 个月的随机假对照刺激阶段和 11 个月的持续开放刺激阶段。在第一阶段，患者接受 2 周的"开"刺激，然后接受 2 周的"关"刺激，或者顺序颠倒。出于伦理上的原因，作者在 11 个月后转入了一项开放性研究。在 11 个月的随访中，发现6名患者中有4名患者的ADAS-cog评分不变或改善。PET扫描显示，在12个月的随访中，4名患者中有3名葡萄糖代谢增加。整体生活质量（QoL）方面，2名患者的QoL增加，2名患者的QoL没有变化，2名患者的QoL下降。

1年后，同一组研究者对2名轻度AD患者（61岁和67岁）进行了另一项研究（Kuhn等，2015a，b）。经过26个月的随访，1名患者的ADAS-cog的评分维持不变，MMSE评分甚至得到了改善。另1名患者在治疗的第1年表现出整体改善，但在26个月后ADAS-cog评分略变差。作者认为，NBM-DBS可调节胆碱能的输入，对于不是特别晚期的AD患者，通过ADAS-cog和MMSE评分可看出其认知得到了长足的改善。

七、精神分裂症

精神分裂症是一种精神疾病，常分为阳性和阴性症状，全世界人口的终生患病率约为0.5%（Simeone等，2015）。阳性的症状表现为妄想、幻觉和思维紊乱，而阴性的症状则包括缺乏动力、无欲、社交问题等（Torres-Gonzalez等，2014）。药物干预治疗主要可以减少精神分裂症的阳性症状，而阴性症状则较难治疗。尽管如此，20%的患者对治疗有抗性，高达75%的患者复发（Smith等，2010）。病理生理学认为，两种较为明显的异常在精神分裂症中起着关键作用。第一种是纹状体多巴胺（D_2）受体的增加，第二种是前额叶皮质（PFC）的GABA能功能的降低。这就是为什么研究人员正考虑通过靶向作用于腹侧被盖区（VTA）、海马或内侧隔核等输入结构来调节纹状体；直接靶向作用于联合纹状体和（或）腹侧纹状体（包括NAC）；或靶向作用于基底节输出结构，如黑质网状部（SNr）和（或）苍白球内侧部（GPi）（Klein等，2013；Perez等，2013；Ma和Leung，2014；Bikovsky等，2016；Gault等，2018）。

到目前为止，只有2个病例报告发表，这些病例选择的治疗靶点是NAC（Plewnia等，2008；Corripio等，2016）。

1名51岁强迫症及精神分裂症患者，通过右侧NAC-DBS进行治疗（Plewnia等，2008）。刺激参数设置为频率130Hz，脉冲宽度60μs，电压4.5V。作者报告了此例病例的DBS显著减少了患者的强迫行为，在6个月、1年和2年的随访时其心理社会功能均得到了改善。然而，DBS并不能改善精神分裂症患者的主要阴性症状。在另一个病例研究中，1名46岁的精神分裂症患者接受双侧NAC-DBS，并在130Hz、脉冲宽度60μs和2.5V参数下行单极（左侧）刺激。DBS治疗4周后，患者阳性症状减少62%，阴性症状改善33%（Corripio等，2016）。患者随后接受双侧刺激，但出现静坐不能症状。在切换回单侧刺激后，患者阴性症状复发，而阳性症状仍比基线水平有所改善。

因此，DBS有可能调节精神分裂症中可能受到干扰的特定环路，因此，它可能是一种有前景的新治疗策略。然而，这种方法对于精神分裂症的治疗是相对较新的，到目前为止，只有很少的临床研究开始评估其效果。关键的问题是，有严重症状的患者是否有能力同意DBS临床试验，在该试验中，风险可以估计，但收益未知。

八、结论

患有成瘾、亨廷顿病、阿尔茨海默病、神经性厌食症、微意识状态和精神分裂症的患者在试验性病例研究或初步临床试验中接受了DBS。将DBS应用于这些疾病的基本原理是调节功能失调的神经结构或环路。虽然这些适应证的大多数已经被报道有效，但我们要提出3个主要的问题。

第一，DBS的作用机制仍不清楚，因此我们无法从这些研究中得出任何结论。了解DBS的确切机制，不仅有助于我们找到更好的治疗方案，更有助于DBS的改善和升级。因此，首先研究DBS的确切作用机制，以提高疗效和减少不良反应，然后将其应用于合适的神经精神疾病是至关重要的（Herrington 等，2016）。第二，尽管 DBS 治疗新的精神类疾病的适应证正在探索中，但是我们希望避免严重的精神病总是可以用 DBS 治疗的刻板认知。过于将问题简单化，认为单一的结构或环路的功能障碍是导致诸如精神分裂症或神经性厌食症等复杂精神疾病的原因。因此，DBS 的有效性可能主要是减少与 DBS 作用部位相关的特定症状，而不是进行整体治疗。第三，我们认为在神经退行性疾病中进行 DBS 时应谨慎。由于脑萎缩和疾病进展，DBS 可能会导致无法预见的不良反应或无效。此外，应考虑电极位置的变化和长期的病理生理变化。因此，即使在植入后多年，DBS 患者也必须进行密切的随访和监测（Martinez-Ramirez 等，2014）。

参考文献

[1] Bernat JL. Chronic consciousness disorders. Annu Rev Med. 2009;60:381–92.

[2] Bernat JL. The natural history of chronic disorders of consciousness. Neurology. 2010;75:206–7.

[3] Bikovsky L, Hadar R, Soto-Montenegro ML, et al. Deep brain stimulation improves behavior and modulates neural circuits in a rodent model of schizophrenia. Exp Neurol. 2016;283:142–50.

[4] Bird ED. Chemical pathology of Huntington's disease. Annu Rev Pharmacol Toxicol. 1980;20:533–51.

[5] Bird ED, Spokes EGS, Iversen LL. Dopamine and noradrenaline in post-mortem brain in Huntington's disease and schizophrenic illness. Acta Psychiatr Scand. 1980;61(S280):63–73.

[6] Bodell LP, Keel PK. Current treatment for anorexia nervosa: efficacy, safety, and adherence. Psychol Res Behav Manag. 2010;3:91–108.

[7] Bonelli RM, Gruber A. Deep brain stimulation in Huntington's disease. Mov Disord. 2002;17:429–30.

[8] Chudy D, Deletis V, Almahariq F, et al. Deep brain stimulation for the early treatment of the minimally conscious state and vegetative state: experience in 14 patients. J Neurosurg. 2018;128:1189.

[9] Corripio I, Sarró S, McKenna PJ, et al. Clinical improvement in a treatment-resistant patient with schizophrenia treated with deep brain stimulation. Biol Psychiatry. 2016;80:e69–70.

[10] de Jong BM. 'Complete motor locked-in' and consequences for the concept of minimally conscious state. J Head Trauma Rehabil. 2013;28:141–3.

[11] Degenhardt L, Charlson F, Ferrari A, et al. The global burden of disease attributable to alcohol and drug use in 195 countries and territories, 1990-2016: a systematic analysis for the Global Burden of Disease Study 2016. Lancet Psychiatry. 2018;5:987–1012.

[12] Edwards TC, Zrinzo L, Limousin P, et al. Deep brain stimulation in the treatment of chorea. Mov Disord. 2012;27:357–63.

[13] Favaro A, Ferrara S, Santonastaso S. The spectrum of eating disorders in young women: a prevalence study in a general population sample. Psychosom Med. 2003;65:701–8.

[14] Feigin VL, Abajobir AA, Abate KH, et al. Global, regional, and national burden of neurological disorders during 1990-2015: a systematic analysis for the Global Burden of Disease Study 2015. Lancet Neurol. 2017;16:877–97.

[15] Fontaine D, Deudon A, Lemaire JJ, et al. Symptomatic treatment of memory decline in Alzheimer's disease by deep brain stimulation: a feasibility study. J Alzheimers Dis. 2013;34:315–23.

[16] Gault JM, Davis R, Cascella NG, et al. Approaches to neuromodulation for schizophrenia. J Neurol Neurosurg Psychiatry. 2018;89:777–87.

[17] Gonçalves-Ferreira A, do Couto FS, Rainha Campos A, et al. Deep brain stimulation for refractory cocaine dependence. Biol Psychiatry. 2016;79:e87–9.

[18] Gossop M, Stewart D, Browne N, et al. Factors associated with abstinence, lapse or relapse to heroin use after residential treatment: protective effect of coping responses. Addiction. 2002;97:1259–67.

[19] Graybiel AM. The basal ganglia. Trends Neurosci. 1995;18:60–2.

[20] Guarda AS. Treatment of anorexia nervosa: insights and obstacles. Physiol Behav. 2008;94:113–20.

[21] Hamani C, McAndrews MP, Cohn M, et al. Memory enhancement induced by hypothalamic/fornix deep brain stimulation. Ann Neurol. 2008;63:119–23.

[22] Hebb MO, Garcia M, Gaudet P, et al. Bilateral stimulation of the globus pallidus internus to treat choreathetosis in Huntington's disease: technical case report. Neurosurgery. 2006;58:E383.

[23] Herrington TM, Cheng JJ, Eskandar EN. Mechanisms of deep brain stimulation. J Neurophysiol. 2016;115:19–38.

[24] Hescham S, Lim L, Jahanshahi A, et al. Deep brain stimulation in dementia-related disorders. Neurosci Biobehav Rev. 2013;37(10 Pt 2):2666–75.

[25] Hoek HW, van Hoeken D. Review of the prevalence and incidence of eating disorders. Int J Eat Disord. 2003;34:383–96.

[26] Jahanshahi AR, Vlamings R, van Roon-Mom WM, et al. Changes in brainstem serotonergic and dopaminergic cell populations in experimental and clinical Huntington's disease. Neuroscience. 2013;238:71–81.

[27] Joel D. Open interconnected model of basal ganglia-thalamocortical circuitry and its relevance to the clinical syndrome of Huntington's disease. Mov Disord. 2001;16:407–23.

[28] Klein J, Hadar R, Götz T, et al. Mapping brain regions in which deep brain stimulation affects schizophrenia-like behavior in two rat models of schizophrenia. Brain Stimul. 2013;6:490–9.

[29] Krack P, Hariz MI, Baunez C, et al. Deep brain stimulation: from neurology to psychiatry? Trends Neurosci. 2010;33:474–84.

[30] Kuhn J, Moller M, Treppmann JF, et al. Deep brain stimulation of the nucleus accumbens and its usefulness in severe opioid addiction. Mol Psychiatry. 2014;19:145–6.

[31] Kuhn J, Hardenacke K, Lenartz D, et al. Deep brain stimulation of the nucleus basalis of Meynert in Alzheimer's dementia. Mol Psychiatry. 2015a;20:353–60.

[32] Kuhn J, Hardenacke K, Shubina E, et al. Deep brain stimulation of the nucleus basalis of Meynert in early stage of Alzheimer's dementia. Brain Stimul. 2015b;8:838–9.

[33] Laxton AW, Tang-Wai DF, McAndrews MP, et al. A phase I trial of deep brain stimulation of memory circuits in Alzheimer's disease. Ann Neurol. 2010;68:521–34.

[34] Ligot N, Krystkowiak P, Simonin C, et al. External globus pallidus stimulation modulates brain connectivity in Huntington's disease. J Cereb Blood Flow Metab. 2011;31:41–6.

[35] Lipsman N, Lam E, Volpini M, et al. Deep brain stimulation of the subcallosal cingulate for treatment-refractory anorexia nervosa: 1 year follow-up of an open-label trial. Lancet Psychiatry. 2017;4:285–94.

[36] Lozano AM, Lipsman N. Probing and regulating dysfunctional circuits using deep brain stimulation. Neuron. 2013;77:406–24.

[37] Lozano AM, Fosdick L, Chakravarty MM, et al. A phase II study of fornix deep brain stimulation in mild Alzheimer's disease. J Alzheimers Dis. 2016;54:777–87.

[38] Ma J, Leung LS. Deep brain stimulation of the medial septum or nucleus accumbens alleviates psychosis-relevant behavior in ketamine-treated rats. Behav Brain Res. 2014;266:174–82.

[39] Martens HCF, Toader E, Decre MMJ, et al. Spatial steering of deep brain stimulation volumes using a novel lead design. Clin Neurophysiol. 2011;122:558–66.

[40] Martinez-Ramirez D, Morishita T, Zeilman PR, et al. Atrophy and other potential factors affecting long term deep brain stimulation response: a case series. PLoS One. 2014;9:e111561.

[41] Masters CL, Bateman R, Blennow K, et al. Alzheimer's disease. Nat Rev Dis Primers. 2015;1:15056.

[42] Moro E, Lang AE, Strafella AP, et al. Bilateral globus pallidus stimulation for Huntington's disease. Ann Neurol. 2004;56:290–4.

[43] Moruzzi G, Magoun HW. Brain stem reticular formation and activation of the EEG. Electroencephalogr Clin Neurophysiol. 1949;1:455–73.

[44] Müller UJ, Voges J, Steiner J, et al. Deep brain stimulation of the nucleus accumbens for the treatment of addiction. Ann N Y Acad Sci. 2013;1282:119–28.

[45] Nestler EJ, Barrot M, DiLeone RJ, et al. Neurobiology of depression. Neuron. 2002;34:13–25.

[46] Oudijn MS, Storosum JG, Nelis E, et al. Is deep brain stimulation a treatment option for anorexia nervosa? BMC Psychiatry. 2013;13:277.

[47] Pelloux Y, Baunez C. Deep brain stimulation for addiction: why the subthalamic nucleus should be favored. Curr Opin Neurobiol. 2013;23:713–20.

[48] Perez SM, Shah A, Asher A, et al. Hippocampal deep brain stimulation reverses physiological and behavioural deficits in a rodent model of schizophrenia. Int J Neuropharmacol. 2013;16:331–1339.

[49] Plewnia C, Schober F, Rilk A, et al. Sustained improvement of obsessive-compulsive disorder by deep brain stimulation in a woman with residual schizophrenia. Int J Neuropsychopharmacol. 2008;11:1181–3.

[50] Price JL, Drevets WC. Neurocircuitry of mood disorders. Neuropsychopharmacology. 2009;35:192.

[51] Purpura KP, Schiff ND. The thalamic intralaminar nuclei: a role in visual awareness. Neuroscientist. 1997;3:8–15.

[52] Sankar T, Chakravarty MM, Bescos A, et al. Deep brain stimulation influences brain structure in Alzheimer's disease. Brain Stimul. 2015;8:645–54.

[53] Schiff ND, Giacino JT, Kalmar K, et al. Behavioural improvements with thalamic stimulation after severe traumatic brain injury. Nature. 2007;448(7153):600–3.

[54] Sieradzan KA, Mann DM. The selective vulnerability of nerve cells in Huntington's disease. Neuropathol Appl Neurobiol. 2001;27:1–21.

[55] Simeone JC, Ward AJ, Rotella P, et al. An evaluation of variation in published estimates of schizophrenia prevalence from 1990–2013: a systematic literature review. BMC Psychiatry. 2015;15:193.

[56] Smith T, Weston C, Lieberman J. Schizophrenia (maintenance treatment). Am Fam Physician. 2010;82:338–9.

[57] Smith GS, Laxton AW, Tang-Wai DF, et al. Increased cerebral metabolism after 1 year of deep brain stimulation in Alzheimer disease. Arch Neurol. 2012;69:1141–8.

[58] Spielberger S, Hotter A, Wolf E, et al. Deep brain stimulation in Huntington's disease: a 4-year follow-up case report. Mov Disord. 2012;27:806–7.

[59] Sussman S, Lisha N, Griffiths M. Prevalence of the addictions: a problem of the majority or the minority? Eval Health Prof. 2011;34:3–56.

[60] Temel Y, Cao C, Vlamings R, et al. Motor and cognitive improvement by deep brain stimulation in a transgenic rat model of Huntington's disease. Neurosci Lett. 2006;406:138–41.

[61] Tony R. Wang, Shayan Moosa, Robert F. Dallapiazza, et al. Deep brain stimulation for the treatment of drug addiction. Neurosurgical Focus. 2018;45(2):E11.

[62] Torres-Gonzalez F, Ibanez-Casas I, Saldivia S, et al. Unmet needs in the management of schizophrenia. Neuropsychiatr Dis Treat. 2014;10:97–110.

[63] Turnbull IM, McGeer PL, Beattie L, et al. Stimulation- of the basal nucleus of Meynert in senile dementia of Alzheimer's type. A preliminary report. Appl Neurophysiol. 1985;48:216–21.

[64] Vedam-Mai V, Martinez-Ramirez D, Hilliard JD, et al. Post-mortem findings in Huntington's deep brain stimulation: a moving target due to atrophy. Tremor Other Hyperkinet Mov. 2016;6:372.

[65] Vigo D, Thornicroft G, Atun R. Estimating the true global burden of mental illness. Lancet Psychiatry. 2016;3:171–8.

[66] Vlamings R, Benazzouz A, Chetrit J, et al. Metabolic and electrophysiological changes in the basal ganglia of transgenic Huntington's disease rats. Neurobiol Dis. 2012;48:488–94.

[67] Vonsattel JP, Myers RH, Stevens TJ, et al. Neuropathological classification of Huntington's disease. J Neuropathol Exp Neurol. 1985;44:559–77.

[68] Zeef D, Schaper F, Vlamings R, et al. Deep brain stimulation in Huntington's disease: the current status. Open Neurosurg J. 2011;4:7–10.

[69] Zhou H, Xu J, Jiang J. Deep brain stimulation of nucleus accumbens on heroin-seeking behaviors: a case report. Biol Psychiatry. 2011;69:e41–2.

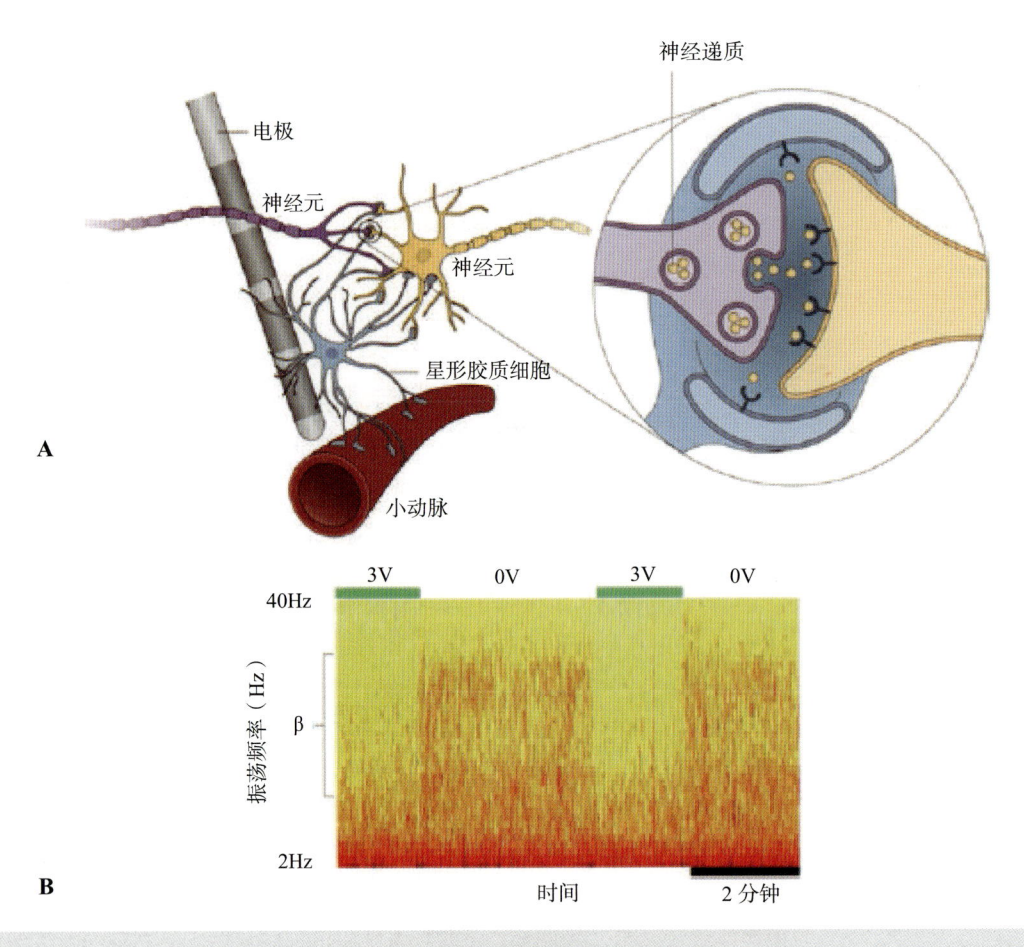

▲ 脑深部电刺激机制示意图

A. 刺激后神经递质释放，引起钙离子浓度变化，随后释放神经胶质递质，进而影响突触可塑性，并使小动脉扩张，局部血流增加。B. 脑深部电刺激（DBS）引起丘脑底核局部场电位变化。在3V刺激时，β波段的活性快速下降，刺激停止时恢复 [经许可转载，引自 Lozano et al. Nature Reviews Neurology, 15, pages 148–160 (2019)]